CLINICAL CARDIOVASCULAR THERAPEUTICS

Series editors

Henry A. Punzi, M.D.

Clinical Associate Professor
Texas Women's University
Denton, Texas;
Medical Director
Trinity Hypertension and Diagnostic Research Center
Carrollton, Texas

Walter Flamenbaum, M.D.

Clinical Professor of Medicine
Mount Sinai School of Medicine
New York, New York;
President
Health and Sciences Research, Inc.
Englewood, New Jersey

CLINICAL CARDIOVASCULAR THERAPEUTICS

Series editors
Henry A. Punzi, M.D.
Walter Flamenbaum, M.D.

Volume 2

Cardiac Arrhythmias: A Practical Approach

editor

Gerald V. Naccarelli, M.D.

Associate Professor of Medicine
Vice Chairman, Division of Cardiology
Director, Clinical Electrophysiology
University of Texas Medical School at Houston
Houston, Texas

FUTURA

Futura Publishing
Company, Inc.
Mount Kisco, NY
1991

Copyright 1991
Futura Publishing Company, Inc.

Published by
Futura Publishing Company, Inc.
2 Bedford Ridge Rd., P.O. Box 330
Mount Kisco, New York 10549

Clinical Cardiovascular Therapeutics ISSN # : 1045-8417
ISBN# : 0-87993-373-9

Every effort has been made to ensure that the information in this
book is as up to date and as accurate as possible at the time of
publication. However, due to the constant developments in medicine,
neither the author, nor the editor, nor the publisher can accept any
legal or any other responsibility for any errors or omissions that may
occur.

Printed in the United States of America.

Contributors

Masood Akhtar, M.D.
Professor of Medicine, Associate Director, Cardiology; Director, Clinical Electrophysiology, Mt. Sinai Medical Center, University of Wisconsin School of Medicine, Milwaukee, Wisconsin

Boaz Avitall, M.D., Ph.D.
Assistant Professor of Medicine, University of Wisconsin Medical School, Milwaukee, Wisconsin

David G. Benditt, M.D.
Associate Professor of Medicine, Director, Cardiac Electrophysiology, University of Minnesota School of Medicine, Minneapolis, Minnesota

Ellison Berns, M.D.
Assistant Professor of Medicine, Director, Clinical Electrophysiology, University of Connecticut Health Center and St. Francis Hospital and Medical Center, University of Connecticut School of Medicine, Farmington, Connecticut

Anil K. Bhandari, M.D.
Associate Clinical Professor, University of California School of Medicine, Director, Electrophysiology Laboratory, Good Samaritan Hospital, Los Angeles Cardiology Associates, Los Angeles, California

Paul G. Colavita, M.D.
Consultant Cardiologist, The Sanger Clinic, P.A., Charlotte, North Carolina

Anne H. Dougherty, M.D.
Assistant Professor of Medicine, Director, Cardiac Pacing, University of Texas Medical School, Houston, Texas

John M. Fedor, M.D.
The Sanger Clinic, P.A., Charlotte, North Carolina

David Fitzgerald, M.D.
Assistant Professor of Medicine, Director, Clinical Electrophysiology, Bowman-Gray School of Medicine, Winston-Salem, North Carolina

John J. Gallagher, M.D.
Director, Electrophysiology Services, Department of Cardiac Laboratories, Carolinas Medical Center/Carolinas Heart Institute, The Sanger Clinic, P.A., Charlotte, North Carolina

Arthur Garson, Jr., M.D.
Professor of Pediatrics and Medicine, Chief of Pediatric Cardiology, Baylor College of Medicine, Houston, Texas

Mary Ann Goldstein, M.D.
Pediatric Cardiologist, Emergency Medicine, Children's Hospital, Minneapolis, Minnesota

Charles C. Gornick, M.D.
Assistant Professor of Medicine, VA Med Ctr, Cardiology Section, Minneapolis, Minnesota

Leonard N. Horowitz, M.D.
Clinical Professor of Medicine, University of Pennsylvania School of Medicine, Co-Director, Philadelphia Heart Institute, Presbyterian Medical Center, Philadelphia, Pennsylvania

Mohammad Jazayeri, M.D.
Assistant Professor of Medicine, University of Wisconsin School of Medicine, Milwaukee, Wisconsin

Lawrence S. Klein, M.D.
Assistant Professor of Medicine, Indiana University School of Medicine, Indianapolis, Indiana

Bruce Kleinman, M.D.
Assistant Professor of Medicine, Director, Department of Anesthesiology, Loyola University Medical School, Maywood, Illinois

Steven P. Kutalek, M.D.
Assistant Professor of Medicine, Clinical Cardiac Electrophysiology, Likoff Cardiovascular Institute, Hahnemann University, Philadelphia, Pennsylvania

Ralph Lazzara, M.D.
George Lynn Cross Research Professor, Natalie O. Warren Professor of Medicine, Chief, Cardiovascular Section, University of Oklahoma Health Sciences Center, Oklahoma City, Oklahoma

James E. Lowe, M.D.
Associate Professor of Surgery, Duke University School of Medicine, Durham, North Carolina

John H. McAnulty, M.D.
Professor of Medicine, Division of Cardiology, Oregon Health Sciences University, Portland, Oregon

Daniel J. McCormick, D.O.
Clinical Assistant Professor of Medicine, Hahneman University/ Likoff Cardiovascular Institute, Philadelphia, Pennsylvania

William M. Miles, M.D.
Associate Professor of Medicine, Director of Clinical Electrophysiology, Indiana University School of Medicine, Krannert Institute of Cardiology, Indianapolis, Indiana

Simon Milstein, M.D.
Assistant Professor of Medicine, Division of Cardiology, University of Minnesota Hospital, Minneapolis, Minnesota

Gerald V. Naccarelli, M.D.
Associate Professor of Medicine, Vice Chairman, Division of Cardiology, Director, Clinical Electrophysiology, University of Texas Medical School, Houston, Texas

Jean Nappi, Pharm.D.
Professor of Clinical Pharmacy, University of Houston, College of Pharmacy, Houston, Texas

Brian Olshansky, M.D.
Assistant Professor of Medicine, Division of Cardiology, Loyola University Medical Center, Maywood, Illinois

Douglas L. Packer, M.D.
Assistant Professor of Medicine, Division of Cardiovascular Diseases, St. Mary's Hospital Complex, Mayo Foundation, Rochester, Minnesota

James C. Perry, M.D.
Assistant Professor of Medicine, Associate in Pediatric Cardiology, Baylor College of Medicine, Houston, Texas

R. Steven Porter, Pharm.D.
Assistant Professor of Medicine, Director, Cardiovascular Pharmacology, Hahneman Hospital/Likoff CV Institute, Philadelphia, Pennsylvania

Eric N. Prystowsky, M.D.
Consulting Professor of Medicine, Duke University School of Medicine, Director, Clinical Electrophysiology Laboratory, St. Vincent's Hospital, Indianapolis, Indiana

Walter J. Reyes, M.D.
University of Minnesota, Minneapolis, Minnesota

Robert L. Rinkenberger, M.D.
Plano, Texas

Philip T. Sager, M.D.
Assistant Professor of Medicine, Director of Clinical Electrophysiology, Wadsworth VA Medical Center, Los Angeles, California

Benjamin J. Scherlag, Ph.D.
Professor of Medicine, Research Career Scientist, Department of Veterans Affairs, Oklahoma City, Oklahoma

Jay G. Selle, M.D.
Chief, Vascular Surgical Service, Department of Thoracic, Cardiac, and Vascular Surgery, The Sanger Clinic, P.A., Charlotte, North Carolina

Robert H. Svenson, M.D.
Director of Laser and Applied Technology, Carolinas Heart Institute, The Sanger Clinic, P.A., Charlotte, North Carolina

Patrick J. Tchou, M.D.
Associate Professor of Medicine, Division of Cardiology, University of Pittsburgh School of Medicine, Pittsburgh, Pennsylvania

Paul J. Troup, M.D.
Associate Professor of Medicine, University of Wisconsin Medical School, Sinai Campus, Arrhythmia Service, Milwaukee, Wisconsin

Stephen C. Vlay, M.D.
Associate Professor of Medicine, Director, The Stony Brook Arrhythmias Study and Sudden Death Prevention Center, Director, The Coronary Care Unit, State University of New York, Stony Brook, New York

David J. Wilber, M.D.
Assistant Professor of Medicine, Director, Electrophysiology Laboratory, Loyola University Medical School, Maywood, Illinois

Deborah Wolbrette, M.D.
Fellow, Division of Cardiology, University of Texas Medical School, Houston, Texas

Samuel H. Zimmern, M.D.
The Sanger Clinic, P.A., Charlotte, North Carolina

Foreword

It is a pleasure for me to be able to write a few words at the beginning of this arrhythmia book. While several texts have been published recently that encompass a wide area of cardiac electrophysiology, none have been devoted solely to a practical approach to arrhythmia management. A book that is written for the practicing clinician, cardiology fellow, internist, and clinical cardiologist is definitely needed. Dr. Naccarelli should be congratulated for securing experts in all areas to author the various chapters. The text includes practical discussions on approaches to understanding mechanisms of arrhythmias, recognizing, evaluating, and treating supreventricular and ventricular tachyarrhythmias and bradyarrhythmias in a variety of settings for adult and pediatric patients. Further, there are comprehensive discussions about pharmacological, electrical, and ablative therapy of cardiac arrhythmias. Timely publication by Futura has delivered an up-to-date resource that will help the clinician make management decisions for patients with cardiac arrhythmias. I can recommend this book for all doctors taking care of patients with these problems and I am pleased to write this enthusiastic foreword.

Douglas P. Zipes, M.D.
Krannert Institute of
Cardiology
Indianapolis, Indiana

Introduction

Sudden cardiac death remains the number one killer in the world. Over 1,000 patients die suddenly every day in the United States and over 80–90% of these deaths occur secondary to a ventricular tachyarrhythmia. The association of arrhythmias and sudden cardiac death have remained the biggest challenge in cardiovascular medicine. Over the last 25 years, advances in therapeutic testing, including Holter monitoring, event recorders, signal-averaged ECGs, tilt-table testing, and intracardiac electrophysiology studies have increased our ability to evaluate patients with brady- and tachyarrhythmias. In addition, newer antiarrhythmic drugs and advances in cardiac pacing, implantable defibrillators, cardiac mapping, and both surgical and catheter ablation techniques have improved our ability to treat and even cure patients with dysrhythmic syndromes.

The present volume was written to provide a review of major dysrhythmic syndromes and the role of diagnostic and therapeutic techniques in the field of cardiac electrophysiology. Each chapter is complementary yet somewhat independent, so that a specific aspect of cardiac electrophysiology may be reviewed. Although the current state of the art may be useful to cardiac electrophysiologists, the text has been written to be a useful source for cardiologists, electrophysiology fellows, cardiology fellows, internists, and family physicians.

This book represents the second volume of a four-part series covering all the major aspects of cardiology. As editor, my task was made easier by the outstanding ability of the multiple contributors to this volume. This book would not have been possible without the help of many people, including Henry Punzi, M.D., and Walter Flamenbaum, M.D., who helped edit and organize the *Clinical Cardiovascular Therapeutics Series*; Steven Korn, Jacques Strauss, Dawn Yardis, and Linda Shaw from Futura Publishing Company, who provided the professionalism to follow this project through to its end-point; and Peggy Casteel, my secretary, who handled the various administrative aspect of this book with her usual professionalism. I appreciate the teaching and support of my past mentors and past and present chairmen. Finally, I owe the most thanks to my wife, Terry, and my children, Michele and Matthew, who have always been supportive of my medical and academic endeavors.

Gerald V. Naccarelli, M.D.

Contents

Chapter 1

Anatomy of Cardiac Conduction System: Basic Concepts in Cardiac Electrophysiology

David Fitzgerald, Benjamin J. Scherlag, and Ralph Lazzara

Basic Electrophysiology of the Conduction System

Cardiac cells can be excited from their resting state to generate an action potential in response to an appropriate (threshold) stimulus. The basis of this excitability is determined by properties of the cell membrane that restrict movement of ions between the intracellular and the extracellular space.[1] Special protein channels embedded in the phospholipid bilayer of the cell membrane governed by voltage and messengers allow selective transport of ions, thus maintaining ionic distributions in the resting state and determining the ionic movements that underlie excitation and recovery.[2]

Negatively charged organic ions (primarily charged structural proteins in the cytoplasm) are present in the intracellular fluid. These anions cannot cross the cell membrane and, thus, are restricted to the intracellular space. Positively charged ions (cations) are required to counterbalance the negative charge and maintain electrical neutrality. Sodium and potassium are the predominant cations present in the cell and

From Naccarelli GV (ed): *Cardiac Arrhythmias: A Practical Approach.* Mount Kisco, NY, Futura Publishing Co., Inc., © 1991.

extracellular fluid that can be distributed across the membrane to neutralize the anionic charge.[3]

In the resting state, sodium conductance across the membrane is very low and any sodium leak into the interior results in activation of a sodium-potassium pump. This pump is associated with the cell membrane and, in an energy-consuming process, transports three sodium ions out of the cell in exchange for two potassium ions.[4] The pump maintains an osmotic balance between the cell and the extracellular fluid. As a result of this pump, intracellular sodium concentration is low and intracellular potassium concentration is high.

Since sodium is effectively excluded from the interior of the resting cell, potassium, which is conducted across the cell membrane, accumulates in the cell to offset the charge effect of the organic anions. This results in a large concentration gradient for potassium across the cell membrane. Potassium will distribute itself across the membrane based on chemical forces (concentration differences) and electrical forces (charge) that result in an electrochemical equilibrium and a membrane potential of approximately -90 millivolts (potential difference between extracellular fluid as ground and intracellular fluid). If, indeed, potassium is the only ion moving across the cell membrane, the Nernst equation ($E = RT/ZF \times \ln [C]_o/[C]_i$ where R = gas constant, T = absolute temperature, Z = valence of ion, F = Faraday constant, ln = natural log, $[C]_o$ and $[C]_i$ = extracellular and intracellular concentration of ion) using potassium concentration across the membrane, should describe the equilibrium potential of the cell. If the intracellular concentration of potassium is 150 mM and the extracellular concentration is 4–5 mM, the Nernst equation predicts an equilibrium potential for potassium of -86 mV, which is very near the resting potential of the cell.[5] Since the membrane is not strictly impermeable to sodium and other ions, the Goldman Constant Field equation takes into account the effect of other ions on membrane potential.[6]

In cardiac tissues, an appropriate stimulus will decrease the membrane potential to a threshold level resulting in a sudden rapid depolarization followed by repolarization back to the resting potential. This represents an action potential. Two types of action potentials have been described for cardiac cells as illustrated in Figure 1.[7] Fast response action potentials are found in cells of the atria, His-Purkinje system, and ventricles. Resting potential is in the range of -80 to -95 mV. In response to a stimulus, the membrane is depolarized to the threshold voltage of the sodium channel (-60 mV), causing sodium channels to open, admitting a rapid influx of sodium ions into the cell, the fast sodium current

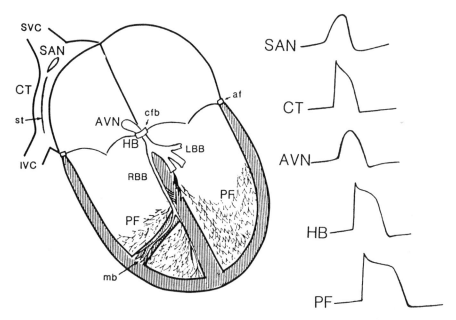

Figure 1. Schematic diagram of the action potential morphologies of the different areas of the specialized conduction system. SVC = superior vena cava; SAN = sinoatrial node; IVC = inferior vena cava; AVN = atrioventric- ular node; HB = His bundle; cfb = central fibrous body; LBB = left bundle branch; RBB = right bundle branch; PF = Purkinje fibers; mb = moderator band; af = annulus fibrosis; CT = cristae terminalis; ST = specialized tracts. (Adapted from F Netter: Ciba Collection of Medical Illustrations, Vol. 5, The Heart, Section II, Plate 11, p 49, 1969.)

(I_{Na}). The upstrokes of action potentials generated by this sodium current generally (Phase 0) have a maximal velocity of 100–500 volts/second. Over 1–5 msec, the cell depolarizes from -90 to approximately $+30$ mV. As the intracellular sodium accumulates and the potential becomes more positive, sodium conductance decreases. Toward the termination of the upstroke calcium channels open, and the calcium current (I_{si}) enters the cell. Inactivation of the sodium current results in a brief period (10–20 msec) of early rapid repolarization (Phase 1). A transient outward current may also contribute to this phase in some cells. The membrane potential changes from $+30$ mV to 0.

A plateau phase (Phase 2) ensues due to a decrease in potassium conductance out of the cell (inward rectification-potassium can enter the cell easier than leaving), and incomplete inactivation of I_{si} inward and I_{Na}, resulting in an equilibrium phase near zero lasting approximately

100 msec. Delayed opening of potassium channels causes increasing outward flow of potassium ions (i_K) which hastens repolarization (Phase 3). This brings the cell back to the resting potential (Phase 4).

Slow response action potentials are found in cells of the sinus and atrioventricular nodes.[3,7] The resting potential of these cells is in the range of -50 to -70 mV. The upstrokes of the action potentials are mediated by the slow inward calcium current with threshold at approximately -50 to -40 mV. The upstrokes of the action potentials are relatively slow with maximal velocities of 1–15 volts per second. Phase 1 is absent and Phase 2 is abbreviated. Phase 4 is characterized by spontaneous diastolic depolarization (automaticity in the sinus node).

Cardiac cells capable of impulse formation (automaticity) can be found throughout the cardiac conduction system including the sinus node, atrioventricular node, His bundle, and upper bundle branches.[8] Additionally, cells in the atrium (along the crista terminalis and near the coronary sinus os) and in the distal Purkinje network and ventricles, can display automatic behavior under certain conditions. Although the action potential configuration of these cells may differ, they are all characterized by spontaneous Phase 4 diastolic depolarization.

The intrinsic firing rate of pacemaker cells is determined by the slope of diastolic depolarization and the maximum diastolic potential of the cell. These features are shown in Figure 2. The faster rates of diastolic depolarization are found in sinoatrial nodal cells which constitute the dominant pacemaker. Cells with slower rates of diastolic depolarization are latent or subsidiary pacemakers. In Figure 3 are illustrated transmembrane potentials from a sinus node pacemaker and a Purkinje pacemaker. The faster firing rate of the dominant pacemaker may result in the conducted impulse activating subsidiary pacemakers before they can manifest significant diastolic depolarization. With default of the dominant pacemaker, a hierarchy of latent pacemakers becomes manifest with more proximal automatic tissues (atrium and atrioventricular node) becoming active before more distal tissues (His bundle, Purkinje fibers, bundle branches, and peripheral tissues).[9,10]

There is a delay in the appearance of a latent pacemaker that is a function of antecedent duration and rate of the dominant pacemaker. This is known as overdrive suppression.[11] The presumed mechanism of this suppression is thought to be secondary to a relative hyperpolarization of the subsidiary pacemakers by the dominant pacemaker. The faster rate of discharge of the dominant pacemaker exposes the slower subsidiary pacemakers (with fast response action potentials) to a relative sodium load with each action potential. The increase in intracellular

potential (mv)

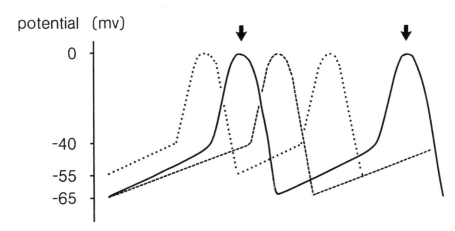

Figure 2. Schematic diagram of the influence of the slope of diastolic depolarization and difference between maximal diastolic potential and threshold on rate of spontaneous discharge. The membrane potentials with interrupted lines illustrate the effect of a decrease in the slope of diastolic
depolarization in slowing the rate of spontaneous firing. The dotted potentials
illustrate the faster rate of discharge in cells with the same slope of diastolic
depolarization as the baseline action potentials (dark-lined) but with a more
positive maximal diastolic potential. Threshold potential for all cells is −40
millivolts (mv).

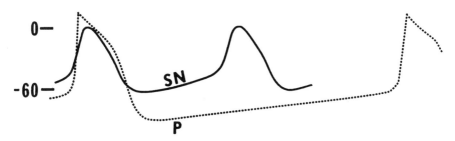

Figure 3. Comparison of the difference between a slow upstroke calcium
channel-mediated action potential of the sinus node (SN) and a fast upstroke
sodium channel-mediated action potential of a Purkinje fiber (P). Note the
more negative potentials and the slower rate of spontaneous discharge of
the P compared to the SN.

sodium activates the electrogenic sodium-potassium pump (three sodium ions exchanged for two potassium ions) creating a net loss of positive charge and a relative hyperpolarization. Upon cessation of the dominant pacemaker, the resting potential of the escape pacemaker is more negative and takes a longer time to reach threshold.

The mechanism of suppression of subsidiary pacemakers may differ based on the location of the subsidiary pacemaker. The atria have an extensive network of autonomic nerve endings that are stimulated by atrial contraction to release acetylcholine and epinephrine. The effects of acetylcholine are more prominent and may be responsible for the delayed appearance of higher subsidiary pacemakers due to effects on membrane conductance of potassium.[8]

The ionic currents involved in the pacemaker potential have been a subject of great interest over the years and have recently been reviewed.[12,13] In studies of Purkinje fibers, Weidman postulated that the pacemaker current was secondary to a decline in membrane conductance of an outward potassium current coupled with a background inward leak current.[14] Voltage clamp studies of the rabbit sinoatrial node area have identified several potassium currents and the slow inward calcium current as possible sources of spontaneous diastolic depolarization.[16] Unfortunately, the functional role of these currents is not so clear because the voltage clamp can cause changes in extracellular potassium concentration in multicellular preparations which might affect membrane conductance.

More recently, techniques have evolved for single cell voltage clamp analysis of sinoatrial cells.[16-18] Although these studies assure voltage uniformity in the preparation and reduce the effects of external potassium accumulation or depletion, single cell analysis has other limitations. There are technical difficulties associated with differentiating the small currents generated by a single cell from the background noise level. The effects of changes in the intracellular ionic concentration secondary to diffusion from the microelectrode solution after impalement are more prominent in single cell preparations compared to multicellular preparations. Changes in the resistance of the system during an experiment can markedly alter the results. Nevertheless, new insights are being obtained using this technique.

In sinus nodal tissue, various currents have been identified. A time- and voltage-dependent outward potassium current (I_K) showing inward rectification is activated on depolarization beyond -50 mV. This current has been well described in multicellular preparations and more recently in single cells.[19-21] The current is important for repolarization of the action potential and a gradual decay in this current leads to an accumulation of positive ions in the cell. Brown and colleagues estimate that I_K may contribute to 80% of the diastolic depolarization in rabbit sinoatrial nodal cells.[22]

The slow inward calcium current is activated during the latter part of the pacemaker potential.[15] Single cell analysis has allowed separation of this current into different components.[23] The more commonly described calcium current is that flowing through L-type channels (I_{CaL}). It is probably responsible for the action potential upstroke of nodal cells. It is activated at -40 mV (which is the threshold for the upstroke of the action potential of sinoatrial nodal cells) and has a large amplitude. Any contribution of this current to diastolic depolarization would occur very late in diastole.

A lower threshold calcium current with activation in the range of -50 mV has been identified in atrial and ventricular cells where its contribution to overall depolarization is very small (less than 5%). In the rabbit sinoatrial node, this current (I_{CaT}) may be responsible for 20% of the current density of I_{si}.

Both calcium channels are blocked by cadmium and cobalt. Gallopamil and nifedipine block I_{CaL} with no effect on I_{CaT} while nickel and tetramethin block I_{CaL} with no effect on I_{CaT}. The effects of these different agents on channel function suggest they are separate channels. Block of I_{CaL} prolongs the cycle length and causes a decrease in the slope of the pacemaker depolarization. The initial phase of depolarization is not affected. The I_{CaT} is not responsive to adrenergic stimulation.

An inward current (I_f) has been identified when sinoatrial nodal cells are hyperpolarized from -60 to -90 mV.[24-26] This current is fully activated at potentials more negative than the maximum diastolic potential of sinoatrial or AV nodal cells in multicellular preparations under normal conditions. However, disaggregated sinus node cells, atrial, and His-Purkinje cells have more negative resting potentials and I_f is probably an important component of the pacemaker current in these cells.

The channel for I_f is nonspecific, carrying either sodium or potassium ions. Cesium blocks this channel and changes the frequency of firing, but does not eliminate diastolic depolarization. This channel is augmented by catecholamines and may become important in the sinoatrial node during conditions of enhanced adrenergic tone.

Other currents may contribute to portions of the pacemaker potential. A transient outward current carrying potassium or sodium has been identified in cells of the rabbit AV node and atrium.[27,28] There is no evidence at present that this is directly involved in pacemaker activity.

The sodium-calcium exchanger transports calcium from the cell in exchange for sodium into the cell in a ratio of three sodium ions for one calcium ion.[29] This net inward current could contribute to diastolic depolarization, but a role in the pacemaker current is not clear. The sodium-potassium exchanger is another ion exchange current that may have a role in the genesis of the pacemaker current.[30] It would be expected to generate an outward current and inhibit diastolic depolarization as potassium is transported into the cell. In slow response tissues where calcium predominantly mediates the upstroke of the action potential, intracellular sodium content should remain rather constant. Therefore, sodium-potassium pump activity should be relatively constant. The role of this ion pump in automatic cells with fast upstroke action potentials requires further investigation.

Finally, a background inward leak current has been proposed that would tend to raise the resting negative membrane potential to more positive levels.[24,31] The nature of this leak is presumed to be mediated by sodium ions, in view of their role as the predominant extracellular cation. The mechanism of the leak, that is, whether through a specific ion channel, via an electrogenic ion pump, or across the lipid portion of the membrane, is not known. The leak current would be expected to be greater in cells with more negative membrane potentials (fast response tissues) compared to cells with more positive membrane potentials (slow response tissues). The role of this leak current in pacemaker activity is not known. The various currents thought to be important in pacemaker function are depicted in Figure 4.

Adrenergic tone increases the slope of diastolic depolarization and speeds the rate of spontaneous discharge. The mechanism is probably multifactorial, with an increase in calcium channel conductance, an increase in electrogenic ion pump activity, and an increase in I_f.

In summary, present concepts of the pacemaker current suggest that it results from an interaction of several currents rather than from a single current. It is based on a slow decay in outward potassium conductance during diastole which causes a gradual rise in membrane potential. This leads to the participation of other ion channels (I_{si}), which further raise the membrane potential to threshold. The role of other channels (I_f) and ion pumps may be important in latent pacemakers with more negative resting potentials or under unusual metabolic conditions. Autonomic influences on these channels may be important in modulating heart rate.

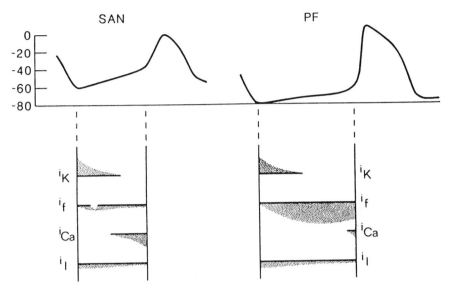

Figure 4. Comparison of currents operative in pacemaker potential in sinoatrial nodal cells and Purkinje fibers. i_K = potassium current; i_f = pacemaker current; i_{Ca} = calcium; i_l = background inward current.

The Sinus Node and Atria

The sinoatrial node is located beneath the epicardium of the upper right atrium in the sulcus terminalis between the base of the right atrial appendage and the superior vena cava.[32] Grossly, it is an elongated structure that averages 5 mm in width by 15 mm in length and 1.5 mm in depth. Microscopically, it appears as a wedge-shaped collection of small cells embedded in dense collagen tissue. Small clusters of round cells are arranged in interweaving bundles around a central artery. The bundles assume a more parallel orientation towards the periphery of the node. At the margin of the node, nodal cells gradually blend with larger atrial myocardial cells.[33,34]

At least two distinct cell types are found in the sinus node: nodal and transitional cells. The nodal cells are believed to be the pacemaker cells. They are arranged in clusters in the body of the node and are in contact only with other nodal cells or with transitional cells. Nodal cells are small (5 to 10 μm) and round, with a large nucleus and empty cytoplasm. Myofibrils are scant and small mitochondria are randomly oriented throughout the cells. Unlike working myocardial cells, the usual end-to-end cellular connections via intercalated discs are absent. Instead, nodal cells are in contact with each other along all aspects of their plasma membrane with only simple intercellular connections characterized by a rare nexus or desmosome.[35,36]

Transitional cells surround the clusters of nodal cells and contact atrial myocardial cells at the periphery of the node. These cells are more elongated and have increased amounts of myofibrils and mitochondria which are oriented longitudinally in the cytoplasm. Transitional cells appear to have more myofibrils towards the periphery of the node so that the outermost layer resembles normal atrial myocardial cells. Intercellular connections are simple near the center, but demonstrate increasing complexity at the margin of the node where intercalated disks are found.[34]

In man, the blood supply of the sinus node is either a branch of the right coronary artery (55%) or a branch of the left coronary artery (45%). A dual blood supply may occasionally be found.[37] A rich supply of adrenergic and cholinergic nerve fibers is found in the sinoatrial node.[38] Parasympathetic ganglia in the epicardium near the sinus node contribute postganglionic fibers which are predominantly related to the right vagus node.[40] With regard to sympathetic control, stimulation of the right stellate ganglion produces a sinus tachycardia while stimulation of the left stellate ganglion can produce shifts in the sinoatrial pacemaker complex.[40,41]

There is debate over the origin of the sinoatrial pacemaker complex. Bleeker and co-workers found that groups or clusters of sinoatrial nodal cells rather than a single cell were responsible for the initiation of pacemaker activity in rabbits.[42] Clusters of leading pacemakers cells occupied an area of 0.1 mm^2 in the central portion of the sinus node and consisted of approximately 5,000 cells. Toward the periphery of the node, sinus nodal cells had a slower rate of diastolic depolarization. In contrast, Boineau and co-workers mapped the epicardial atrial activation sequence in dogs.[43,44] They found multiple areas of early activation over a 40-mm area of the right atrium in a region that could include the sinus node, but also included atrial tissue outside of the sinus node. Two or three areas could excite simultaneously, although there were shifts in the order of activation at different heart rates. All sites of early activation were located along the crista terminalis. At faster heart rates, sites in the node or at more cranial locations were dominant. During slower rates, more caudal sites were dominant. These findings suggested a multicentric origin of the atrial pacemaker complex and functional differentiation according to heart rates.

More recently, epicardial maps of atrial activation in patients with Wolff-Parkinson-White syndrome undergoing operative mapping have demonstrated one or two areas of early atrial activation during sinus rhythm. Sites of early activation were near the location of the sinoatrial node. Shifts in pacemaker site were seen with various interventions confirming a multicentric origin of the atrial pacemaker complex in man.[45]

Until recently, it was accepted that the pacemaker region was the region that discharged at the fastest rate. The multicentric origin of the pacemaker complex raises questions regarding the validity of this hypothesis. Studies in isolated tissues have shown that the discharge rate of a group of synchronous pacemaker cells is different from the intrinsic rate of the fastest or even the slowest cell and does not necessarily equal the mean of all of the frequencies in the group.[46,47] From these studies, the concept has evolved that the sinus node may consist of several populations of pacemaker cells all firing at different rates. Because they are electrically coupled, the faster groups can entrain the slower groups, resulting in an overall rate somewhere in an intermediate range. Rather than conduction of the dominant pacemaker impulse to subsidiary pacemakers in the sinus node, each pacemaker group has a dynamic influence on neighboring groups, depending on the degree of electrical coupling.[48,49] The overall sinus rate may be a composite of all pacemaker populations and may reflect mutual entrainment.

The simple intercellular connections in the sinus node may be adequate to allow transmission of the pacemaker impulse through sinus nodal cells. The large areas of membrane-to-membrane apposition could act to conserve a weak excitatory current and synchronize changes in membrane potential among neighboring cells. The increasing complexity of the intercellular connections towards the periphery of the node may compensate for the decrease in membrane apposition and may facilitate transmission of the weak excitatory current to the atrial myocardium, where cellular connections are more typically end-to-end. In a similar fashion, the decrease in intercellular connections towards the center of the node may act as a protective mechanism to block extraneous impulses from entering the node and resetting it.[50]

The sinoatrial nodal impulse is transmitted through the atrial myocardium to the atrioventricular node. Anatomists postulated three internodal tracts on the basis of light microscopy: the anterior internodal tract, the middle internodal tract, and the posterior internodal tract.[51]

Although cells with different functional characteristics in the area of the proposed pathways have been identified, there has been no evidence of special anatomical characteristics of cells or tissues in these distributions.[52-54] Lesions created in the regions of these proposed tracts do not affect the speed of conduction of the sinus impulse to the atrioventricular node. Current thoughts on sinoatrial-AV nodal conduction focus on the orientation of the atrial muscle bundles around the openings of the superior vena cava, inferior vena, cava, fossa ovalis, and coronary sinus ostium and the role of tissue anisotropy as primary determinants of conduction pattern.[56,57]

Autonomic innervation of the atria shows both sympathetic and parasympathetic components. Interestingly, both sympathetic and parasympathetic stimulation shorten the atrial action potential duration and atrial muscle refractory periods.[58] Hence, both sympathetic and parasympathetic stimulation may be arrhythmogenic in the atrium.[59]

Potassium channels activated by acetylcholine exist in atrial cells and hasten repolarization during muscarinic stimulation. These channels mediate the hyperpolarization and reduced the rate of diastolic depolarization observed with muscarinic stimulation.

The AV Node and His-Purkinje System

The AV node, the common bundle, its branches and terminal fibers were discovered in reverse order of their normal activation. In 1845, Purkinje described the ramifying fibers that connected the bundle branches to ventricular muscle;[60] in 1893, His[61] and Kent[62] independently published their findings of a muscular connection between the atria and ventricles; and in 1906, Tawara[63] characterized the structure of the AV node that was a continuation of the common AV bundle. In 1907, Keith and Flack completed the discovery of the major portions of the specialized conduction system of the heart with the anatomical description of the sinoatrial node.[64]

In the normal heart, the AV node and His-Purkinje system comprise a continuous system for the passage of the cardiac impulse which enters at the AV node via multiple atrial inputs and leaves via the arborizations of the left and right bundle branches to excite regular working muscle of the ventricles. The structural-functional relationships in the human heart are based mainly on anatomical studies done in man and clinical electrophysiological reports from catheterization laboratories. Much of the information on the basic electrophysiology of the AV conduction system has relied on studies performed on other mammalian species such as rabbit and dog. Significant differences in structure and function may exist among species, but the dog appears to resemble the human rather closely.[65–67]

Anatomically, the AV node lies embedded in the low atrial septum with the coronary sinus slightly superior and posterior and the membranous septum inferior and anterior (Fig. 5). It is generally described as an "ovoid" structure, 5–6 mm long, 3 mm high, and 1–2 mm wide.[65,68] Histologically, the AV node appears as a plexus of loosely interwoven cells separated by many interstitial spaces. James and Scherf,[66] from electron micrographs, identified four different cell types composing the AV node in man: (1) "P" cells similar to those found in the sinus node have been suggested as representing the sites of automatic function in both nodes; (2) elongated, star-shaped cells with multiple connections to each other (the majority of cells in the AV node); (3) some myocardial cells with myofibrils and mitochondrial more akin to working myocardium; and (4) Purkinje cells which are found in the anterior positions of the node at its juncture with the common bundle.

Automaticity, as a property in the AV node was questioned in the 1960s[69] and the 1970s.[70] However, recent animal experiments have provided strong evidence that two distinct pacemakers are operative in the AV node and His bundle with the rate of the former being consistently faster than the latter.[71,72]

Through certain portions of the mammalian AV node (N-region) conduction as slow as 0.01 to 0.05 meters/sec has been found.[73] In the 1970s, studies utilizing His bundle recordings in man clearly established that the AV node (A-H interval) represented the site of slow conduction in the passage of the cardiac impulse from atria to ventricles.[74] With incremental atrial pacing, Wenckebach type second-degree AV block can be induced. Atrial premature beats with variable coupling can be used to test AV nodal refractoriness (Fig. 6). Such AV function curves show remarkable similarities in the dog[75] and in man.[76] These curves indicate in man and in dog that as atrial premature stimuli (A_2) are more closely coupled to the last of several successive atrial paced beats (A_1), the conduction time through the AV node (A_2–H_2 interval) becomes progressively longer until AV nodal refractoriness causes block. Commonly in both species at very short A_1–A_2 intervals, there is a marked prolongation of the A_2–H_2 interval which forms a portion of a discontinuous curve. This has been used as evidence for a functional duality of conduction in the normal AV node, e.g., the existence of a fast and a slow pathway. These findings can explain reentrant echo beats, as well as

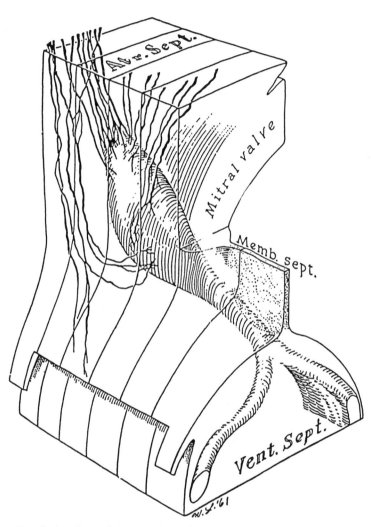

Figure 5. A drawing of the portion of the AV junction in the human heart containing the AV node within the atrial septum, the His bundle within the membranous septum, and the right and left bundle branches arising from the His bundle. Also included are AV bypass fibers from the atria which terminate in ventricular septal muscle at the base of the tricuspid valve. (With permission from James TN: Morphology of the human atrioventricular node, with remarks pertinent to its electrophysiology. Am Heart J 62:756–771, 1961.)

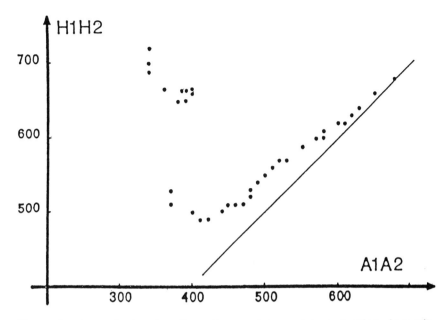

Figure 6. A graph showing discontinuous intranodal conduction. At a critical A_1–A_2 cycle, sudden lengthening of the H_1–H_2 responses is observed, reflecting a functional dual conduction pathway between the atrium and His bundle. (With permission from Puech P, Victor J: Clinical electrophysiological investigation. In: The Cardiac Arrhythmias, Arrhythmia Working Group of the French Cardiac Society, Puech P, Slama R (eds). Corbière RMDP and Roussel-UCLAF, Mt. Kisco, NY, Futura Publishing Co., 1979, pp 31–35.)

reciprocal beats that can be induced in normal hearts. A greater and more extensive anatomical and/or functional dissociation of such alpha and beta pathways may, in part, account for AV nodal reentrant arrhythmias in man.

This duality in AV nodal conduction is also seen in its response to specific types of drugs. For example, Class I antiarrhythmic agents which have sodium channel blocking properties only effect antegrade AV nodal conduction, to a very small extent, whereas calcium channel blockers, such as verapamil, potently inhibit AV nodal conduction. These findings suggest that cells of the AV node may contain both fast and slow channels as do ordinary myocardial cells, but that the slow channels may be more important in the AV node for antegrade propagation.[77]

Both basic and clinical studies have shown distinct responses of the canine AV nodal and His bundle pacemakers to various cardioactive agents. For example, AV nodal pacemakers show gradual and significant depression of the mean heart rate (from 94/min to 52/min) in response to cumulative (nontoxic) doses of cardiac glycosides, whereas, the same dose regimen does not significantly alter His bundle automaticity.[78] Clinical studies have shown that atropine causes acceleration of nodal rhythms but His bundle rhythms show little if any response.[79]

The His bundle is composed of longitudinally arranged, broad, rectangular cells coming directly out of the AV node.[67,80] The gross structure measures 1–1.2 cm in length and 1–2 mm in diameter and sits astride the crest of the interventricular septum. It courses initially through the central fibrous body (penetrating portion) with the branching portion lying within the membranous septum. According to Rosenbaum et al., "the branching portion extends from the point where the bundle starts to emit the most posterior fibers of the left bundle branch to the point which marks the origin of the right bundle branch and the most anterior fibers of the left bundle branch."[67]

Conduction velocity in the human His bundle has been estimated to be 1.5 meter/sec.[81] Although multiple interconnections have been noted between the cells of the common bundle,[79,82] the functional capability implied by these connections has been questioned. On the basis of ample collagen partitions seen between longitudinal strands of Purkinje cells comprising the common bundle, electrophysiological "partitioning" of impulses has been inferred by some[83,84] to produce functional longitudinal dissociation in the normal heart. This concept presumes the existence of separate, independent pathways from the common bundle to the peripheral Purkinje fiber.[84] A preponderance of evidence in the normal dog heart has shown that abundant functional connections in the His bundle are responsible for the concurrent excitation of sites in the peripheral His-Purkinje system when any individual His bundle cell is stimulated.[85,86] However, it has been shown that in the damaged His bundle, right or left bundle branch block can occur probably due to focal obstruction of impulse propagation to either left or right bundle branches.[87,89]

The vascularization of the AV node and His bundle is characterized by its duality much the same as the blood supply to the sinoatrial node. In man, the AV nodal artery arises as the initial branch off of the posterior descending portion of the right coronary artery. In the dominant left coronary anatomy in the dog, the AV nodal artery penetrates the crux of the heart as the first perforator arising from the posterior descending portion of the left circumflex artery. In man,[65] complete obstruction or ligation of this vessel has been shown to be innocuous in its effect supposedly due to the existence of collateral supply from other penetrating branches of the posterior descending and anastomotic flow from the first major perforator coming off the proximal left anterior descending coronary artery. In the dog, the caliber and origin of the first septal perforator from the left main coronary artery classifies the anterior septal artery as the major contributor to the summit of the interventricular septum.

The right bundle branch is essentially a continuation of the His bundle and traverses from the anterior tricuspid valve area to the base of the papillary muscle mainly subendocardially. At the base of the papillary muscle, branches of Purkinje fibers are given off through which early septal activation occurs at the same time as the cardiac impulse spreads across the chamber to activate the free wall by way of the moderator band. Conduction velocity in the right bundle reaches velocities of 2.0–2.5 meter/sec in the distal bundle and its arborizations. The upper septal portion is separated from the adjacent myocardium by a thin connective tissue layer and branches from the fascicle to myocardium have been noted only rarely.[82]

Vascularization of the right bundle has been described in great detail,[82] but the vasculature whose obstruction is most associated with bundle branch block patterns on the ECG are the initial branches arising from the posterior descending of the right coronary artery and the first septal perforator from the left anterior descending artery.

The left bundle branch originates at the branching portion of the common bundle as a flat sheet of subendocardial Purkinje fibers starting as a "neck," 2–14 mm wide, and diverging down the left side of the interventricular system as a subendocardial fan with myriad interconnections.[90] The anatomical basis of the various ECG patterns of hemiblocks may be envisioned as the left bundle having a bifascicular structure, with two independent and separate divisions, anterior and posterior, which account for the left anterior and left posterior hemiblock ECG patterns commonly seen in intraventricular conduction defects.[67]

Several subsequent anatomical and functional studies concluded that there is a prominent "central" division of the left bundle system[91] with multiple interconnections between both the anterior and the posterior radiations. Lesions in this central division do not appear to induce characteristic ECG changes since this region serves more as a connecting network to synchronize activation of anterior septal-free wall and posterior septal-free wall of the left ventricle. In both experimental studies in the dog and histopathological studies in man, it appears that large areas of the anterior and posterior border fibers of the left bundle need to be impaired to produce the characteristic ECG changes of left anterior and posterior hemiblock.[91]

A profuse interconnecting network of subendocardial Purkinje fibers extends throughout both ventricles. This network connects with ordinary ventricular myocardium via transitional fibers also in the subendocardial layers. There is little evidence for appreciable penetration of Purkinje fibers into the ventricular walls toward the epicardium in man. The Purkinje network becomes sparse near the base and the upper septum and is most dense near the apex in both ventricles.

Propagation of the excitation wavefront in the ventricles proceeds from the subendocardial Purkinje network toward the epicardium and base of the heart through ordinary myocardial cells at a slower conduction velocity than that in the His-Purkinje system. Recently there has been renewed interest in the old observation[93] that conduction is more rapid in the direction parallel to the longitudinal axis of the fiber bundles than in the transverse direction. Interest in the phenomenon of anisotropic conditions has been rekindled by studies of the atrial myocardium, which demonstrated that more rapid longitudinal conduction was associated with lesser upstroke velocities of action potentials than the slower transverse conduction, and that the safety factor was lower in the longitudinal direction, i.e., block was more likely to occur in the direction of most rapid conduction. These observations implied that anisotropic properties might play a role in the formation of arcs (interfaces) of functional block and zones of slow conduction necessary for the formation of re-entry circuits. They predicted that interfaces of block most likely would be aligned perpendicular to the long axes of the fibers, since block would occur in that direction, and that very slow conduction would be more likely in a direction transverse to the long axis. Later studies in ventricular myocardium indicate that block is more likely to occur in the direction transverse to the longitudinal axes of the fibers, the same direction as slow conduction.[95] Those observations fit better with the observed configuration of functional re-entry circuits in the myocardial syncytium in which slow conduction around the edges of an interface of block proceeds in the same direction in which block occurred to form the interface. The role of anisotropic conduction in the formation of re-entry circuits in normal and abnormal myocardium is under active investigation.

Recent interest has focused on differences in the configuration of action potentials of myocytes near the endocardium compared with those near the epicardium.[96] The subepicardial myocytes contain a prominent phase one and notch before the plateau thought to be due to a transient outward current of potassium, i_{TO}, which appears to be greatly reduced or absent in subendocardial myocytes. This current is more prominent at slower rates and serves to reduce the overshoot and delay of the plateau. It has been suggested that these differences might be important in various differential responses including supernormal conduction in subepicardial layers but not in subendocardial layers, different responses to pharmacological agents, greater sensitivity of the action potentials of subepicardial myocytes to ischemia, and more pronounced responses of action potential durations of subepicardial myocytes to rate.

Recent studies have disclosed the presence of ATP-sensitive potassium channels in cardiac myocytes.[97] These channels activate when ATP drops to low levels, causing outward flow of potassium ions at membrane potentials more positive than the potassium equilibrium potential. The decreased duration of action potentials in acute ischemia may be related in part to the activation of these channels.

Arrhythmia Mechanisms

The classification of arrhythmia mechanisms shown in Table 1 accommodates recently observed phenomena.[98] The prerequisites for re-entry incorporated in the familiar ring model include slow conduction, undirectional block, and an inexcitable barrier separating conduction pathways. In the archetypical models of re-entry, the barrier is a fixed

Table 1
Mechanisms of Tachyarrhythmias*

Disorders of Impulse Propagation
    Re-entry
    Reflection
Disorders of Impulse Generation
    Enhanced normal automaticity
    Abnormal automaticity
    Afterdepolarizations
        Delayed
        Early

* Adapted from reference 98.

region of inexcitability in the center of the circuit, and slow conduction is uniform along the circuit. In the earliest biological models of re-entry studied systematically—rings dissected from jellyfish mantles—the unidirectional block could be produced by repetitive perturbations (pressure) that blocked in one direction, presumably due to refractoriness, but conducted from the other direction.[99] Thus the idea of time-dependent rather than constant unidirectional block was introduced.

Contemporary models of re-entry usually involve the concept of time-dependent unidirectional block depending on refractoriness in a setting of heterogeneous refractory properties.[100] Real re-entry circuits often form when a premature excitation propagates to a segment of the circuit that is refractory but can find another segment excitable because of disparate refractory periods in the segments. The Wolff-Parkinson-White syndrome is a well-studied example of re-entry forming when appropriately timed premature impulses encounter time-dependent unidirectional block in the accessory pathway yet conduct through the AV node because the accessory pathway usually has a longer refractory period than the AV node. However, there are also examples in this syndrome of constant unidirectional block in accessory pathways.

Studies in the 1970s[101] demonstrated that the barrier necessary for a stable circuit to form need not be fixed but could be functional—an interface of refractory and excitable tissue dynamically alternating during a single circuit. This interface-barrier, like unidirectional block, can be time-dependent, needing premature excitation for the refractory barrier to form. Thus, a quantum of progress in the understanding of re-entry occurred with the realization that the essential elements of a circuit could form in a continuous syncytium of conducting tissue.

There has been debate over the relative importance of heterogeneous refractoriness versus anisotropic conduction in the formation of interface-barriers and segments of slow conduction. According to one camp, the interface forms where there is a steep gradient of increasing refractory periods.[102] The other camp relates the interface and slow conduction to the anisotropic properties of the myocardium accentuated by disease which attenuates intercellular communications.[103] Slow conduction occurs in the direction of most sparse intercellular connections. The interface may represent a finite, narrow region of very slow conduction rather than block. Recent data derived from ischemically damaged epicardium overlying myocardial infarction appear to favor the idea that the interface represents a barrier to conduction imposed by refractory tissue, as originally proposed in the "leading circle" model of Alessie.[101]

As our understanding of the complex processes of ionic flow across the sarcolemma has increased, it has become obvious that the oscillatory behavior generally and simplistically labeled automaticity can have a variety of underlying ionic mechanisms with critical dependence on the level of membrane potential as well as other factors. The phrase "abnormal automaticity" has been used to refer to oscillatory firing occurring as less negative ranges of membrane potential as opposed to "normal automaticity" occurring at diastolic potentials -90 to -60 mV. However, the normal automaticity of the SA node appears to occur at diastolic potentials of -60 to -40 mV in vivo.

Arrhythmogenic foci of abnormal or enhanced normal automaticity are time-honored hypothetical constructs. Their existence in the heart in vivo is difficult to prove as a general case or in a specific instance. The issue is further complicated by the phenomena of oscillatory firing related to afterdepolarizations which when persistent may be indistinguishable from automatic firing. The accepted distinction between automatic oscillation and oscillation due to afterdepolarizations is that the former is self-sustaining and the latter always requires a triggering excitation incited by an independent mechanism, e.g., a propagated impulse.

After depolarizations, transient depolarizing shifts of membrane potential, are classified as delayed when they occur after the completion of repolarization,[104] and early when they occur during repolarization. Delayed afterdepolarization (DAD) occurs when cardiac cells are loaded with calcium, such as by treatment with cardiac glycosides, leading to repetitive release from the loaded sarcoplasmic reticulum, which in turn generates depolarizing transsarcolemmal current flow.[105] The ionic mechanisms for early afterdepolarizations (EAD) are not well defined, and it is likely that the phenomena classified as EAD may reflect multiple mechanisms. In the past two decades, these phenomena have been the focus of intensified study as possible arrhythmogenic mechanisms. DAD or EAD are prime suspects for some digitoxic and adrenergic tachyarrhythmias, certain ventricular tachycardias sensitive to beta-blockers and calcium channel blockers, multifocal atrial tachycardias, and the long QT syndromes.

References

1. Fozzard HA: Cardiac muscle: excitability and passive electrical properties. Prog Cardiovasc Dis 19:343, 1977.

2. Hille B: Ionic channels in nerve membranes. Prog Biophys Mol Biol 21:3, 1971.
3. Sperelakis N: Origin of the cardiac resting potential. In: Berne RM, et al. (eds), Handbook of Physiology: The Cardiovascular System. Bethesda, Maryland, American Physiological Society, 1979, p 187.
4. Thomas RC: Electrogenic sodium pump in nerve and muscle cells. Physiol Rev 52:563, 1972.
5. Hoffman BF, Cranefield PF: Electrophysiology of the Heart. New York, NY, McGraw Hill, 1960, pp 30–32.
6. Goldman DE: Potential, impedance, and rectification in membranes. J Gen Physiol 27:27, 1943.
7. Carmeliet E, Vereecke J: Electrogenesis of the action potential and automaticity. In: Berne RM, et al. (eds), Handbook of Physiology: The Cardiovascular System. Bethesda, Maryland, American Physiological Society, 1979, p 269.
8. Vassalle M: Cardiac automaticity and its control. In: Levy MN, Vassalle M (eds), Excitation and Neural Control of the Heart. Bethesda, Maryland, American Physiological Society, 1982.
9. Randall WC, Wehrmacher WH, Jones SV: Hierarchy of supraventricular pacemakers. J Thorac Cardiovasc Surg 82:797, 1981.
10. Hope RR, Scherlag BJ, El Sherif N, Lazzara R: Hierarchy of ventricular pacemakers. Circ Res 39:883, 1976.
11. Vassalle M: Electrogenic suppression of automaticity in sheep and dog Purkinje fibers. Circ Res 27:361, 1970.
12. Noble D: The surprising heart: A review of recent progress in cardiac electrophysiology. J Physiol (London) 353:1, 1984.
13. Giles W, Van Ginnekin A, Shibata EF: Ionic currents underlying cardiac pacemaker activity: a summary of voltage-clamp data from single cells. In: Nathan R (ed), Cardiac Muscle: The Regulation of Excitation and Contraction. Orlando, Florida, Academic Press, 1986, pp 1–27.
14. Draper MH, Weidman S: Cardiac resting and action potentials recorded with an intracellular electrode. J Physiol (London) 115:74, 1951.
15. Brown HF: Electrophysiology of the sinoatrial node. Physiol Rev 62:505, 1982.
16. Neher E, Sakman V: Single channel currents recorded from membranes of denervated frog muscle fibers. Nature (London) 260:799, 1976.
17. Hamill OP, Marty A, Neher E, et al: Improved patch clamp techniques for high-resolution current recording from cell and cell-free membrane patches. Pflügers Arch Gen Physiol 391:85, 1981.
18. Hume JR, Giles W: Ionic currents in single isolated bullfrog atrial cells. J Gen Physiol 81:153, 1983.
19. Noble D, Tsien RW: Outward membrane currents activated in plateau range of potential in cardiac Purkinje fibers. J Physiol (London) 200:205, 1969.
20. Callewaert E, Carmeliet E, Vereecke J: Single cardiac Purkinje cells: general electrophysiology and voltage-clamp analysis of the pacemaker current. J Physiol (London) 349:643, 1984.
21. Shibata EF, Giles WR: Ionic currents in isolated cardiac pacemaker cells from bullfrog sinus venosus. Proc Int Union Physiol Sci 15:76, 1983.

22. Brown HF, Kimura J, Noble SJ: The relative contribution of various time-dependent membrane currents to pacemaker activity in sinoatrial node. In: Bouman LN, Jongsma HJ (eds), Cardiac Rate and Rhythm. The Hague, Martinus Nijhoff, 1982, pp 53–68.
23. Hagiwara N, Irisawa H, Kamejani M: Contribution of two types of calcium currents to pacemaker potential of rabbit sinoatrial nodal cells. J Physiol (London) 395:233, 1988.
24. Brown HF, Giles WR, Noble SJ: Membrane currents underlying activity in frog sinus venosus. J Physiol (London) 271:783, 1977.
25. Noma A, Yanagihara K, Irisawa H: Inward current activated during hyperpolarization in the rabbit sinoatrial node cell. Pflügers Arch 385:11, 1977.
26. DiFrancesco D, Ojeda C: Properties of the current i_f in the sinoatrial node of the rabbit compared with those of i_{K2} in Purkinje fibers. J Physiol (London) 308:353, 1980.
27. DiFrancesco D: A new interpretation of the pacemaker current in calf Purkinje fibers. J Physiol (London) 314:359, 1981.
28. Giles W, van Ginneken A: A transient outward current in isolated cells from crista terminalis of rabbit heart. J Physiol (London) 368:243, 1985.
29. Eisner DA, Lederer WJ: Na-Ca exchange: stoichiometry and electrogenicity. Am J Physiol 248:C189, 1985.
30. Shibata EF, Momose Y, Giles W: An electrogenic Na^+/K^+ pump current in individual bullfrog atrial myocytes. Biophys J 45:136a, 1984.
31. DiFrancesco D, Noble D: A model of cardiac electrical activity incorporating ionic pumps and concentration changes (abstract). Phil Trans R Soc London 307:353, 1985.
32. Keith A, Flack M: The form and nature of the muscular connections between the primary divisions of the vertebrate heart. J Anat Physiol 41:172, 1987.
33. James TN: The sinus node. Am J Cardiol 40:965, 1977.
34. Bouman LN, Jongsma HJ: Structure and function of the sinoatrial node: a review. Eur Heart J 7:94, 1986.
35. James TN, Sherf L, Fine G, et al: Comparative ultrastructure of the sinus node in man and dog. Circulation 34:139, 1966.
36. Masson-Pevet M, Bleeker WK, Gas D: The plasma membrane of leading pacemaker cells in the rabbit sinus node: a qualitative and quantitative ultrastructural analysis. Circ Res 45:621, 1979.
37. James TN: Anatomy of the Coronary Arteries. Hagerstown, Maryland, Harper and Row, 1961, pp 103–131.
38. Levy MM, Marti PJ: Neural control of the heart. In: Berne RM, et al. (eds), Handbook of Physiology: The Cardiovascular System. Volume 1, The Heart. Bethesda, Maryland, American Physiological Society, 1979, p 581.
39. Ardell JL, Randall WC: Selective vagal innervation of the sinoatrial and atrioventricular nodes in the canine heart. Am J Physiol 251:H764, 1986.
40. MacKaay AJC, Opthof T, Bleeker WK, et al: Interaction of adrenaline or acetylcholine on cardiac pacemaker function: functional inhomogeneity of rabbit sinoatrial node. J Pharmacol Exp Ther 214:417, 1980.
41. Ardell JL, Randall WC, Cannon WJ, et al: Differential sympathetic regulation of automatic, conductile and contractile tissues of the canine heart. Am J Physiol 255:H1050, 1988.

42. Bleeker WK, MacKaay AJC, Masson-Pevet M, et al: Functional and morphological organization of the rabbit sinus node. Circ Res 46:11, 1980.
43. Boineau JP, Scheussler RB, Mooney CR, et al: Multicentric origin of the atrial depolarization wave: the pacemaker complex. Circulation 58:1036, 1978.
44. Boineau JP, Scheusser RB, Hackel DV, et al: Widespread distribution and rate differentiation of the atrial pacemaker complex. Am J Physiol 239:H406, 1980.
45. Boineau JP, Canavan TE, Schuessler RB, et al: Demonstration of a widely distributed atrial pacemaker complex in the human heart. Circulation 77:1221, 1988.
46. Ypey DL, Clapham DE, De Haan RL: Development of electrical coupling and action potential synchrony between paired aggregates of embryonic heart cells. J Membr Biol 51:75, 1979.
47. Veenstra RD, De Haan RL: Electrotonic interactions between aggregates of chick embryo cardiac pacemaker cells. Am J Physiol 250:H453, 1986.
48. Jalife J: Mutual entrainment and electrical coupling as mechanisms for synchronous firing of rabbit sinoatrial pacemaker cells. J Physiol (London) 356:221, 1984.
49. Delmar M, Jalife J, Michaels DC: Effects of changes in excitability and intercellular coupling on synchronization in the rabbit sinoatrial node. J Physiol (London) 370:127, 1986.
50. Joyner RW, Van Capelle JL: Propagation through electrically coupled cells: how a small SA node drives a large atrium. Biophys J 50:1157, 1986.
51. James TN: The connecting pathways between the sinus node and the AV node and between the right and the left atrium in the human heart. Am Heart J 66:498, 1963.
52. Paes de Carvalho A, de Mello WC, Hoffman BF: Electrophysiological evidence for specialized fiber types in the rabbit atrium. Am J Physiol 196:483, 1959.
53. Hogan PM, Davis LD: Evidence for specialized fibers in the canine right atrium. Circ Res 23:387, 1968.
54. Sherf L, James TN: Fine structure of cells and their histologic organization within the internodal pathways of the heart: clinical and electrocardiographic implications. Am J Cardiol 44:345, 1979.
55. Spach MS, Leiberman M, Scott JG, et al: Excitation sequence of the atrial septum and the AV node in isolated heart of the dog and rabbit. Circ Res 29:156, 1971.
56. Becker AE, Bouman LN, Janse NJ, et al: Functional anatomy of the cardiac conduction system. In: Harrison DC (ed), Cardiac Arrhythmias: A Decade of Progress. Boston, G.K. Hall, 1981, pp 3–24.
57. Roberts DE, Hirsch LT, Scher AM: Influence of cardiac fiber orientation on wave front voltage, conduction velocity, and tissue resistivity in the dog. Circ Res 44:701, 1979.
58. Zipes DP, Mihalich JM, Robbins GT: Effect of selective vagal and stellate ganglion stimulation on atrial refractoriness. Cardiovasc Res 8:647, 1974.
59. Coumel P, Attuel P, Lecerc JF: Arhythmie auriculaires d'origine vagale ou catecholergique. Effets compares du traitement beta-bloquer et phenomene d' echappement. Arch Mal Coeur 75:373, 1982.

60. Purkinje JE: Mikroskopisch-neurologische beobachtungen. (citado por 45) Arch Anat Physiol Wissen Med 12:281, 1845.
61. His W Jr: Die tatigkeit des embryonalen herzens und deren bedentung fur die leher von der herzbewegung beim erwach senen. Arch Med Klin Leipzig, 1893.
62. Kent AFS: Researches on the structure and function of the mammalian heart. J Physiol 14:233, 1893.
63. Tawara S: Des reizleitung des saugetier-herzens. Jena, Fischer. Eine anatomisch-histobogische studie uber das atrioventrikular bundle und die Purkinjesche fäden, 1906.
64. Keith A, Flack M: The form and nature of the muscular connections between the primary division of the vertebrate heart. J Anat Physiol 41:172, 1907.
65. Rossi L: Histopathology of cardiac arrhythmias. Casa Editrice Ambrosiana, Milan, 1978, Chapter II.
66. James TN, Sherf L: Ultrastructure of the human atrioventricular node. Circulation 37:1049, 1968.
67. Rosenbaum MB, Elizari MV, Lazzari JO: The Hemiblocks Tampe Tracings, 1970, Chapter II.
68. Brechenmacher C: Anatomy and histology of the conduction pathways. In: Puech P, Slama R (eds), The Cardiac Arrhythmias. Corbiere RMDP and Roussel-UCLAF, 1979, pp 13–19.
69. Hoffman BF, Cranefield PF: The physiological basis of cardiac arrhythmias. Am J Med 37:670, 1964.
70. Damato AN, Lau SH: His bundle rhythms. Circulation 40:527, 1969.
71. Tse WW: Evidence of presence of automatic fibers in the canine atrioventricular node. Am J Physiol 225:716, 1973.
72. Tse WW: Effect of epinephrine on automaticity of the canine atrioventricular node. Am J Physiol 229:34, 1975.
73. Woods WT, Sherf L, James TN: Structure and function of specific regions in the canine atrioventricular node. Am J Physiol 243:H41, 1982.
74. Damato AN, Lau SH, Helfant RH, et al: A study of heart block in man using His bundle recordings. Circulation 39:297, 1969.
75. Hoffman BF, Moore EN, Stuckey JH, et al: Functional properties of the atrioventricular conduction system. Circ Res 13:308, 1963.
76. Wit AL, Weiss MB, Berkowitz WD, et al: Patterns of atrioventricular conduction in the human heart. Circ Res 27:345, 1970.
77. Irisarwa H, Noma A, Matsuda H: Electrogenesis of the pacemaker potential as revealed by atrioventricular nodal experiments. In: Sperelakis N (ed), Physiology and Pathophysiology of the Heart. Boston, Kluwer Academic Publishers, Chapter 6, 1984.
78. Scherlag BJ, Abelleira JL, Narula OS, et al: The differential effects of ouabain on sinus, A-V nodal, His bundle and idioventricular rhythms. Am Heart J 81:227, 1971.
79. Narula OS, Narula JT: Junctional pacemakers in man: Response to overdrive suppression with and without parasympathetic blockade. Circulation 57:880, 1978.
80. James TN, Sherf L, Urthaler F: Fine structure of the bundle-branches. Br Heart J 36:1, 1974.

81. Katz AM: Physiology of the Heart. New York, Raven Press, 1977, Chapter 15.
82. Lev M: The conduction system. In: Gould SE (ed). Pathology of the Heart and Blood Vessels. Springfield, Illinois, Charles C. Thomas, 1968, Chapter 6.
83. Sciacca A, Sangiorgi M: Trouble de la conduction intraventriculaire du a la lesion du tronc commun du faiseau de His. Acta Cardiol 2:486, 1967.
84. Sherf L, James TN: New electrocardiographic concept: synchronized sino-ventricular conduction. Dis Chest 55:127, 1969.
85. Lazzara R, Yeh BK, Samet P: Functional transverse interconnections within the His bundle and the bundle branches. Circ Res 32:509, 1973.
86. Lazzara R, Yeh BK, Samet P: Functional transverse interconnections within the His bundle and the bundle branches. Circ Res 32:509, 1973.
87. Bailey JC, Anderson GJ, Pippenger D, et al: Re-entry within the isolated canine Bundle of His. Am J Cardiol 32:808, 1973.
88. Narula OS: Longitudinal dissociation in the His bundle. Circulation 56:996, 1977.
89. El-Sherif N, Amat-y-Leon F, Schonfeld C, et al: Normalization of bundle branch block patterns by distal His bundle pacing. Circulation 57:465, 1978.
90. Scherlag BJ, El-Sherif N, Hope RR, et al: The significance of dissociation of conduction in the canine His bundle: electrophysiological studies in vivo and in vitro. J Electrocardiol 11:343, 1978.
91. Wenckebach KF, Winterberg H: Die unregelmassige Herztatigkeit. Verlag von Wilhem Engelmann, Leipzig, 1927.
92. Kulbertus HE, Demoulin JCP: Pathophysiologic basis of concept of left hemiblock. In: Wellens HJJ, Lie KI, Janse MJ (eds), The Conduction System of the Heart. The Netherlands, HE Stenfert Kroese BV-Leiden, 1976, Chapter 16.
93. Sano T, Takayama N, Shimamoto T: Directional difference of conduction velocity in cardiac ventricular syncytium studied by microelectrodes. Circ Res 7:262, 1959.
94. Spach MS, Kootsey JM: The nature of electrical propagation in cardiac muscle. Am J Physiol 244:H, 1983.
95. Delgado C, Steinhaus B, Delmar M, et al: Directional differences in excitability and margin of safety for propagation in sheep ventricular epicardial muscle. Circ Res 67:97, 1990.
96. Litowsky S, Antzelevitch C: Transient outward current prominent in canine ventricular epicardium but not endocardium. Circ Res 62:116, 1988.
97. Heidbuchel H, Vereecke J, Carmeliet E: Three different potassium channels in human atrium: contribution to the basal potassium conductance. Circ Res 66:1277, 1990.
98. Hoffman BF, Cranefield PF: The physiological basis of cardiac arrhythmias. Am J Med 37:670, 1964.
99. Mayer AG: Rhythmical pulsation in scyphomedusae. Publication 47 of the Carnegie Institution 1906, pp 1–66.
100. Janse MJ: Re-entry rhythms. In: Fozzard HA (ed), The Heart and Vascular System. New York, Raven Press, 1986, pp 1203–1233.
101. Allessie MA, Bonke FIM, Schopman FJG: Circus movement in rabbit atrial muscle as a mechanism of tachycardia. Circ Res 41:9, 1977.

102. Gough WM, Mehra R, Restivo M, et al: Reentrant ventricular arrhythmias in the late myocardial infarction period in the dog. Circ Res 57:432, 1985.
103. Dillon SM, Allessie MA, Ursell PC, et al: Influences of anisotropic tissue structure in reentrant circuits in the epicardial border zone of subacute canine infarcts. Circ Res 63:182, 1988.
104. Tsien RW, Kass RS, Weingart R: Cellular and subcellular mechanism of cardiac pacemaker oscillations. J Exp Biol 81:205, 1979.
105. Cranefield PF: Action potentials, afterpotentials and arrhythmias. Circ Res 41:415, 1977.

Chapter 2

Noninvasive Cardiac Evaluation of Patients with Arrhythmias

Gerald V. Naccarelli,
Anne H. Dougherty, and
Robert L. Rinkenberger

Introduction

In patients who have cardiac arrhythmias, noninvasive cardiac testing can be used to define the quality and quantity of arrhythmia, identify patients who may be at risk for sudden death, and document associated underlying cardiovascular disease. In this chapter we will review the indications, usefulness, and limitations of various noninvasive cardiac procedures including echocardiography, radionuclide angiocardiography, stress testing, long-term electrocardiographic monitoring, and signal-averaging techniques in managing patients who have arrhythmias.

Echocardiography

All patients with complex ventricular arrhythmias should have some form of noninvasive assessment of their cardiac status. M-mode and 2-dimensional echocardiographic abnormalities that may be documented in patients with arrhythmias include: segmental left ventricular

From Naccarelli GV (ed): *Cardiac Arrhythmias: A Practical Approach*. Mount Kisco, NY, Futura Publishing Co., Inc., © 1991.

wall motion abnormalities consistent with coronary artery disease, serious valvular stenosis or regurgitation, mitral valve prolapse, hypertrophic obstructive cardiomyopathy, chamber dilatation and left ventricular dysfunction associated with dilated cardiomyopathy, pericardial disease, intracardiac tumors, arrhythmogenic right ventricular dysplasia, and congenital heart defects.[1-7] Doppler studies give us the ability to noninvasively quantitate valvular stenoses and regurgitation and also to identify intracardiac shunts.

Echocardiography can be useful in documenting chamber dilatation, global or segmental left ventricular dysfunction, and the presence of ventricular aneurysms.[8] The presence of left ventricular dysfunction within any ventricular arrhythmia subclass may increase that patient's risk for sudden death and influence the necessity for prophylactic treatment.[9-11] Documentation of serious left ventricular dysfunction provides a useful screen for avoidance of antiarrhythmic drugs that have marked negative inotropy. M-mode echocardiography, cardiac Doppler, and nuclear techniques can be useful in screening for patients with diastolic left ventricular dysfunction.[12]

Echocardiography may also be useful in documenting cardiac abnormalities associated with the Wolff-Parkinson-White syndrome,[13] such as hypertrophic obstructive cardiomyopathy, atrial septal defect, mitral valve prolapse,[14] and Ebstein's anomaly.[15] The presence of Ebstein's anomaly should increase one's suspicion of the presence of a right-sided accessory atrioventricular (AV) connection.

In patients with a history of atrial fibrillation, echocardiography can measure the left atrial size which may predict drug response in this group of patients. Medical therapy is less likely to prevent recurrences or revert atrial fibrillation to sinus rhythm in patients who have a markedly dilated left atrium.[16] Echocardiography is also useful in screening for anomalies associated with atrial fibrillation such as rheumatic mitral disease, mitral valve prolapse, and hypertrophic or ischemic cardiomyopathy.

In the patient who has syncope of undetermined etiology, an echocardiogram can be useful in screening for anatomical cardiac abnormalities.[17] However, in patients with a normal physical examination and no history suggestive of organic heart disease, the diagnostic yield from echocardiography is low. Conversely, in the patient with a systolic murmur suggestive of left ventricular outflow tract obstruction, an echocardiogram can be diagnostic. Echocardiographic findings that can aid in the diagnosis in the patient with syncope include hypertrophic obstructive cardiomyopathy, left atrial myxoma, and thickening of the aortic valve leaflets with doming suggestive of aortic stenosis.

Radionuclide Angiocardiography

Radionuclide angiocardiography is a noninvasive test used for the quantitative assessment of global and regional left ventricular performance. Ejection fraction can be measured using the first pass technique, or the gated cardiac blood pool imaging technique.[18]

Radionuclide angiocardiography quantitates left ventricular systolic pump performance. Ejection fraction is calculated by measuring a change in radioactive counts within the left ventricle at end-diastole and end-systole. Normal ejection fractions are greater than or equal to 50%. Ejection fraction measurements by nuclear techniques have been found to be accurate, reproducible ($\pm 6\%$),[18] and correlate well with angiographically measured ejection fraction (R = .92). In a patient who has atrial fibrillation with a rapid ventricular response or frequent spontaneous ventricular ectopic activity, gating of heart beats may be inaccurate, leading to quantitative errors in the measurement of ejection fraction.[19]

Radionuclide angiocardiography is an excellent method for evaluating ventricular wall motion. This technique is useful in determining segmental or regional left ventricular hypokinesis, akinesis, or dyskinesis,[20] and can be used to screen for patients with left ventricular dysfunction who may be at increased risk for sudden and nonsudden death. Therefore, radionuclide angiocardiography is useful in risk stratification of patients post-myocardial infarction in whom depressed ejection fractions are associated with an enhanced mortality (Fig. 1). The presence of left ventricular dysfunction may be useful in determining which patients need prophylactic treatment. In addition, it may be useful in identifying patients in whom antiarrhythmic drugs with negative inotropic activity should be avoided.

Exercise stress tests using a bicycle ergometer and cardiac blood pool imaging before and during stress can be used to screen for coronary artery disease. In normal subjects, the left ventricular ejection fraction will increase by at least 6% during stress.[21] In contrast, the left ventricular performance of ischemic patients may show no increase or actually decrease during exercise. In addition, patients with exercise-induced ischemia may develop localized ischemic wall motion abnormalities. The use of exercise gated studies is more sensitive and specific than electro-

POSTMYOCARDIAL INFARCTION
RISK STRATIFICATION

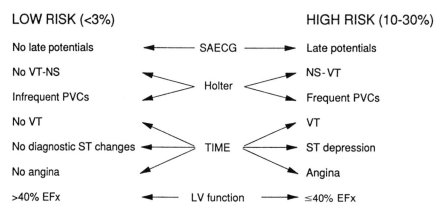

Figure 1. Role of ejection fraction (EFx), presence of nonsustained VT on Holter (NS-VT), latent ischemia and signal averaging (SAECG) in risk stratification of post-myocardial infarction patients. VT = ventricular tachycardia; NS = nonsustained; PVCs = preventricular contractions; EFx = ejection fraction; SAECG = signal-averaging electrocardiogram.

cardiographic stress tests in the diagnosis of coronary artery disease and approaches stress thallium testing in predictive accuracy.[22]

Radionuclide angiocardiography has the advantage of being an accurate, noninvasive means of quantitating left ventricular function. Quantitatively, this technique is more accurate than echocardiography. In addition, technically acceptable studies are easier to obtain compared to echocardiography in patients who have chronic obstructive pulmonary disease and in obese patients.

Because there is close electromechanical coupling of mechanical events, nuclear techniques utilizing phase analysis have been used as a noninvasive means of mapping myocardial contraction sequences. These techniques have been used to map the location of accessory AV connections[23] and initiating areas of ventricular tachycardia (VT).[24]

Exercise Stress Testing

The exercise stress test is the most commonly used noninvasive technique for the detection of latent coronary artery disease. Since exertion induces myocardial ischemia by causing myocardial oxygen demand to exceed supply, the exercise stress test can provoke an electrocardiographic change suggestive of myocardial ischemia.

Our stress test protocol starts with a baseline 12-lead electrocardiogram and blood pressure. Heart rate and blood pressure are monitored throughout the exercise test and recovery periods. Before starting the stress test, we obtain an electrocardiogram after hyperventilation is obtained in a standing position to screen for labile ST-T wave segment changes. The stress test is usually performed with the patient on a treadmill, although a bicycle ergometer can also be used. Depending on the stress protocol, the rate and incline of the treadmill is increased at 2- to 3-minute intervals. The stress test is continued until the patient achieves a target heart rate that is greater than 85% of the predicted maximum heart rate for that patient's age and sex. Occasionally, the patient is exercised only to a maximum predetermined heart rate. For example, in the early phase after myocardial infarction, we rarely allow a patient to exceed a heart rate of 120 beats/minute.[25] The exercise stress test is usually terminated before this target heart rate if the patient develops marked hypotension, long runs of ventricular tachycardia, or marked ST segment depression.[26] In addition, the stress test may be terminated because of severe chest pain or exhaustion.

We define a positive exercise stress test result (i.e., positive for ischemia) as greater than 1 mm of horizontal or downsloping ST segment depression occurring 80 msec after the J-point (Fig. 2). Although increasing the criteria for a positive result to 2 mm of ST segment depres-

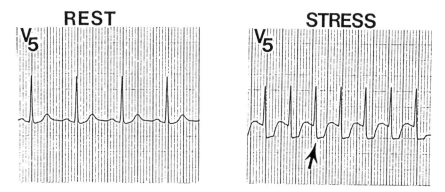

Figure 2. ECG lead V_5 at rest (left) and during stress (right) demonstrating >1 mm horizontal ST segment depression (arrow) associated with chest pain diagnostic of a positive stress test. (Reproduced with permission.[145])

sion will increase the specificity, this adjustment will also reduce the sensitivity of the test. According to Baye's theorem, the sensitivity and specificity of stress testing depends largely on the pretest likelihood of coronary artery disease as determined by history and physical examination.[22,27,28] The magnitude of ST segment depression, the level of exercise at which ST segment depression occurs, and the persistence of ST segment abnormalities in the recovery phase all provide an index of the severity of coronary artery disease.[29–31] Additional criteria for a positive result that add to the sensitivity of the stress test include the development of hypotension, inverted U waves, typical anginal chest pain, or ventricular arrhythmias.[32]

Nuclear techniques, such as thallium stress testing, will also increase the sensitivity and specificity of the exercise stress test.[22,32] In addition to screening for patients with coronary artery disease, stress testing with or without thallium is also useful in screening for reversible areas of ischemia in patients with known coronary artery disease after myocardial infarction, angioplasty, or coronary artery bypass surgery. Newer techniques such as Spect imaging or dipyridamole positron emission tomography may be more accurate than earlier techniques.

Exercise stress testing is also used for evaluating an individual's physical condition and New York Heart Association functional status.[33] This application of the stress test is useful for the patient who has valvular heart disease, especially mitral stenosis, since the patient's functional status is often used in determining the timing of prosthetic heart valve replacement. In cardiac rehabilitation programs, the presence of angina dyspnea, or exercise-aggravated arrhythmia at a certain reproducible workload can be useful in limiting physical activity to a prescribed level.

Stress testing has been found to be useful for risk stratification of patients after a myocardial infarction (Fig. 1).[22,27,34–36] Several studies have shown that the occurrence of exercise-induced angina, exercise-induced ventricular arrhythmia, or exercise-induced diagnostic ST segment changes 1–2 weeks after myocardial infarction is predictive of future anginal events, myocardial infarction, and sudden death.[34,36] Patients found to have exercise-induced ischemia appear to be in a high-risk category. These patients should be strongly considered for prophylactic beta-blocker protection or early cardiac catheterization with appropriate treatment to alter this natural history.[9]

Interpretation of a positive stress-test result is limited in patients who have baseline ST segment abnormalities because of the increased frequency of false-positive tests. Such patients would include those taking digitalis, patients with bundle branch block, patients with left ventricular hypertrophy with associated ST-T wave changes, and patients with overt Wolff-Parkinson-White syndrome.[32] Female patients with mitral valve prolapse syndrome also may have ST segment shifts during stress testing that represent a false-positive response.[32] In order to minimize the frequency of false-positive responses in these subgroups, we routinely recommend a stress thallium test to improve specificity.

Stress Testing for the Patient with Arrhythmias

In patients with arrhythmias, stress testing may be useful in documenting arrhythmias by withdrawing vagal tone, increasing sympathetic tone and circulating catecholamines, and inducing ischemic arrhythmias. The stress test also screens for concomitant coronary artery disease. In addition, during stress testing some patients may have a ventricular tachyarrhythmia related to ischemia (Fig. 3). In patients with this finding, cardiac catheterization followed by appropriate management of the obstructive coronary disease should be considered in conjunction with appropriate antiarrhythmic therapy.

During stress testing, patients are monitored for 10–15 minutes. Therefore, ventricular ectopy, couplets, and ventricular tachycardia can be more frequently identified than on routine electrocardiogram and rhythm strips, which have a shorter monitoring period.[37,38] If the quantitation of the patient's exercise-induced arrhythmias must be accurate, continuous electrocardiographic monitoring using a trendscriber has been found to be superior to intermittent monitoring.[39] Some newer treadmill machines can store a record of arrhythmias that are noted during exercise. These tracings can then be reviewed after completion of the test.

Although exercise induction of sustained ventricular tachycardia in patients with a prior history of sustained ventricular tachycardia is less than 10%, stress testing is useful in identifying patients with exercise-induced or exercise-aggravated ventricular tachycardia (Fig. 4).[40–42] Frequently, these patients are young and have no evidence of serious organic heart disease. There is some variability in the occurrence of VT during exercise. We prefer to see VT occur on at least two sequential treadmills before using it as a sole marker of therapy assessment. In six patients with exercise-induced ventricular tachycardia, the QRS morphology of the tachycardia was usually of a left bundle branch block form.[40] Mapping of the tachycardia showed the earliest activation in the

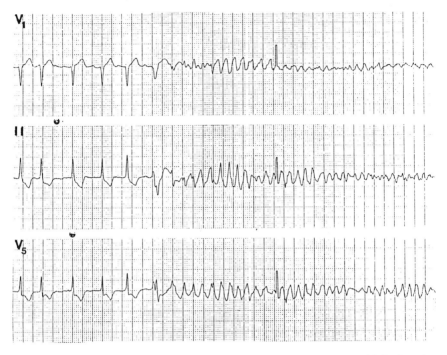

Figure 3. Exercise-induced ventricular fibrillation associated with ischemia (ST depression). On cardiac catheterization, the patient had obstructive left main coronary artery disease. (Reproduced with permission.[146])

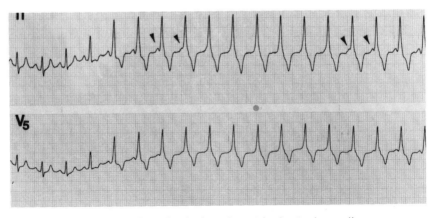

Figure 4. Exercise-induced ventricular tachycardia.

area of the right ventricular outflow tract, when ventricular tachycardia was not induced by programmed stimulation. Therefore, stress test results can be an important marker of the patient's electrical instability and the only method available to guide therapy through serial drug studies. We then use serial stress testing after drug therapy is begun to determine whether a drug is effective in preventing recurrences of exercise-induced ventricular tachycardia.

Although the mechanism of this tachycardia remains controversial, the sympathetic nervous system appears to be causative, in that stress testing increases adrenergic tone and beta-blockers frequently are effective in controlling the arrhythmia. Recent data show that circulating norepinephrine levels are no higher at the time of recurrence of tachycardia during exercise in these patients than they are in control patients.[43] These data suggest that the myocardium of patients with exercise-induced ventricular tachycardia may be more sensitive to circulating norepinephrine. This finding, plus the inability to induce these patients' ventricular tachycardia during programmed stimulation, suggests that the mechanism of the tachycardia may not be reentrant.

Although the presence of exercise-induced ventricular tachycardia may be pathological, it should be kept in mind that about one-third of normal subjects may develop various ventricular arrhythmias in response to exercise.[44] Studies have demonstrated that ventricular ectopy is more likely to occur at faster heart rates in normal subjects, but these findings are usually limited to the occurrence of premature ventricular complexes (PVCs).[45] The induction of ventricular tachycardia during stress testing is rare in normal patients. In comparison, in over 50% of patients who have coronary disease, PVCs develop in response to exercise testing.[45] In this group, PVCs often occur in the early recovery period. Ventricular ectopy appears to be more reproducible in patients with coronary artery disease.[44,46]

In many patients, stress testing provides useful information that can be used in a complementary fashion to Holter monitoring and EP testing since stress testing is the only method of the three which induces physiological changes that may trigger arrhythmias or modify antiarrhythmic drug activity. In several studies, catecholamines have been shown to reverse beneficial effects of antiarrhythmic drugs.[47,48] In addition, presumed adequate suppression of arrhythmia as assessed by Holter monitoring may be noted during drug treatment yet stress testing may reveal persistent repetitive ventricular activity. In fact, with IC agents, stress testing appears to screen for proarrhythmia with the new appearance of incessant sustained VT.[49,50]

Stress Testing in SVT Patients

Stress testing has had minimal use in the screening of patients with supraventricular arrhythmias since exercise-induced supraventricular arrhythmias are rarely seen. However, in patients with overt Wolff-Parkinson-White syndrome, the loss of the delta wave at low levels of exercise has correlated with a long refractory period of the accessory AV connection in the antegrade direction.[51] Thus, stress testing may be useful in the noninvasive risk stratification of patients with this syn-

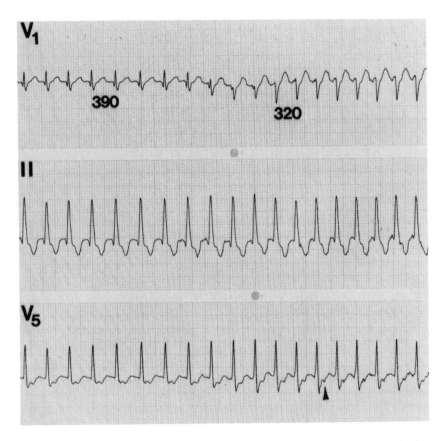

Figure 5. Exercise-induced orthodromic paroxysmal supraventricular tachycardia (cycle length of 320 ms) in a patient with overt preexcitation. Serial testing resulted in effective suppression of the above on a combination of propranolol plus encainide.

drome. Although premature auricular contractions (PACs) occur in up to 40% of patients during stress testing, the induction of sustained supraventricular tachycardia (SVT) is rare (1–3%) (Fig. 5). In a patient with a previous history of sustained SVT, the incidence of SVT during exercise is less than 15%. If SVT is reproducibly induced by exercise in the control state, serial stress testing can be performed to judge efficacious antiarrhythmic drug trials. In patients with atrial fibrillation and flutter, assessment of rate response control via drugs can be made including screening for the occurrence of atrial flutter with 1:1 AV nodal conduction.

Stress Testing in Syncope

Stress testing may also be useful for patients who are suspected of having arrhythmias causing dizziness or syncope. It has been reported that Holter monitoring is superior to treadmill testing in detecting arrhythmias in patients with syncope;[52] however, the treadmill test can slightly increase the diagnostic yield in this group of patients.

Long-term Electrocardiographic Recordings

Electrocardiographic recording to document a patient's arrhythmia has had widespread application as a noninvasive tool in cardiology.[53] A patient's arrhythmia may be documented by a simple electrocardiogram; however, the use of techniques with longer monitoring periods (rhythm strips, trendscription, stress testing, and Holter monitoring) increases the likelihood of documenting the arrhythmia.[38] Although trendscription had been used as a means to screen patients and to conduct serial drug studies,[54,55] most investigators prefer longer monitoring periods.

Since the original description by Holter in the 1950s,[56,57] Holter monitoring, or continuous ambulatory electrocardiographic monitoring, has been a useful technique for patients with cardiac arrhythmias. Lightweight battery-powered recorders are worn continuously for 24 or more hours. One can record one- or two-lead electrocardiographic data, which can then be analyzed. We prefer a two-lead system since it is more sensitive in documenting ST segment abnormalities, identifying aberrancy, and screening out artifactual abnormalities.[58] The leads usually used are modifications of leads V_1 and V_5.[59] We prefer this lead system since the modified V_1 lead often gives easily recognizable P waves, and is helpful in differentiating right from left bundle branch block. The second electrocardiographic channel can also be utilized to record simultaneous atrial activity in patients with arrhythmias that are difficult to interpret. This can be performed by having the patient swallow an esophageal bipolar pill electrode that can record atrial activity on the second channel.[60] The ambulatory recorders can be either cassette or reel-to-reel and can be attached to a belt or a shoulder strap. Cassette tapes are lighter and more compact, but reel-to-reel tapes have a better signal-to-noise ratio. Signals may be AM or FM analog signals. In some systems, the recorder converts the signal to a digital format for storage. Recorders have a clock and event marker buttons so that electrocardiographic events can be accurately correlated with the timing of patient's symptoms. All patients are instructed in the use of a diary in which they can record the time of symptoms, as well as their activity and medication taken.

In addition to the recorder, the ambulatory electrocardiographic system also includes a scanner. The components of the scanner vary depending on the manufacturer.[59,61] Basically, there is a playback system that permits rapid review of the recorder tape. Tapes can be scanned at up to 120 times real time and slowed to real time when careful analysis is necessary. A technician reviews the scan on an oscilloscope display unit. The scanner also has a data analysis system built into it. Most new systems have a computer-based analysis system with only a very small error in the quantitative analysis of the data. With some units, the information on the recorder tape is dumped onto a hard disk. The computer analyzes all the different types of beats, and the technician interacts with the system and correctly classifies the beats. The computer then reanalyzes and quantitates the numbers of PVCs and PACs and runs of tachycardia. Most scanning units print out data in a trend or graph format and give a 24-hour display of the minimum and maximum heart rate and the total numbers of normal beats, PVCs, and PACs and quantitate the number of couplets and runs of tachycardia. Tables of the hourly counts of PACs and PVCs and a trend graph of the hourly heart rate and ST segment changes are recorded. Once the computer-based system has scanned and analyzed the record with the technician's input, data are compiled along with representative printout strips as preprogrammed. Printout strips are determined by certain preset criteria and include representative ectopic beats, runs of brady- or tachyarrhythmia (Figs. 6, 7), and electrocardiograms (either normal or abnormal) that occur during patient's symptoms. The technician can interact with the system to print out additional strips that are felt to be informative. Full

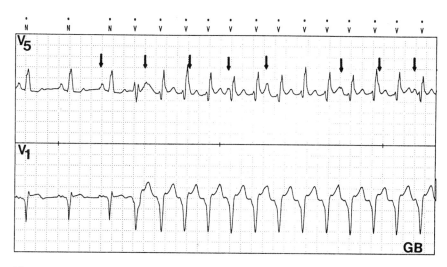

Figure 6. Simultaneously recorded modified leads V_5 and V_1 demonstrating the onset of ventricular tachycardia noted during a Holter recording.

disclosure formats with compressed size and slower recording speeds are also available.

During the interpretation, the physician must correlate the data from these reports with the total clinical picture since it is common for 24-hour monitoring to show abnormalities even in patients with normal

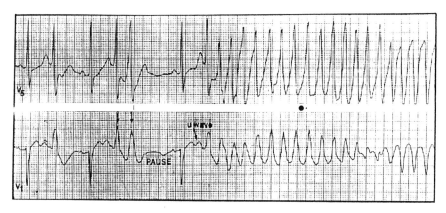

Figure 7. Holter recording demonstrating pause-dependent ventricular tachycardia (torsades de pointes).

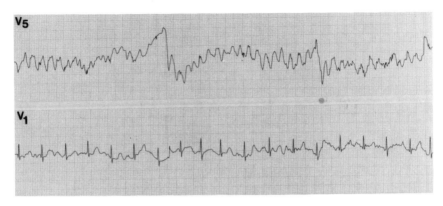

Figure 8. Artifact during Holter monitoring simulating ventricular fibrillation in V_5. Diagnosis of sinus rhythm confirmed in lead V_1.

cardiac function. Electrocardiographic abnormalities including marked sinus bradycardia (less than 40 beats/min), sinus pauses, PACs and PVCs,[62] transient Wenckebach AV block during sleep, and short runs of atrial tachycardia have been recorded in various normal populations.[62–65] These normal variants must be kept in mind so that normal subjects who experience them are not inappropriately treated. Physicians who interpret Holter monitoring results must be aware of artifacts that either are due to electrical or mechanical malfunction that can cause pseudobradyarrhythmia, pseudotachyarrhythmia, or false AV block[59,61] (Fig. 8). Poor electrode placement, broken lead wires and patient's cables, jamming of the tape, and defective batteries can cause these abnormalities. The use of two electrocardiographic leads is helpful in identifying these spurious results.[62] Indications for Holter monitoring are listed in Table 1.

Table 1
Indications for Holter Monitoring

---

1. Evaluation of suspected or known cardiac rhythm disorders
2. Evaluation of symptoms suggestive of an arrhythmic disorder
3. Evaluation of clinical syndromes in which arrhythmias may increase the risk of sudden death
4. Evaluation of pacemaker function
5. Evaluation of chest pain

Holter Monitoring—Spontaneous Variability

Determination of Drug Effect

Ambulatory monitoring is used primarily for evaluating cases of suspected cardiac rhythm disturbances. Since these arrhythmias can be episodic, detection of complex ventricular arrhythmias will vary, depending on the duration of the recording. A 24-hour Holter recording permits the recording of cardiac rhythm during both sleep and awake states. Thus, the variation of arrhythmias during waking hours and during physical and mental stress can be demonstrated. Sleep has usually been associated with a marked decrease in PVC frequency. An examination of the effectiveness of 1 to 48 hours of recording in patients with coronary artery disease and normal subjects indicates that the most malignant type of ventricular ectopic activity was recorded in over 95% of patients by 36 hours, compared to a diagnostic yield of 58–84% when only 24 hours of recording was performed.

Holter monitors are used in a serial fashion to judge the efficacy of antiarrhythmic drug treatment. However, one must keep in mind that because of the spontaneous variability of a patient's arrhythmia, this approach may be limited. Figure 9 shows the variability in PVC frequency in a cardiac arrest patient who underwent 2 consecutive days of Holter monitoring while not taking antiarrhythmic drugs. Although the patient had frequent ventricular ectopic activity during the first 24 hours, a marked decrease in arrhythmia occurred spontaneously on the second day.

Spontaneous variability can mimic antiarrhythmic drug effect[68] and make the physician think that the arrhythmia has been controlled. Similarly, patients may have a low frequency of spontaneous ventricular ectopic activity between very serious spells of life-threatening ventricular tachycardia. In this group of patients, serial comparison of drug-treated recordings may be limited. In a group of patients with hypertrophic cardiomyopathy, nonsustained VT present on control Holter was not present in 50% on repeat monitoring.[69] In two recent studies, frequent spontaneous ventricular ectopic activity was noted in only 25–50% of patients with a history of sustained ventricular tachyarrhythmias.[70,71] It has been reported that two-thirds of patients who had survived an out-of-hospital cardiac arrest did not have the presence of even nonsustained VT on continuous electrocardiographic monitoring (Fig. 10).[72] Others have demonstrated that Holter monitoring detected arrhythmias suitable for serial testing in 50% of 43 patients with sustained

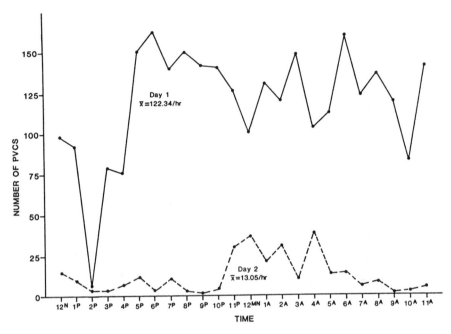

Figure 9. Variability in PVC frequency noted in a patient with a history of sustained VT. Note marked variability over 2 consecutive days of recording off antiarrhythmic therapy. (Reproduced with permission.[145])

VT and coronary artery disease (CAD) while EP studies induced VT in 82% (p = .003).[73] In patients with infrequent spontaneous ectopy and sustained ventricular tachyarrhythmia, serial Holter monitoring alone is not adequate to evaluate treatment efficacy. Therefore, invasive electrophysiological study should be strongly considered as part of the evaluation in these cases. In patients who have more frequent ectopy during their control Holter recordings, serial comparisons of recording were shown to be a reliable method in treating patients with potentially lethal[74] and life-threatening ventricular arrhythmias.[75]

Pooled data suggest that an 83% reduction in the number of PVCs over a 24-hour period can define drug effect.[76,77] In patients with post-myocardial infarction, variability is even more marked and drug effect may require in excess of a 95% reduction in PVCs.[78] In the Cardiac Arrhythmia Pilot Study (CAPS),[79] 37% of placebo patients had more than a 70% suppression of PVCs on repeat Holter due to spontaneous variability in this population. Drug effect only defines a statistically sig-

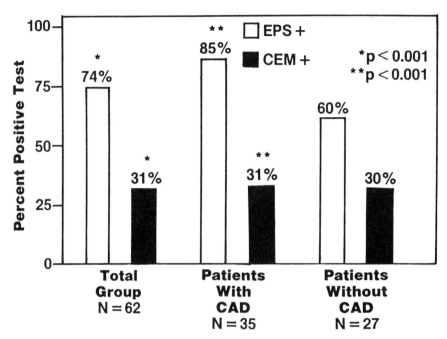

Figure 10. Presence of nonsustained VT on Holter compared to inducible VT/VF during EP study in cardiac arrest patients. EPS = electrophysiological study; CEM = continuous electrocardiographic monitoring; CAD = coronary artery disease. (Adapted from Skale, et al.[72])

nificant reduction in the number of antiarrhythmic events caused by an antiarrhythmic drug. Drug effect is not synonymous with drug effectiveness, that is, an end-point reached after drug therapy that predicts no further life-threatening recurrence of arrhythmia. Although in pooled data, the above end-point (83% reduction in PVCs in 24 hours) is valid, in an individual patient the end-point of drug effect is variable and depends on the density of the baseline arrhythmia. In addition, long-term is worse than short-term reproducibility.[80] It has been demonstrated that patients frequently met efficacy criteria 1 year after drug withdrawal based on repeat 24-hour Holter recordings.[81] More variability has been noted in coronary than in noncoronary patients.[82] During chronic antiarrhythmic therapy, substantial variability in arrhythmia frequency occurs.[83] Partial, but not complete, suppression of significant arrhythmia during drug therapy may be misinterpreted as drug effectiveness. If longer monitoring periods are used before and after drug treatment, a correction factor for some of the spontaneous variability of the arrhythmia can be made. With this factor, a smaller reduction in baseline arrhythmia frequency can define drug effect.

As mentioned above, it is important not to confuse drug effect with drug effectiveness; however, criteria for drug effectiveness are not well defined. In one study, a 100% reduction in spontaneously occurring runs of ventricular tachycardia, a 90% reduction in ventricular couplets, and at least a 50% reduction in the number of PVCs over 24 hours seemed to be predictive of a good therapeutic response in high-risk patients with baseline high-density arrhythmia.[75] Other proposed criteria for drug effectiveness include a 70–80% reduction in PVCs and a 90–100% reduction in runs of ventricular tachycardia.[79] However, these criteria were associated with a higher incidence of sudden cardiac death in the Cardiac Arrhythmia Suppression Trial (CAST) study.[84]

Noninvasive Versus Invasive Testing

Several studies have shown limitations in the Holter approach in that many patients who appear to have drug effectiveness by Holter recording may still have their ventricular tachycardia induced by programmed stimulation.[85–87] Therefore, there appears to be a lack of concordance between Holter monitoring and electrophysiological testing for this end-point.

Some controversy exists as to the superiority of noninvasive versus invasive electrophysiology methods in predicting adequate drug efficacy in patients with sustained ventricular tachyarrhythmias. A marked decrease in sudden death has been observed in patients with high-risk ventricular arrhythmias solely stratified by noninvasive monitoring. This study is somewhat flawed in that entry criteria included "high-density" arrhythmia. As mentioned earlier, up to two-thirds of patients with sustained ventricular tachyarrhythmias have inadequate baseline arrhythmia to use Holter monitoring as the sole method of predicting drug response.

Some comparative data between the usefulness of noninvasive versus invasive testing exist. Many of these studies are limited by their retrospective nature. In a comparison of both techniques in patients with hemodynamically significant ventricular tachycardia, electrophysiological testing was effective in predicting long-term follow up and Holter monitoring was not.[88] Unfortunately, in this analysis, the predictiveness was based on discharge testing with baseline testing not performed in all patients. In a nonrandomized study, it was shown that Holter monitoring and electrophysiological studies were discordant in 50% of patients with sustained ventricular tachycardia;[89,90] all patients in this study had frequent PVCs (≥30/hr) and inducible ventricular tachycardia on baseline electrophysiological study. This discordance is usually due to "assessed efficacy" by Holter, but not programmed electrical stimulation. This study demonstrated that inefficacy as determined by programmed stimulation does not preclude a good outcome if Holter efficacy is achieved.

In the only randomized comparison of Holter monitoring versus electrophysiological testing in patients with sustained ventricular tachyarrhythmias (Fig. 11), "presumed drug efficacy" by Holter criteria were easier to attain; however, the recurrence rate was high in the Holter group suggesting that "presumed" did not equal "true" drug efficacy by noninvasive criteria.[91] These findings are primarily weakened by the small patient population randomized to this study. Because of this, a large-scale multicenter trial (ESVEM—electrophysiological study versus

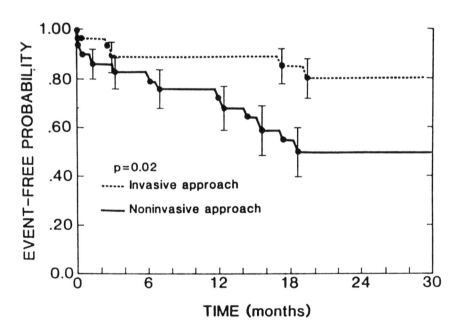

Figure 11. Superiority of serial electrophysiological testing vs. Holter monitoring in predicting VT recurrence during serial drug therapy. (Reproduced with permission from Mitchell, et al.[91])

electrocardiographic monitoring)[92] is ongoing. In this study, baseline studies must show both frequent PVCs on Holter (10 PVCs/hr) and sustained ventricular tachycardia induced during control electrophysiological study. After baseline, patients are randomized to one of two wings of drug therapy (guided by electrophysiological testing or Holter monitoring). The final data report from the ESVEM study may clear the above controversy.

Holter Diagnosis of Proarrhythmia

Holter monitors are frequently used as part of diagnostic studies to determine whether a new cardioactive drug has either antiarrhythmic or proarrhythmic effects.[93] Because of spontaneous variability, these studies are often limited and should be viewed with caution. Studies that have used longer monitoring periods may be more accurate; however, determining proarrhythmia by noninvasive techniques remains controversial since inefficacy may be misconstrued as proarrhythmia. The Cardiac Arrhythmia Pilot Study published criteria for spontaneous proarrhythmia.[79] Increases in PVCs used to define a proarrhythmia are related to the frequency of PVCs on baseline control Holter monitoring. These criteria are flawed due to marked variability in patients' arrhythmias from day to day. Using these criteria, 3% of placebo patients in the CAPS trial had proarrhythmia.

As a general rule, we consider a proarrhythmic response to have occurred when the patient develops new ventricular tachycardia or ventricular fibrillation that had not been previously documented, develops a new incessant, noncardiovertible ventricular tachycardia, or converts from nonsustained to sustained ventricular tachycardia, or has spontaneous torsades de pointes. Increases in spontaneous PVC counts are not life-threatening; therefore, we do not consider these to be a clinically important proarrhythmic response.

Summary: Holter Monitoring for Ventricular Arrhythmias

Holter monitoring has the advantage of being a noninvasive test with widespread availability. In addition, it may serve as the only useful marker of electrical instability in patients who cannot have their ventricular tachycardia reproduced by programmed stimulation and in patients whose treatment is based primarily on the result of noninvasive tests. Disadvantages of Holter monitoring include: the problem of spontaneous variability of arrhythmias; the fact that some patients have little ectopy between severe, life-threatening episodes of tachyarrhythmias; and the difficulty in defining an end-point for drug effectiveness.

Ambulatory Recording: Other Indications

Holter monitors may also be used for screening patients with symptoms (dizziness, presyncope, syncope) suggestive of sinus node or AV node conduction problems. Although Holter monitoring can frequently establish the temporal correlation between symptoms and the occurrence of an arrhythmia (Fig. 12), Holter recording can be helpful in a negative correlative sense (i.e., occurrence of symptoms during normal sinus rhythm). Several studies[94–96] demonstrated that symptoms occurred in 17–47% of patients during Holter monitoring, however 15–39% have no significant arrhythmia during symptoms. Correlation of symptoms and simultaneous electrocardiographic abnormalities ranged from 2% to 13% in these studies and 22% overall in a review of seven studies.[53] Thus, up to 78% of patients may have nondiagnostic Holters.

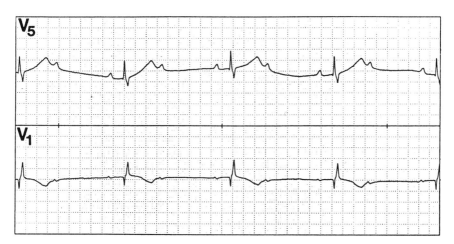

Figure 12. Symptomatic (dizziness) bradycardia secondary to 2:1 AV block with baseline right bundle branch block noted during Holter monitoring of a modified lead V_5 (top) and lead V_1 (bottom). Electrophysiological testing confirmed presence of block distal to bundle of His.

Therefore, in patients who have recurrent symptoms in the absence of electrocardiographic abnormalities, a workup for nonarrhythmic causes of syncope should be considered.[17] Despite the above limitations, Holter recordings do appear to be more sensitive than stress testing in identifying arrhythmic abnormalities in patients with a history of syncope.

Holter monitoring can be useful in correlating episodes of chest pain with diagnostic ST segment abnormalities. Reel-to-reel recorders have better frequency responses for analyzing ST segment shifts. However, since only two electrocardiographic leads are recorded, major ST segment changes can occur in leads that are not being monitored. In addition, frequent changes of ST segments can be noted in normal subjects during changes of position or hyperventilation. Therefore, we obtain baseline supine and standing tracings and tracings with hyperventilation at the beginning of the recording, as we do in treadmill testing. We have also found Holter monitoring to be limited in the patient with typical effort angina. However, patients who have atypical angina from coronary spasm may have frequent episodes of chest pain that are not routinely induced with stress and may occur at any time of the day. Holter monitoring may be more useful in screening for ST segment elevation and arrhythmias during a typical chest pain in this group of patients.[98] Other studies have demonstrated asymptomatic electrocardiographic abnormalities during Holter monitoring in patients having silent myocardial ischemia.[27,99,100]

Holter recordings are also used to screen patients who have clinical syndromes in which the presence of an arrhythmia may increase the risk of sudden death. Such situations include the period after myocardial infarction,[101–103] congestive heart failure and dilated cardiomyopathy,[10,11,104–108] hypertrophic obstructive cardiomyopathy,[109] and the congenital prolonged QT syndrome (see Figs. 7–9).[110] In risk-stratification of post-infarction patients, late in-hospital arrhythmias have prognostic significance and are used in conjunction with depressed ejection fraction stress testing and abnormal signal-averaged electrocardiography (Fig. 1). Patients with benign profiles (all factors negative) have a 3% 1-year post-infarction mortality compared to a 15% 1-year mortality when all factors are positive. Several studies have shown that Holter monitoring is superior to treadmill testing in screening for arrhythmias in patients with coronary artery disease including post-myocardial infarction patients[111] and in patients with hypertrophic obstructive cardiomyopathy. Holter recordings may also be useful in screening for arrhythmias in patients with the mitral valve prolapse syndrome[112] and in those recovering from coronary artery bypass surgery.[113] Holter mon-

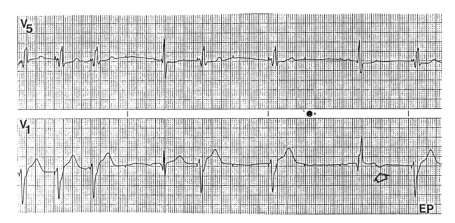

Figure 13. Pacemaker malfunction noted during Holter monitoring with failure of pacemaker capture and failure to sense (arrow).

itoring can also be used to screen patients with symptomatic or asymptomatic Wolff-Parkinson-White syndrome.[51,114] In contrast, Holter monitoring is not very sensitive in identifying high-risk patients with bifascicular block.[115]

Patients who have suspected pacemaker malfunction may also require long-term monitoring to document an intermittent episode of failure to capture or failure to sense (Fig. 13).[116] These abnormalities and oversensing problems may be easily documented during ambulatory monitoring.

Use of Holter Monitoring in Supraventricular Arrhythmias

Little attention has been paid to the use of Holter monitoring in patients with supraventricular arrhythmias, partly due to technological problems in accurately assessing the frequency of PACs and runs of supraventricular tachycardia. Patients with paroxysmal supraventricular tachycardia often have little spontaneous atrial ectopic activity between paroxysms of tachycardia. In our experience, sustained SVT will be documented on random Holter in <10% of patients. Because of this, Holter monitoring has had limited use in the management of these cases. Event recorders may have more usefulness in patients with paroxysmal atrial tachycardias.[117] Holter monitoring may be useful in noninvasively documenting frequent PACs or short runs of atrial tachycardia that can act as markers of these patients' arrhythmia. In patients with Wolff-Parkinson-White syndrome, Holter recordings can screen for intermittent preexcitation and atrial arrhythmias.

In patients with paroxysmal AV node or AV re-entry, complete therapeutic efficacy requires 100% abolition of tachycardia recurrence on repeated Holter monitoring after treatment. Partial efficacy can be defined as marked reduction in the number of electrocardiographically documented runs of tachycardia or shorter, slower episodes of tachycardia after antiarrhythmic or surgical treatment.[118] In patients with atrial fibrillation, Holter monitoring may be useful in determining if the atrial fibrillation is chronic or paroxysmal, in defining the minimum, average, and maximum R-R interval, and ruling out coexisting ventricular arrhythmias and sick sinus syndrome.

Holter recordings may be most useful in the patient with incessant supraventricular tachycardia who has tachycardia for more than 10% of the day. These patients can often be treated by means of a noninvasive approach. Complete efficacy of drug treatment can be defined as a 100% reduction in the episodes of tachycardia; partial efficacy can be defined as a reduction of tachycardia to less than 5% of the day.[110]

Noncontinuous Forms of Electrocardiographic Recording

In patients who have rare episodes of arrhythmia, even several days of Holter monitoring may not be sufficient to document the arrhythmia or symptoms. In these patients, a noncontinuous form of ambulatory recording may be more useful.[119–121] Several different types of recorders are available. Recorders that can be intermittently activated by an event such as bradycardia or tachycardia or activated by the patient during symptoms can be worn for 24–72 hours in an attempt to document the suspected arrhythmia. These devices may also record representative strips at preset points in time. The devices are limited by minimal storage capabilities. We have had patients who have filled up the tape with routine strips and had symptoms that could not be recorded because no tape storage was available.

Transient symptomatic event recorders that can electrocardiographically record an arrhythmia during symptoms have memory capability and can record up to 30 seconds of information until the patient has access to a telephone. These devices can convert the electrocardiographic signal to a noise signal that can be transmitted over the telephone. Audiotone signals are then converted back to electrocardiographic signals at a central station. Most companies have nurses or technicians available to interpret the strips immediately, and several hospitals have set up interactive stations so that proper treatment can be rapidly initiated for serious arrhythmias. Transient symptomatic event recorders can also be used to document arrhythmia recurrences in patients who have been treated with an antiarrhythmic agent and also to screen high-risk patients for arrhythmias after myocardial infarction. Although those recorders may be useful for patients with infrequent symptoms, they are limited by their short storage capabilities.

Using telephone transmitters, it has been documented that nearly 80% of patients who were sudden death survivors had ventricular tachycardia transmitted after serial electrophysiological testing.[121] Improved survival was noted compared to patients who did not use the transmitters. These observations suggest that early diagnosis of residual arrhythmia results in prompt treatment and efficient access to the medical care system.

Some patient-activated event recorders have a short period of pre-event memory. Thus, the initiating sequence of a tachycardia can be electrocardiographically documented. In addition, this memory is useful in documenting short episodes of self-terminating tachycardia. With loop recorders,[122] sinus rhythm has frequently resumed by the time the patient has activated the device (e.g., post-syncope or implantable defibrillator discharge). However, due to the memory loop, any arrhythmia that occurred in the immediate preactivation period will be recorded. Loop recorders have also been useful in recording the initiation and termination sequence of tachyarrhythmias.

Signal-Averaging Techniques

Signal averaging is a signal processing technique which has been applied to record microvolt signals at body surface. With this technique, noninvasive recordings of the His-bundle[123] and screening of high-risk arrhythmia patients for "late potentials" have been performed.

Signal averaging facilitates the detection of late potentials[124] which are felt to represent fragmented electrical activity, including (1) low amplitude activity (1–20 mV); (2) activity that is continuous within the QRS complex; (3) activity that may be 20–60 msec in duration; and (4) activity that persists well into the ST segment (Fig. 14). These potentials seem to reflect asynchronous depolarization within damaged but surviving

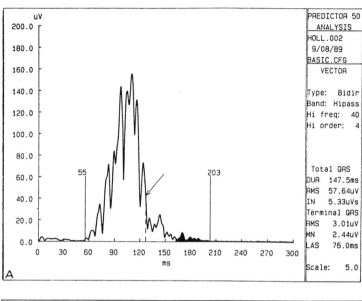

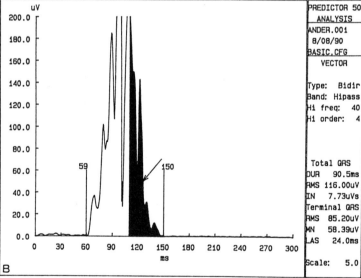

Figure 14. (A) Presence of late potential in a patient with a history of sustained VT. (B) Normal SAECG in a syncopal patient. DUR = duration; RMS = root mean square; IN = integral; MN = mean; LAS = low amplitude signals.

myocardium predominantly at the border of a scar and are not seen on routine surface electrocardiograms, although they can be recorded directly by catheter or intraoperative mapping. The presence of these signals has been associated with the development of re-entry forms of ventricular tachycardia and are felt to be a marker for a ventricular arrhythmia substrate. The ability to screen patients who may be at risk for developing sustained ventricular tachycardia noninvasively makes signal averaging attractive. Late potentials cannot be detected with ordinary cardiac monitors because the signal intensity of the late potential measured at the body surface is small compared to the QRS complex and is obscured by background noise (myoelectric potentials and respiratory artifacts). Since noise is random, late potentials can be distinguished from noise using signal-enhancing techniques.

The presence of a late potential can be seen as a low amplitude waveform that persists beyond the end of the QRS complex (Fig. 14). Many criteria exist to define the presence of a late potential. These vary depending on the filter settings and technique. Common criteria[125,126] include: (1) root mean square (RMS) voltage in the last 40 msec of QRS <20 microvolts, (2) total filtered duration of QRS >120 msec, and (3) LAS$_{40}$ <38 msec (the terminal QRS complex (Fig. 14, arrow) remains below 40 μV for more than 38 msec).

Late potentials are not abolished after administration of antiarrhythmic therapy. In fact, the duration of the late potential may increase during antiarrhythmic therapy, suggesting a further slowing of conduction through the affected myocardium. The presence or absence of late potentials or drug-induced changes in morphology of the late potential have not been predictive of antiarrhythmic efficacy.

A limitation of signal averaging techniques is that patients with bundle branch block or intraventricular conduction delays are not considered good candidates since prolongation of the QRS may obscure the late potential at the terminal portion of the QRS complex.

Acquisition and analyses of a signal-averaged electrocardiogram is demonstrated in Fig. 15.[129] By repetitively averaging the QRS signal taken from the three orthogonal Frank lead system, random noise components are attenuated in intensity by a factor equal to the square root of the number of sample beats acquired. Typically, 200–400 beats are sampled. A smaller number of beats can be averaged depending on the noise level.

After the signal-averaged ECG is obtained, high-pass filtering (time-domain analyses, 25 to 100 Hz; we use 40 Hz) is used to minimize interference of large-amplitude, low-frequency signals. Simson has de-

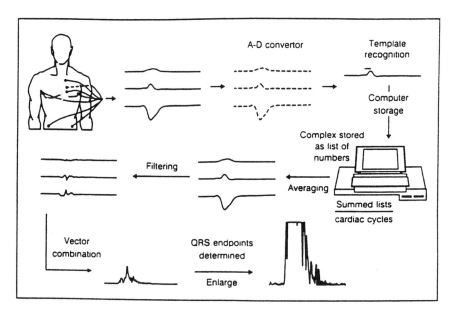

Figure 15. Diagram detailing acquisition and processing of SAECG. (Reproduced with permission from Vatterott, et al.[129])

veloped a bidirectional digital filter that minimizes artifact from "ringing" after a large signal ends.[130,131] After filtering out low-frequency components which make up the majority of energy in the QRS, the X, Y, and Z leads are summed into a vector. This vector magnitude is termed the filtered QRS complex. The amplitude is then calculated by the computer using the root mean square method.

Although the above time domain analysis is most commonly used, others[132,133] have popularized Fast Fourier Transform (FFT) analysis. In this technique, the signal is mathematically broken down into its fundamental and harmonic frequencies. A plot of amplitude versus frequency is made.

Clinical Studies with Signal Averaging

Although commonly present, the presence of late potentials is of minimal use in patients with documented sustained ventricular tachyarrhythmias. In patients with ventricular tachycardia, prolonged high-frequency low-amplitude signals are typically seen at the end of the QRS.

The average voltage in the last 40 msec of the QRS was a major discriminator (p < .001) between patients with arrhythmia and normals, since more than 90% of the ventricular tachycardia group but less than 10% of the normal subjects will have high-frequency signals of less than 25 mV in the last 40 msec of the QRS. Abnormal late potentials are powerful independent markers for ventricular tachycardia. The vast majority of patients with sustained ventricular tachyarrhythmias and dilated cardiomyopathy have an abnormal signal-averaged ECG.[134] Late potentials have also been described in patients with arrhythmogenic right ventricular dysplasia.

Surgical ablation of electrically abnormal areas of myocardium in patients with late potentials and sustained ventricular tachycardia can result in abolishment of both late potentials and sustained ventricular tachycardia.[135] In patients who could not have ventricular tachycardia induced after endocardial excision, late potentials decreased from 71% preoperatively to 33% postoperatively. Even in those patients who have persistent postsurgical late potentials with successful abolishment of clinical sustained ventricular tachycardia, the morphology of the post-surgery late potentials is altered.

Clinical Indications for Signal Averaging

The clinical uses of signal averaging include:[124,129] (1) risk stratification of patients with nonsustained ventricular tachycardia, (2) risk stratification of post-myocardial infarction patients, and (3) screening of syncope patients.

Late potentials as a predictor of sustained ventricular tachycardia in patients with clinical nonsustained ventricular tachycardia have been studied.[136,137] Signal averaging may be a useful tool for screening patients with nonsustained ventricular tachycardia who should undergo invasive electrophysiological study. The induction of sustained VT is more common in patients who have late potentials. In one study,[136] two-thirds of the patients with a history of nonsustained VT and late potentials had sustained VT induced by programmed stimulation, while approximately 10% of patients without inducible VT had late potentials.

It has also been shown that post-myocardial infarction populations at risk for sustained ventricular tachycardia could be reliably screened by the presence of late potentials.[138] Delayed activity may be a marker for the substrate (slowed conduction) necessary for re-entrant ventricular tachycardia. The prolonged electrical activity that they represent may

99666666

66666666666666666

66666666666666

66666666666666

reflect areas of myocardium that are critical to the maintenance of a ventricular tachycardia circuit. Abnormal signal-averaged ECGs are noted in over 70% of patients with a previous myocardial infarction who have sustained monomorphic VT induced by programmed stimulation compared to less than 16% of similar patients without inducible VT. Although late potentials are usually noted in patients with sustained ventricular tachycardia who have had a previous myocardial infarction, they are less commonly noted in ventricular fibrillation patients.[139]

In healed post-myocardial infarction populations, location of the myocardial infarction influences the ability of the late potentials to predict sustained ventricular tachycardia in nonsustained ventricular tachycardia populations. Late potential characteristics in myocardial infarct patients are superior to anterior myocardial infarction patients to differentiate patients with nonsustained ventricular tachycardia into those with and those without inducible sustained ventricular tachycardia as determined by programmed electrical stimulation. The difference in predictability based on infarct location may be due to relative activation of damaged or ischemic myocardium to the QRS complex. Normal late activation or damaged posterobasal segments of the left ventricle (because of an inferior myocardial infarction) may result in late potentials produced toward the end of the QRS allowing for easier identification at the terminal portion of the QRS complex of late potentials in contradistinction to anterior myocardial infarction where the damaged area of myocardium is activated relatively early and late potentials may not persist long enough to be noted after signal averaging.

The presence of late potentials in the early post-myocardial infarction period has not been shown to be useful in predicting early cardiac arrhythmias since late potentials appear to be intermittently present during this time, possibly reflecting the changing substrate evolving during the immediate post-myocardial infarction period. Continuous sampling of late potentials during the early post-myocardial infarction has not been well studied.

The use of late potentials in the late post-myocardial infarction populations has shown considerable promise in predicting the probability of a cardiac event in the post-infarction period. In a comparison of late potentials with Holter and radionuclide ventriculography in the late post-myocardial infarction population, the presence of a late potential and an EF <40% identified patients with a 34% probability of arrhythmic events.[125] In patients with no late potential and normal left ventricular function, the risk of arrhythmic events was 4%. Thus, the absence of a late potential may be more useful clinically. In the presence of relatively normal left ventricular function and infrequent ventricular ectopy as assessed by Holter recording, a group of patients with a sudden death rate of <3–4% at 1 year can be identified. Multivariate regression showed presence of late potential in the early post-myocardial infarction period was independent of ejection fraction predicting ventricular arrhythmias. Others have reported similar findings.[126]

In reviewing these studies, over 30% of patients with left ventricular dysfunction and late potentials had sustained VT or sudden cardiac death. In a retrospective study of 98 patients who had recurrent sustained ventricular tachycardia and 76 patients without ventricular tachycardia after a myocardial infarction, an abnormal signal-averaged ECG was found in 90% of the ventricular tachycardia group and in only 30% of the group without ventricular tachycardia.[140] When combined with frequent PVCs and left ventricular dysfunction, 18 patients with all three prognostic variables had VT while only 1 of 18 without any of these variables had ventricular tachycardia.

Data now exist that successful thrombolysis with reperfusion during acute myocardial infarction is associated with a lower incidence of late potentials.[141,142] This is not surprising since salvage of ischemic myocardium by opening an occluded coronary artery should be associated with less electrical damage, an improved ejection fraction, and an improvement in post-infarction prognosis.

Role of Signal Averaging in Syncope

Several studies[143,144] have reported the role of signal averaging in predicting which patients with syncope of undetermined etiology will have sustained ventricular tachycardia induced by programmed stimulation. An abnormal signal-averaged ECG (positive for late potentials) is predictive of the induction of sustained ventricular tachycardia in over 70% of cases. Therefore, signal averaging may be a useful screen in syncopal patients since the yield of inducible tachycardia will be higher in late potential positive patients. More importantly, a negative predictive accuracy of 97% has been demonstrated.[129]

References

1. Feigenbaum H, et al: Role of echocardiography in patients with coronary artery disease. Am J Cardiol 37:775, 1976.

2. Gramiak R, Shah PM: Echocardiography of the normal and diseased aortic valve. Radiology 96:1, 1974.
3. Henry WL, et al: Measurement of mitral valve orifice area in patients with echocardiography. Circulation 51:837, 1975.
4. Weyman AE, et al: Cross-sectional echocardiography in assessing the severity of valvular aortic stenosis. Circulation 52:828, 1975.
5. DeMaria AN, et al: The variable spectrum of echocardiographic manifestations of the mitral valve prolapse syndrome. Circulation 50:33, 1974.
6. Manyari DE, Duff HJ, Kostuk WJ, et al: Usefulness of noninvasive studies for diagnosis of right ventricular dysplasia. Am J Cardiol 57:1147, 1986.
7. Shah PM, et al: Role of echocardiography in diagnostic and hemodynamic assessment of hypertrophic subaortic stenosis. Circulation 44:891, 1971.
8. Moynihan PF, Parisi AF, Feldman CL: Quantitative detection of regional left ventricular contraction abnormalities by two-dimensional echocardiography. I. Analysis of methods. Circulation 63:752, 1981.
9. Epstein SE, Palmeri ST, Patterson RE: Evaluation of patients after acute myocardial infarction: indications for cardiac catheterization and surgical intervention. N Engl J Med 307:1487, 1982.
10. Follansbee WP, Michelson EL, Morganroth J: Nonsustained ventricular tachycardia in ambulatory patients: characteristics and association with sudden cardiac death. Ann Intern Med 92:741, 1980.
11. Wilson JR, Schwartz JS, St. John Sutton M, et al: Prognosis in severe heart failure: relation to hemodynamic measurements and ventricular ectopic activity. J Am Coll Cardiol 2:403, 1983.
12. Dougherty AH, Naccarelli GV, Gray EL, et al: Congestive heart failure with normal systolic function. Am J Cardiol 54:778, 1984.
13. Gallagher JJ, et al: Wolff-Parkinson-White syndrome: the problem, evaluation, and surgical correction. Circulation 51:767, 1975.
14. Drake CE, Hodsden JE, Sridharan MR, et al: Evaluation of the association of mitral valve prolapse in patients with Wolff-Parkinson-White type ECG and its relationship to the ventricular activation pattern. Am Heart J 109:83, 1985.
15. Smith WM, Gallagher JJ, Kerr CR, et al: The electrophysiological basis and management of symptomatic recurrent tachycardia in patients with Ebstein's anomaly of the tricuspid valve. Am J Cardiol 49:1223, 1982.
16. Henry WL, et al: Relation between echocardiographically determined left atrial size and atrial fibrillation. Circulation 53:273, 1976.
17. Naccarelli GV: Evaluation of the patient with syncope. Med Clin North Am 5:1211, 1984.
18. Wackers FJTh, et al: Multiple-gated cardiac blood pool imaging for left ventricular ejection fraction: validation of the technique and assessment of variability. Am J Cardiol 43:1159, 1979.
19. Pitt B, Strauss WH: Evaluation of ventricular function by radioisotope techniques. N Engl J Med 296:1097, 1977.
20. Okada RD, Kirshenbaum HD, Kushner FG, et al: Observer variance in the qualitative evaluation of left ventricular wall motion and the quantitation of left ventricular ejection fraction using rest and exercise multigated blood pool imaging. Circulation 61:128, 1980.

21. Borer JS, et al: Real-time radionuclide cineangiography in the noninvasive evaluation of global and regional left ventricular function and rest and during exercise in patients with coronary artery disease. N Engl J Med 296:839, 1977.

22. Epstein SE: Implications of probability analysis on the strategy used for noninvasive detection of coronary artery disease: role of single or combined use of exercise electrocardiographic testing, radionuclide cineangiography and myocardial perfusion imaging. Am J Cardiol 46:491, 1980.

23. Botvinick E, Frais M, O'Connell W, et al: Phase image evaluation of patients with ventricular preexcitation syndromes. J Am Coll Cardiol 3:799, 1984.

24. Swiryn S, Pavel D, Byron E, et al: Sequential regional phase mapping of radionuclide-gated biventriculograms in patients with sustained ventricular tachycardia: close correlation with electrophysiological characteristics. Am Heart J 103:319, 1982.

25. DeMaria AN, Amsterdam EA, Vismara LA: Arrhythmias in the mitral valve prolapse syndrome: prevalence, nature, and frequency. Ann Intern Med 84:656, 1976.

26. Bruce RA: Methods of exercise testing. Am J Cardiol 33:715, 1974.

27. Cohn PF: Silent myocardial ischemia: to treat or not to treat? Hosp Pract 18:125, 1983.

28. Rifkin RD, Hood WB: Bayesian analysis of electrocardiographic exercise stress testing. N Engl J Med 297:681, 1977.

29. Goldman S, Tselos S, Cohn K: Marked depth of ST-segment depression during treadmill exercise testing: indicator of severe coronary artery disease. Chest 69:729, 1976.

30. Goldschlager N, Selzer A, Cohn K: Treadmill stress tests as indications of presence and severity of coronary artery disease. Ann Intern Med 85:277, 1976.

31. Kattus AA: Exercise electrocardiography: recognition of the ischemic response, false positive and negative patterns. Am J Cardiol 33:721, 1974.

32. Ellestad MH, Couke BM, Greenberg PS: Stress testing: clinical application and predictive capacity. Prog Cardiovasc Dis 21:431, 1979.

33. Bruce RA: Exercise testing for evaluation of ventricular function. N Engl J Med 296:671, 1977.

34. Cohn PF: The role of noninvasive cardiac testing after an uncomplicated myocardial infarction. N Engl J Med 309:90, 1983.

35. Multicenter Postinfarction Research Group: Risk stratification and survival after myocardial infarction. N Engl J Med 309:331, 1983.

36. Theroux P, et al: Prognostic value of exercise testing soon after myocardial infarction. N Engl J Med 301:341, 1979.

37. Jelinek MV, Lown B: Exercise stress testing for exposure of cardiac arrhythmia. Prog Cardiovasc Dis 6:497, 1974.

38. Lown B: Cardiovascular collapse and sudden cardiac death. In: Braunwald E (ed), Heart Disease: A Textbook of Cardiovascular Medicine, Vol. 2. Philadelphia, WB Saunders, 1984.

39. Antman E, Graboys TB, Lown B: Continuous monitoring for ventricular arrhythmias during exercise tests. JAMA 241:2802, 1979.

40. Palileo EV, Ashley WW, Swiryn S, et al: Exercise provocable right ventricular outflow tract tachycardia. Am Heart J 104:185, 1982.
41. Woelfel A, Foster JR, Simpson RJ, et al: Reproducibility and treatment of exercise-induced ventricular tachycardia. Am J Cardiol 53:751, 1984.
42. Wu D, Kou HC, Hung JS: Exercise-triggered paroxysmal ventricular tachycardia: a repetitive rhythmic activity possibly related to afterdepolarization. Ann Intern Med 95:410, 1981.
43. Sokoloff N, Spielman SR, Greenspan AM, et al: Plasma norepinephrine in exercise-induced ventricular tachycardia. J Am Coll Cardiol 8:11, 1986.
44. Blackburn H, et al: Premature ventricular complexes induced by stress testing. Am J Cardiol 31:441, 1973.
45. McHenry P, et al: Comparative study of exercise-induced ventricular arrhythmias in normal subjects and patients with documented coronary artery disease. Am J Cardiol 37:609, 1976.
46. Faris SV, et al: Prevalence and reproducibility of exercise-induced ventricular arrhythmias during maximal exercise testing in normal men. Am J Cardiol 37:617, 1976.
47. Akhtar M, Niazi I, Naccarelli GV, et al: Role of adrenergic stimulation in reversal of drug effects in supraventricular tachycardia. Am J Cardiol 62:45L, 1988.
48. Morady F, Kau WH, Kadish AH, et al: Antagonism of quinidine's electrophysiological effects by epinephrine in patients with ventricular tachycardia. J Am Coll Cardiol 12:388, 1988.
49. Falk RH: Flecainide-induced ventricular tachycardia and fibrillation in patients treated for atrial fibrillation. Ann Intern Med 111:107, 1989.
50. Anastasiou-Nana MI, Anderson JL, Stewart JR, et al: Occurrence of exercise-induced and spontaneous wide complex tachycardia during therapy with flecainide for complex ventricular arrhythmias: a probable proarrhythmic effect. Am Heart J 113:1071, 1987.
51. Klein GJ, Gulamhusein SS: Intermittent preexcitation in the Wolff-Parkinson-White syndrome. Am J Cardiol 52:292, 1983.
52. Boudoulos HG, Schaal SF, Lewis RP: Superiority of 24-hour outpatient monitoring over multi-stage exercise testing for the evaluation of syncope. J Electrocardiol 12:103, 1979.
53. DiMarco JP, Philbrick JT: Use of ambulatory electrocardiographic (Holter) monitoring. Ann Intern Med 113:53, 1990.
54. Graboys TB, Lown B: Abbreviated ECG monitoring for exposing ventricular ectopic activity. Cardiovasc Med 4:794, 1979.
55. Lown B, Matta RJ, Besser HW: Programmed trendscription: a new approach to electrocardiographic monitoring. JAMA 232:39, 1975.
56. Holter NJ: Radioelectrocardiography: a new technique for cardiovascular studies. Ann NY Acad Sci 65:913, 1957.
57. Holter NJ: New method for heart studies. Science 134:1214, 1961.
58. Kennedy HL, Underhill SJ, Warbasse JR: Practical advantages of two-channel electrocardiographic Holter recordings. Am Heart J 91:882, 1976.
59. Kennedy HL: Ambulatory Electrocardiography Including Holter Recording Technology. Philadelphia, Lea & Febiger, 1981.
60. Jenkins JM, Wu D, Arsbaecher RL: Computer diagnosis of supraventricular

and ventricular arrhythmias: a new esophageal technique. Circulation 60:977, 1979.

61. Morganroth J: Ambulatory Holter electrocardiography: choice of technologies and clinical uses. Ann Intern Med 102:73, 1985.
62. Sobotka PA, et al: Arrhythmias documented by 24-hour continuous ambulatory electrocardiographic monitoring in young women without apparent heart disease. Am Heart J 101:753, 1981.
63. Fleg JL, Kennedy HL: Cardiac arrhythmias in a healthy elderly population: detection by 24-hour ambulatory electrocardiography. Chest 81:302, 1982.
64. Brodsky M, Wu D, Denes P, et al: Arrhythmias documented by 24-hour continuous electrocardiographic monitoring in 50 male medical students without apparent heart disease. Am J Cardiol 39:390, 1977.
65. Kostis JB, Moreyra AE, Natorajan N, et al: Ambulatory electrocardiography: what is normal? Am J Cardiol 43:420, 1979 (abstract).
66. Gardin JM, Belic N, Singer DH: Pseudodysrhythmias in ambulatory ECG monitoring. Arch Intern Med 139:809, 1979.
67. Kennedy HL, Underhill SJ: Frequent or complex ventricular ectopy in apparently healthy subjects. Am J Cardiol 38:141, 1976.
68. Winkle RA: Antiarrhythmic drug effect mimicked by spontaneous variability of ventricular ectopy. Circulation 57:1116, 1978.
69. Mulrow JP, Healy MJ, McKenna WJ: Variability of ventricular arrhythmias in hypertrophic cardiomyopathy and implications of treatment. Am J Cardiol 58:615, 1986.
70. Lal R, Chapman PD, Naccarelli GV, et al: Short- and long-term experience with flecainide acetate in the management of refractory life-threatening ventricular arrhythmias. J Am Coll Cardiol 6:772, 1985.
71. Sokoloff N, Spielman SR, Greenspan AM, et al: Utility of ambulatory electrocardiographic monitoring for predicting recurrence of sustained ventricular tachyarrhythmias in patients receiving amiodarone. J Am Coll Cardiol 7:938, 1986.
72. Skale BT, Miles WM, Heger JJ, et al: Survivors of cardiac arrest: prevention of recurrence by drug therapy as predicted by electrophysiological testing or electrocardiographic monitoring. Am J Cardiol 57:113, 1986.
73. Swerdlow CD, Peterson J: Prospective comparison of Holter monitoring and electrophysiological study in patients with coronary artery disease and sustained ventricular tachyarrhythmias. Am J Cardiol 56:577, 1985.
74. Hoffman A, Schutz E, White R, et al: Suppression of high-grade ventricular ectopic activity by antiarrhythmic drug treatment as a marker for survival in patients with chronic coronary artery disease. Am Heart J 107:1103, 1984.
75. Graboys TB, et al: Long-term survival of patients with malignant ventricular arrhythmias treated with antiarrhythmic drugs. Am J Cardiol 50:437, 1982.
76. Michelson EL, Morganroth J: Spontaneous variability of complex ventricular arrhythmias detected by long-term electrocardiographic recording. Circulation 61:690, 1980.
77. Morganroth J, et al: Limitations of routine long-term electrocardiographic monitoring to assess ventricular ectopic frequency. Circulation 53:408, 1978.

78. Pratt CM, Theroux P, Slymen D, et al: Spontaneous variability of ventricular arrhythmias in patients at increased risk of sudden death after acute myocardial infarction: consecutive ambulatory electrocardiographic recordings of 88 patients. Am J Cardiol 59:178, 1987.
79. CAPS Investigators: The cardiac arrhythmia pilot study (CAPS). Am J Cardiol 57:91, 1986.
80. Toivonen L: Spontaneous variability in the frequency of ventricular premature complexes over prolonged intervals and implications for antiarrhythmic treatment. Am J Cardiol 60:608, 1987.
81. Pratt CM, Delclos G, Wierman AM, et al: The changing baseline of complex ventricular arrhythmias: a new consideration in assessing long-term antiarrhythmic drug therapy. N Engl J Med 313:1444, 1985.
82. Pratt CM, Slymen DJ, Wierman AM, et al: Analysis of the spontaneous variability of ventricular arrhythmias: consecutive ambulatory electrocardiographic recordings of ventricular tachycardia. Am J Cardiol 56:67, 1985.
83. Anderson JL, Anastasiou-Nana MI, Menlove RL, et al: Spontaneous variability in ventricular ectopic activity during chronic antiarrhythmic therapy. Circulation 82:830, 1990.
84. The Cardiac Arrhythmia Suppression Trial Investigators: Preliminary report: Effect of encainide and flecainide on mortality in a randomized trial of arrhythmia suppression after myocardial infarction. N Engl J Med 321:406, 1989.
85. Ezri MD, Huang SK, Denes P: The role of Holter monitoring in patients with recurrent sustained ventricular tachycardia: an electrophysiological correlation. Am Heart J 108:1229, 1984.
86. Heger JJ, Prystowsky EN, Jackman WM, et al: Comparison between results obtained from electrocardiographic testing, exercise testing and ambulatory ECG recording. In: Wenger NK, Mock MB, Ringquist I (eds), Ambulatory Electrocardiographic Recording. Chicago, Medical Publishers Inc. pp 379–389, 1981.
87. Kim SG, Seiden SW, Matos JA, et al: Discordance between ambulatory monitoring and programmed stimulation in assessing efficacy of Class IA antiarrhythmic agents in patients with ventricular tachycardia. J Am Coll Cardiol 6:539, 1985.
88. Platia EV, Reid PR: Comparison of programmed electrical stimulation and ambulatory electrocardiographic (Holter) monitoring in the management of ventricular tachycardia and ventricular fibrillation. J Am Coll Cardiol 4:493, 1984.
89. Kim SG, Seiden SW, Felder SD, et al: Is programmed stimulation of value in predicting the long-term success of antiarrhythmic therapy for ventricular tachycardias. N Engl J Med 315:356, 1982.
90. Kim SG: The management of patients with life-threatening ventricular tachyarrhythmias: programmed stimulation or Holter monitoring (either or both)? Circulation 76:1, 1987.
91. Mitchell LB, Duff HJ, Manyari DE, et al: A randomized clinical trial of the noninvasive and invasive approaches to drug therapy of ventricular tachycardia. N Engl J Med 317:1681, 1987.
92. The ESVEM Investigators: The ESVEM trial. Electrophysiologic study vs.

electrocardiographic monitoring for selection of antiarrhythmic therapy of ventricular tachyarrhythmias. Circulation 79:1354, 1989.

93. Morganroth J: Flecainide: its proarrhythmic effect and expected changes on the surface electrocardiogram. Am J Cardiol 53:89B, 1984.

94. Zeldis SM, et al: Cardiovascular complaints: correlation with cardiac arrhythmias on 24-hour electrocardiographic monitoring. Chest 78:456, 1980.

95. Clark PA, Glasser SP, Spoto E: Arrhythmias detected by ambulatory monitoring: lack of correlation with symptoms of dizziness and syncope. Chest 77:722, 1980.

96. Gibson TC, Heitzman MR: Diagnostic efficacy of 24-hour electrocardiographic monitoring for syncope. Am J Cardiol 53:1013, 1984.

97. Crawford MA, et al: Limitations of continuous ambulatory electrocardiogram monitoring for detecting coronary artery disease. Ann Intern Med 89:1, 1978.

98. Guazzi M, et al: Continuous electrocardiographic recording in Prinzmetal's variant angina pectoris: a report of 4 cases. Br Heart J 32:611, 1970.

99. Gottlieb SO, et al: Silent ischemia as a marker for unfavorable outcomes in patients with unstable angina. N Engl J Med 314:1214, 1986.

100. Armstrong WF, Morris SN: The ST segment during ambulatory electrocardiographic monitoring. Ann Intern Med 98:249, 1983.

101. Anderson KP, DeCamilla J, Moss AJ: Clinical significance of ventricular tachycardia (3 beats or longer) detected during ambulatory monitoring after myocardial infarction. Circulation 57:890, 1978.

102. Bigger JT, Weld FM, Rolnitzky LM: The prevalence and significance of ventricular tachycardia detected by ambulatory ECG recording in the late hospital phase of acute myocardial infarction. Am J Cardiol 48:815, 1981.

103. Kotler MN, et al: Prognostic significance of ventricular ectopic beats with respect to sudden death in the late post-infarction period. Circulation 49:959, 1973.

104. Chakko CS, Gheorghaide M: Ventricular arrhythmias in severe heart failure: incidence, significance, and effectiveness of antiarrhythmic therapy. Am Heart J 109:497, 1985.

105. Francis GS: Development of arrhythmias in the patient with congestive heart failure: pathophysiology, prevalence and prognosis. Am J Cardiol 57:3B, 1986.

106. Huang SK, Messer JV, Denes P: Significance of ventricular tachycardia in idiopathic dilated cardiomyopathy: observations in 35 patients. Am J Cardiol 51:507, 1983.

107. Maskin CS, Siskind SJ, LeJemtel TH: High prevalence of nonsustained ventricular tachycardia in severe congestive heart failure. Am Heart J 107:896, 1984.

108. Meinertz T, Hofmann T, Kasper W, et al: Significance of ventricular arrhythmias in idiopathic dilated cardiomyopathy. Am J Cardiol 53:902, 1984.

109. McKenna WJ, Chetty S, Oakley CM, et al: Exercise electrocardiographic and 48-hour ambulatory electrocardiographic monitor assessment of arrhythmia on and off beta-blocker therapy in hypertrophic cardiomyopathy. Am J Cardiol 43:420, 1979 (abstract).

110. Schwartz PJ, Periti M, Malliani A: The long QT syndrome. Am Heart J 89:378, 1975.

111. DeBusk RF, Davidson DM, Houston N, et al: Serial ambulatory electrocardiography and treadmill testing after uncomplicated myocardial infarction. Am J Cardiol 45:547, 1980.
112. Winkle RA, et al: Arrhythmias in patients with mitral valve prolapse. Circulation 52:73, 1975.
113. Price JE, Vismora LA, Amsterdam EA, et al: Evaluation of ventricular arrhythmias post-coronary bypass surgery: decreased prevalence following hospital discharge determined by ambulatory ECG-monitoring. Am J Cardiol 39:269, 1977 (abstract).
114. Force T, Graboys TB: Exercise testing and ambulatory monitoring in patients with preexcitation syndrome. Arch Intern Med 141:88, 1981.
115. McAnulty SH, Rahimtoola SH, Murphy ES: A prospective study of sudden death in "high-risk" bundle branch block. N Engl J Med 299:209, 1978.
116. Bleifer SB, et al: Diagnosis of occult arrhythmias by Holter electrocardiography. Prog Cardiovasc Dis 16:569, 1974.
117. Pritchett ELC, et al: Electrocardiogram recording by telephone in antiarrhythmic drug trials. Chest 81:473, 1982.
118. Naccarelli GV, Dougherty AH, Berns E, et al: Assessment of antiarrhythmic drug efficacy in the treatment of supraventricular arrhythmias. Am J Cardiol 58:31C, 1986.
119. Hasin Y, David D, Rogel S: Transtelephonic adjustment of antiarrhythmic therapy in ambulatory patients. Cardiology 63:243, 1978.
120. Tuttle WB, Schoenfeld CD: ECG phone monitoring of the convalescing MI patient. Primary Cardiol Clin 1:13, 1984.
121. Chadda KD, Harrington D, Kushnik H, et al: The impact of transtelephonic documentation of arrhythmia on morbidity and mortality rates in sudden death survivors. Am Heart J 112:1159, 1986.
122. Brown AP, Dawkins KD, Cavies JG: Detection of arrhythmias: use of a patient-activated ambulatory electrocardiogram device with a solid-state memory loop. Br Heart J 58:251, 1987.
123. Flowers NC, Shvartsman Y, Kennelly BM, et al: Surface recording of His-Purkinje activity on an every-beat basis without digital averaging. Circulation 63:948, 1981.
124. Berbari EJ, Scherlag BJ, Hope RR, et al: Recording from the body surface of arrhythmogenic ventricular activity during the ST segment. Am J Cardiol 41:697, 1978.
125. Kuchar DL, Thorburn CW, Sammel NL: Prediction of serious arrhythmic events after myocardial infarction: signal-averaged electrocardiogram, Holter monitoring and radionuclide ventriculography. J Am Coll Cardiol 9:531, 1987.
126. Gomes JA, Winters SL, Stewart D, et al: A new noninvasive index to predict sustained ventricular tachycardia and sudden death in the first year after myocardial infarction: based on signal-averaged electrocardiogram, radionuclide ejection fraction and Holter monitoring. J Am Coll Cardiol 10:349, 1987.
127. Lindsey BD, Markham J, Schechtman KM, et al: Identification of patients with sustained ventricular tachycardia by frequency analysis of signal-averaged electrocardiograms despite the presence of bundle branch block. Circulation 77:122, 1987.

128. Buckingham TA, Thessen CC, Stevens RN, et al: Effect of conduction defects on the signal-averaged electrocardiographic detection of late potentials. Am J Cardiol 61:1265, 1988.
129. Vatterott PJ, Hammill SC, Bailey KR, et al: Signal-averaged electrocardiography: a new noninvasive test to identify patients at risk for ventricular arrhythmias. Mayo Clin Proc 63:931, 1988.
130. Simson MB, Untereker WJ, Spielman SR, et al: Relation between late potentials on the body surface and directly recorded fragmented electrograms in patients with ventricular tachycardia. Am J Cardiol 51:105, 1983.
131. Simson MB, Kanovsky MS, Dresden CA: Signal averaging methods to select patients at risk for lethal arrhythmias. Cardiovasc Clin 15:145, 1985.
132. Cain ME, Ambos HD, Witkowski FX, et al: Fast Fourier transform analysis of signal-averaged electrocardiograms for the identification of patients prone to sustained ventricular tachycardia. Circulation 69:711, 1984.
133. Cain ME, Ambos HD, Markham J, et al: Quantification of differences in frequency content of signal-averaged electrocardiographs in patients with compared to those without ventricular tachycardia. Am J Cardiol 55:1500, 1985.
134. Poll DS, Marchlinski FE, Falcone RA, et al: Abnormal signal-averaged electrocardiograms in patients with non-ischemic congestive cardiomyopathy: relationship to sustained ventricular tachyarrhythmias. Circulation 72:1308, 1986.
135. Simson MB, Untereker W, Spielman SR, et al: Relation between late potentials on the body surface and directly recorded fragmented electrograms in patients with ventricular tachycardia. Am J Cardiol 51:105, 1983.
136. Turitto G, Fontaine JM, Ursell SN, et al: Value of the signal-averaged electrocardiogram as a predictor of the results of programmed stimulation in nonsustained ventricular tachycardia. Am J Cardiol 61:1272, 1988.
137. Winters SL, Stewart D, Targonski A, et al: Role of signal averaging of the surface QRS complex in selecting patients with nonsustained ventricular tachycardia and high grade ventricular arrhythmias for programmed ventricular stimulation. J Am Coll Cardiol 12:1481, 1988.
138. Simson MB: Use of signals in the terminal QRS complex to identify patients with ventricular tachycardia after myocardial infarction. Circulation 64:235, 1981.
139. Breithardt G, Borggrefe M: Pathophysiological mechanisms and clinical significance of ventricular late potentials. Eur Heart J 7:364, 1986.
140. Kanovsky MS, Falcone RA, Dresden CA, et al: Identification of patients with ventricular tachycardia after myocardial infarction: signal-averaged electrocardiogram, Holter monitoring and cardiac catheterization. Circulation 70:264, 1984.
141. Gang ES, Lew AS, Hong M, et al: Decreased incidence of ventricular late potentials after successful thrombolytic therapy for acute myocardial infarction. N Engl J Med 321:712, 1989.
142. Breithardt G, Borgreffe M: Late potentials as predictors of risk after thrombolytic treatment? Br Heart J 64:174, 1990.
143. Kuchar DL, Thorburn CW, Samme NL: Signal-averaged electrocardiogram for evaluation of recurrent syncope. Am J Cardiol 58:949, 1986.
144. Gang ES, Peter T, Rosental ME, et al: Detection of late potentials on the

surface electrocardiogram in unexplained syncope. Am J Cardiol 58:1014, 1986.

145. Naccarelli GV, Nishikawa A, Giebel RA: Patient assessment: laboratory studies. In: Comprehensive Cardiac Care, Andreoli KG, Zipes DP, Wallace A, et al. (eds), St Louis, CV Mosby Co., pp 58–81, 1987.

146. Naccarelli GV, Dougherty AH, Rinkenberger RL: Noninvasive evaluation of the patient with cardiac arrhythmia. In: Clinical Management of Arrhythmias: Practice Guide. Vlay SC (ed), Boston, Little, Brown & Co., pp 198–220, 1988.

Chapter 3

Indications for Electrophysiological Testing in Patients with Cardiac Arrhythmias

Robert L. Rinkenberger,
Gerald V. Naccarelli, and
Anne H. Dougherty

Introduction

The first intracardiac recordings of a His bundle electrocardiogram was performed in 1968.[1,2] Early recordings were used to record local cardiac electrograms in an attempt to evaluate atrioventricular conduction.[3] These studies gained clinical application in patients with conduction disturbances and bradycardia. The development of programmed electrical stimulation expanded the clinical application of intracardiac recordings in providing diagnostic information regarding tachycardias and assisting in determining forms of therapy. The procedure has become widely available and can be indispensable in evaluating and treating certain types of cardiac arrhythmias. The technique of programmed electrical stimulation involves pacing the atrium or ventricle at different rates and the introduction of critically timed premature stimuli by means of a programmable stimulator.[4] Local cardiac electrical

From Naccarelli GV (ed): *Cardiac Arrhythmias: A Practical Approach*. Mount Kisco, NY, Futura Publishing Co., Inc., © 1991.

activity can be recorded by catheter techniques to determine electrical activation sequences and to help locate sites of tachycardia origin.

The application of programmed electrical stimulation allows a more dynamic evaluation of sinus node and atrioventricular conduction in addition to the initiation and termination of tachycardias. Electrophysiological (EP) procedures have been informative in understanding the mechanisms of tachycardias and have led to therapeutic approaches for arrhythmia management, including serial antiarrhythmic drug testing, electrophysiologically guided surgical procedures, antitachycardia pacing, the implantable automatic defibrillator, and catheter ablation procedures. The test is a cardiac catheterization procedure involving the

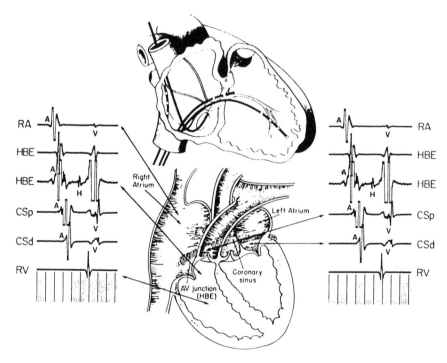

Figure 1. Sites of catheter placement and example of intracardiac recordings obtained during electrophysiological studies. Multipolar catheters can be placed for purposes of simultaneous electrogram recording and pacing in the high right atrium, His bundle area, right ventricular apex, and coronary sinus. RA = right atrium; HBE = His bundle recording; H = His bundle potential; CSp = proximal coronary sinus; CSd = distal coronary sinus; RV = right ventricle; V = ventricular activation; A = atrial activation.

percutaneous introduction of several multipolar catheters for the purpose of recording electrograms and pacing the heart at a variety of intracardiac sites.[5] Examples of catheter placement and intracardiac electrograms are shown in Figures 1 and 2.

Extrastimulation involves the introduction of timed premature impulses after a series of normal or paced impulses, beginning first with long coupling intervals, then shortening the coupling intervals until the tissue is refractory to the signal. Specific stimulation protocols or sequence of stimulation are used for the different clinical situations that can be evaluated by these techniques.

Electrophysiological testing has a lower risk and complication rate compared to more general cardiac catheterizations for coronary and valvular heart disease. The complication rate has been reported as low as

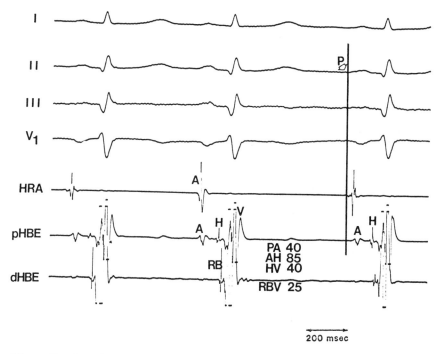

Figure 2. Spontaneous surface and intracardiac recordings in sinus rhythm. The PA interval measures conduction time from the high to low right atrium, the AH through the AV node, and the HV distal to the AV node through the His-Purkinje system. In some patients, right bundle (RB) potentials can be recorded from a distal His bundle lead (dHBE). Same abbreviations as in Figure 1. (Reproduced with permission from Naccarelli GV, Jackman WM.[37])

Table 1
Major Complications of Clinical Cardiac Electrophysiological
Studies*
(n = 8545 studies in 4015 patients)

Complications	n	% Studies	% Patients
Death	5	0.06	0.12
Cardiac perforation	19	0.22	0.5
Major hemorrhage	4	0.05	0.1
Arterial injury	8	0.1	0.2
Major venous thrombosis	20	0.23	0.5

* Adapted from Horowitz LN.[6]

0.7%, and is summarized in Table 1. Most of the complications were related to unexpected mechanical aspects of the study and not to electrophysiological stimulation or the induction of arrhythmias. Venous thrombosis is the most common complication. The complication rate is low since, except for the cases of left ventricular mapping, electrophysiological studies require only venous puncture and right heart catheterization. Although cardioversion for an induced hemodynamically unstable tachycardia is occasionally necessary, serious complications are

Table 2
Indications for Electrophysiological Studies

1. Assessment of suspected sinus node dysfunction
2. Assessment of suspected AV nodal or His-Purkinje conduction disturbances
3. Diagnosis, serial study of supraventricular tachycardia
4. Wolff-Parkinson-White syndrome
5. Diagnosis, serial study of ventricular tachycardia and out-of-hospital cardiac arrest not associated with a myocardial infarction.
6. Differential diagnosis of wide QRS tachycardia
7. Syncope of undetermined etiology
8. Mapping for catheter or surgical ablation
9. Pacemaker, antitachycardia pacemaker, and implantable defibrillator prescription

uncommon. Indications for invasive electrophysiological testing are listed in Table 2.

Sinus Node Dysfunction

Abnormalities of the sinus node involve a spectrum of symptoms and electrocardiographic findings, including sinus bradycardia, sinus pauses, sinus arrest, sinoatrial exit block, and tachycardia-bradycardia syndrome. Clinical symptoms can vary and are often intermittent. Chronic sinus bradycardia is generally the earliest finding with progressive changes into more significant sinus node abnormalities. The initial step in approaching patients with suspected sick sinus syndrome is to consider the physiological and pharmacological causes of sinus bradycardia. Exacerbating drugs should be discontinued. Hypothyroidism should be ruled out. Ambulatory monitoring with documentation of electrocardiographic abnormalities and correlation with symptoms is the most useful diagnostic technique for establishing the presence of sick sinus syndrome. Exercise testing can occasionally be helpful in assessing sinus node chronotropic function and carotid sinus massage may identify patients with sinus node dysfunction and carotid sinus hypersensitivity.

Electrophysiological Methods for Assessing Sinus Node Function

Electrophysiological methods of assessing sinus node automaticity include evaluating sinus node response to the introduction of premature atrial stimuli and rapid overdrive pacing. Rapid overdrive pacing is the most commonly used method to assess sinus node automaticity. This involves pacing the high right atrium for 30–60 seconds at several rates between 100 and 150 beats per minute and recording sinus recovery time following termination of atrial pacing. The interval between the last paced response and the first spontaneous sinus node response is measured as the sinus node recovery time (SNRT) (Fig. 3). Because of variation in spontaneous sinus rate, the spontaneous cycle length prior to pacing is subtracted from SNRT to determine the corrected SNRT (CSNRT). Normal CSNRT values are less than 525 msec. Occasionally, following cessation of pacing, the first return cycle is normal in duration, but the subsequent cycles may be prolonged, termed a secondary pause.

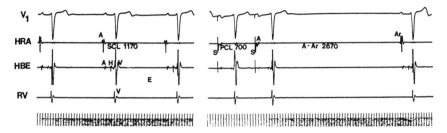

Figure 3. Surface lead V_1 and intracardiac leads demonstrating resting sinus rhythm on left at spontaneous cycle length of 1170 msec and prolonged sinus node recovery time of 2670 msec after termination of high right atrial pacing on right (corrected sinus node recovery time of 1500 msec). Same abbreviations as in Figure 1. (Reproduced with permission from Naccarelli GV, Jackman WM.[37])

Abnormal values for CSNRT have been documented in 30–90% of patients with sick sinus syndrome; therefore, the absence of an abnormal CSNRT does not exclude the diagnosis of sick sinus syndrome. However, a markedly abnormally long CSNRT is a strong indicator of sinus node dysfunction.[7,8]

Other methods have been used to evaluate sinus node function, including sinus node response to premature stimuli (sinoatrial conduction time) and direct catheter measurement of SACT; however, these methods are less sensitive indicators of sinus node dysfunction. The sensitivity of the SACT for detecting sinus node dysfunction is about 50%.

Electrophysiological testing is generally not required, nor is electrophysiological testing routinely indicated in asymptomatic patients with sinus node abnormalities. Electrophysiological testing is indicated when the diagnosis is suspected, but cannot be confirmed by ambulatory recordings. In patients with sinus node dysfunction, other conduction abnormalities may exist. Electrophysiological investigation aids in the proper prescription of pacemakers for these patients.

Atrioventricular Conduction System Dysfunction

Patients with documented symptomatic AV block generally do not require electrophysiology studies to judge the need for permanent pacing. In asymptomatic patients, the site of block, AV nodal versus infranodal block, may be important to establish because of prognostic implications. Patients with infranodal block (Mobitz II block) more commonly progress to complete heart block and require pacemaker implantation than patients with AV nodal block (Mobitz I block). Symptoms associated with Mobitz I block would be an indication for pacing. The asymptomatic patient may not require pacing since escape mechanisms are usually very adequate.[9] Generally, the site of AV block can be determined from a careful analysis of the surface ECG prior to the onset of block analyzed in conjunction with the presence or absence of bundle branch block. When this cannot be adequately determined by surface recordings, electrophysiological recording may be indicated.

In Mobitz I AV block with narrow QRS, the block is usually at the level of the AV node; less commonly, it may be within the His bundle. In type I AV block with a wide QRS complex, the block may be AV nodal, within or below the His bundle. Mobitz II block is usually within or below the His bundle and is most often associated with a bundle branch block (Fig. 4). The prognosis of patients depends on the site of block. AV nodal block, in general, has a good prognosis; however, untreated Mobitz II has a poor prognosis.

The normal intraventricular conduction system is trifascicular, consisting of a right bundle branch and two divisions of the left bundle branch. Bifascicular block refers to block in two divisions of the con-

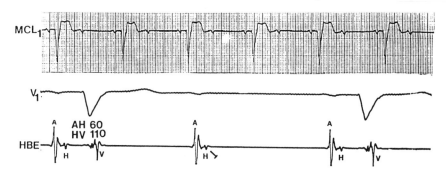

Figure 4. Example of distal His bundle block (Mobitz II) in a patient presenting with congestive heart failure and 2:1 AV conduction associated with a left bundle branch block (lead V_1). The PR interval of conducted impulses on the surface ECG is normal as well as conduction through the AV node as measured by the AH interval of 60 msec (normal less than 120 msec). Conduction below the AV node is markedly abnormal with an HV interval of 110 msec in conducting impulses (normal 35 to 55 msec) and block following His bundle activation following every other normal sinus impulse. A permanent pacemaker is indicated.

duction system, i.e., right bundle branch block and a division of the left bundle branch. Electrophysiological testing generally is not indicated in asymptomatic patients with bifascicular block or left bundle branch block. Measurement of the HV interval (conduction in the remaining fascicle) has not been useful to predict future development of heart block. Patients with bifascicular block and prolonged HV interval (>55 msec) are at slightly higher risk of developing complete heart block, but the incidence is low (2–3% per year). The HV interval has a high sensitivity (82%); however, it has a low specificity (63%) for predicting the development of complete AV block.[11–13] In some symptomatic patients, however, marked HV prolongation of >100 msec is associated with a high incidence of progression to complete heart block. Rapid atrial pacing may help identify significant distal disease. The sensitivity of distal His block induced by atrial pacing is low, but its predictive value for development of complete AV block is high. Many patients with bifascicular block and syncope will have induced sustained VT at EP study as the cause of their symptoms.

Supraventricular Tachycardia

The mechanism of a supraventricular tachycardia can be correctly identified in many instances by a careful analysis of the surface ECG. This process begins by correctly identifying atrial activity during the tachycardia and determining its relationship or potential relationship to the QRS complex. Events at the initiation of tachycardia, as well as changes in rate and/or AV relationship during the tachycardia, are very useful in identifying the most likely mechanism of the tachycardia. Electrophysiological testing, however, may be necessary to identify or confirm the mechanism and can be extremely useful in determining appropriate treatment of the tachycardia.

Electrophysiological testing is most useful in evaluating patients with AV nodal re-entrant tachycardia and tachycardia associated with accessory pathways.[15,16] Re-entrant arrhythmias are more commonly initiated by these techniques and various responses to physiological maneuvers, pacing, and drugs are determined (Fig. 5). The test is generally not of value in judging potential effective antiarrhythmic treatment in patients with primary atrial tachycardias. Localizing the site of origin of an ectopic atrial tachycardia via mapping is indicated when an ablative approach to treatment is considered. Pacing termination and serial drug

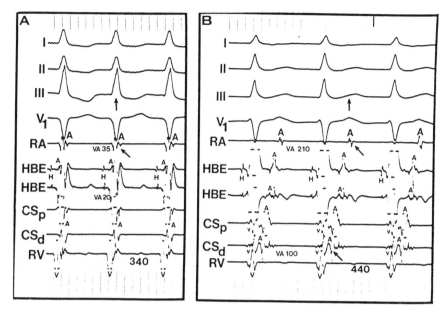

Figure 5. Examples of arrhythmia mechanisms determined by electrophysiological testing in patients with supraventricular tachycardias. (A) AV nodal re-entrant tachycardia demonstrating retrograde activation of the atria during tachycardia occurring inside the QRS complex. (B) Re-entrant tachycardia using a concealed left-sided accessory pathway demonstrating retrograde atria activation during tachycardia beginning the left atrial (CS$_d$ recording). Documentation of the mechanism is useful in planning and evaluating antiarrhythmic therapy. Same abbreviations as in Figure 1.

testing is generally not of value in patients with arrhythmias where automaticity is the basic mechanism.

It is common for patients with paroxysmal supraventricular tachycardia to have sporadic attacks. Empirical drug therapy may take months to evaluate. If the re-entrant supraventricular tachycardia can be initiated in a controlled state, a drug may be given, and an attempt made to reinitiate the tachycardia or determine the influence of the drug on the conduction pathway involved in the tachycardia. If supraventricular tachycardia cannot be reinitiated, the drug is usually successful in preventing recurrent episodes of tachycardia, although induction of supraventricular tachycardia may not preclude a good clinical response in some instances. Dual AV nodal pathways in patients with AV nodal tachycardia can be demonstrated and the characteristics of antegrade and retrograde conduction determined. The pathways involved may respond differently to antiarrhythmic drugs and, in the individual patient, some drugs may be shown to be ineffective in producing a significant electrophysiological response.[17,18] Drug response may be evaluated in patients with AV nodal re-entrant tachycardia as well as other forms of therapy, such as antitachycardia devices.

Supraventricular tachycardia may also involve the presence of accessory AV connections. Patients with accessory pathways may have a delta wave on the surface ECG, indicating the presence of antegrade conduction, or pathways may conduct in the retrograde conduction only (concealed accessory pathways), evident only during episodes of supraventricular tachycardia or during ventricular pacing. In both situations, accessory pathways may participate in a re-entrant circuit. Patients with antegrade accessory pathway conduction may have rapid conduction to the ventricle during atrial fibrillation or atrial flutter, depending on the electrophysiological character of the accessory. Electrophysiological testing is the most useful method for evaluating the risk of atrial fibrillation prior to and after drug treatment, and is helpful in determining the influence of drugs in retrograde conduction.

In patients with accessory pathways, an electrophysiological study may be informative in several ways (Tables 3, 4). The decision to perform an electrophysiology study in patients with the Wolff-Parkinson-White (WPW) syndrome is generally based on individual patient presentation and consideration of certain therapeutic approaches. The issue of whether asymptomatic patients with WPW syndrome should be studied remains controversial. The major concern is the potential risk in patients with rapidly conducting accessory pathways for sudden death. Electro-

---

Table 3
Diagnostic and Clinically Useful Information Obtained During
Electrophysiological Testing in Patients with Accessory Pathways

---

1. Determining the mechanism of the tachycardia especially if wide QRS tachycardias are present
2. Confirmation of the presence of an accessory pathway and its participation in a re-entrant circuit
3. Determining the location and number of accessory pathways in surgical or ablation candidates
4. Determining the risk of atrial fibrillation
5. Evaluation of the response to antiarrhythmic drugs or antitachycardia devices to control arrhythmias

Table 4
Indications for Electrophysiological Studies in the Patient with
Wolff-Parkinson-White Syndrome

1. Spontaneous episodes of atrial fibrillation, especially with rapid ventricular response
2. Episodes of paroxysmal supraventricular tachycardia if:
   a. Empirical therapy has been unsuccessful
   b. Noninvasive evaluation cannot exclude an accessory pathway with a short refractory period
   c. Associated with organic heart disease (HOCM, Ebstein's anomaly, CAD)
3. Patient prefers surgery or ablation for treatment
4. Asymptomatic patients with family history of life-threatening arrhythmias, sports participation, or high-risk occupations, in whom knowledge of electrophysiological characteristics of the accessory pathway may help guide therapy

physiological techniques may establish the diagnosis of WPW syndrome and provide useful information regarding the number, location, and character of accessory connections. In addition, the response of accessory pathway tissue to drug therapy may be instrumental in selecting other forms of therapy for the patient.

Serial Drug Testing in Patients with Supraventricular Tachycardias

In patients with WPW syndrome who have orthodromic tachycardia utilizing the AV node and accessory pathway, prevention of induction of tachycardia will generally predict long-term drug efficacy. Complete block of anterograde conduction over the accessory pathway, marked lengthening of the anterograde refractory period of the accessory pathway, and a marked reduction in the ventricular response during atrial fibrillation are predictive of a therapeutic drug response. AV nodal re-entry is less well studied in terms of drug response, but current data suggest that drug efficacy may be predicted by response in the electrophysiological laboratory in selected patients with AV nodal reentrant tachycardia. The addition of isoproterenol may add to the predictive accuracy of serial drug testing in SVT. Prevention of pacing induction of atrial fibrillation may predict long-term response in some patients; however, the technique is not widely accepted for that purpose. Other primary atrial arrhythmias, such as ectopic atrial tachycardia or multifocal atrial tachycardia, are not inducible by these techniques.

Wide QRS Tachycardia

Wide QRS complex tachycardia is a common clinical problem. Appropriate management of the patient is dependent upon an accurate diagnosis of the type of tachycardia. There are four basic mechanisms of wide QRS tachycardias listed in Table 5. Although the surface ECG can provide valuable clues regarding the mechanism of a wide complex tachycardia at times, frequently a correct distinction cannot be made between supraventricular tachycardia with aberrancy and ventricular tachycardia.[20,21]

Intracardiac recordings and atrial pacing can be extremely important in establishing the correct diagnosis. In the majority of supraventricular tachycardias, the atrial rate either equals or exceeds the ventricular rate. Atrioventricular (AV) dissociation has been the most reliable criterion to distinguish between supraventricular tachycardia with aberrancy and ventricular tachycardia (Fig. 6). AV dissociation, however, may not be recognized on the surface ECG or 1:1 retrograde conduction to the atria can occur. In practice, although the criterion of AV dissociation is useful, it has limitations since it can be identified on surface ECGs in only a small percentage of patients with ventricular tachycardia. Only the presence of AV dissociation or intermittent failure of retrograde conduction during antidromic AV reciprocating tachycardia can exclude an accessory pathway as a mechanism of tachycardia. The ECG patterns of tach-

---

Table 5
Mechanisms of Wide QRS Tachycardias

---

1. Supreventricular tachycardia associated with pre-existing bundle branch block
2. Supraventricular tachycardia associated with functional or rate-related aberrant conduction
3. SVT associated with conduction to the ventricle over an accessory connection
4. Ventricular tachycardia

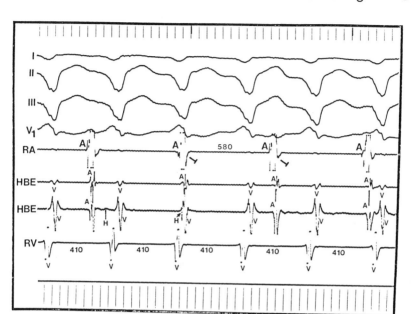

Figure 6. Intracardiac recordings in a patient presenting with a wide QRS tachycardia. Intracardiac recording confirms the diagnosis as ventricular tachycardia. The right atrial electrograms (RA) demonstrate AV dissociation. The His bundle electrogram (HBE) demonstrated His bundle activation (H) occurring inside the QRS complex intermittently associated with atrial activation and at other times associated retrograde with ventricular activation. The QRS rate (410 msec) remains constant.

ycardias with ventricular activation related to an accessory connection cannot be distinguished from ventricular tachycardias originating from the bore of the left ventricle by ECG morphology alone.

Analysis of atrial activation sequence and timing during the tachycardia is important as well as the response of His bundle deflection and atrial activation and timing in response to timed premature ventricular stimuli during the tachycardia. During tachycardia, an HV interval equal to or exceeding the HV interval recorded during sinus rhythm would be consistent with a supraventricular tachycardia. Catheter position is critical for demonstration of this relationship; however, the absence of the ability to record His deflection does not alone establish proof of ventricular tachycardia. Thus, dynamic changes during the tachycardia can be essential for the proper diagnosis.

The differential diagnosis of wide complex arrhythmias can be difficult and requires a very comprehensive electrophysiological study as well as a detailed analysis of the surface electrocardiogram. Major indications for study of patients with wide complex tachycardias include patients with symptomatic tachycardias where the diagnosis is uncertain and necessary for correct treatment. Likewise, patients with preexcitation syndrome and wide QRS tachycardia are candidates for electrophysiological study to differentiate orthodromic supraventricular tachycardia with aberrancy, preexcited supraventricular tachycardia, ventricular tachycardia, and nodoventricular conduction (Mahaim).

Ventricular Tachycardia

Electrophysiological testing has been shown to be useful in determining the type of management of patients with sustained ventricular tachycardia and out-of-hospital cardiac arrest not associated with acute myocardial infarction.[23-28] The goals of electrophysiological testing in patients with ventricular tachycardia include: (1) to reproduce the clinical arrhythmia and confirm the diagnosis of a wide QRS tachycardia; (2) to evaluate the efficacy of pharmacological and/or electrical treatment of the tachycardia; (3) to localize the site of origin of the ventricular tachycardia prior to catheter or surgical ablation.

Induction of ventricular tachycardia depends upon both the type of heart disease and whether the clinical arrhythmia is sustained (greater than 30 seconds in duration) or nonsustained (three impulses in duration up to 30 seconds).[24,29] It is important that the induced arrhythmia is the same or similar to the patient's spontaneous arrhythmia. In patients with coronary artery disease, the induction of ventricular tachycardia is more likely than in patients without coronary artery disease (e.g., cardiomyopathy, mitral valve prolapse, primary electrical disease).[24,29] The induction of ventricular tachycardia is most common in patients with sustained ventricular tachycardia (Table 6).

The role of electrophysiological testing in the diagnosis and evaluation of patients with congenital or acquired forms of prolonged QT interval syndrome is less clear and apparently limited. These patients are generally noninducible, although information regarding dynamic changes in the QT interval with drugs or maneuvers may be beneficial in some patients. Such studies, however, have not been demonstrated to have predictive value. The analysis of monophasic action potential recordings is an investigational technique that may prove helpful.

Table 6
Frequency of Ventricular Tachycardia by
Programmed Electrical Stimulation*

	CAD	Non-CAD
Sustained VT	95%	70%
Survivor cardiac arrest	85%	60%
Nonsustained VT	80%	35%

* Adapted from Naccarelli GV, et al.[24] and from Prystowsky EN, et al.[29]

CAD = coronary artery disease; VT = ventricular tachycardia.

Serial Electrophysiological Testing in Patients with Ventricular Tachycardia

Induction of ventricular tachycardia during a control study allows the patient to be evaluated on antiarrhythmic drugs to identify which drug or drug combination prevents induction or markedly changes the induced ventricular tachycardia. If ventricular tachycardia remains non-inducible, patients have about an 80% chance of doing well; however, if ventricular tachycardia is still induced (with the exception of amiodarone) approximately 80% of patients will have a recurrence within 1 year of discharge. If the induced tachycardia is considerably slower compared to the baseline arrhythmia, the patient will be less symptomatic if tachycardia occurs. In addition, continued inducibility despite several antiarrhythmic drug trials can help select candidates for nonpharmacological therapy. Figure 7 demonstrates our evaluation protocol in patients with sustained ventricular tachycardia or ventricular fibrillation.

The usefulness of repeat electrophysiological testing in assessing efficacy of amiodarone remains controversial.[30,31] Inability to induce ventricular tachycardia in a patient receiving amiodarone when previously inducible is highly predictive of long-term efficacy. Approximately 60% of patients receiving amiodarone have the ability to have ventricular tachycardia induced during electrophysiological testing despite therapy with amiodarone, and yet they do well clinically long-term. More difficult induction of tachycardia after amiodarone appears to predict partial efficacy on amiodarone or other drugs.[31] Patients with hemodynamically compromising ventricular tachycardia should proceed to nonpharmacological or combination antiarrhythmic therapy.

VENTRICULAR TACHYCARDIA

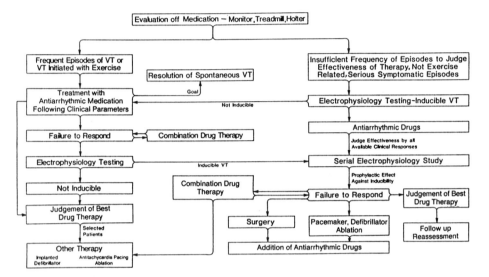

Figure 7. Algorithm for evaluating and treating patients with sustained ventricular tachyarrhythmias.

Although serial electrophysiological testing has an important role in the management of patients with recurrent sustained ventricular tachycardia, its application in patients with nonsustained ventricular tachycardia is controversial. Inducibility is less common in this group, and in some studies, left ventricular dysfunction is a better predictor of survival. In some instances, electrophysiology testing can identify patients whose nonsustained ventricular tachycardia becomes worse while receiving antiarrhythmic drugs. The induction of sustained ventricular tachycardia in these patients may be associated with a worse prognosis. The presence of an abnormal signal-averaged electrocardiogram may identify patients who are likely to have sustained ventricular tachycardia induced by programmed stimulation.[32] More data concerning nonsustained ventricular tachycardia must be obtained before specific recommendations can be made.

Out-of-Hospital Cardiac Arrest

Ventricular fibrillation is the most common arrhythmia documented at the time of sudden cardiac death. Patients resuscitated from cardiac arrest without a new Q-wave myocardial infarction are at high risk for recurrent sudden death. The recurrence rate may be as high as 30–45%, within 1 to 2 years, although these numbers may improve because of aggressive therapy of the underlying heart disease. In the absence of antiarrhythmic drug therapy, ventricular tachyarrhythmias can be initiated in 60–85% of patients resuscitated from cardiac arrest. Patients with coronary artery disease have a higher frequency of tachycardia induction than do those without coronary disease (Table 6).

A number of studies have demonstrated good predictive value of serial electrophysiological-pharmacological testing in survivors of cardiac arrest. A recent study by Ruskin and colleagues demonstrated that inducible ventricular arrhythmias can be documented in nearly 80% of patients tested and that noninducibility of ventricular tachycardia during drug treatment predicted a favorable result.[26] During a follow-up period of 21 months, cardiac arrest recurred in 12% of patients in whom inducible arrhythmias had been suppressed, in 33% in whom inducible arrhythmias still occurred, and in 17% of patients in whom arrhythmias could not be induced at the control study. Although some patients whose arrhythmia remains inducible may not have recurrent episodes, those patients still inducible prior to discharge are at significantly higher risk for recurrent cardiac arrest and sudden death, estimated at 23% at 1 year and 30% at 3 years. Most investigators feel that electrophysiological testing in this group provides a method for selecting treatment options such as drugs, surgery, or devices that reduce the risk of recurrent cardiac arrest. Because of the high risk of sudden death in these patients and the unreliability of noninvasive testing, we recommend serial electrophysiological testing for all of these patients. Therapy can be individualized, depending on the results of testing. Patients with cardiac arrest occurring only within the first 48 hours of acute myocardial infarction are not initial candidates for electrophysiological studies. Noninducibility during the baseline study in survivors of cardiac arrest is associated with a variable prognosis. Patients with a low ejection fraction and no reversible cause of the arrhythmia remain at high risk for recurrent cardiac arrest.[28]

Syncope

Patients commonly present to their physician with syncope. Arrhythmias causing syncope are usually intermittent and may be difficult to diagnose. Table 7 lists the abnormal electrophysiological findings that

---

Table 7

Abnormal Electrophysiological Findings Associated with Syncope

---

1. Sinus Node Dysfunction
   a. Prolonged sinus node recovery time
   b. Prolonged sinoatrial conduction time
   c. Secondary pauses
2. Abnormalities of AV Conduction
   a. Markedly prolonged AV nodal effective refractory period
   b. Abnormally slow 1:1 maximal AV nodal conduction
   c. Markedly prolonged HV interval
   d. Block distal to the bundle of His at slow atrial pacing rates
3. Induced Tachyarrhythmias
   a. Supraventricular tachycardias with a rapid rate
   b. Presence of a rapidly conducting accessory pathway
   c. Sustained ventricular tachycardia

---

have been documented in patients experiencing syncope. From the electrophysiological standpoint, the purpose of the study is to assess sinus node dysfunction, the presence of AV nodal or infranodal dysfunction, and the induction of supraventricular, as well as ventricular, tachycardia. Ventricular tachycardia is the most common abnormality documented.[33–35] Induction of sustained monomorphic ventricular tachycardia or documentation of significant sinus node or infranodal block may have diagnostic value. Induction of a specific mechanism of SVT associated with hypotension may also be clinically important. Induction of nonsustained ventricular tachycardia, polymorphic ventricular tachycardia, or atrial fibrillation may be nonspecific. Clinical description of the event can be helpful in determining the most likely cause. In some situations, the etiology can be readily apparent and specific therapy indicated. From an arrhythmic standpoint, the most important aspect is to document the symptoms during electrocardiographic recordings. If the noninvasive evaluation has not revealed an etiology despite repeated Holter monitors, an electrophysiology study should be considered (Fig. 8).

In patients with organic heart disease, the diagnostic yield from electrophysiological studies is quite high (60% abnormal findings). However, the yield is low (26% abnormal findings) in patients with normal ECGs and no definite evidence of organic heart disease. Because of possible false negative responses, failure to initiate an arrhythmia does not

EVALUATION OF POSSIBLE ARRHYTHMIC SYNCOPE

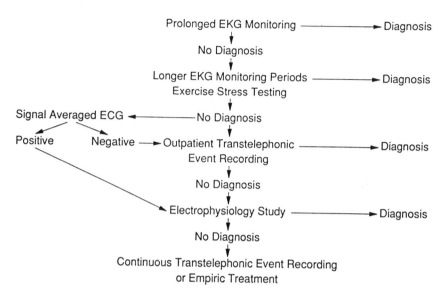

Figure 8. Flow diagram of recommended approach to evaluation of patients with possible arrhythmic syncope.

exclude an arrhythmia as a cause of the patient's syncope. Likewise, some of the abnormalities documented during an electrophysiological study may not completely explain the patient's syncope. Therapy based on the results of electrophysiological testing have been shown to prevent symptoms in over 80% of patients. Such results, however, must be weighted against the probability of recurrence. In syncope patients who have had normal EP studies, the prognosis is better with a low incidence of mortality, possibly because obvious, major dysrhythmic abnormalities have been excluded.

Patients who have recurrent syncope not documented by multiple Holter records, event records, or exercise testing should have an electrophysiology study. If the study is normal or inconclusive and arrhythmia symptoms are still suspected, continued effort to document the arrhythmia should be made. Thus, patients with unexplained syncope and structural heart disease are the most likely candidates to benefit from testing.

One potentially useful application of the signal-averaged ECG is in the identification of the patient with unexplained syncope who may have had ventricular tachycardia as a cause of syncope. In an evaluation of 250 patients with syncope, late potentials were demonstrated in 16 of 22 patients with ventricular tachycardia, and no late potentials in 110 of 114 patients in syncope were related to other causes.[36] This demonstrates that presence of late potentials has a sensitivity of 73%, a specificity of 89%, and a predictive accuracy of 55%. A positive study in patients with unexplained syncope has been shown to be 85% sensitive and 94% specific in identifying patients with inducible VT undergoing electrophysiological testing. When abnormal late potentials are found, especially in a patient with syncope, structural heart disease may help to select those patients who should undergo invasive electrophysiological studies.

Patients with Unexplained Palpitations

Long-term ambulatory recording is the most useful method to document an arrhythmia associated with palpitations. Patients with palpitations whose pulse rate is known to be greater than 150 bpm in whom ECG documentation has not been possible may be considered for electrophysiological testing.

Nonpharmacological Therapy of Arrhythmias: Role of Electrophysiology Studies

Surgical and catheter ablative techniques are other treatment options in patients with supraventricular tachycardia, ventricular tachycardia, and WPW syndrome.[19] Prior to ablation, the patient requires an electrophysiological study to identify the site and number of accessory pathways, atrial or ventricular tachycardia focus, etc. Intraoperative epicardial and endocardial mapping is also done at the time of surgical ablation to confirm the location of the accessory pathway or arrhythmia focus. Post-ablation testing is important to confirm successful treatment.

Electrophysiology studies are useful in defining the need and best type of permanent pacemaker prescription. Preoperative, intraoperative, and postoperative electrophysiology studies are required to properly prescribe an implantable defibrillator or antitachycardia pacemaker, study drug-device interactions, determine acceptable termination sequences and defibrillation thresholds and assess the efficacy and electronics of the implanted generator.

References

1. Scherlag BJ, Helfant RH, Damato AN: A catheterization technique for His bundle stimulation and recording in the intact dog. J Appl Physiol 25:425, 1968.
2. Sherlag BJ, Lau SH, Helfant RH, et al: Catheter technique for recording His bundle activity in man. Circulation 39:13, 1969.
3. Narula OS, Scherlag BJ, Samet P, et al: Atrioventricular block: localization and classification by His bundle recording. Am J Med 50:146, 1975.
4. Scheiman MM, Morady F: Invasive cardiac electrophysiologic testing: the current state-of-the-art. Circulation 67:1169, 1983.
5. Hammill SC, Sugrue DD, Gersh BJ, et al: Clinical intracardiac electrophysiology testing: technique, diagnostic indications and therapeutic uses. Mayo Clin Proc 61:478, 1986.
6. Horowitz LN: Safety of electrophysiologic studies. Circulation 73:(2)28, 1986.
7. Mandel WH, Hayakawa H, Danzig R, et al: Evaluation of sino-atrial node function in man by overdrive suppression 44:59, 1971.
8. Breithardt G, Speigel L, Loogen F: Sinus node recovery time and calculated sinoatrial conduction time in normal subjects and patients with sinus node dysfunction. Circulation 56:43, 1977.
9. Strasberg B, Amat-y-Leon F, Dhingra RC, et al: Natural history of chronic second-degree atrioventricular nodal block. Circulation 63:1043, 1981.
10. Dhingra RC, Denes P, Wu D, et al: The significance of second-degree atrioventricular block and bundle branch block. Circulation 49:638, 1974.
11. Dhingra RC, Palileo E, Strasberg B, et al: Significance of the HV interval in 517 patients with chronic bifascicular block. Circulation 64:1265, 1981.
12. Dhingra RC, Wyndham C, Amat-y-Leon F, et al: Incidence and site of atrioventricular block in patients with chronic bifascicular block. Circulation 59:238, 1979.
13. Scheinman M, Weiss A, Kunkel F: His bundle recordings in patients with bundle branch block and transient neurologic symptoms. Circulation 48:322, 1973.
14. Rinkenberger RL, Naccarelli GV: Evaluation and treatment of narrow complex tachycardias. Crit Care Clin 5(3):569, 1989.
15. Wu D, Amat-y-Leon F, Simpson RJ Jr, et al: Electrophysiologic studies with multiple drugs in patients with atrioventricular reentrant tachycardias utilizing an extra nodal pathway. Circulation 56:727, 1977.
16. Bauernfeind RA, Wyndham CR, Dhingra RC, et al: Serial electrophysiologic testing of multiple drugs in patients with atrioventricular nodal reentrant paroxysmal tachycardia. Circulation 62:1341, 1980.
17. Morady F, Sledge C, Shen E, et al: Electrophysiologic testing in the management of patients with the WPW syndrome and atrial fibrillation. Am J Cardiol 51:1623, 1983.

18. Rinkenberger RL, Naccarelli GV, Miles WM, et al: Encainide for atrial fibrillation associated with Wolff-Parkinson-White syndrome. Am J Cardiol 62:26L, 1988.
19. Morady F: A perspective on the role of catheter ablation in the management of tachyarrhythmias. PACE 11:98, 1988.
20. Wellens HJ, Bar FWH, Lie KI: The value of the electrocardiogram in the differential diagnosis of a tachycardia with a widened QRS complex. Am J Med 64:27, 1978.
21. Rinkenberger RL, Naccarelli GV: Evaluation and acute treatment of wide complex tachycardias. Crit Care Clin 5(3):599, 1989.
22. Akhtar M: Retrograde conduction in man. PACE 4:548, 1981.
23. Mitchell LB, et al: A randomized clinical trial of the noninvasive and invasive approaches to drug therapy of ventricular tachycardia. N Engl J Med 317:1681, 1987.
24. Naccarelli GV, Prystowsky EN, Jackman WM, et al: Role of electrophysiologic testing in managing patients who have ventricular tachycardia unrelated to coronary artery disease. Am J Cardiol 50:165, 1982.
25. Skale BT, Miles WM, Heger JJ, et al: Survivors of cardiac arrest: prevention of recurrence by drug therapy as predicted by electrophysiologic testing or electrocardiographic monitoring. Am J Cardiol 57:113, 1986.
26. Ruskin JN, DiMarco JP, Garan H: Out-of-hospital cardiac arrest: electrophysiologic observations and selection of long-term antiarrhythmic therapy. N Engl J Med 303:607, 1980.
27. Morady F, Scheinman MM, Hess DS, et al: Electrophysiologic testing in the management of survivors of out-of-hospital cardiac arrest. Am J Cardiol 51:85, 1983.
28. Wilber DJ, Garan H, Kelly E, et al: Out-of-hospital cardiac arrest: role of electrophysiologic testing in prediction of long-term outcome. N Engl J Med 318:19, 1987.
29. Prystowsky EN, Miles WM, Evans JJ, et al: Induction of ventricular tachycardia during programmed electrical stimulation: analysis of pacing methods. Circulation 73(2):32, 1986.
30. Kadish AH, Marchlinski FE, Josephson ME, et al: Amiodarone: correlation of early and late electrophysiology studies with outcome. Am Heart J 112:1134, 1986.
31. Naccarelli GV, Fineberg NS, Zipes DP, et al: Amiodarone: risk factors for recurrence of symptomatic ventricular tachycardia identified at electrophysiologic study. J Am Coll Cardiol 6:814, 1985.
32. Winters SL, Stewart D, Targonski A, et al: Role of signal averaging of the surface QRS complex in selecting patients with nonsustained arrhythmias for programmed ventricular stimulation. J Am Coll Cardiol 12:1481, 1988.
33. Olshansky B, Mazuz M, Martins JB: Significance of inducible tachycardias in patients with syncope of unknown origin: a long-term followup. J Am Coll Cardiol 5:216, 1985.
34. Teichman SL, Felder SD, Matos JA, et al: The value of electrophysiology studies in syncope of undetermined origin: report of 150 cases. Am Heart J 110:469, 1985.
35. Akhtar M, Shenasa M, Denker S, et al: Role of cardiac electrophysiology

studies in patients with unexplained recurrent syncope. PACE 6:192, 1983.

36. Kuchar DL, Thorburn CW, Sammel NL: Signal averaged electrocardiogram for evaluation of recurrent syncope. Am J Cardiol 58:949, 1986.
37. Naccarelli GV, Jackman WM: Invasive electrophysiology. In: Weeks L (ed), Advanced Cardiovascular Nursing. Boston, Blackwell Scientific Publications, Inc., pp 515–549, 1986.

Chapter 4

Ventricular Arrhythmias: Recognition and Treatment

Leonard N. Horowitz

Introduction

Ventricular arrhythmias occur frequently, both in patients without identifiable structural or functional heart disease and in patients with organic heart disease of all types. In some patients, these arrhythmias present no apparent risk, while in others they cause significant morbidity and mortality. It has long been assumed that in some, if not many patients, antiarrhythmic therapy was desirable and indeed indicated for the reduction of this morbidity and mortality. While the indications for antiarrhythmic therapy continue to be debated, it is clear that the appropriate treatment of patients with ventricular arrhythmias requires an assessment of the type and the severity of the arrhythmia and a clinical assessment of the type and severity of the underlying heart disease. This assessment allows a clinical classification of ventricular arrhythmias which is useful in considering the indications for antiarrhythmic therapy and the method of approach used in selecting and monitoring therapy.

A commonly used classification system of ventricular arrhythmias separates them into three groups: benign, prognostically significant, and malignant ventricular arrhythmias. It must be emphasized that this classification system creates three distinct categories in what is actually a spectrum of patients with ventricular arrhythmias. Thus, the classification system is imperfect; however, it does have clinical utility.

From Naccarelli GV (ed): *Cardiac Arrhythmias: A Practical Approach.* Mount Kisco, NY, Futura Publishing Co., Inc., © 1991.

Benign Ventricular Arrhythmias

While ventricular premature complexes (VPC) are not uncommon in the general population, they are more often found in association with significant organic heart disease.[1] VPCs do occur in individuals without organic heart disease or with cardiac abnormalities that are of negligible significance (e.g., mitral valve prolapse without mitral regurgitation). When ventricular arrhythmias do occur in this setting, they are usually infrequent, and repetitive forms such as couplets and unsustained ventricular tachycardia (VT) are uncommon. In a study of normal individuals, VPC frequency was found to be less than 100/day (or less than 5/hour) and repetitive forms were not present.[2] Thus, the presence of ventricular arrhythmia at levels greater than these can be considered "abnormal." The presence of ventricular arrhythmias exceeding these limits can be considered statistically abnormal, although the presence of even frequent ventricular premature complexes in the absence of clinical evidence of or major risk factors for heart disease is associated with a minimal incidence of arrhythmic death.[3,4] Even repetitive VPCs and unsustained VT in individuals without organic heart disease are not associated with an increased risk of arrhythmic morbidity or sudden cardiac death and are therefore prognostically insignificant.[5]

Ventricular arrhythmia may also be detected during exercise testing. VPCs have been reported to occur in 5% to 34% of normal subjects.[6–8] Repetitive forms of ventricular arrhythmia are less commonly noted during exercise testing in normal individuals but have been reported in 1% to 3% of subjects.[6–9] As with ambient ventricular ectopy, cardiac morbidity and mortality is minimal in individuals with exercise-induced ventricular arrhythmia but with no evidence of heart disease.[9]

It therefore appears that VPCs, even if frequent and repetitive, in apparently healthy individuals without risk factors for heart disease can be considered benign.

Despite their benign prognosis, VPCs, ventricular couplets, and runs of unsustained VT may produce symptoms. These are generally modest in severity. Occasionally, lifestyle-limiting symptoms may occur and despite the benign prognosis, antiarrhythmic therapy may be considered.

Prognostically Significant Ventricular Arrhythmias

In patients with organic heart disease, most notably coronary artery disease, ventricular arrhythmias are associated with a significant risk of subsequent cardiac mortality. Early epidemiologic studies showed that VPCs detected with a 12-lead electrocardiogram were associated with an increased risk of sudden death in patients with coronary artery disease.[10,11] Subsequently, it was shown that frequent and repetitive ventricular premature complexes, detected by long-term ambulatory electrocardiographic monitoring, are associated with an increased risk of death in post-infarction patients.[12-14] Post-infarction patients with a VPC frequency of greater than 6–10/hour in the early weeks following myocardial infarction have a 15% to 20% mortality in the first post-infarction year. In comparison, patients without ventricular ectopy or less frequent VPCs have a mortality rate of approximately 7% to 10% in the first post-infarction year. Patients with repetitive forms of ventricular ectopy have an even higher mortality, approximately 25% in the same time interval. The presence of unsustained VT portends an even worse prognosis. In this latter group, mortality may exceed 30% in the first post-infarction year and 50% in the first 3 years after myocardial infarction.[8,15,16]

Most of the data supporting the relationship between prognosis and ventricular ectopy in patients with coronary artery disease has been collected in patients with recent myocardial infarction. The presence of ventricular ectopy in patients with coronary artery disease and remote myocardial infarction similarly increases the risk of cardiac mortality.[17] Ventricular arrhythmias have been shown to be associated with an increased risk of death in patients with other forms of heart disease, including congestive and hypertrophic cardiomyopathy and congenital heart disease.[7-10]

The risk associated with ventricular arrhythmias in patients with organic heart disease is modulated by left ventricular function. The influence of left ventricular function, as measured by symptoms of congestive heart failure or ejection fraction, has previously been a point of considerable controversy. Initial studies suggested that the association between mortality and complex ventricular arrhythmias was independent of left ventricular function;[12,13] however, others questioned this.[21] Recent large studies have confirmed that the risk associated with VPCs is independent of the presence and extent of left ventricular dysfunction.[14,22,23] Moreover, the risks associated with ventricular ectopy and left ventricular dysfunction are additive and the prognostic significance of a specific frequency and severity of ventricular arrhythmia increases as the level of left ventricular function decreases.

Further Evaluation of Risk in Patients with Prognostically Significant Ventricular Arrhythmias

Patients with prognostically significant ventricular arrhythmias comprise a large group of patients with a varying risk of cardiac mortality and sudden death. In this group, the risk increases as the frequency and complexity of ventricular arrhythmia increases. In addition, the risk increases as left ventricular function, as measured by the presence of congestive heart failure or objectively by ejection fraction, decreases. Thus, some patients with prognostically significant ventricular arrhythmia have a prognosis which is only minimally worse than patients with benign ventricular arrhythmias. An example of such a patient might be one with a remote myocardial infarction, ventricular premature complexes, and a left ventricular ejection fraction of 0.40. On the other hand, other patients with prognostically significant ventricular arrhythmia may have a prognosis almost as poor as patients with malignant ventricular arrhythmia (infra vide). Such patients have frequent unsustained VT and poor left ventricular function. Further evaluation may be of some utility in further evaluating the risk in such patients.

The signal-averaged electrocardiogram is a technique that detects delayed myocardial depolarization (late potentials) which provide the substrate for sustained ventricular tachyarrhythmias.[24] Late potentials detected by the signal-averaged electrocardiogram are commonly present in patients with malignant ventricular arrhythmias.[25] More recently, the presence of late potentials on the signal-averaged electrocardiogram has been shown to identify post-infarction patients who will subsequently develop malignant ventricular tachyarrhythmias.[26,27]

The combination of the signal-averaged electrocardiogram with an assessment of left ventricular function and Holter monitoring data provide even greater power in discriminating patients at very high risk from lower risk patients. Signal-averaged electrocardiogram and the left ventricular ejection fraction have predicted the occurrence of malignant ventricular arrhythmias with a sensitivity of 80% and a specificity of 89%. Multivariate analysis has shown, moreover, that the late potential detected by signal-averaged electrocardiography is an independent variable predicting mortality and malignant arrhythmia. Therefore, the presence of late potentials in a signal-averaged electrocardiogram increases the risk associated with prognostically significant ventricular arrhythmias and places the patient closer in the spectrum of patients with ventricular arrhythmias to patients with malignant arrhythmias.

Provocative tests have been suggested to discriminate between lower and higher risk patients with prognostically significant ventricular arrhythmias. Exercise testing has been shown to be useful, particularly in patients with coronary artery disease. In patients with recent myocardial infarction, the first year mortality rate is significantly increased by the presence of exercise-provoked VPCs.[28,29] The utility of exercise testing in patients with chronic coronary artery disease and other forms of heart disease is more controversial. While some[9] have shown a relationship between exercise-induced ventricular arrhythmia and prognosis in coronary artery disease patients without recent myocardial infarction, other have challenged this[30] and a definitive conclusion is not yet warranted.

Electrophysiological techniques, including programmed electrical stimulation, are useful in evaluating and managing patients with sustained VT and other malignant ventricular arrhythmias.[31] Moreover, it has been shown that in patients with unsustained VT and decreased left ventricular function, sustained monomorphic VT can be induced by programmed electrical stimulation.[32] Thus, it has been suggested that electrophysiological testing may be useful in identifying patients with prognostically significant arrhythmia who are at the highest risk for developing malignant ventricular arrhythmia.

The role of electrophysiological testing in risk stratification has been controversial for many reasons. Differences in patient selection and protocol variability are the major contributing factors in the controversy. Several studies have enrolled patients with recent myocardial infarction and results have been disparate. In two studies, patients with inducible ventricular arrhythmia had a 30% to 32% mortality rate, whereas mortality rates in patients without inducible arrhythmia ranged from 2% to 4%.[33,34] In other studies, however, no significant difference in survival or the occurrence of malignant arrhythmia was found between patients with and without inducible ventricular arrhythmias.[35,36] In one of these latter studies,[36] patients without significant ventricular ectopy were studied and this result may not be applicable to risk stratification of patients with prognostically significant ventricular arrhythmia. Conclusions in patients with recent myocardial infarction remain uncertain at present.

Data are less controversial in patients with coronary artery disease and remote myocardial infarction. The use of electrophysiological testing in patients with unsustained VT and left ventricular dysfunction (ejection fraction of less than 0.40) has been useful in identifying high- and low-risk subsets within the group of patients with prognostically significant arrhythmia.[37,38] Klein and Machell[38] reported that monomorphic VT was inducible in 22 of 40 patients with coronary artery disease and unsustained VT. Nine of these patients subsequently developed a clinical episode of sustained ventricular tachyarrhythmia. In 18 patients in whom no VT was inducible, no spontaneous clinical episodes of arrhythmia occurred. Electrophysiological testing thus may be useful in further substratifying patients with prognostically significant arrhythmias.

The symptoms experienced by patients with prognostically significant arrhythmias are similar to those encountered in patients with benign ventricular arrhythmias. Since the arrhythmias in the two groups are the same, namely VPCs, ventricular couplets, and unsustained VT, there is no significant difference in symptoms produced by them. No increase in risk of death or sustained arrhythmia has been found in patients with symptomatic prognostically significant arrhythmias compared to those patients in whom these arrhythmias produced no symptoms.

Malignant Ventricular Arrhythmias

Unlike patients with benign or prognostically significant arrhythmias in which the arrhythmias are VPCs and unsustained VT, which may or may not be symptomatic, patients with malignant ventricular arrhythmias have symptomatic, hemodynamically significant, sustained VT, or ventricular fibrillation. The vast majority of these patients have significant organic heart disease and left ventricular dysfunction is common. In patients with malignant ventricular arrhythmia, the first episode of sustained arrhythmia is associated with a greater than 50% mortality. In patients who survive their initial episode, there is a 40% to 80% mortality within 1 year if appropriate therapy is not provided.[39,40]

An appreciation of the prognostic significance of ventricular arrhythmias has led to a classification system of ventricular arrhythmias which is based on their prognosis. The prognosis is related primarily to the types of arrhythmia and the clinical setting in which they occur. Arrhythmias are classified across the spectrum from benign to malignant (Table 1). This classification serves as a useful framework within which

Table 1
Classification Scheme of Ventricular Arrhythmias

	Benign	Prognostically Significant	Malignant
Risk of Sudden Death	minimal	moderate (variable)	high
Type of Arrhythmia	VPC VC UNVT	VPC VC UNVT	SUSVT VFIB (VPC, VC, UNVT, common)
Organic Heart Disease	none or minimal	yes (variable severity)	yes (usually severe)
Symptoms	none to moderately severe	none to moderately severe	typically severe
Rationale for Therapy			
Symptom Relief	yes	yes	yes
Prevention of Sudden Death	no	not substantiated	yes

SUSVT = sustained ventricular tachycardia.
UNVT = unsustained ventricular tachycardia.
VC = ventricular couplets.
VPC = ventricular premature complexes.

to consider the indications for treatment and the methods for assessing therapy.

Goals of Therapy of Ventricular Arrhythmias

The goals of therapy in the treatment of ventricular arrhythmias are well defined. They include prevention of sudden cardiac death and elimination of symptoms. Infrequently, arrhythmias that do not pose a risk of sudden death do have hemodynamic significance and their suppression is necessary (Table 2).

If the patient is not at increased risk of death, it therefore follows

---

Table 2
Goals of Therapy in Managing Ventricular Arrhythmias

---

1. Elimination or amelioration of symptoms
2. Prevention of sudden death and life-threatening sustained ventricular tachyarrhythmias
3. Suppression of hemodynamically significant but not life-threatening arrhythmias (e.g., ventricular bigeminy producing a low effective heart rate)

---

that the usual indication for antiarrhythmic therapy is elimination of symptoms. Therefore, if the patient is asymptomatic and the arrhythmia does not place the patient at increased risk, there is no indication for antiarrhythmic therapy.

Who to Treat?

The decision to treat ventricular arrhythmia must include a consideration of the risk-to-benefit ratio. Such a decision depends upon the clinician's informed judgment about the patient's anticipated clinical course and a comprehensive knowledge of the efficacy and adverse effects of antiarrhythmic drugs. The clinician should consider the cost of the therapy (including not only the cost of the drug, but also the attendant tests required to manage its administration) as well as the potential adverse effects of the agent.

The adverse effects of antiarrhythmic drugs include nonspecific whole body as well as organ-specific adverse effects, interactions with other drugs, and depression of left ventricular function. Probably the most important adverse effect to be considered, however, is proarrhythmia, which may be life-threatening. The patient, the arrhythmia, and the anticipated antiarrhythmic drug must be considered in assessing the potential risk of proarrhythmia.

In patients with benign ventricular arrhythmias, the risk of sudden death is essentially absent. These patients, typically with VPCs and even unsustained VT, generally have normal ventricular function and insignificant organic heart disease. In such patients, the only rationale for treatment is elimination or amelioration of symptoms. It should be emphasized that since such patients are not at risk of sudden death, it is not logical to treat them to prevent this syndrome.

Patients with prognostically significant arrhythmias form the largest group of patients with ventricular arrhythmias. The decision to treat ventricular arrhythmias in this group is complicated. Not only does the risk of sudden death vary considerably within this group, it is not yet clear that suppression of ambient ventricular arrhythmia results in a reduction in the risk of sudden death. While some studies have shown a reduction in mortality in patients with prognostically significant arrhythmias,[41,42] others have shown no benefit.[43] The preliminary results of the CAST provide further data which question the advisability of treating asymptomatic prognostically significant ventricular arrhythmia. In the Cardiac Arrhythmia Suppressive Trial (CAST), suppression of prognostically significantly arrhythmias was associated with a two- to threefold increase in mortality, presumably due to proarrhythmic events. There was, however, no evidence of reduction in mortality due to suppression of the arrhythmia.

A consensus regarding therapy in patients with prognostically significant arrhythmias does not exist. Although prevention of sudden death by antiarrhythmic therapy has been shown in several small non-randomized studies, no statistically rigorous study in a large number of patients has shown conclusively that antiarrhythmic therapy has been beneficial in reducing mortality in such patients. While many physicians choose to treat patients with prognostically significant arrhythmias, it must be emphasized that one cannot be certain that suppression of ventricular premature complexes or unsustained ventricular tachycardia (VT) will translate into prevention of sudden death.

I favor further risk stratification in such patients to identify a higher risk subset of patients with prognostically significant arrhythmias in whom the risks of antiarrhythmic therapy are justified. In the asymptomatic patient with frequent and complex ventricular premature contractions (VPCs) or unsustained VT, a thorough clinical evaluation should be undertaken. A 24-hour ambulatory electrocardiographic monitor should be obtained to fully characterize the type and frequency of arrhythmia. Left ventricular function should be assessed, preferably by radionuclide angiography. In patients with unsustained VT and significant left ventricular dysfunction (ejection fraction less than 0.40), a signal-averaged electrocardiogram should be obtained. If the signal-averaged electrocardiogram is abnormal, electrophysiological studies should be seriously considered, particularly in patients with coronary artery disease and previous myocardial infarction.

The risk of a malignant ventricular arrhythmia occurring spontaneously is significant in patients in whom sustained monomorphic VT is induced with one to three ventricular extrastimuli and therapy is warranted in these patients. The interpretation of induced ventricular fibrillation is somewhat more controversial. Initiation of ventricular fibrillation in patients without a history of malignant ventricular arrhythmia is uncommon with one or two ventricular extrastimuli. Although this may be a low sensitivity stimulation protocol, its specificity is high and therapy is warranted if polymorphic VT or ventricular fibrillation is initiated with one or two ventricular extrastimuli.

The treatment of patients with malignant ventricular arrhythmias is universally accepted as appropriate. The indications for treatment of patients with malignant arrhythmias includes both elimination of symptoms as well as prevention of sudden death.

How to Guide Therapy

The selection and monitoring of antiarrhythmic therapy have become quite complex. The number of available agents has increased over the past decade as have the technologies available for evaluating patients with ventricular arrhythmias. A thorough knowledge of both is required to optimally manage the patient. The techniques to be discussed are outlined in Table 3.

Table 3
Techniques Employed in Selecting and Guiding Antiarrhythmic
Therapy

Noninvasive, passive
    History
    Physical examination
    Electrocardiographic monitoring
    Plasma drug concentration monitoring
    Ambulatory electrocardiographic (Holter) monitoring
    Transtelephonic electrocardiographic monitoring
Noninvasive, provocative
    Exercise stress testing
Invasive, provocative
    Electrophysiological testing (programmed electrical stimulation)

Clinical Evaluation

Clinical evaluation of patients with ventricular arrhythmias is the initial step in selecting and monitoring therapy. Selection of the initial antiarrhythmic drug to be used should be made after a careful consideration of the patient's past medical history, concomitant medical disorders, history of allergies and drug sensitivities, and a clinical evaluation of cardiac function. Once antiarrhythmic therapy has been initiated, the patient should be carefully evaluated by history and physical examination to detect efficacy and toxicity of the regimen. While efficacy is not usually assessed by history and physical examination because the arrhythmias are typically paroxysmal, when the primary indication for therapy is elimination of symptoms, the history is ideal for establishing efficacy. Careful attention should be paid to the history and physical examination in eliciting evidence of toxicity of antiarrhythmic agents, including nonspecific effects, organ-specific toxicities, reduction in left ventricular function, and symptoms compatible with worsening of the arrhythmia.

Plasma Concentration Monitoring

Monitoring of plasma antiarrhythmic drug concentrations can be a useful method of guiding therapy. Plasma concentration monitoring can be used to document compliance to the antiarrhythmic regimen, to alter drug dosage to maintain a stable antiarrhythmic effect in the presence of a changing clinical condition, to detect and manage possible drug interactions, and to assess potential drug adverse effects.

To be useful, plasma concentration monitoring requires that a reliable relationship exist between a drug's pharmacological (and hopefully toxic) effect and the plasma concentration of the agent. Moreover, it assumes that the measurement of plasma concentration is performed with accurate and reproducible tests so that changes from one measurement to another are significant.

It has been suggested that the term "plasma concentration monitoring guidelines" be used to describe the plasma concentration range within which efficacy is most likely and toxicity least likely. This term should replace the term "therapeutic range," as this latter term implies that most if not all patients will be effectively treated if the plasma concentration of the drug is maintained within that range. This of course is not so and efficacy may be infrequent even when the agent is used within its plasma concentration guidelines. Moreover, it should be emphasized that a drug may be effective when its plasma concentration is below the guideline and may not be toxic when it is above the upper limit of the guideline. An individual patient's clinical situation must be fully considered in assessing the antiarrhythmic regimen.

Monitoring plasma concentration at interval evaluations confirms compliance with therapy. In addition, if significant alterations in plasma concentration occur, in addition to questioning compliance, the physician may assess absorption of the agent, hepatic and renal function which influence metabolism and elimination of the agent, and potential drug interactions. For those agents and adverse effects that are concentration-related, measurement of the plasma concentration may allow determination of whether a specific event is related to drug toxicity. In assessing the risk of increasing the dose of a specific antiarrhythmic agent, a plasma concentration in the lower range of the plasma concentration guideline might suggest that increasing the dose is of potential value in increasing efficacy with an acceptably low risk of producing toxicity. On the other hand, if the plasma concentration is in the upper range of the plasma concentration guideline, such an increase may not be justified.[44]

Plasma concentration monitoring guidelines have significant limitations. First and foremost is that maintaining a plasma concentration within the appropriate plasma concentration guideline does not guarantee antiarrhythmic efficacy. A specific drug may simply be ineffective in an individual patient. Many antiarrhythmic drugs have metabolites, some of which are active and contribute to antiarrhythmic efficacy and toxicity. Monitoring must take these into account. In addition, several antiarrhythmic drugs have stereoisomers and these may have different effects. Currently, monitoring does not take these differences into account. Monitoring plasma concentrations measures the total amount of drug in the plasma and does not differentiate free from protein-bound drug. Since the free, unbound drug is the portion that produces the pharmacological effect and significant changes in protein binding occur, significant pharmacological effects may occur without a change in the plasma concentration.

Plasma concentration monitoring guidelines and routine monitoring of plasma concentration are useful in monitoring therapy with procainamide, disopyramide, lidocaine, amiodarone, and phenytoin. Monitoring is of limited value in assessing therapy with quinidine, tocainide, mexiletine, bretylium, encainide, propafenone, and moricizine.[44] The utility of plasma concentration monitoring guideline for flecainide is uncertain. While concentrations in excess of 0.1 μg/mL are associated with toxicity, such levels are infrequently reached with present dosing guidelines, and efficacy and toxicity are not reliably differentiated at plasma concentrations less than 0.1 μg/mL.

Plasma concentration monitoring guidelines are useful in managing patients on antiarrhythmic therapy when these data are correlated with the clinical status of the patient and objective evidence of antiarrhythmic efficacy. Therapy should not be guided solely by plasma drug concentration.

Twelve-Lead Electrocardiogram

The resting 12-lead electrocardiogram contains approximately 15 to 45 seconds of cardiac rhythm monitoring and is thus useless in assessing suppression or aggravation of arrhythmia. It is, however, useful in monitoring the effects of antiarrhythmic drugs on the electrophysiological function of the heart. The electrocardiogram is relatively easily obtained and is standardized. It is available for immediate evaluation in contrast to plasma antiarrhythmic drug concentrations. The electrocardiogram can be used to monitor effects of antiarrhythmic drugs on pacemaker function (sinus as well as ectopic pacemakers), AV conduction system function, and conduction and repolarization in myocardial tissue. The effect on sinus rate and the rate of subsidiary pacemakers is easily evaluated with the electrocardiogram. Many antiarrhythmic drugs may effect the PR interval and such alterations may be due to either AV nodal or His-Purkinje depression or both. Marked changes in sinus rate and AV conduction intervals may presage significant sinus node depression or AV block.

Most of the commonly employed antiarrhythmic agents have the potential for slowing conduction within the myocardium. This is generally appreciated as a widening of the QRS complex. This is most marked with the IC antiarrhythmic agents but can be seen under certain circumstances with other drugs. Certain drugs, particularly the class IA and class III drugs, have significant effects on myocardial repolarization and affect the QT (or more specifically, JT interval) of the electrocardiogram.

Monitoring of the electrocardiogram adds little to the assessment of efficacy of antiarrhythmic regimens. Certainly, simply quantifying an arrhythmia during the brief time period of monitoring afforded by the electrocardiogram is of no utility. The relationship between effects on the electrocardiogram and efficacy of a variety of antiarrhythmic drugs is modest at best.[45]

The greatest utility of electrocardiographic monitoring is to detect impending drug toxicity. Marked increases in QRS duration may be associated with the development of incessant VT or high-grade AV block. Similarly, marked prolongation of the QT interval, especially during treatment with IA drugs, suggests a propensity to developing torsades de pointes.[45]

The electrocardiogram is an easily obtained measure of overall drug effect. Because of its simplicity and its ready availability, it provides a useful technique for monitoring antiarrhythmic drug effect.

Ambulatory Electrocardiographic (Holter) Monitoring

The advent of continuous ambulatory electrocardiographic monitoring pioneered by Norman J. Holter has had a major impact on the selection and monitoring of antiarrhythmic therapy. A variety of protocols have been proposed for the use of Holter monitoring in the assessment of antiarrhythmic therapy. In general, these protocols include a baseline recording made in the absence of antiarrhythmic therapy when the patient is clinically stable and factors that are known to influence the frequency of ambient ventricular arrhythmia have been eliminated or treated. Thus, myocardial ischemia, congestive heart failure, and electrolyte disturbances are corrected and eliminated to the extent that that is possible. Antiarrhythmic therapy is then instituted and monitoring is repeated. The American Heart Association has established technical criteria for appropriate Holter monitoring and these should be met by any system used in evaluating antiarrhythmic therapy.[46]

The standard length of recording Holter monitors has generally been considered 24 hours. This includes one full diurnal cycle, periods of sleep, and normal daily activity. While longer periods of recording do increase the yield of detected arrhythmias, it does not appear that this increase is worth the time and expense.

A major limitation in the use of Holter monitoring is the spontaneous variability of ambient ventricular arrhythmias that is now commonly appreciated.[47,48] The frequency of VPCs and unsustained VT varies substantially from hour to hour and between successive 24-hour recordings. This day-to-day variability may in fact mimic actual antiarrhythmic drug effect. Criteria have been proposed that take into account

Table 4
Criteria for Efficacy in Holter Monitoring

	VPC Suppression (% from baseline) to Identify Efficacy		
	VPC	VC	UNVT
Morganroth[1,2]	>84	>75	>65
Sami[3]	>65		
Graboys[4]	>50	>90	100
Pratt[5]	>78	>83	>77

Based on comparison of a 24-hour baseline and 24-hour on-drug Holter recording.
UNVT = unsustained ventricular tachycardia.
VC = ventricular couplet.
VPC = ventricular premature complexes.
[1] Moganroth et al: Circulation 58:408, 1978.
[2] Michelson et al: Circulation 61:690, 1980.
[3] Sami et al: Circulation 62:1172, 1980.
[4] Graboys et al: Am J Cardiol 50:437, 1982.
[5] Pratt et al: Am J Cardiol 56:67, 1985.

this variability so that true drug effect and efficacy can be determined (Table 4).

The variability of repetitive forms of ventricular ectopy, ventricular couplets, and unsustained VT show even more marked spontaneous variability than that of VPCs. Moreover, the variability of unsustained VT frequency increases as the frequency of unsustained VT increases.[48]

Holter monitoring can also be employed to detect proarrhythmic responses to antiarrhythmic therapy. The increase in frequency of VPCs and repetitive forms of ventricular ectopy while statistically significant has not been shown conclusively to increase the likelihood of a more serious form of proarrhythmia such as torsades de pointes or incessant VT. Statistically significant increases in the frequency of these unsustained events can be detected by Holter monitoring but the identification of the more virulent forms of proarrhythmia does not require Holter monitoring, as they are often symptomatic and routine electrocardiography or telemetric monitoring is sufficient.

Repeated or sequential Holter monitoring is frequently impractical and may be of modest utility in evaluating patients with symptomatic but infrequent arrhythmias. For such patients, transtelephonic electrocardiographic monitoring is ideal. A variety of devices are available that are connected to the patient by ECG leads or are applied at the time of symptoms. These devices typically record 30 to 120 seconds of electrocardiographic data during symptomatic episodes and can transmit the electrocardiographic data by telephone line to a receiving station that prints the electrocardiogram. These devices have been used both diagnostically and to evaluate symptoms during chronic drug therapy.

Exercise Stress Testing

Exercise stress testing is a noninvasive provocative technique that can be useful in assessing antiarrhythmic therapy. As already mentioned, exercise testing can provoke ventricular arrhythmias, typically VPCs and unsustained VT, in many patients with ventricular arrhythmia, and in patients with sustained ventricular tachyarrhythmias, these arrhythmias are frequently noted during exercise testing. In some patients, ventricular arrhythmias appear to be catecholamine-induced and exercise testing may be the only way in which to evaluate such arrhythmias.

Exercise testing may be particularly useful in evaluating reversal of antiarrhythmic effects by catecholamines and catecholamine- or exercise-induced proarrhythmia. Because the electrophysiological effects of catecholamines generally antagonize the effects of antiarrhythmic agents,[49] the provocation of ventricular arrhythmia during exercise testing therefore indicates a lack of efficacy of the tested regimen. Exercise testing may be a useful adjunctive technique when combined with Holter monitoring. In addition, patients who have undergone electrophysiological testing may also benefit from exercise testing to assess the effects of exercise on the antiarrhythmic regimen.

Exercise testing is also important in evaluating potential proarrhythmic effects of antiarrhythmic drugs. The effects of increases in heart rate and the rate-dependent slowing of conduction produced by some antiarrhythmic drugs may be obvious only during exercise.

The major limitation of exercise testing in the evaluation of arrhythmias is the spontaneous variability of arrhythmias induced by exercise testing. Reproducibility of arrhythmia between a baseline and a second exercise test is lowest in patients with VPCs and no cardiac disease, and is highest in patients with sustained ventricular tachyarrhythmias and heart disease. The arrhythmias typically induced by exercise, however, are not sustained and include VPCs and unsustained VT. Reproducibility is approximately 50% to 80%.[49] When used in combination with ambulatory monitoring, exercise testing appears to add significantly to the detection and evaluation of arrhythmias.

Since exercise testing is a provocative technique, its safety should be considered. In general, the safety of exercise has been assessed in patients with ischemic heart disease and the complications have been related to myocardial ischemia and/or infarction. With regard to monitoring antiarrhythmic therapy, however, complications related to provoking serious arrhythmias should be considered. The safety of exercise testing in patients with ventricular arrhythmia has been carefully evaluated.[50] Serious arrhythmic complications were noted in approximately 10% of patients and occurred in slightly more than 2% of studies. These included induced sustained VT or ventricular fibrillation. No deaths, myocardial infarction, or other significant morbidity were noted. Exercise testing appears to be a relatively safe procedure and when balanced with the risk of failing to identify serious proarrhythmia, the infrequent complications are acceptable.

Invasive Electrophysiological Studies

The use of noninvasive techniques, including Holter monitoring and exercise testing, have been most often applied to the evaluation and treatment of patients with benign and prognostically significant arrhythmias. Increasingly, invasive electrophysiological testing has been used to evaluate therapy for patients with malignant ventricular arrhythmias. Approximately 25% of patients with malignant ventricular arrhythmias do not have ambient ventricular ectopy and thus noninvasive, passive monitoring techniques are of no value in such patients. Moreover, the use of reduction in the frequency of VPCs and unsustained VT has not been shown to predict suppression of malignant ventricular arrhythmias in all studies.[43,51]

The use of electrophysiological testing is based on the reproducible initiation of VT or fibrillation by programmed electrical stimulation. It is hypothesized that this technique allows assessment of the arrhythmogenic milieu, which allows initiation and maintenance of the malignant ventricular arrhythmia. Drugs that suppress the initiation of ventricular arrhythmia by programmed electrical stimulation are thought to have altered the arrhythmogenic milieu such that the arrhythmia can no longer be initiated or sustained. Many studies have confirmed that the chronic use of drugs that prevent initiation of malignant arrhythmia by programmed stimulation is associated with infrequent recurrence of sustained arrhythmia and a substantial reduction in the sudden and all-cause mortality in these patients.[52-54]

In patients with previous clinical episodes of malignant ventricular arrhythmia unrelated to intercurrent or readily corrected conditions (e.g., electrolyte disturbance, uncontrolled congestive heart failure or myocardial ischemia, etc.), VT can be induced in over 90% of patients with organic heart disease. A variety of stimulation protocols have been proposed. Many investigators now recommend that the stimulation protocol should be selected according to the indications for the study.[55] In patients with clinically documented sustained VT or fibrillation, an aggressive stimulation protocol including multiple extrastimuli and several ventricular pacing sites should be employed. In patients without documented sustained ventricular tachyarrhythmias, such as patients with syncope of undetermined etiology or unsustained VT, fewer extrastimuli and possibly fewer stimulation sites should be used, as this latter study has higher specificity, although sensitivity may be sacrificed.

Electrophysiological testing has been found to be quite reproducible and VT can be reproducibly induced in 80% to 95% of patients.[55] Because the induction of sustained arrhythmia is reproducible, the criterion for effectiveness (ability to prevent initiation of sustained arrhythmia) has been accepted to be initiation of 5 to 15 complexes during drug therapy.[52-55]

The predicted accuracy of antiarrhythmic evaluation using programmed electrical stimulation is very good. As previously noted, freedom from recurrent sustained ventricular tachyarrhythmias and survival are significantly greater in patients in whom previously inducible arrhythmias were no longer inducible on antiarrhythmic therapy that is continued chronically.[51-55] On the contrary, patients treated with agents that failed to prevent initiation of the arrhythmia have a much poorer prognosis with a high mortality rate and incidence of recurrent arrhythmia. Electrophysiological testing may also be helpful in identifying serious forms of proarrhythmia.[56] While still controversial, it appears that the conversion of inducible unsustained VT to inducible sustained VT by antiarrhythmic therapy is a clinically significant form of proarrhythmia. The significance of other criteria, such as induction of arrhythmia with fewer extrastimuli or shortening of the tachycardia cycle length by drugs, remains unproved.

Isoproterenol may be used during electrophysiological testing to assess reversibility of a regimen's antiarrhythmic effect by catecholamine stimulation and potentially to evaluate the proarrhythmic effect of a drug in clinical situations characterized by high adrenergic tone. Preliminary studies have suggested that if the antiarrhythmic effect of a regimen is reversed by isoproterenol infusion during programmed electrical stimulation, the long-term prognosis is worsened and the likelihood of recurrent arrhythmia is increased.[57]

Like exercise testing, programmed electrical stimulation and electrophysiological testing are provocative techniques with the potential for significant morbidity and mortality. In general, the morbidity and mortality of electrophysiological testing is about half that reported for angiographic cardiac catheterization. Death has been reported rarely and generally occurs in patients with severe arrhythmia and heart disease.[58] Vascular complications are infrequent. Cardioversion is frequently required during electrophysiological-pharmacological evaluation of therapy in patients with malignant ventricular arrhythmia.[58] Electrophysiological testing is generally safe, however, and the risks should be compared to the potential benefits of increased survival in patients with malignant ventricular arrhythmias.

Which Techniques Should be Used for Which Patients

In patients with benign ventricular arrhythmias, the goal of therapy is elimination of symptoms. Therefore, antiarrhythmic therapy should be selected so as to achieve this goal with minimum risk of toxicity. Antiarrhythmic therapy should be monitored by noninvasive techniques. The history is sufficient to document elimination of symptoms. Typical examination combined with electrocardiographic monitoring are simple and important techniques for identifying potential toxicity. Holter monitoring and exercise testing are important in detecting proarrhythmic effects and are not particularly important in this group in assessing efficacy, as the actual reduction in arrhythmia is less important than elimination of symptoms. Plasma drug concentration monitoring may be useful in certain situations.

In patients with prognostically significant arrhythmias, antiarrhythmic therapy should be monitored by noninvasive techniques in all patients. History, physical examination, electrocardiographic monitoring, Holter monitoring, and exercise testing all are useful in evaluating efficacy and toxicity. Plasma drug concentration monitoring is again useful with selected drugs and in certain clinical situations. The use of invasive techniques in this group of patients continues to be controversial. Particularly in patients with extensive heart disease, left ventricular dysfunction and unsustained VT, electrophysiological testing appears to be beneficial in stratifying patients according to risk of malignant ventricular arrhythmia and evaluating pharmacological therapy in those patients at risk of developing malignant ventricular arrhythmias.[38]

In patients with malignant ventricular arrhythmias, electrophysiological evaluation is the principal method of evaluating antiarrhythmic efficacy. Noninvasive techniques are also important in identifying toxicity and proarrhythmia. Holter monitoring and exercise testing are also often useful adjunctive techniques for evaluating partially effective regimens. Noninvasive techniques assume greater importance in those patients with malignant ventricular arrhythmias in whom sustained arrhythmias cannot be induced by programmed stimulation.

References

1. Hinkle LE, Carver ST, Stevens M: The frequency of asymptomatic disturbances of cardiac rhythm and conduction in middle-aged men. Am J Cardiol 24:629, 1969.
2. Kostis JB, McCrone K, Moreyra AE, et al: Premature ventricular complexes in the absence of identifiable heart disease. Circulation 63:1351, 1981.
3. Hinkle LE, Carver ST, Argyros DC: The prognostic significance of ventricular premature contractions in healthy people and in people with coronary heart disease. Acta Cardiol 43:5, 1974.
4. Rudstein M, Wolloch L, Gubner RS: Mortality study of the significance of extrasystole in an insured population. Circulation 44:617, 1971.
5. Kennedy HL, Whitlock JA, Sprauge MK, et al: Long-term follow-up of asymptomatic healthy subjects with frequent and complex ventricular ectopy. N Engl J Med 312:193, 1985.
6. McHenry PL, Fisch C, Jordan JW: Cardiac arrhythmia observed during maximal exercise testing in clinically normal men. Am J Cardiol 39:331, 1978.
7. Jelinek MV, Lown B: Exercise stress testing for exposure of cardiac arrhythmia. Prog Cardiovasc Dis 16:497, 1974.
8. Poblete PF, Kennedy HL, Cavalis DG: Detection of ventricular ectopy in patients with coronary heart disease and normal subjects by exercise testing and ambulatory monitoring. Chest 74:402, 1978.
9. Califf RM, McKinnis RA, McNeer F, et al: Prognostic value of ventricular arrhythmias associated with treadmill exercise testing in patients studied with cardiac catheterization for suspected ischemic heart disease. J Am Coll Cardiol 2:1060, 1983.
10. Chiang BN, Perlman LV, Ostrander LD Jr, et al: Relationship of premature systoles to coronary heart disease and sudden death in the Tucumseh epidemiology study. Ann Intern Med 70:1159, 1969.

11. Coronary Drug Project Research Group: Prognostic importance of premature beats following myocardial infarction. JAMA 233:1116, 1973.
12. Ruberman W, Weinblatt E, Goldberg JD, et al: Ventricular premature beats and mortality after myocardial infarction. N Engl J Med 297:750, 1977.
13. Moss AJ, Davis HT, DeCamilla J, et al: Ventricular ectopic beats and their relationship to sudden and nonsudden cardiac death after myocardial infarction. Circulation 60:998, 1978.
14. Bigger JT Jr, Fleiss JL, Kleiger R, et al: The relationship between ventricular arrhythmias, left ventricular dysfunction and mortality in the two years after myocardial infarction. Circulation 69:250, 1984.
15. Bigger JT Jr, Francis MW, Rolnitzky LN: Prevalence, characterization and significance of ventricular tachycardia ($\geq$3 complexes) detected with ambulatory electrocardiographic recording in the late hospital phase of acute myocardial infarction. Am J Cardiol 48:816, 1981.
16. Anderson KD, DeCamilla J, Moss AJ: Clinical significance of ventricular tachycardia (3 beats or longer) detected during ambulatory monitoring after myocardial infarction. Circulation 57:890, 1978.
17. Meinertz T, Hofmann T, Kasper W, et al: Significance of ventricular arrhythmias in idiopathic dilated cardiomyopathy. Am J Cardiol 53:902, 1984.
18. Unverferth DV, Magorien RD, Moeschberger ML, et al: Factors influencing the one-year mortality of dilated cardiomyopathy. Am J Cardiol 54:147, 1984.
19. Maron BJ, Savage DD, Wolfson JK, et al: Prognostic significance of 24 hour ambulatory electrocardiographic monitoring in patients with hypertrophic cardiomyopathy: A prospective study. Am J Cardiol 48:252, 1981.
20. Vetter VL, Horowitz LN: Electrophysiologic residua and sequelae of surgery for congenital heart defects. Am J Cardiol 50:588, 1982.
21. Califf RM, McKinnis RA, Burks J, et al: Prognostic implications of ventricular arrhythmias during 24-hour ambulatory monitoring in patients undergoing cardiac catheterization for coronary artery disease. Am J Cardiol 50:23, 1982.
22. Tofler GH, Stone PH, Muller JE, et al: Prognosis after cardiac arrest due to ventricular tachycardia or ventricular fibrillation associated with acute myocardial infarction (The MILIS Study). Am J Cardiol 60:755, 1987.
23. Greene HL, Reid PR, Schaeffer AH: The repetitive ventricular response in man: a predictor of sudden death. N Engl J Med 299:729, 1978.
24. Simson MB, Untereker WJ, Spielman SR, et al: Relation between late potentials on the body surface and directly recorded fragmented electrograms in patients with ventricular tachycardia. Am J Cardiol 51:105, 1983.
25. Gomes JA, Winters SL, Stewart D, et al: A new noninvasive index to predict sustained ventricular tachycardia and sudden death in the first year after myocardial infarction. J Am Coll Cardiol 10:343, 1987.
26. Kuchar DL, Thorburn CW, Sammel NL: Prediction of serious arrhythmic events after myocardial infarction: signal-averaged electrocardiogram, Holter monitoring and radionuclide ventriculography. J Am Coll Cardiol 9:531, 1987.
27. Winters SL, Stewart D, Targonski A, et al: Role of signal averaging of the surface QRS complex in selecting patients with nonsustained ventricular tachycardia and high-grade ventricular arrhythmias for programmed ventricular stimulation. J Am Coll Cardiol 12:1481, 1988.

28. Weld FM, Chu KL, Bigger JT, et al: Risk stratification with low level exercise testing two weeks after myocardial infarction. Circulation 64:306, 1981.
29. Henry RL, Kennedy GT, Crawford MH: Prognostic value of exercise-induced ventricular ectopic activity for mortality after acute myocardial infarction. Am J Cardiol 59:1251, 1987.
30. Sami M, Chaitman B, Fisher L, et al: Significance of exercise-induced ventricular arrhythmia in stable coronary artery disease: A Coronary Artery Surgery Study project. Am J Cardiol 54:1182, 1984.
31. Prystowsky EN: Antiarrhythmic therapy for asymptomatic ventricular arrhythmias. Am J Cardiol 61:102A, 1988.
32. Spielman SR, Greenspan AM, Kay HR, et al: Electrophysiologic testing in patients at high risk for sudden cardiac death: nonsustained ventricular tachycardia and abnormal ventricular function. J Am Coll Cardiol 6:31, 1985.
33. Hamer A, Vohra J, Hunt D, et al: Prediction of sudden death by electrophysiologic studies in high-risk patients surviving acute myocardial infarction. Am J Cardiol 50:223, 1982.
34. Denniss AR, Richards DA, Cody DV, et al: Prognostic significance of ventricular tachycardia and fibrillation induced at programmed stimulation and delayed potentials detected on the signal-averaged electrocardiogram of survivors of acute myocardial infarction. Circulation 74:731, 1986.
35. Roy D, Marchand E, Theroux P, et al: Programmed ventricular stimulation in survivors of an acute myocardial infarction. Circulation 72:487, 1985.
36. Marchlinski FE, Buxton AE, Waxman HL, et al: Identifying patients at high risk of sudden death after myocardial infarction: value of the response to programmed stimulation, degree of ventricular ectopic activity and severity of left ventricular dysfunction. Am J Cardiol 52:1190, 1983.
37. Gomes JAC, Hariman RI, Kang PA, et al: Programmed electrical stimulation in patients with high-grade ventricular ectopy: electrophysiologic findings and prognosis for survival. Circulation 70:43, 1984.
38. Klein RC, Machell C: Use of electrophysiologic testing in patients with nonsustained ventricular tachycardia: prognostic and therapeutic implications. J Am Coll Cardiol 14:155, 1989.
39. Cobb LA, Werner JA, Trobaugh GB: Sudden cardiac death. II. Outcome of resuscitation, management and future directions. Modern Concepts Cardiovasc Dis 49:37, 1980.
40. Graboys TB, Lown B, Podrid PJ, et al: Long-term survival of patients with ventricular arrhythmia treated with antiarrhythmic drugs. Am J Cardiol 50:437, 1982.
41. Hoffmann A, Schutz E, White R, et al: Suppression of high-grade ventricular ectopic activity by antiarrhythmic drug treatment as a marker for survival in patients with chronic coronary artery disease. Am Heart J 107:1103, 1984.
42. Blevins RD, Zerin NZ, Frumin H, et al: Arrhythmia control and other factors related to sudden death in coronary disease patients at intermediate risk. Am Heart J 111:638, 1986.
43. The Cardiac Arrhythmia Suppression Trial (CAST) Investigators: Preliminary report: effects of encainide and flecainide on mortality in a randomized trial of arrhythmia suppression after myocardial infarction. N Engl J Med 321:406, 1989.

44. Woosley RL: Role of plasma concentration monitoring in the evaluation of response to antiarrhythmic drugs. Am J Cardiol 62:9H, 1988.
45. Roden DM: Role of the electrocardiogram in determining electrophysiologic end-points of drug therapy. Am J Cardiol 34H–38H, 1988.
46. Sheffield LT, Berson A, Bragg-Remschel D, et al: Recommendations for standards of instrumentation and practice in the use of ambulatory electrocardiography. Circulation 72:824, 1985.
47. Morganroth J, Michelson EL, Horowitz LN, et al: Limitations of routine long-term electrophysiologic monitoring to assess ventricular ectopic frequency. Circulation 58:408, 1978.
48. Pratt CM, Slymen DJ, Wierman AM, et al: Analysis of the spontaneous variability of ventricular arrhythmias: consecutive ambulatory electrocardiographic recordings of ventricular tachycardia. Am J Cardiol 56:67, 1985.
49. Podrid PJ, Venditti FJ, Levine PA, et al: The role of exercise testing in evaluation of arrhythmias. Am J Cardiol 62:24H, 1988.
50. Young D, Lampert S, Graboys TB, et al: Safety of maximal exercise testing in patients at high risk for ventricular arrhythmia. Circulation 70:184, 1984.
51. Mitchell LB, Duff HJ, Manyari DE, et al: A randomized clinical trial of the noninvasive and invasive approaches to drug therapy of ventricular tachycardia. N Engl J Med 317:1681, 1987.
52. Swerdlow CD, Winkle RA, Mason JW: Determinants of survival in patients with ventricular tachyarrhythmias. N Engl J Med 308:1436, 1983.
53. Rae AP, Greenspan AM, Spielman SR, et al: Antiarrhythmic drug efficacy for ventricular tachyarrhythmias associated with coronary artery diseases assessed by electrophysiologic studies. Am J Cardiol 55:1494, 1985.
54. Waller TJ, Kay HR, Spielman SR, et al: Reduction in sudden death and total mortality by antiarrhythmic therapy evaluated by electrophysiologic drug testing: criteria of efficacy in patients with sustained ventricular tachyarrhythmia. J Am Coll Cardiol 10:83, 1987.
55. Kuchar DL, Garan H, Ruskin JN: Electrophysiologic evaluation of antiarrhythmic therapy for ventricular arrhythmias. Am J Cardiol 62:39H, 1988.
56. Rae AP, Kay HR, Horowitz LN, et al: Proarrhythmic effects of antiarrhythmic drugs in patients with malignant ventricular arrhythmias evaluated by electrophysiologic testing. J Am Coll Cardiol 12:131, 1989.
57. Jazayeri MR, Van Wyhe G, Avitall B, et al: Isoproterenol reversal of antiarrhythmic effects in patients with inducible sustained ventricular tachyarrhythmias. J Am Coll Cardiol 14:705, 1989.
58. Horowitz LN, Kay HR, Kutalek SP, et al: Risks and complications of clinical cardiac electrophysiologic studies: a prospective analysis of 1,000 consecutive patients. J Am Coll Cardiol 9:1261, 1987.

Chapter 5

Sudden Cardiac Death

Stephen C. Vlay

Definition, Mechanism

Sudden cardiac death (SCD) is defined as a nonviolent, nontraumatic death due to cardiac causes. Sudden cardiac death is unexpected, usually instantaneous, and uniformly fatal within an hour of the terminal symptoms. If the event is unwitnessed, it is necessary for the patient to have been seen alive during the prior 24 hours to classify it as a sudden cardiac death.

This event continues to assume a major role in the annual cardiovascular mortality in the United States with an estimated 250,000–500,000 sudden cardiac deaths. No age, gender, occupation, or socioeconomic group is spared. A major economic impact results from loss of income, ability to provide for the needs of the family, and the financial requirement to partially offset these losses. The personal impact on the surviving family is also devastating.

The mechanism of SCD involves a ventricular tachyarrhythmia (VT), ventricular tachycardia degenerating into ventricular fibrillation (VF), in over 80–90% of cases. Less common, bradycardia or complete heart block leading to asystole results in sudden cardiac death. The ability to perform cardiopulmonary resuscitation (CPR) has allowed many victims of sudden cardiac arrest to survive and undergo further evaluation and treatment, leading to a greater understanding of complex mechanisms and interactions involved.

CPR is becoming more widely learned, a skill beneficial to the entire community. It should be learned by medical and paramedical personnel,

From Naccarelli GV (ed): *Cardiac Arrhythmias: A Practical Approach.* Mount Kisco, NY, Futura Publishing Co., Inc., © 1991.

selected family members of patients with cardiac disease, and capable members of the general public. CPR has the best chance of success when started early and performed properly. Guidelines for basic and advanced life support were published by the National Conference on Cardiopulmonary Resuscitation and Emergency Cardiac Care (JAMA 255:2905–2992) and should be reviewed by all physicians and personnel involved in the care of critically ill patients.

Epidemiology

A review of the etiology of the cardiac and vascular causes of sudden death indicates that the majority of adult patients have underlying coronary artery disease with or without myocardial infarction. Cardiomyopathy and cardiomyopathic states resulting from valvular heart disease comprise the next most frequent categories. Rarely patients will have primary electrical instability with little or no detectable heart disease.

The Framingham Study indicated that half the deaths in men and 64% in women occur in the absence of overt or known coronary heart disease.[2] This underscores the importance of silent heart disease and silent ischemia, as well as its early detection. The individual most likely to be a victim of sudden cardiac death is a male over the age of 45 years. When affected, women are more likely to be older (≥65 years). Infrequently, sudden cardiac death occurs in younger individuals. Studies also indicate an increased frequency of sudden death in the morning hours (6 AM–noon), a time factor still incompletely understood but possibly related to activation of neurohormonal systems, platelet aggregability,[5] other circadian rhythms, and the variability of ventricular arrhythmias.

In patients with known coronary artery disease (CAD) with acute myocardial infarction, 18% of men and 24% of women suffer sudden cardiac death (Framingham data).[2] Left ventricular dysfunction is a major risk factor for SCD in patients with overt CAD. In those without overt CAD, the cardiac risk factors become important.

In the pediatric population, the incidence of sudden death ranges from 1.3 to 8.5/100,000 in several reported series, although not all are necessarily cardiac.[6,7] Possible risk factors include coronary artery anomalies, congenital heart disease, dysfunction of the sinus and atrioventricular nodes, prolonged QT syndromes, accessory pathway conduction in patients with Wolff-Parkinson-White (WPW) syndrome, exercise-associated and nonvasodepressor syncope, familial history of sudden cardiac death or hypertrophic cardiomyopathy, and patients with ventricular arrhythmias after repair of tetralogy of Fallot.

The Equation for Sudden Cardiac Death

SUDDEN CARDIAC DEATH = ANATOMIC SUBSTRATE + TRIGGER FACTOR

Sudden cardiac death is a function of an anatomical substrate, either structural or electrical, and a trigger factor that precipitates the final malignant arrhythmia. Therapy should be directed at both as it may not be possible to completely neutralize either variable alone.

Trigger Factors

While some trigger factors may be obvious, others may be subtle or unrecognized. Perhaps these latter factors may explain sudden cardiac death in patients whose anatomical/electrical substrate remains unchanged. Thus it becomes important to carefully review all of the various possibilities.

Mechanical

Patients with indwelling pulmonary artery catheters or temporary pacemakers may have mechanical irritation of the right ventricular outflow tract leading to ventricular tachycardia. Needless to say, this is not the usual case.

Electrolyte Disturbance

Quite commonly, abnormalities of potassium, magnesium, and calcium, whether low or high, may lead to ventricular tachycardia/fibrillation. In particular, patients receiving diuretics lose significant amounts of potassium and magnesium which may be difficult to replace in an acute setting.

Metabolic Abnormalities

These include acidosis/alkalosis (which may further exacerbate the electrolyte disorder) and hypoxia.

Systemic Disorders

Systemic disorders such as anemia (causing hypoxia), fever, infection, sepsis, dehydration, hypovolemia, hypotension, hypertension, and hyperthyroidism may all exacerbate metabolic abnormalities and electrolyte disturbances.

Drug Toxicity

Many drugs have been implicated in SCD.

Digitalis

Particularly in the presence of hypokalemia, digitalis toxicity may result in ventricular tachycardia. In the majority of cases, digitalis toxicity may be managed by holding the digoxin and treating with lidocaine as necessary. Cases of massive overdose may be treated with Fab fragment antibodies.

Type 1 Antiarrhythmic Drugs

Quinidine and disopyramide have been most often implicated in the exacerbation of ventricular tachyarrhythmias, but it is important to remember that *all* of these drugs have the potential to cause sudden cardiac death. Drugs that prolong the QT interval (type 1A) may result in torsades de pointes (twisting of the points), a type of VT particularly difficult to treat. Some of the type 1C drugs (e.g., flecainide) may further depress left ventricular function by virtue of their negative inotropic effect and further exacerbate VT/VF.

Tricyclic Antidepressants and Phenothiazines

Tricyclic antidepressants and phenothiazines may also be implicated in the exacerbation of ventricular arrhythmias. It is important to note that imipramine is also considered a type 1A antiarrhythmic agent.

Myocardial Ischemia

Unquestionably, myocardial ischemia is responsible for at least some episodes of VT/VF resulting in sudden cardiac death. Myocardial ischemia may result in diastolic dysfunction and ventricular irritability, as well as further exacerbating local metabolic and biochemical abnormalities. It must again be emphasized that myocardial ischemia may be "silent"[8] as well as cause typical or atypical chest pain. The role of platelet aggregation in the genesis of myocardial ischemia may also be important as may be the local effects of prostaglandins, serotonin, and bradykinin.

Neural Stimulation

The role of autonomic nervous system and central neural stimulation may be critical in certain cases of sudden cardiac death.[9] Excess sympathetic tone seems detrimental and enhanced vagal tone partially protective. Stimulation of the left stellate ganglion, the recipient of most of the afferent sympathetic reflex nerve fibers, results in prolongation of the QT interval and reduction in the VT threshold. Ablation of this ganglion increases the threshold for VT.[10,11] Direct or indirect vagal stimulation results in an antifibrillatory effect.[12] An indirect effect of vagal tone on ventricular vulnerability is achieved by opposing increased adrenergic tone.

Laboratory work has suggested that stimulation of the hypothalamus may result in ventricular ectopy or ventricular tachycardia.[13] Efferent sympathetic pathways arising from the hypothalamus, midbrain, and adjacent structures eventually arrive at the heart via the stellate ganglia and cardiac sympathetic nerves.

Thus the brain-nervous system-heart interaction is complex and incompletely understood. Unquestionably, nervous system influence may act as a trigger factor and may be more important in the presence of an anatomical substrate for cardiac arrhythmias.

Emotional Stress and Psychosocial Factors

Emotional stress and psychosocial factors are often overlooked but may potentially trigger physiological events via activation of the sympathetic nervous system. Numerous studies have documented a variety of psychosocial stresses, anger, anxiety, and depression prior to an episode of sudden cardiac death.[9] While there may not be a specific relationship between a psychological/psychiatric disorder and a cardiac disease, there seems little doubt that an emotional flare-up may stimulate the autonomic nervous system and thus act as a trigger factor for a subsequent cardiac event such as VT/VF. Relationships between anxiety levels and recurrent arrhythmias have been recently investigated in patients with the automatic internal cardioverter defibrillator (AICD).[14] At baseline, these high-risk patients have elevated traits (baseline tendencies) and states of anxiety. After AICD implant, the state of anxiety (i.e., the current level) decreases although the trait is unchanged.

These variables respresent some of the known triggers of malignant ventricular tachyarrhythmias. There may be many more, particularly operational at the cellular level. One must endeavor to minimize the known risk factors, a task difficult in itself.

Anatomical Substrates

In the majority of patients who suffer sudden cardiac death, left ventricular dysfunction of varying degree is present. It is well recognized that an elevated left ventricular end-diastolic pressure and a low ejection fraction are variables predictive of a poor outcome. Ventricular ectopy is frequently present in these conditions and may be a marker for the anatomical substrate or serve as the final mechanism if it becomes sustained and hemodynamically embarrassing. Nevertheless, the presence of nonsustained ventricular tachycardia may have different meaning in varying underlying substrates.

Coronary Artery Disease

CAD still represents the most common underlying substrate, with or without myocardial infarction. A variety of studies and multivariate analyses have identified variables predictive of survival in addition to left ventricular end-diastolic pressure and ejection fraction. These include: prior myocardial infarction, number of diseased vessels, proximal left anterior descending artery disease, high risk as characterized by New York Heart Association functional class, left ventricular aneurysm, extensive regional wall motion abnormalities, easy inducibility and failure to achieve arrhythmia suppression at electrophysiology study, frequent and complex ventricular ectopic activity, prolonged HV interval, and male gender.[15-20]

It has been pointed out that procrastination before seeking medical attention maybe a contributory factor to sudden cardiac death.[21] With acute myocardial infarction, 15–45% of the deaths occur within the first hour with a lower incidence of ventricular fibrillation thereafter. In addition, out-of-hospital deaths are more likely to be arrhythmic (88%) and in-hospital deaths are more likely due to failure to maintain the circulation (71%).[22]

Pathologically, a wide spectrum of findings has been described in victims of sudden cardiac death including the presence or absence of coronary thrombus, minimal to extensive coronary artery disease, and ventricular scarring.[23-25] Increased heart weight and myocardial hypertrophy are additional factors that may place the patient at risk. Thus there is no single set of anatomical findings in patients with coronary artery disease characteristic of sudden cardiac death. Certainly the more severe the findings, the greater the risk of cardiac death, but *sudden* cardiac death may be partially dictated by the presence of known or unknown trigger factors.

Cardiomyopathy

Abnormalities of heart muscle and its contractility constitute a major substrate for congestive heart failure and/or sudden cardiac death. Ischemic cardiomyopathy related to coronary artery disease is common and was considered above. Among the nonischemic cardiomyopathies included are dilated congestive, hypertrophic, those related to valvular heart disease with pressure-volume overload, and a variety related to infiltrative, infectious, or occult causes.

Ventricular ectopy may be common in these disorders of heart muscle but may have different significance depending on the variety. Contractility may be extremely poor (congestive), enhanced (hypertrophic), or relatively unaffected. Thus there is no common finding regarding contractility as all of those conditions may be associated with sudden cardiac death. In the discussion of each of these entities, potential mechanisms will be mentioned as will potential therapies. Unfortunately, most medical therapies for patients with recurrent VT in these conditions have been disappointing.

Dilated Congestive Cardiomyopathy

In this disorder of cardiac muscle, global and regional contractility become progressively more impaired, leading to congestive heart failure. The etiology is generally unknown although some cases are preceded by myocarditis. Throughout its course, dilated congestive cardiomyopathy is associated with ventricular ectopy and nonsustained ventricular tachycardia (VT).[26] In those patients with asymptomatic nonsustained VT, there is no evidence to suggest improved survival with antiarrhythmic drug therapy, which may not even be able to eradicate Lown grade 4B ectopy. Patients with symptomatic sustained VT may benefit from electrophysiology study with suppression of inducible VT, indicating a beneficial response from antiarrhythmic drugs. Noninducible patients may be more difficult to manage. The ultimate outcome often is related to the deterioration of left ventricular function.

Hypertrophic Cardiomyopathy

This familial disorder (autosomal dominant with varying degrees of penetrance) is quite often the cause of sudden cardiac death in young athletes who have not been adequately evaluated before participating in strenuous physically demanding sports. Hypertrophic cardiomyopathy is characterized by impaired diastolic filling and hypercontractile systolic function. In some patients, there is actual obstruction to aortic outflow. The presence of nonsustained asymptomatic VT in these patients is associated with an increased risk of sudden cardiac death.[27,28]

Death in this disorder may be caused by hemodynamic compromise (hypotension, obstruction to outflow, pulmonary edema), myocardial infarction, asystole, or ventricular tachycardia/fibrillation). Rarely, some patients with hypertrophic cardiomyopathy may have, in addition, Wolff-Parkinson-White syndrome with associated tachyarrhythmias requiring treatment. Risk factors for sudden cardiac death include death in other family members from this disorder, syncope, severe dyspnea, young age, high ejection fraction, large end-systolic volume, and low ventricular peak filling rate.

Cardiomyopathy Related to Valvular Heart Disease

Valvular heart disease may result in abnormal left ventricular function due to chronic pressure-volume overload. Perhaps the most likely factors to affect the left ventricle include mitral regurgitation and aortic stenosis or aortic regurgitation. In aortic stenosis, sudden cardiac death may be hemodynamic, resulting from obstruction to aortic outflow, congestive heart failure, or pulmonary edema. Due to calcification of the valvular structures and conduction system, heart block may occur and cause a fatal outcome from a bradyarrhythmia or reduction in cardiac output. Symptomatic ventricular arrhythmias may occur in any of these three valvular disorders. Atrial arrhythmias are most likely to occur in mitral regurgitation or when the aortic disorders cause left ventricular failure with increased left atrial pressures.

Patients with prosthetic valves may suffer left ventricular dysfunction during cardiac surgery leading to cardiomyopathy or possibly experience a late complication such as prosthetic valvular dysfunction, endocarditis, or thrombosis. Thus, in cardiomyopathies related to valvular disease, cardiac death may be electrical or mechanical, cardiac or noncardiac, and sudden or nonsudden.

Other Cardiomyopathies

In North America, the aforementioned cardiomopathies are most common. In South America, *Chagas disease* may result in extensive scarring of the myocardium. Chagas disease is a result of infection with a parasite, *Trypanosoma cruzi,* and clinically may be manifest by atrial arrhythmias, malignant ventricular tachyarrhythmias, and sudden cardiac death.

Sarcoidosis may affect the heart by infiltration of the myocardium with sarcoid granulomata. While overall contractility may not be impaired, these islands may become irritable foci, resulting in ventricular tachyarrhythmias that may be extremely difficult to control with antiarrhythmic drugs. For these patients, electronic devices such as the automatic internal cardioverter defibrillator may be more advantageous than futile surgical attempts at local excision of granuloma. *Amyloid* is another infiltrative cardiomyopathy resulting in congestive heart failure and arrhythmias.

Unusual varieties of cardiomyopathies may involve the right ventricle. A paper thin dilated right ventricle with hemodynamic and electrical abnormalities is known as *Uhl's anomaly.* Another difficult to control ventricular arrhythmia is known as *arrhythmogenic right ventricular dysplasia.*

Focal cardiomyopathies may exist, explaining sudden cardiac arrest in individuals with otherwise apparently normal coronary arteries and left ventricular function. Myocardial biopsy in some of these individuals has demonstrated lymphocytic infiltration, indicating an inflammatory process such as myocarditis.[29] In fact, this process may provide an explanation for the rare cases of SCD in patients with mitral valve prolapse. Although patients with mitral valve prolapse may have atypical chest pain, atrial arrhythmias, and/or ventricular arrhythmias, the cause and effect relationship between these rare cases of mitral valve prolapse and fatal ventricular fibrillation has not been conclusively demonstrated to everyone's satisfaction. The incidence of mitral valve prolapse is so high that one might expect more cases of sudden cardiac death if it was truly responsible. Still one cannot completely exclude the possibility that the papillary muscle tugging on the ventricular myocardium could cause ventricular tachycardia in isolated cases. Nevertheless, it is the bias of this author that at least some of the rare cases of SCD associated with mitral valve prolapse are coincidental.

Congenital and Other Rare Cardiac Abnormalities

Among the congenital cardiac anomalies associated with SCD, one includes abnormalities of the coronary arteries. Rarely they will arise from the pulmonary trunk rather than the aorta, arise from an abnormal location in the aorta with compression, or possibly have a single coronary artery that supplies the entire myocardium. In these situations, hypoxia and myocardial ischemia are the most likely precipitating causes of SCD. Congenital malformation of the cardiac chambers (e.g., transposition of the great vessels, tetralogy of Fallot, septal defects) may similarly result in sudden cardiac death in certain patients. Patients with ventricular arrhythmias after repair of tetralogy of Fallot represent another high-risk group.

Mechanical Abnormalities Causing Sudden Cardiac Death

Although not directly related to disease of the myocardium, certain mechanical catastrophes may cause SCD. Pericardial tamponade with rapid accumulation of fluid in the pericardial sac compressing contractility will result in death if not promptly relieved by pericardiocentesis. Abnormalities such as atrial myxoma interrupt the flow of blood intermittently. Rarely sudden death occurs. Rare causes of myocardial infarction such as dissection or embolism are mechanical events leading to secondary myocardial events.

Nutritional Abnormalities Associated with Sudden Cardiac Death

Liquid protein diets have been implicated in SCD.[30] The precipitating event may have been related to abnormalities of electrolytes. Severe fasting and deificiency of trace elements may also have been contributory although the prolongation of the QT interval may be the primary abnormality. Some patients with anorexia nervosa have suffered SCD.[31]

Electrical Substrates

Prolonged QT Syndrome

This syndrome may be acquired or congenital and is often overlooked. Acquired syndromes are often caused by physicians prescribing type 1A antiarrhythmic drugs (quinidine, disopyramide, procainamide), tricyclic antidepressants (imipramine is also a type 1A drug), or phenothiazines. Consequently, it is important that the physician pay attention to the QT interval before and after prescribing the drug.

Congenital syndromes have been described. The Romano-Ward syndrome is autosomal dominant. The Jervell-Lange-Nielsen syndrome is autosomal recessive and is associated with deafness. Thus, a family history of sudden death is important and must be elucidated in the history.

The QT interval may be transiently prolonged during myocardial infarction. Hypocalcemia or hypokalemia are metabolic disturbances that prolong the QT interval. Autonomic dysfunction as a result of disease of the central or peripheral nervous system may also prolong the QT interval.

Pre-Excitation Syndromes

Ventricular pre-excitation, particularly in WPW syndrome, may result in a very rapid ventricular response, often faster than 300 bpm and may degenerate into ventricular fibrillatrion. WPW syndrome is characterized by atrioventricular bypass tracts (bundle of Kent), which may be single or multiple. It is important to remember that not all individuals with WPW syndrome are at high risk for SCD. The highest risk is associated with a short effective refractory period of the bypass tract and a very short R-R interval during a rapid tachyarrhythmia. Therapy for symptomatic patients with WPW syndrome includes antiarrhythmic drugs, but surgical approaches may be more advantageous in providing a permanent disruption of the tract. Other pre-excitation syndromes include Mahaim fibers (fascicular-ventricular pathways) and James fibers (atrio-Hisian pathways). The latter may be manifest as atrial arrhythmias as part of the Lown-Ganong-Levine syndrome.

Degeneration of the Conduction System

Inflammation, infiltration, fibrosis, and degeneration of any or all parts of the conduction system may result in bundle branch block, heart block, bradyarrhythmias, and asystole. As mentioned earlier, tachyarrhythmias are the mechanisms of the majority of SCD with bradyarrhythmias playing only a minor role. Degeneration of the conduction system is a common indication for permanent pacing and is sometimes known as Lenegre's disease. Calcification of the cardiac conduction system, or Lev's disease, is more common in older individuals. All of these processes may occur in the absence of significant coronary artery disease or left ventricular dysfunction. Specific involvement of the cardiac nerves manifest as ganglionitis, viral or hereditary neuropathy, or neurotoxic injury are other rare possibilities.

One must be aware that patients may have more than one problem. Implanting a permanent pacemaker may keep conduction intact but will not protect against ventricular tachyarrhythmias if that problem is also present but unsuspected.

Patients without Apparent Anatomical or Electrical Substrates

In every series of patients with ventricular tachycardia, ventricular fibrillation, and sudden cardiac death, 1–3% of the patients will exhibit no identifiable anatomical or electrical substrate and a distinct absence of known trigger factors. Possible explanations include a lack of sophistication in our methods of detection, an early stage of disease with few manifestations, or a mechanism not yet identified. Some investigators are extremely suspicious about the role of neural influences in such cases. The other major concern is that of an unexpected focal myocarditis that may or may not be identifiable by biopsy. Note that myocardial biopsy is not considered a routine part of the evaluation. Recently a syndrome of SCD occurring in young Southeast Asians during the early morning hours has been described.[32] Again, autopsies have been unrevealing. Sudden infant death syndrome is another intriguing disease. As this time it is unclear whether the involvement of the heart has a primary role.

The group of patients without apparent or electrical substrates presents the greatest therapeutic challenge to the physician. There is no ischemia or heart failure to treat. Trigger factors are unclear. Electrophysiological testing is quite often nondiagnostic due to lack of inducibility despite continued risk for sudden cardiac death. In these individuals thought to be at continued risk, electronic devices such as the automatic internal cardioverter defibrillator may offer the greatest benefit.

Sudden Cardiac Death: The Approach in the 1990s

SCD has been an ongoing challenge confronting cardiology.[33] Have we met the challenge? Partially. There are still goals left to achieve.

The Survivor of Sudden Cardiac Arrest

This individual deserves a comprehensive evaluation. The next episode may not have an outcome as fortunate. It is imperative to learn as much as possible about these individuals to base therapy on the anatomical substrate and possible trigger factors. There is no substitute for cardiac catheterization and electrophysiological testing. Even those arrhythmia specialists who believe in a noninvasive approach are willing to concede this point for survivors of sudden cardiac arrest. Antiarrhythmic therapy is guided by the result of electrophysiological studies (EPS) and may include drugs, devices, or surgery.

Patients Identified at EPS as Being at High Risk for SCD

If these individuals have not had a clinical episode of sudden cardiac arrest, some physicians may find it more difficult to justify aggressive invasive therapeutic procedures. Nevertheless, this may represent a form of risk stratification. If we are to make an impact on the devastating mortality rate associated with sudden cardiac death, it is imperative to identify those individuals at risk before the first episode, which may be the last. It may be possible to define this population with the help of multivariate equations taking into account a variety of electrophysiological, anatomical, and clinical variables. Patients identified at high risk may be subjects for future trials comparing routine follow-up with protection by antiarrhythmic drugs or electronic devices. Future directions will be determined by the results of these trials if they ever are performed.

Surgical Techniques for Ventricular Tachyarrhythmias

Surgical techniques for ventricular tachyarrhythmias range from aneurysmectomy to blind resection to EPS-guided resection. Localization of the arrhythmia or tachycardia zone resulted in better results with fewer recurrent ventricular tachyarrhythmias. Initially performed with subendocardial resection by scalpel or surgical scissors, ablation can now be performed with a cryoprobe or laser. These latter techniques have enabled the resection of areas previously inaccessible including parts of the papillary muscle and thin sections of the intraventricular septum.

Nonsurgical Techniques for Arrhythmia Ablation

Catheter ablation involves the application of direct current from an external defibrillator through a pacing electrode to an area of myocardium. Most successful with ablation of the atrioventricular node and uncommonly successful in ablation of some accessory pathways, its utility in ventricular tachycardia has been extremely limited. It is possible that further refinement of mapping techniques and new electrodes will allow more success but expectations should be modest. Recently, some investigators have reported initial trials of chemical ablation with instillation of alcohol into distal myocardial segments via selective injection into coronary artery segments. Certainly appealing in terms of avoiding operative morbidity or mortality, its efficacy and potential adverse effects remains to be determined.

Electronic Devices for Ventricular Tachyarrhythmias

The electronic device with the greatest contribution to reducing SCD remains the automatic internal cardioverter defibrillator (AICD). The annual mortality rate for survivors of sudden cardiac arrest, 25–40%, has been reduced to 2–5% once the AICD has been implanted.[34] The defibrillator is much more appealing than antitachycardia pacemakers or transvenous cardioverters, which have the potential to accelerate the VT to ventricular fibrillation without the ability to defibrillate them. Nevertheless, there is a tremendous potential for improvement. Currently, the implantation of the AICD requires thoracotomy (even if limited) to attach one or two electrodes to the myocardium. Clinical research trials are underway using a transvenous electrode-subcutaneous electrode configuration. If successful, this type of system would allow the device to be implanted with less risk in those deserving patients with poor left ventricular and pulmonary function who could not tolerate thoracotomy.

The ability to combine antitachycardia pacing with AICD might permit termination of malignant ventricular tachyarrhythmias without depleting the AICD battery. Presently, the AICD pulse generator has a life span of $1\frac{1}{2}$–$2\frac{1}{2}$ years or 75–100 discharges, whichever comes first. Obviously, more discharges will result in faster battery depletion. The addition of antitachycardia pacing should prolong the life of the system before replacement is necessary. Rarely, after defibrillation, bradyarrhythmias appear before resumption of sinus rhythm. Backup pacing would prevent hemodynamic compromise until sinus rhythm is restored and could easily be part of the antitachycardia pacing system.

Future devices should be programmable in terms of the VT rate necessary to trigger the AICD, the ability to add or delete the probability density function as part of the arrhythmia detection algorithm, and the energy delivered to allow for maximal protection as well as preservation of battery life. Certainly longer battery life and smaller battery size would also be desirable.

Finally, telemetry would permit documentation of the arrhythmia shocked by the AICD, allowing verification of its appropriateness, as well as providing the ability to monitor the integrity of the sensing and defibrillating electrodes.

Public Education and Programs

CPR has been learned by medical and paramedical personnel, police, firemen, family members of patients with heart disease, and increasing members of the general public. This educational process must be supported, encouraged, and expanded. For those suffering sudden cardiac arrest, the immediate institution of CPR may make the difference between life and death.

Recently, automatic external defibrillators have been introduced, allowing their application to victims of sudden cardiac arrest even if the rescuer may not be fully trained in CPR. The installation of these devices in public places such as office buildings, department stores, supermarkets, etc. may allow rescue before arrival of the paramedics.

Antiarrhythmic Drugs

The search for the "silver bullet" of antiarrhythmic drugs has been disappointing. While certain new drugs may offer additional advantages, toxicities will remain a problem. Correct application of current drugs, alone or in combination, may have more to offer than expecting a miracle in the future.

These considerations represent some of the future directions in the prevention of sudden cardiac death. First, one must identify the patient at risk, evaluate the anatomical substrate, and eliminate potential trigger factors. There is no substitute for a comprehensive evaluation and aggressive medical/surgical intervention as appropriate for the individual patient.

References

1. Roberts WC: Sudden cardiac death: definitions and causes. Am J Cardiol 57:1411, 1986.
2. Kannel WB, Schatzkin A: Sudden death: lessons from subsets in population studies. J Am Coll Cardiol 5:141B, 1985.
3. Muller JE, Ludmer PL, Willich SN, et al: Circadian variation in the frequency of sudden cardiac death. Circulation 75:131, 1987.
4. Willich SN, Levy D, Rocco MB, et al: Circadian variation in the incidence of sudden cardiac death in the Framingham Heart Study Population. Am J Cardiol 60:801, 1987.
5. Tofler GH, Brezinski D, Schafer AI, et al: Concurrent morning increase in platelet aggregability and the risk of myocardial infarction and sudden cardiac death. N Engl J Med 316:1514, 1987.
6. Driscoll DJ, Edwards WD: Sudden unexpected death in children and adolescents. J Am Coll Cardiol 5:118B, 1985.
7. Garson A, et al: Ventricular arrhythmias and sudden death in children. J Am Coll Cardiol 5:130B, 1985.

8. Cohn PF: Silent Myocardial Ischemia and Infarction. New York, Marcel Dekker, Inc., 1986.
9. Fricchione GL, Vlay SC: Psychiatric and neurologic aspects of arrhythmia evaluation and management. In: Vlay SC (ed), Manual of Cardiac Arrhythmias: A Practical Guide to Clinical Management. Little Brown & Co., 1988, pp. 421–434.
10. Schwartz P, Stone H: The role of the autonomic nervous system in sudden coronary death. Ann NY Acad Sci 382:162, 1982.
11. DeSilva R: Central nervous system risk factors for sudden cardiac death. Ann NY Acad Sci 382:143, 1982.
12. Lown B, Verrier R: Neural activity and ventricular fibrillation. N Engl J Med 294:1165, 1976.
13. Talman W: Cardiovascular regulation and lesions of the central nervous system. Ann Neurol 220:71, 1979.
14. Vlay SC, Olson LC, Fricchione GL, et al: Anxiety and anger in patients with ventricular tachyarrhythmias: responses after automatic internal cardioverter defibrillator implantation. PACE 12:366, 1989.
15. Weaver WD, et al: Angiographic findings and prognostic indicators in patients resuscitated from sudden cardiac death. Circulation 54:895, 1976.
16. Swerdlow CD, Winkle RA, Mason JW: Determinants of survival in patients with ventricular tachyarrhythmias. N Engl J Med 308:1436, 1983.
17. Spielman SR, et al: Predictors of the success or failure of medical therapy in patients with chronic recurrent sustained ventricular tachycardia: a discriminant analysis. J Am Coll Cardiol 1:401, 1983.
18. Swerdlow CD, et al: Clinical factors predicting successful electrophysiologic-pharmacologic study in patients with ventricular tachycardia. J Am Coll Cardiol 1:409, 1983.
19. Vlay SC, et al: Relationship of specific coronary lesions and regional left ventricular dysfunction to prognosis in survivors of sudden cardiac death. Am Heart J 108:1212, 1984.
20. Vlay SC, et al: Anatomic substrate and clinical outcome in survivors of sudden cardiac death: a multivariate analysis. Cardiovasc Rev Rep 7:861, 1986.
21. Goldstein S, Moss AJ, Green W: Sudden death in acute myocardial infarction: relationship to factors affecting delay in hospitalization. Arch Intern Med 129:720, 1972.
22. Hinkle LE, Thaler HT: Clinical classification of cardiac deaths. Circulation 65:457, 1982.
23. Roberts WC, Jones AA: Quantitation of coronary arterial narrowing at necropsy in sudden coronary death: analysis of 31 patients and comparison with 25 control subjects. Am J Cardiol 44:39, 1979.
24. Warnes CA, Roberts WC: Sudden coronary death: relation of amount and distribution of coronary narrowing at necropsy to previous symptoms of myocardial ischemia, left ventricular scarring and heart weight. Am J Cardiol 54:65, 1984.
25. Warnes CA, Roberts WC: Sudden coronary death: comparison of patients with those and coronary thrombus at necropsy. Am J Cardiol 54:1206, 1984.
26. Follansbee WP, Michelson EL, Morganroth J: Nonsustained ventricular

tachycardia in ambulatory patients: Characteristics and association with sudden cardiac death. Ann Intern Med 92:741, 1980.

27. Savage DD, et al: Prevalence of arrhythmias during 24-hour electrocardiographic monitoring and exercise testing in patients with obstructive and nonobstructive hypertrophic cardiomyopathy. Circulation 59:866, 1979.

28. McKenna WJ, et al: Prognosis in hypertrophic cardiomyopathy: role of age and clinical electrocardiographic and hemodynamic features. Am J Cardiol 47:532, 1981.

29. Sugruee DD, et al: Cardiac histologic findings in patients with life-threatening ventricular arrhythmias of unknown origin. J Am Coll Cardiol 4:952, 1984.

30. Isner J, et al: Sudden, unexpected death in avid dieters using the liquid-protein-modified-fast diet. Circulation 60:1401, 1979.

31. Isner J, et al: Anorexia nervosa and sudden death. Ann Intern Med 102:49, 1985.

32. Otto CM, et al: Ventricular fibrillation causes sudden death in Southeast Asian immigrants. Ann Intern Med 100:45, 1984.

33. Lown B: Sudden cardiac death: the major challenge confronting contemporary cardiology. Am J Cardiol 43:313, 1979.

34. Mirowski M: The automatic implantable defibrillator. An overview. J Am Coll Cardiol 6:461, 1985.

Additional References

Myerburg RJ: Key References: risk factors and epidemiology, pathology and pathophysiology. Circulation 64:1070, 1984.

Myerburg RJ: Key references: clinical, intervention, survival, neurophysiologic and psychophysiologic factors, and miscellaneous. Circulation 64:1291, 1984.

Vlay SC: Manual of Cardiac Arrhythmias: A Practical Guide to Clinical Management. Boston, Little Brown & Co., 1988.

Kulbertus HE, Wellens HJJ: Sudden Death. Boston, Martinus Nijhoff, 1980.

Chapter 6

Supraventricular Tachycardias: Recognition and Treatment

David G. Benditt, Walter J. Reyes,
Charles C. Gornick, Mary Ann Goldstein,
and Simon Milstein

Introduction

The supraventricular tachycardias (SVT) encompass a variety of rhythm disturbances, including those which are primarily of atrial origin, those arising from electrophysiological abnormalities within or adjacent to the atrioventricular (AV) node, and others due to re-entry utilizing accessory conduction tissue (accessory connections).[1-5] Table 1 summarizes preferred terminology for the variety of arrhythmias that comprise the supraventricular tachycardias.[5,6] In general, nonspecific designations such as paroxysmal atrial tachycardia (PAT) or paroxysmal junctional tachycardia are no longer useful. Similarly, although eponyms may be of interest historically, their use is discouraged. Thus, even such eponyms as Wolff-Parkinson-White syndrome and Lown-Ganong-Levine syndrome are not as useful as they once might have been, given improved understanding of the diverse pathophysiology of

Dr. Goldstein is a recipient of the Kenneth N. Rosen Fellowship of the North American Society of Pacing and Electrophysiology (NASPE). Dr. Reyes was supported in part by the Minnesota Medical Foundation Electrophysiology Research Fund.

From Naccarelli GV (ed): *Cardiac Arrhythmias: A Practical Approach.* Mount Kisco, NY, Futura Publishing Co., Inc., © 1991.

Table 1
Supraventricular Tachycardias

Preferred Terminology	Definition or Conventional Terminology
1. Orthodromic reciprocating (re-entrant) tachycardia	RT in which conduction in the antegrade (AV) direction uses the AV node-His bundle axis and conduction in the retrograde (VA) direction uses one or more accessory AV connections
2. Antidromic reciprocating (re-entrant) tachycardia	RT in which conduction in the antegrade connection occurs over an accessory connection and conduction in the retrograde (VA) direction uses either the AV node-His bundle or an additional accessory AV connection
3. Reciprocating tachycardia due to re-entry within the AV node	RT in which the critical elements of the re-entry circuit appear to be restricted to the region of the AV node
4. "Incessant" AV reciprocating tachycardia	"Persistent" or "permanent" form of junctional reciprocating tachycardia (PJRT)
5. Pre-excited QRS complex tachycardias	Tachycardias with a prolonged QRS complex in which ventricular activation appears to be primarily the result of conduction in the antegrade (AV) direction over an accessory connection or bypass tract
6. Wide QRS complex tachycardias	Tachycardias with a prolonged QRS complex due to underlying or functional bundle branch block, ventricular activation due to AV conduction over an accessory connection or bypass tract, or ventricular tachycardia
7. Normal QRS complex tachycardias	Tachycardia in which the QRS complex is of normal duration

RT = reciprocating tachycardia
AV = atrioventricular
VA = ventriculoatrial

arrhythmias in these patients. The term *pre-excitation syndromes*, with subsequent specific designation of the electrophysiological substrate, is preferred.

Mechanisms

Abnormal automaticity and re-entry continues to be the mechanisms associated with most clinical supraventricular arrhythmias. Triggered automaticity may also occur on rare occasions (e.g., digitalis toxicity). Reflection, although well established experimentally, has yet to be established as playing a role in spontaneous supraventricular tachyarrhythmias.

Re-entry is the most common basis for paroxysmal and sustained supraventricular tachyarrhythmias (Fig. 1). In order for re-entry to take place, a circuit made up of excitable tissues capable of conducting an electrical impulse must be present. This circuit must comprise two separate anatomical or functional pathways, one of which exhibits transient or permanent unidirectional block while the other manifests sufficiently slow conduction so that the impulse propagating over it is capable of re-entering the blocked pathway from the opposite direction. As a result, the potential for continuous repetitive activation of cardiac tissues by the circulating electrical impulse is set up. In fact, once initiated, the re-entry impulse will be able to continue to travel around the circuit as long as the time taken to traverse the circuit (i.e., the cycle length of the resulting tachycardia) exceeds the longest refractory period of the participating cardiac tissues. The leading edge of the tachycardia always encounters excitable tissue.

The concept of a re-entry circuit provides a useful model to explain many tachycardias. However, the pathways that comprise the re-entry circuit are not necessarily well-defined anatomical structures. Even in the classic re-entry arrhythmias associated with accessory AV connections (Table 2), the accessory connection only comprises a small portion of the re-entry circuit. The bulk of the circuit is made up of atrial, ventricular, and specialized conduction system tissues (Fig. 2). In other rhythm disturbances where re-entry is also almost certainly the mechanism (e.g., atrial flutter, tachycardia due to re-entry within the AV node), the elements of the circuit are less well defined.

Primary Atrial Tachycardias

Re-entry probably predominates as the basis for most primary atrial tachycardias,[3,4] including atrial fibrillation and flutter, sinus node re-

REENTRY : Basic Concepts

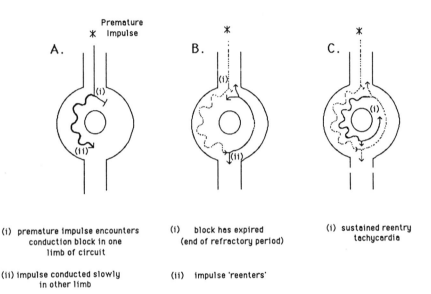

(i) premature impulse encounters conduction block in one limb of circuit

(ii) impulse conducted slowly in other limb

(i) block has expired (end of refractory period)

(ii) impulse 'reenters'

(i) sustained reentry tachycardia

Figure 1. Schematic illustration depicting the basic concept of re-entry arrhythmias. The requirements for re-entry are the presence of an electrically excitable circuit, slow conduction in one portion of the circuit, and unidirectional conduction block in another element of the circuit. In A, a premature impulse enters the circuit from above and encounters conduction block in one limb of the circuit (i) and conducts slowly in the other limb of the circuit (ii). In B, the unidirectional block has expired in the right hand half of the circuit and consequently the slowly conducted impulse is able to re-enter the right hand half of the circuit in the retrograde direction. In C, the sequence is repeated and re-entry is sustained. See text for the discussion.

entry, and many so-called "ectopic atrial tachycardias." Atrial fibrillation and atrial flutter are the subjects of a separate chapter and will not be discussed here.

Sinus Node Re-entrant Tachycardia

Definitive substantiation of re-entry within the sinus node region is extremely difficult to obtain experimentally and virtually impossible

Table 2
Anatomical Terminology Describing Substrates in the
Pre-excitation Syndromes

Anatomical Terminology	Previous Terminology
Accessory AV connection	Kent bundle (in septum Paladino tract)
Atriofascicular bypass tract	Atrio-Hisian fiber
Nodoventricular connection	Mahaim fiber
Fasciculoventricular connection	Mahaim fiber

in the clinical setting (Fig. 3).[7] Therefore, despite numerous clinical reports describing tachycardias that may be the result of this mechanism,[15,16] the topic remains controversial.

Demonstration that precisely timed premature atrial beats could reproducibly induce a subsequent atrial depolarization exhibiting the features of a spontaneous sinus impulse, but occurring earlier than expected, provided the initial indirect evidence favoring occurrence of re-entry within the sinus node region in man. It was based upon these observations that clinical criteria for diagnosis of sinus node re-entry were developed[9] and may be summarized as follows (Fig. 4): (1) the morphology of the P waves generated by the re-entrant cycles is identical to those of sinus beats; (2) the intracardiac sequence of atrial activation of re-entrant cycles is identical to that of sinus impulses; (3) the re-entry phenomenon is reproducible; and (4) the tachycardia is usually relatively slow (110 to 140 beats/min), with the tachycardia cycle length often exhibiting wide fluctuations.[14] Further, the episodes are typically brief, but when they are sustained, the tachycardia can be terminated by atrial premature stimuli.

During atrial extrastimulus testing in the electrophysiology laboratory, the phenomenon of apparent sinus node re-entry has been reported in 9–17% of patients.[15,17] However, in only about 1% of patients does the induced sinus node re-entry tachycardia appear to correspond to the spontaneous tachyarrhythmia in that individual. Our own experience is comparable. On the other hand, in a smaller series of 65 patients undergoing electrophysiological studies for paroxysmal supraventricular tachycardia, a surprisingly frequent incidence of clinically significant sinus node re-entrant tachycardia (16.9%) has been observed. The latter experience appears to be the exception.

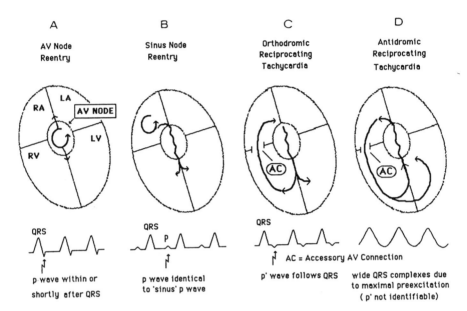

Figure 2. Schematics illustrating various forms of supraventricular re-entry arrhythmias and their resulting electrocardiograms. In A, typical AV node re-entrant tachycardia is illustrated. The re-entry circuit lies within the AV node and the resulting atrial and ventricular activations occur virtually simultaneously. Thus, on surface electrocardiogram, the atrial activation (P wave) is usually buried within the QRS complex or follows very shortly after the QRS. In B, sinus node re-entry is illustrated as a re-entry circuit within the region of the right atrium closely adjacent to the sinus node and perhaps incorporating a portion or all of the sinus node tissue itself. The resulting electrocardiogram reveals a P wave virtually identical to that of the sinus P wave. In C, a re-entrant tachycardia using an accessory AV connection (AC) is illustrated. This tachycardia is commonly referred to as orthodromic reciprocating tachycardia, and it is evident that both supraventricular and ventricular tissue are important parts of the re-entrant circuit. Since atrial activation follows the ventricular activation in this tachycardia, the surface ECG usually shows the P wave following the QRS complex. In D, antidromic reciprocating tachycardia is schematically illustrated in which the re-entry circuit utilizes an accessory AV connection (AC) in the antegrade (atrioventricular) direction. Since this tachycardia sequence results in abnormal ventricular activation due to maximal pre-excitation, the QRS morphology is wide and bizarre. This tachycardia may be difficult to distinguish from a ventricular tachycardia.

SINOATRIAL REENTRY TACHYCARDIA

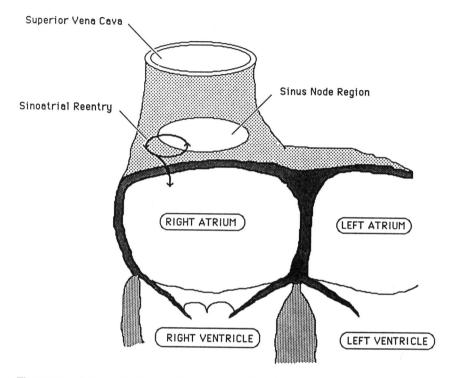

Figure 3. Schematic illustration showing the site of re-entry for arrhythmias resulting in sinoatrial re-entry tachycardia. In this illustration, the re-entry circuit is shown to encompass a portion of the sinus node region along with a portion of the right atrium. In other circumstances, the re-entry circuit may be solely within the sinus node region or alternatively may utilize only atrial tissue in close proximity to the sinus node region. These possible mechanisms cannot be differentiated clearly in the electrophysiology laboratory.

Other Primary Atrial Tachycardias

Re-entry is probably the most common mechanism of atrial tachycardias. In its macro-re-entry form (encompassing large segments of atrial tissue), these tachycardias may be similar to atrial flutter, both in mechanism and in atrial rate. In their micro-re-entry form, they may be indistinguishable from automatic tachycardias of focal origin such as may occur due to triggered automaticity. Multifocal atrial tachycardias

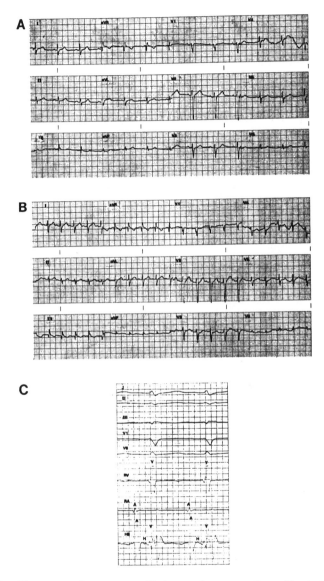

Figure 4. Electrocardiograms and intracardiac recordings illustrating sinus node re-entrant tachycardia. (A) Baseline 12-lead electrocardiogram during sinus rhythm. (B) 12-lead electrocardiogram recorded during an episode of paroxysmal tachycardia. Note that during this tachycardia, the P wave morphology is identical to that recorded in sinus rhythm. (C) Electrocardiograms and intracardiac recordings obtained during the episode of tachycardia illustrated in panel B. Note that the high right atrial recording (RA) precedes the atrial electrogram at the low septal right atrium as recorded on the His bundle electrode (HB).

(MAT) (presumably a result of abnormal automaticity) and the accelerated junctional rhythm (junctional tachycardia) associated with digitalis toxicity (presumably due to triggered automaticity) are probable exceptions to the otherwise dominance of re-entry mechanisms.

In general, primary atrial arrhythmias are characterized by the presence of concomitant disease processes such as chronic pulmonary disease, atrial septal defect, previous atrial surgery, an unstable hemodynamic state, or drug toxicity. However, if these factors do not appear to be present, the possibility of a subclinical cardiomyopathy should be entertained.[18]

Tachycardia Due to Re-entry Within the AV Node (AV Node Re-entry Tachycardia)

AV node re-entry tachycardia is believed to be the most common form of paroxysmal supraventricular tachycardia in adults, accounting for approximately 60% of patients undergoing electrophysiological study for SVT. The substrate for this arrhythmia is presumed to be functional longitudinal dissociation of conduction properties within the AV node itself (although participation of atrionodal [intranodal] bypass tracts has not been entirely excluded) (Fig. 5). Electrophysiological testing using intracardiac recordings and extrastimulus techniques can often demonstrate this longitudinal dissociation (so-called "dual AV nodal pathways") (Fig. 6) and identify the electrophysiological differences among the elements of the circuit that permit re-entry to occur. Most commonly, dual AV nodal pathways comprise a "fast" pathway with a relatively long refractory period and a "slow" pathway with a relatively short refractory period. These pathways, probably along with segments of atrial tissue in the vicinity of the AV node, form the re-entry circuit. Under appropriate conditions, a premature atrial or ventricular extrasystole will be blocked in the fast pathway due to its usually relatively long refractory period, but will be conducted slowly over the slow pathway with its shorter refractory period. After having reached the far end of the slow pathway, the refractoriness of the fast pathway having expired will permit the impulse to re-enter the fast pathway in the opposite direction. Thus, the electrical circuit has been completely traversed. Under appropriate conditions, this circular movement could be maintained for prolonged periods of time, resulting in sustained tachycardia.

It should be pointed out that there is no evident physiological reason for fast pathways to necessarily exhibit long refractory periods, while

AV NODE REENTRY

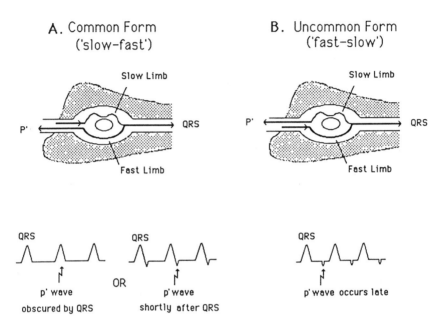

A. Common Form ('slow-fast')

Slow Limb

P' ⟶ QRS

Fast Limb

B. Uncommon Form ('fast-slow')

Slow Limb

P' ⟵ QRS

Fast Limb

QRS

p' wave obscured by QRS

OR

QRS

p' wave shortly after QRS

QRS

p' wave occurs late

Figure 5. Illustrations depicting two forms of supraventricular tachycardia due to re-entry within the AV node. Both forms of tachycardia rely on the concept of the presence of functional longitudinal dissociation of conduction properties within the AV node itself. In A, the common form of AV node re-entrant tachycardia is illustrated. In this form, the slow limb of the re-entry circuit is utilized for conduction of the cardiac impulse from the atria to the ventricles. The fast limb of the re-entrant circuit conducts the electrical impulse in the retrograde (ventriculoatrial) direction. As a result of this relationship between slow conduction in the antegrade direction and relatively fast conduction in the retrograde direction, atrial activation (P wave) is usually obscured by the QRS complex or occurs shortly after the QRS complex. In B, the uncommon form of AV node re-entry tachycardia is illustrated. In this situation, the fast limb of the re-entry circuit is utilized in the antegrade (atrioventricular) direction and the slow limb is utilized in the ventriculoatrial direction. As a result of the relationship between fast and slow conduction, atrial activation (P wave) occurs well after the inscription of the QRS complex and consequently it is more easily observed on the surface ECG. Differentiation of the later form of AV node re-entrant tachycardia from reciprocating tachycardias utilizing accessory AV connections (see text) necessitates invasive electrophysiological testing.

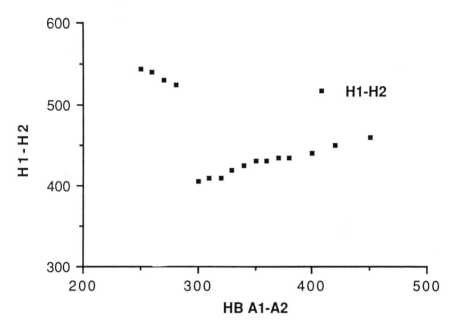

Figure 6. Graph illustrating discontinuous conduction curves indicative of dual AV nodal pathways in a patient with supraventricular tachycardia due to re-entry within the AV node. The ordinate indicates the interval (ms) between the His bundle electrogram (H1) recorded at the end of an atrial pacing sequence and that recorded (H2) for a single subsequent premature atrial beat. The abscissa indicates the interval (ms) between the last paced atrial electrogram during a drive train (A1) and the subsequent premature atrial electrogram (A2) recorded at the low septal right atrial site. Note that as A1-A2 intervals shorten, the H1-H2 initially (at right) interval tends to shorten in a corresponding fashion. However, in an A1-A2 interval of approximately 280 ms there is an abrupt discontinuity in the conduction curve with subsequent H1-H2 intervals being much longer. This discontinuity in the AV node conduction curve has been generally accepted as representing an initial fast conduction pathway with a relatively long refractory period (in this case approximately 290 ms), followed by conduction over a slow pathway which exhibits a somewhat longer refractory period (see text for details).

slow conducting pathways exhibit short refractory periods. However, in those instances in which the reverse occurs, the two pathways would not be readily distinguishable since the fast conducting pathway would always mask the slower one.

In the typical or common form of AV node re-entry (i.e., the slow-fast mechanism described above), both the atria and the ventricles are essentially "innocent bystanders" and are activated almost simultaneously by impulses leaving the AV node in both directions (Fig. 5). Consequently, atrial electrical activity is frequently obscured on the surface ECG by the simultaneously occurring QRS complex. In effect, the R-P' interval during tachycardia (P' refers to the atrial activation during tachycardia, thereby differentiating it from the normal P wave during sinus rhythm) is substantially shorter than the P'-R interval (R-P' < P'-R). On the other hand, a less common form of AV node re-entry tachycardia (uncommon form, atypical form) may be observed. In this case, the direction of the re-entry circuit is reversed, and conduction in the antegrade (AV) direction occurs over the fast pathway. Retrograde conduction occurs over the slow pathway, and consequently atrial activation is not obscured by the QRS (i.e., retrograde P' waves are visible on the ECG because they occur later, after completion of the QRS). In the latter instance, the R-P' interval during tachycardia is long and is often greater than the P'-R interval (R-P' > P'-R) (Fig. 5).

Differentiating the fast-slow uncommon form of AV node re-entry from other tachycardias in which R-P' > P'-R (especially the incessant form of AV reciprocating tachycardia) may be difficult and necessitates invasive electrophysiological testing. Nonetheless, it is useful to pay particular attention to the relationship of R waves and P' waves during supraventricular tachycardias since they may help better clarify the differential diagnosis. Accomplishing this task usually necessitates examination of a 12-lead ECG recording during tachycardia (in order to better identify P' waves), and on occasion may necessitate transesophageal or intra-atrial recordings. Table 3 summarizes the potential diagnostic value of assessing ventriculoatrial timing.

Reciprocating Tachycardias Utilizing Accessory AV Connections

A wide variety of accessory conduction tissues have been described (Fig. 7), and may both result in an ECG picture of ventricular pre-excitation (Fig. 8), as well as participate in paroxysmal tachycardias in man. Accessory AV connections are by far the most common of these, when viewed from the perspective of clinical manifestations.

Accessory AV connections are small (not usually visible by eye) muscular bridges that provide an abnormal electrical pathway between the atria and the ventricles.[6] These connections are congenital anomalies presumably due to inadequate breakdown of electrical continuity be-

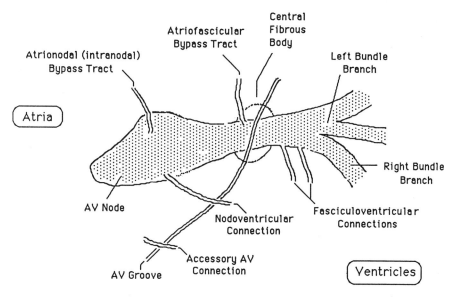

Figure 7. Schematic illustration depicting the wide variety of accessory cardiac conduction tissues that have been identified. The stippled region represents the normal specialized cardiac conduction system (AV node, His bundle, left and right bundle branches). The AV groove, demarcating the boundary between the atria and ventricles, is indicated as is the central fibrous body of the heart. The variety of accessory conduction tissues that have been identified are illustrated. For example, note that accessory AV connections cross the AV groove thereby providing an additional electrical connection between the atria and the ventricles. More than one accessory connection may be present in an individual patient.

tween atria and ventricles during in utero and postnatal development of the AV groove. In conjunction with the normal specialized AV conduction system and/or additional accessory connections, accessory AV connections provide a critical element of the substrate for a re-entry circuit.[5,19,20]

Accessory AV connections may traverse the AV groove almost anywhere along the tricuspid or mitral valve annuli, and in many cases multiple connections may be present.[19,20] In those instances in which the accessory connection exhibits antegrade (i.e., atrioventricular direction) conduction characteristics during sinus rhythm, abnormal ventricular pre-excitation may be observed. Electrocardiographically, the latter is manifest by both a short PR interval and a delta wave (the electrocardiographic hallmarks of Wolff-Parkinson-White syndrome, a

ACCESSORY CONNECTIONS AND TRACTS

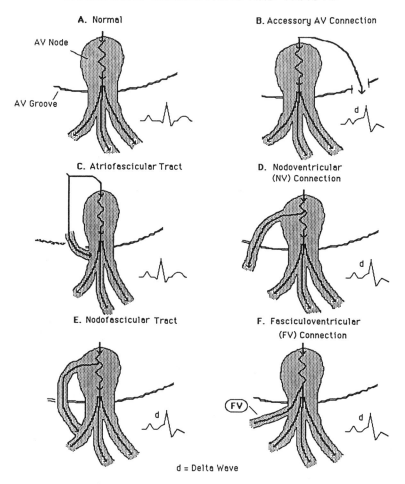

A. Normal

AV Node

AV Groove

B. Accessory AV Connection

d

C. Atriofascicular Tract

D. Nodoventricular (NV) Connection

d

E. Nodofascicular Tract

d

F. Fasciculoventricular (FV) Connection

FV

d

d = Delta Wave

Figure 8. Schematics illustrating the manner in which accessory conduction connections may affect the electrocardiogram. By convention, accessory conduction tissues that insert into myocardium are designated connections whereas accessory conduction tissues that insert into specialized conduction tissue of the heart are designated tracts. Panel A provides a schematic of the normal specialized cardiac conduction system illustrating the AV node, AV groove, and His bundle branch system. The electrocardiogram reveals a normal PR interval and QRS complex. Panel B illustrates an accessory AV connection with conduction occurring both over the AV node-His bundle axis and across the AV groove via the accessory AV connection. Note that the electrocardiogram reveals a delta wave (d) due to pre-excitation of the ventricles resulting from conduction over the accessory AV connection. Panel

subset of the pre-excitation syndromes). In many patients, however, these ECG findings may be subtle or absent due to the connection being far from the sinus node (e.g., left lateral connections) or as a result of preferential conduction over a relatively fast AV node. Furthermore, in many patients with accessory AV connections, ECG findings of overt ventricular pre-excitation are not present due to the fact that the accessory connection is able to conduct only in the retrograde (ventriculoatrial) direction. The latter connections are termed "inapparent" or "concealed." Nonetheless, whether pre-excitation is evident or the accessory connection is concealed, the mechanism of the most common form of tachycardia in these patients (orthodromic AV reciprocating tachycardia) is the same (see below).

Recently, findings in neonates and infants have tended to confirm the frequent occurrence with which accessory connections are present in the developing heart. Indeed, apart from atrial flutter, most paroxysmal supraventricular tachycardias in utero and in neonates and young infants are now believed to be due to re-entry utilizing residual accessory AV connections. Definitive evidence is of course difficult to obtain in very small infants, since multicatheter electrophysiological studies are not readily performed. Nonetheless, transesophageal recordings and careful examination of the ECG in these cases support this contention. Further, as these children grow, susceptibility to re-entrant tachyarrhythmias can often continue to be demonstrated by cardiac stimulation techniques (transesophageal or intracardiac), and not infrequently spontaneous tachycardias recur later in life. In the latter cases, the presence

---

C depicts an atriofascicular tract connecting the atrium to the His bundle or bundle branches. In this case, the electrocardiogram reveals a shortened PR interval due to more rapid conduction from the atria to the His bundle via the accessory tract. The QRS complex is normal since ventricular activation occurs over the normal conduction tissue. This situation is probably a rare cause of short PR intervals in patients. Panel D illustrates a nodoventricular connection arising from the AV node and crossing the AV groove to insert in ventricular myocardium. In this instance, the ventricles are pre-excited and a delta wave is evident on the ECG. Panel E depicts a nodofascicular tract that arises in the AV node and inserts in the His bundle or bundle branches. If the nodofascicular tract inserts into the bundle branches, then relatively early ventricular activation (pre-excitation) will be present and a delta wave may be observed on the ECG. Panel F depicts a fasciculoventricular connection that arises in the His bundle or bundle branches and inserts into the ventricular myocardium. Pre-excitation will be present and consequently a delta wave is evident on the ECG.

of an accessory AV connection can be more readily proven by electro-physiological study.

Orthodromic AV Reciprocating Tachycardia

Orthodromic AV reciprocating tachycardia is a re-entry tachycardia in which the circulating electrical impulse utilizes the AV node in the antegrade (atrioventricular) direction, while the accessory AV connection is a principal element of the retrograde (ventriculoatrial) limb of the circuit. The specialized intraventricular conduction system, ventricular muscle, and atrial muscle comprise the remainder of the re-entry loop. In this setting, a spontaneous premature atrial extrasystole might find itself unable to traverse the accessory AV connection in the antegrade direction (either due to permanent unidirectional block in the connection or due to its exhibiting a relatively long refractory period). However, this same premature beat may be able to conduct to the ventricles slowly over the AV node. After the impulse has penetrated the conduction system and the ventricles, it may find that the refractory period of the accessory AV connection has expired, and that it can now re-enter the atria by conduction over the accessory AV connection in the retrograde (ventriculoatrial) direction. Repetitive circus movement of this type would lead to a sustained tachycardia, usually exhibiting a normal QRS morphology (although the QRS may be wide in the presence of co-existing or functional bundle branch block) (Figs. 9B, 10).

Antidromic AV Reciprocating Tachycardia

In patients with accessory AV connections capable of conducting impulses in the antegrade (AV) direction (e.g., patients with overt pre-excitation), the re-entry circuit may on rare occasion comprise atrioventricular antegrade conduction over the accessory AV connection and ventriculoatrial (retrograde) conduction over the AV node and/or another accessory AV connection (Figs. 9C, 11). In the example of antidromic tachycardia provided in Figure 11, the presence of retrograde His bundle potentials following each ventricular activation suggested that the His bundle-AV node axis comprised a critical portion of the retrograde limb of the re-entry circuit. In other cases, additional accessory AV connections have been shown to contribute to the retrograde limb. Reciprocating tachycardias utilizing an accessory AV connection as the

A. Reentry within AV Node

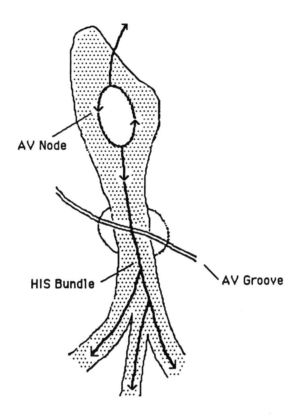

AV Node

HIS Bundle

AV Groove

bundle branches

Figure 9. Schematics depicting various mechanisms of reciprocating tachycardia. (A) Illustration depicting the mechanism of reciprocating tachycardia due to re-entry within the AV node. The stippled region depicts the AV node, His bundle, and bundle branches. The AV groove dividing the atria from the ventricles is indicated. (B) Schematic of the usual mechanism of orthodromic reciprocating tachycardia utilizing an accessory AV connection. In this tachycardia, antegrade atrioventricular conduction occurs through the AV node and bundle branches with retrograde activation of the atria via the accessory AV connection. A macro re-entrant loop is thereby established. (C) Illustration of a rarer form of reciprocating tachycardia in which an accessory AV connection is utilized in the antegrade direction. This so-called "antidromic"

Figure continues

B. Orthodromic RT
using an
Accessory AV Connection

C. Antidromic RT
using an
Accessory AV Connection

D. Antidromic RT
using a
Nodoventricular
Connection

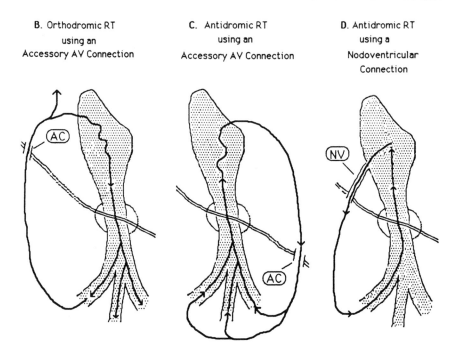

Figure 9. (*Continued*)
tachycardia results in a broad bizarre QRS complex. Retrograde activation
of the atria during this arrhythmia occurs most commonly via the specialized
cardiac conduction system, but in some patients a second accessory AV connection may be utilized. (D) Depiction of the mechanism of tachycardia in
patients using a nodoventricular connection. These tachycardias typically
exhibit a wide QRS complex due to pre-excitation. Most often, the nodoventricular connection inserts into the right ventricle and typically the electrocardiogram exhibits a left bundle branch appearance with left axis deviation.

antegrade limb of a re-entry circuit are termed "antidromic" and their
inscription on the surface ECG is characterized by a broad bizarre QRS
complex due to maximal ventricular preexcitation.

Differentiation of antidromic reciprocating tachycardia from ventricular tachycardia can prove to be exceptionally difficult even during
invasive electrophysiological study. Additionally, determining whether
a tachycardia exhibiting a bizarre, apparently maximally pre-excited QRS
complex is critically dependent on the accessory connection as part of
a re-entrant circuit, or dependent on whether the accessory connection
is purely an "innocent bystander" (such as AV nodal re-entry with an-

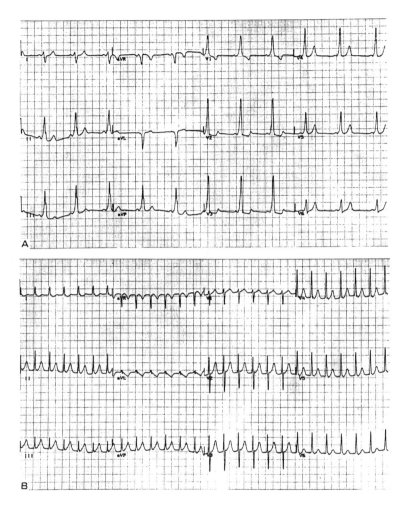

Figure 10. Electrocardiograms illustrating orthodromic reciprocating tachycardia in a patient with pre-excitation syndrome. (A) A 12-lead electrocardiogram revealing a delta wave indicative of pre-excitation syndrome. A left lateral accessory connection was present in this patient. (B) A 12-lead electrocardiogram revealing a normal QRS complex tachycardia, consistent with typical orthodromic reciprocating tachycardia. This patient later underwent successful surgical ablation of the accessory AV connection, with normalization of the QRS complex.

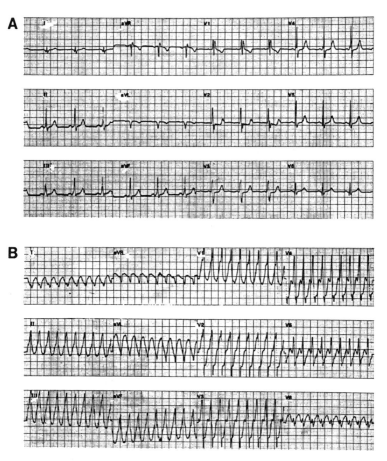

Figure 11. Electrocardiograms illustrating antidromic reciprocating tachycardia in a patient with an accessory AV connection. (A) A 12-lead electrocardiogram in a patient with pre-excitation syndrome and a left lateral accessory AV connection. (B) A 12-lead electrocardiogram revealing a wide QRS complex tachycardia in which the QS pattern in leads I and aVL are most compatible with maximal pre-excitation of the left lateral aspect of the left ventricles due to antegrade conduction over an accessory AV connection. A detailed intracardiac electrophysiological study confirmed that antidromic reciprocating tachycardia utilizing a left lateral accessory AV connection.

tegrade conduction to the ventricles over a "bystander" accessory connection) poses a challenge even to the experienced invasive cardiac electrophysiologist.

Primary Atrial Tachycardias in Patients with Pre-excitation Syndrome

In patients with ventricular pre-excitation, the possibility exists that exceedingly rapid and potentially life-threatening ventricular responses can develop if a primary atrial tachycardia (particularly atrial fibrillation) happens to occur in the presence of an accessory AV connection with a short antegrade refractory period (typically ≤250 ms).[5,20] In this setting, the accessory connection and ventricles are believed to be primarily "innocent bystanders," responding to a rapid atrial rhythm (Fig. 12). However, the presence of accessory AV connections may enhance susceptibility to development of primary atrial tachyarrhythmias in patients with pre-excitation syndrome. Most commonly, repeated bouts of reciprocating tachycardia ultimately lead to degeneration of the atrial rhythm to atrial fibrillation. Alternatively, an accessory AV connection may permit a ventricular extrasystole to impinge upon a vulnerable atrium, thereby initiating a primary atrial tachyarrhythmia. In any event, the patient is potentially exposed to the risk of an extremely rapid ventricular response since the accessory connection essentially bypasses the protection offered by normal individual by the AV node[21] (Fig. 12). Aggressive therapeutic intervention is essential, both in the acute situation and for chronic prophylaxis.

Pre-excitation Variants

Whereas accessory AV connections are relatively common among patients with recurrent supraventricular tachycardias, other less common and more difficult to identify anatomical substrates for pre-excitation and re-entry tachycardias exist[5,20,22] (Fig. 8, Table 2). Accessory nodoventricular and fasciculoventricular connections (formerly termed Mahaim fibers[6]) are probably quite prevalent anatomically in humans but only rarely become clinically relevent. Nodoventricular connections, as their name implies, are small muscle bundles that arise from AV nodal tissue and insert into ventricular myocardium. Similarly, fasciculoventricular connections arise from the His bundle or bundle branches and

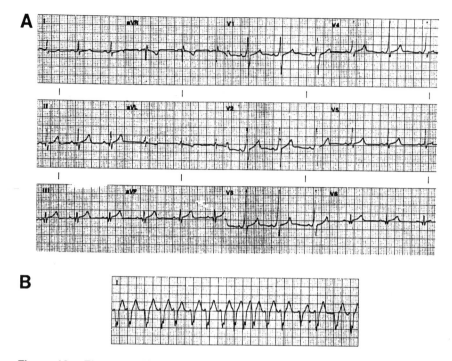

Figure 12. Electrocardiograms illustrating a rapid ventricular response during atrial fibrillation in a patient with pre-excitation syndrome. (A) A 12-lead electrocardiogram in a patient with a left posterolateral accessory AV connection. (B) A rhythm strip revealing an irregularly irregular wide QRS tachyarrhythmia in the same patient. In this instance, the shortest pre-excited R-R interval is approximately 240 ms, a finding that has been suggested to imply increased risk of potential development of ventricular fibrillation.

insert into ventricular myocardium. In both cases, pre-excitation in the form of a short PR and a delta wave on the ECG may be observed.

The manner in which nodoventricular and fasciculoventricular connections participate in re-entry tachycardias remains somewhat speculative. It is believed that these connections are most often "innocent bystanders," resulting in ventricular pre-excitation during either primary atrial tachycardias or conventional reciprocating tachycardias (e.g., re-entrant AV nodal tachycardia with ventricular activation occurring over a "bystander" accessory connection). In only a few instances have nodoventricular connections been implicated in re-entry, and participation of fasciculoventricular connections in re-entry is even more uncertain.

The presence of accessory tracts that arise in the atrium and bypass part (atrionodal) or all (atriofascicular) of the normal AV node and inserting respectively into distal portions of the AV node or into specialized intraventricular cardiac conduction tissue, are well established histologically.[23] These atrionodal (also called intranodal) and atriofascicular tracts may form part of the substrate for reciprocating tachycardia due to re-entry within the AV node in some patients and may account for short PR intervals and enhanced AV node conduction in others.[23–25]

The potential for AV nodal bypass tracts to participate in re-entry tachycardias and provide the substrate for the syndrome of short PR interval, normal QRS complex, and recurrent tachycardia (formerly designated Lown-Ganong-Levine syndrome[26]) is tempting to advocate. However, clinical electrophysiological studies in such patients are not convincing in this regard, and it appears that tachycardia mechanisms in such individuals do not differ from those in patients with normal PR intervals. Perhaps the association of a short PR interval with enhanced AV node conduction may result in development of more rapid tachyarrhythmias and thereby more disconcerting symptoms. Further, antiarrhythmic drug therapy may be less effective in slowing conduction across an enhanced AV node than one exhibiting more typical electrophysiological characteristics.

In a fashion analogous to concealed accessory AV connections, nodoventricular and fasciculoventricular connections and atrionodal and atriofascicular tracts might similarly exhibit unidirectional conduction block and thereby be "concealed." Under such conditions, re-entry tachycardia might still occur yet there would be no overt suspicion of the presence of such connections or tracts based upon conventional ECG observations. Indeed, even detailed intracardiac electrophysiological study might be unable to provide direct evidence substantiating such connections.

Electrocardiographic and Electrophysiological Features

The 12-lead ECG and transesophageal recordings comprise the minimum necessary tools for assessment of supraventricular tachycardias. However, in many instances, substantiation of the diagnosis requires detailed intracardiac electrophysiological study. The necessary personnel qualifications and laboratory facilities required to carry out electrophysiological studies have recently been adequately outlined.[27]

Primary Atrial Tachycardias

The ECG recognition of atrial fibrillation and atrial flutter is usually straightforward and is discussed elsewhere. However, definitive diagnostic substantiation of other re-entrant primary atrial tachycardias (e.g., sinus node re-entry) requires invasive electrophysiological study, especially if the tachycardia manifests a continuous 1:1 AV relationship.[3] As a rule, sinus node re-entry tends to be relatively slow and electrocardiographically exhibits a P-wave morphology essentially identical to those recorded during sinus rhythm (Fig. 4). Other re-entrant primary atrial tachycardias may exhibit atrial rates approaching those of atrial flutter.

Certain atrial tachycardias, especially those associated with long-standing cardiac disease or severe pulmonary disease, are thought to be due to abnormal automaticity. Not infrequently, these tachycardias exhibit multiple P-wave morphologies suggesting a multicentric origin (e.g., multifocal atrial tachycardia). Evidence supporting multifocal abnormal automaticity in these arrhythmias is their somewhat irregular rhythm, resistance to termination by pacing or cardioversion techniques, and demonstration of overdrive suppression in some instances.

Re-entry Within the AV Node

Susceptibility to AV nodal re-entry tachycardia is probably quite common in the population, and when detected in the asymptomatic individual should not be cause for concern. Typically, patients with symptomatic AV nodal re-entry tachycardia have normal hearts. Usually the tachycardia is well tolerated with the main complaint being palpitations. However, lightheadedness and syncope may occur, as might chest pain or shortness of breath in individuals with concomitant coronary artery disease and/or left ventricular dysfunction.

During sinus rhythm, patients with susceptibility to AV node re-entry usually show no specific ECG findings. In rare instances, the presence of two discrete PR interval durations may be observed, suggesting the presence of dual-AV nodal pathway physiology. During tachycardia, the heart rate is typically regular, and for most patients is in the range 150–200 bpm. Faster rates do occur, however. The most distinctive finding during the common form (slow-fast) of AV node re-entry tachycardia is the tendency for retrograde atrial depolarization (P' wave) to be obscured within the QRS complex (see discussion of R-P' timing above)

(Fig. 5). Indeed, identification of atrial activity may not be possible without the aid of a transesophageal or intra-atrial recording. Demonstration of a ventriculoatrial interval (R-P' interval) less than 60 ms is essentially diagnostic of an AV nodal re-entry mechanism.[28] However, ventriculoatrial intervals during both the common (slow-fast) and the uncommon (fast-slow) forms of AV nodal re-entry tachycardia may be longer than 60 ms in many patients. In these latter cases, although retrograde P' waves may become apparent on ECG, only detailed electrophysiological study can differentiate AV nodal re-entry tachycardia from re-entry utilizing an accessory AV connection.

Re-entry Utilizing an Accessory AV Connection

As a rule, patients with accessory AV connections do not exhibit evidence of other structural cardiac disease. Although an association between right-sided accessory AV connections and Ebstein's malformation of the tricuspid valve is important to keep in mind, other previously reported associations between accessory AV connections and mitral valve prolapse or idiopathic hypertrophic subaortic stenosis (IHSS) are probably spurious.

In patients with overt ECG evidence of pre-excitation (i.e., the presence of a short PR interval and delta wave during sinus rhythm), paroxysmal tachycardias are usually due to re-entry utilizing the accessory AV connection(s). However, these patients may also suffer from primary atrial tachycardias (e.g., atrial fibrillation), and like other patients may manifest tachycardias that are entirely unrelated to their pre-excitation syndrome (e.g., AV nodal re-entry tachycardia, ventricular tachycardia). Indeed, among patients with pre-excitation syndrome who undergo surgery for ablation of their accessory AV connections, our experience suggests that approximately 20% also exhibit susceptibility to re-entry within the AV node.

The 12-lead ECG may provide clues suggesting the approximate location of an accessory AV connection in patients with overt pre-excitation.[29] However, there are important limitations. First, as the degree of pre-excitation diminishes (i.e., as the delta wave becomes less obvious), correct interpretation of delta wave polarity becomes more tenuous. Additionally, multiple accessory connections may exist in a given patient, and only the most dominant one may be detected. Finally, body habitus, QRS abnormalities due to concomitant heart disease, and forces generated by atrial repolarization may complicate interpretation of the pre-excitation pattern. Consequently, detailed electrophysiological evaluation is required for definitive diagnosis of the number, location, and type of accessory connections present.

Whether pre-excitation is apparent on surface ECG or the accessory AV connections are concealed, the most common form of tachycardia in this setting is orthodromic reciprocating tachycardia in which antegrade (AV) conduction occurs over the AV node and retrograde conduction occurs via the accessory AV connection(s) (Fig. 9B). The result is usually a regular narrow QRS tachycardia ranging in rates between 150–260 bpm. Unlike AV nodal re-entrant tachycardia, inscription of the retrograde atrial depolarization (P' wave) usually occurs after the QRS complex due to the fact that the re-entry circuit requires ventricular depolarization to be essentially complete before the atria can be accessed by retrograde conduction over an accessory AV connection. Thus, the presence of a retrograde P wave following the QRS complex is suggestive of the participation of an accessory AV connection, but it is not unequivocally diagnostic for reasons discussed above.[5,28]

Apart from timing of retrograde atrial activation, certain other ECG findings during reciprocating tachycardia suggest participation of accessory AV connections. Most importantly, slowing of tachycardia rate and/or prolongation of the ventriculoatrial (VA) interval (i.e., R-P' interval) following development of functional bundle branch block during tachycardia is diagnostic of orthodromic reciprocating tachycardia utilizing an accessory AV connection crossing the AV groove on the same side of the heart as the bundle branch block. Thus, if during the course of sustained tachycardia one observes occurrence of left bundle branch block aberration accompanied by tachycardia slowing and/or ventriculoatrial interval prolongation, one can reasonably suppose participation of a left-sided accessory AV connection in the tachycardia. In fact, the value of this observation is so great that during electrophysiological studies one may induce and terminate many tachycardia episodes in an attempt to observe the effects of functional bundle branch aberration on tachycardia cycle length and/or ventriculoatrial interval on at least on one occasion.

ECG findings in two forms of relatively uncommon reciprocating tachycardia in patients with accessory AV connections deserve special mention. First, during antidromic reciprocating tachycardia, conduction in the atrioventricular direction occurs over the accessory AV connection and retrograde conduction occurs via the AV node and/or additional accessory AV connections (Fig. 9C). The ECG hallmark of this tachycardia is a wide QRS complex due to maximal ventricular pre-excitation.

Electrophysiological studies are essential to diagnose this tachycardia with certainty. The second tachycardia of special note is the "persistent" or "incessant" form of orthodromic AV reciprocating tachycardia. In this instance, a concealed (usually posteroseptal) accessory AV connection that tends to exhibit slow conduction properties participates in the re-entry loop. As a result, retrograde atrial activation is even further delayed than is usually the case with orthodromic reciprocating tachycardia (i.e., the long ventriculoatrial interval results in R-P′ > P′-R). The ECG signature of this arrhythmia is both its relatively incessant nature (often interrupted only briefly by one or two sinus beats with immediate resumption of the tachycardia) and the distinctive long R-P′ interval with retrograde atrial activity usually observed most prominently in the inferior ECG leads (Fig. 13). Electrophysiological studies are essential both to confirm the presence and participation of the accessory AV connection, and to differentiate this tachycardia from both the uncommon form

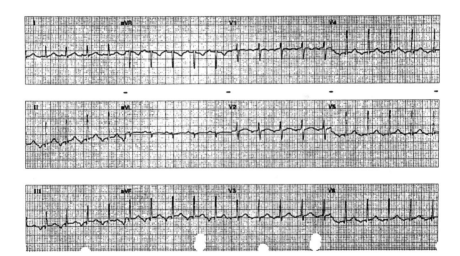

Figure 13. A 12-lead electrocardiogram illustrating the persistent or incessant form of orthodromic AV reciprocating tachycardia. In this tachycardia, a concealed posteroseptal accessory AV connection participates in re-entry. Since accessory AV connections in this condition tend to exhibit relatively slow conduction properties, retrograde activation of the atria is delayed and the P wave occurs quite late. The hallmarks of this tachycardia are its persistent nature, the ratio R-P′ > P′R, and the evident retrograde atrial activation seem most prominently in the inferior ECG leads (II, III, aVF). Prior to recognition of the mechanism of this arrhythmia, it was frequently misdiagnosed as an atrial ectopic tachycardia.

of AV nodal re-entry tachycardia and certain primary atrial tachycardias, which can also manifest R-P' > P'-R (Table 3).

In summary, intracardiac electrophysiological studies are the most effective way of defining the presence, number, location(s), and participation of accessory AV connections in patients with recurrent tachycardias. Additionally, such studies are crucial for identifying the electrophysiological characteristics and response to drug therapy of

---

Table 3
Differential Diagnosis of Supraventricular Tachycardias Based on
Atrial and Ventricular Relationships

Atrial (P') and Ventricular (R) Relationship	Probable Tachycardia Mechanism	Cannot Absolutely Exclude
1. P' buried with R wave	Re-entry within AV node	Accelerated junctional rhythm
2. R-P' < P'-R	Common form ("slow-fast") Re-entry within AV node	Re-entry utilizing accessory connection
3. P'-R > R-P'	Re-entry utilizing concealed accessory connection. If incessant, consider permanent or incessant form of reciprocating tachycardia	Unusual form ("slow-fast") of re-entry within AV node
4. Variable R-P' relation	Primary atrial tachycardia with varying AV conduction time	Re-entry utilizing more than one accessory connection, or re-entry utilizing an accessory connection in conjunction with dual AV nodal pathways

accessory AV connections. In particular, these studies permit assessing the ventricular response resulting from induced atrial risk of excessively rapid heart rate due to conduction over the accessory AV connection in the event that atrial fibrillation occurs spontaneously.

Pre-excitation Variants

Patients with nodoventricular and fasciculoventricular accessory connections may manifest a wide variety of supraventricular tachycardias, but in most cases these accessory connections (especially fasciculoventricular connections) are "innocent bystanders."[22] Electrocardiographically, nodoventricular connections are usually characterized by a distinctive left bundle branch block QRS morphology with left axis deviation. Intracardiac electrophysiological studies are essential to define the presence of nodoventricular and fasciculoventricular connections and determine the role they play in reciprocating tachycardias. However, even in experienced hands, such studies often prove inconclusive.

Patients with the syndrome of a short PR interval, normal QRS complex, and rapid heart beats (previously characterized as Lown-Ganong-Levine syndrome)[26] may be subject to the wide variety of supraventricular tachycardias already described, although heart rates may be somewhat faster than average due to the concomitant presence of enhanced AV nodal conduction in many of these individuals.[24] However, ventricular tachycardia has also been reported as a cause of rapid heart beating in some instances. Consequently, one must avoid pre-judging the nature of the arrhythmia in these individuals and proceed with a careful diagnostic evaluation.

Supraventricular Tachycardia in Infants

Utilizing fetal echocardiography, supraventricular tachycardia can now be recognized in utero and its treatment at this early stage may eliminate one potential cause of fetal distress. Orthodromic reciprocating tachycardia in utero is an important, but often overlooked, cause of hydrops fetalis.

In the neonate and young infant, supraventricular tachycardia is a relatively common arrhythmia. Until recently, the mechanisms of these arrhythmias could not be fully elucidated due to the risks and difficulties of invasive intracardiac electrophysiological studies. However, with the advent of transesophageal recordings and improved invasive electro-physiological techniques, it has been possible to study very young infants.[30–32] Based on these studies, it is evident that orthodromic reciprocating tachycardia utilizing either a concealed or overt accessory AV connection is the most common mechanism of regular narrow QRS tachycardia in neonates and young infants.[32] The tachycardia rates frequently vary between 200 and 320 bpm with ventriculoatrial (VA) intervals on the esophageal electrogram being ≥70 ms. The clinical presentation may vary from relatively benign (fussy infant with little or no congestive heart failure) to a moribund infant (a picture often confused with sepsis). The infant's clinical appearance likely relates to the duration of the tachycardia, the tachycardia rate, and whether other contributory structural heart disease (e.g., Ebstein's anomaly of the tricuspid valve) is present.

Atrial flutter also occurs in neonates and in infants, and may be observed in both normal children and in those with structural or functional cardiac disorders. Further, atrial flutter may be difficult to diagnose by examination of the surface ECG alone, since flutter waves may not be as discrete as in adult patients. Transesophageal recordings may be essential to establish the diagnosis. In infancy, atrial flutter usually results in ventricular rates in the range of 160–220 bpm, which are slower than typical orthodromic reciprocating tachycardia rates in this age group.

Junctional ectopic tachycardia (JET), a relatively rare arrhythmia in adults, has proven to be a challenging problem in the immediate postoperative state in infants and young children undergoing open heart surgery. JET is usually associated with myocardial ischemia/necrosis or a poor hemodynamic situation (e.g., pump failure, unresolved outflow tract obstruction, etc.) and may result in heart rates of 200 bpm or greater.[33] Additionally, the tachycardia seems to be exacerbated by endogenous catecholamines released when the patient is in pain or is febrile. The diagnosis depends on clinical suspicion and may be difficult to establish by ECG alone. Epicardial pacing wires placed at time of surgery may be helpful to ascertain the relationship between atrial and ventricular activity; there may be AV dissociation or 1:1 relationship with retrograde conduction during this tachycardia.

Treatment

Therapy of supraventricular tachycardias comprises both termination of acute episodes and subsequent chronic prophylaxis. Not infrequently, careful examination of a 12-lead ECG obtained during tachycardia will provide sufficient information to initiate a therapeutic program. For example, an irregularly irregular tachycardia with a normal QRS complex is most often atrial fibrillation, and treatment may be directed toward termination of the arrhythmia (usually most effectively accomplished by synchronized DC shock). Alternatively, one may choose to slow the ventricular response either transiently by vagal maneuvers, or in a more prolonged manner by pharmacological intervention (beta-adrenergic blockade, calcium channel blockers, or cardiac glycosides). The latter maneuvers will not typically interrupt atrial fibrillation. On the other hand, a regular tachycardia with a normal QRS complex is most often re-entrant in nature, and may terminate with vagal maneuvers, or during infusion of drugs designed to slow AV node conduction (e.g., beta-blockers, calcium channel blockers). However, in many instances, detailed electrophysiological studies may be needed in order to define the nature of the arrhythmia and the electrical characteristics of the cardiac tissues participating in the arrhythmia, thereby permitting more precise treatment selection.

Basic Principles of Treatment of the Acute Episode

Life-threatening tachyarrhythmias necessitate DC cardioversion. Drug therapy in this situation is usually too slow and may be hazardous. JET is an exception to this rule because it will not respond to DC cardioversion. Optimization of the hemodynamic and metabolic status along with ancillary measures such as the use of hypothermia and certain antiarrhythmic agents are the principal recourses available (see below). In the absence of a life-threatening arrhythmia, treatment of re-entrant tachycardia should be aimed at interrupting conduction at some point in the re-entry loop, usually the weakest link. Obviously information obtained at a previous electrophysiological evaluation can prove useful in managing such patients. In the absence of such information, certain assumptions will have to be made, but will be mandatory to avert an undesirable complication.

Often slow conduction within the AV node is the weakest link in re-entrant supraventricular tachycardias, and even transient alteration of conduction within the AV node by vagal maneuvers (e.g., carotid sinus massage, Valsalva) or by infusion of drugs that manifest a strong negative dromotropic effect (e.g., beta-adrenergic blockers, calcium channel blockers [verapamil, diltiazem], adenosine, marketed in 1990 in the US (Adenocard®, Fujisawa Pharmaceutical Co.) may be sufficient to interrupt the critical timing required for re-entry. Alternatively, in those patients in whom an accessory connection is known to be the weak link in the re-entry circuit, conventional membrane active antiarrhythmic drugs may effectively interrupt conduction and terminate re-entry. Procainamide is the usual choice in North America since it is widely available for parenteral use. In general, parenteral cardiac glycosides or calcium channel blockers are contraindicated in patients in whom pre-excitation may be present (see below). For those arrhythmias in which acute therapeutic interventions cannot be aimed directly at an element of the re-entry circuit (e.g., atrial fibrillation, atrial flutter), therapy may be directed either towards terminating the dysrhythmia (DC cardioversion, atrial or transesophageal pacing) and/or diminishing the ventricular response by autonomic and/or pharmacological interventions. Finally, the treatment choice must be made with due consideration for minimizing potential adverse consequences. Thus, the patient presenting with an irregularly irregular rhythm, broad bizarre QRS complexes, and a rapid ventricular response should raise suspicion of atrial fibrillation in the presence of ventricular pre-excitation. Under these circumstances, administration of either parenteral cardiac glycosides or verapamil is contraindicated, having been demonstrated to accelerate the ventricular rate in some patients.[20,30] Use of DC cardioversion or slow intravenous infusion of procainamide would be less prone to complication. Similarly, in patients with reciprocating tachycardia, an apparently stable hemodynamic state may be the result of peripheral compensatory mechanisms. Consequently, administration of antiarrhythmic drugs which also happen to induce vasodilation (e.g., calcium channel blockers, type 1 antiarrhythmic agents) may overwhelm these compensatory mechanisms and result in abrupt hemodynamic collapse. Therefore, careful evaluation of the clinical arrhythmia and a complete understanding of the potential impact of the various therapeutic alternatives are essential prior to embarking on a treatment course.

Basic Principles of Prophylaxis

Prevention of SVT recurrences is based upon both reducing the number of potential triggering events (usually PVCs, PACs), and diminishing the likelihood of a sustained re-entry circuit being maintained. The former is most effectively achieved by use of conventional type 1 membrane active antiarrhythmic drugs (e.g., quinidine, procainamide, encainide, flecainide; the last two drugs do not presently carry an indication for this use). The latter may be affected by use of beta-adrenergic blockers or calcium channel blockers alone or in combination with membrane-active agents. Cardiac glycosides may also play a role in long-term prophylaxis of re-entrant SVT, but are probably less effective than agents that act more directly on conduction tissue. Cardiac glycosides (even in their oral form) are best avoided in patients with pre-excitation syndrome, since acceleration of antegrade conduction over accessory connections remains a concern.

Treatment of Specific Tachyarrhythmias

Primary Atrial Tachycardias

Management of atrial flutter and fibrillation is detailed elsewhere. However, as noted above, although ventricular response may slow these arrhythmias, they would not be expected to terminate during vagal maneuvers, or with infusion of drugs that slow conduction in the AV node or sinus node regions. As a rule, termination of atrial fibrillation or flutter is best achieved by synchronous DC cardioversion under general anesthetic. Occasionally, infusion of a type 1 antiarrhythmic agent (e.g., procainamide) may be chosen as a means of conversion, although this approach is slower and less effective. In either case, careful consideration should be given to prophylactic anticoagulation prior to proceeding with conversion, especially if the arrhythmia has been present for more than a few days. Sinus node re-entrant tachycardia is only rarely a clinical problem and may be amenable to agents that slow conduction in the sinoatrial junction (e.g., beta-adrenergic blockers, calcium channel blockers) as well as to agents that act directly on the conduction properties of the remainder of the atrium (type 1 antiarrhythmic drugs). The presumed automatic atrial tachycardias (e.g., multifocal atrial tachycardia) are often resistant to conventional antiarrhythmic drug therapy and their treatment depends to a large extent on management of the underlying chronic disease process with which they are most frequently associated.

Surgical or electrode catheter ablation techniques may be helpful in treatment of drug-refractory primary atrial tachycardias. Intraoperative mapping and surgical ablation has proved successful in some patients with ectopic or re-entrant atrial tachycardias arising in the left atrium. On the other hand, similar techniques have been notably unsuccessful for right atrial tachycardias presumably due to a greater propensity to multicentric origins. More commonly, patients with intractable primary atrial arrhythmias may find benefit from electrode catheter ablation of the AV node-His bundle.[34] The latter procedure has largely superseded surgical His bundle ablation and has proved particularly useful in many patients whose medical condition precludes a surgical procedure aimed directly at the arrhythmia.

Antitachycardia cardiac pacing techniques are not widely used in patients with primary atrial tachycardias. However, such techniques may be successful in selected patients with refractory atrial flutter or in individuals with well-defined intra-atrial or sinus node re-entry. In such cases, detailed electrophysiological testing is required. Specialized antitachycardia pacemakers should be prescribed only by physicians experienced in their application and follow-up.

Re-entry Within the AV Node

Susceptibility to AV nodal re-entry tachycardia is usually characterized by dual AV nodal pathway physiology. Since one of these pathways tends to exhibit relatively slow conduction, it is frequently amenable to block by enhancement of vagal tone reflexly (e.g., carotid sinus massage, Valsalva maneuver) or pharmacologically (tensilon, cardiac glycosides), or by cautious intravenous administration of beta-adrenergic (e.g., propranolol 1 mg/kg IV) or calcium channel blocking drugs (e.g., verapamil 5–10 mg IV), or adenosine or adenosine triphosphate (ATP). Alternatively, although less reliably, the so-called fast pathway may be blocked by conventional type 1 antiarrhythmic drugs (e.g., procainamide). Alternatively, transesophageal or intra-atrial pacing, or DC cardioversion are highly effective.

Chronic prophylaxis of AV nodal re-entry tachycardia usually relies on either beta-adrenergic or calcium channel blocking drugs. However, not infrequently it proves necessary to obtain the synergistic effects of treating both limbs of the re-entrant pathway by drug combinations. Thus, both AV nodal blocking drugs and type 1 antiarrhythmic agents are used together. Of note, the use of type 1 antiarrhythmic drugs has the advantage of suppressing premature atrial or ventricular extrasystoles which are the most common initiating events for re-entry tachycardias. Amiodarone (a type 3 drug), while potentially highly effective in this setting, is rarely indicated due to its frequent undesirable long-term side effects.

Surgical treatment for elimination of susceptibility to AV nodal re-entrant tachycardia has recently been described.[35,36] The procedure appears to be effective in skilled hands and may represent an appropriate therapy for patients in whom drug therapy has proved inadequate or in whom the rhythm disturbance results in catastrophic symptoms (e.g., syncope). In addition, implantable antitachycardia pacing systems may be very effective for patients with refractory AV nodal re-entrant tachycardia. Available implantable pacing systems have the capability of utilizing a wide range of pacing techniques to terminate tachycardia (Fig. 14). Selection of the optimal device and pacing modality requires detailed electrophysiological study and should be undertaken only by experienced individuals.

Re-entry Utilizing an Accessory AV Connection

In patients with accessory AV connections, DC cardioversion or atrial pacing techniques are often highly effective for acute termination of reciprocating tachycardia. When pharmacological therapy is selected, it is usually directed at interrupting or altering AV nodal conduction by cautious intravenous infusion of beta-adrenergic or calcium channel blocking drugs. Adenosine and adenosine triphosphate (both investigational at present) may also be highly effective, but are presently restricted to clinical investigation. Alternatively, in certain patients in whom the accessory connections have been determined by electrophysiological study to comprise the "weak link" of the re-entry circuit,

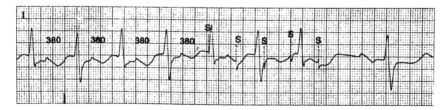

Figure 14. Rhythm strip from a patient with a re-entrant atrial tachycardia that responded to implantation of an automatic antitachycardia pacemaker. In this example, the tachycardia (cycle length 380 ms) is detected by the device and a series of pacing stimuli (S) are automatically inserted based upon a previously determined effective pacing sequence. Sinus rhythm is restored (at right) by interruption of the re-entry circuit by the stimulation sequence.

careful infusion of procainamide may be highly effective. Again, one needs to be aware of the potential for cardiac glycosides and/or verapamil to accelerate conduction over accessory connections. The latter agents should be avoided in the acute treatment of tachycardia where there is doubt regarding the presence of ventricular pre-excitation (e.g., Wolff-Parkinson-White syndrome).

Chronic prophylaxis of orthodromic reciprocating tachycardia may often best be achieved by combined application of drugs aimed at both altering AV nodal conduction (beta-adrenergic blockers, calcium channel blockers) and impeding conduction in the accessory connection (type 1 antiarrhythmic drugs and rarely amiodarone). However, it is possible that excessive conduction slowing may inadvertently enhance susceptibility to development of re-entry, a potential proarrhythmic effect. Consequently, careful electrophysiological evaluation is recommended before embarking upon empiric combined drug regimens.

Patients with pre-excitation syndromes present therapeutic problems of particular importance. First, individuals with atrial fibrillation and rapid conduction in the antegrade direction over accessory AV connections may exhibit potentially life-threatening ventricular responses. Immediate treatment of these individuals is most safely and effectively achieved by DC cardioversion. Alternatively, careful infusion of antiarrhythmic drugs such as procainamide may slow the ventricular response and terminate the atrial arrhythmia. On the other hand, administration of cardiac glycosides or calcium channel blockers such as verapamil are contraindicated as they may accelerate the ventricular response. Additionally, excessively rapid parenteral administration of almost any antiarrhythmic drug may provoke marked hypotension and result in acute hemodynamic deterioration.

Implantable antitachycardia pacemakers may be effective for terminating reciprocating tachycardia in patients with accessory AV connections. However, of special concern in individuals with pre-excitation syndromes is the potential for induction of atrial fibrillation by aggressive atrial pacing techniques. The use of antitachycardia pacing systems for control of arrhythmias in patients with accessory AV connections necessitates careful electrophysiological study and should remain in the hands of experienced individuals.

Surgical ablation of accessory AV connections is now highly successful and is frequently recommended not only for individuals with life-threatening arrhythmias but also for those in whom the tachycardias or the pharmacological treatment result in adverse lifestyle consequences. Detailed intracardiac mapping during electrophysiological study and intraoperative mapping at the time of surgical ablation is essential in order to achieve the outstanding success rate reported for this surgery (Fig. 15). Both open and closed heart surgical techniques have been advocated for accessory connection ablation. The results of both approaches are comparable and the choice of the operative procedure depends primarily on the preference of the surgical team.

Recently, electrode catheter techniques have been developed for transvenous ablation (fulguration) of accessory AV connections in the posteroseptal region.[40] The number of procedures reported is small but the technique appears promising in skilled hands. In essence, the procedure parallels that utilized for AV node-His bundle ablation except that the electrode catheter is positioned in the vicinity of the os of the coronary sinus. At present, accessory connections other than in the region of the posterior septal zone are not readily amenable to this technique. However, development of techniques for recording accessory

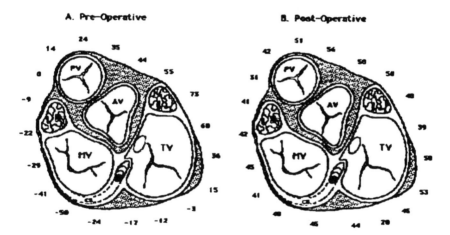

Figure 15. Epicardial activation sequence maps prior to (A) and following (B) surgical ablation of an accessory AV connection in a patient with Wolff-Parkinson-White syndrome. In each panel, the atrioventricular groove of the heart is depicted. In panel A, earliest epicardial activation occurs in a left posterior position (−50 ms with respect to onset of the QRS complex) during atrial pacing. This finding is compatible with the presence of an accessory AV connection crossing the AV groove from the left atrium to the posterior aspect of the left ventricle. In panel B, following surgical dissection of the AV groove using an external approach, the activation sequence of the ventricles is now normalized. The patient has subsequently been free of paroxysmal tachycardias, and the ECG now reveals a normal QRS complex without evidence of ventricular pre-excitation.

connection electrograms,[41] and availability of both new mapping catheters and alternative energy sources make the likelihood of successful ablation of right-sided accessory AV connections increasingly likely.

Pre-excitation Variants

Treatment of tachycardias associated with nodoventricular and fasciculoventricular connections relies primarily upon pharmacological therapy. As a rule, these tachycardias require treatment with membrane-active antiarrhythmic agents and are not adequately controlled by beta-adrenergic blockers or calcium channel blockers alone. Recently, surgical techniques have been developed for ablation of nodoventricular connections. However, the effectiveness of these surgical procedures is unclear and they are not widely available. Implantable antitachycardia pacing systems may prove helpful in patients with particularly difficult to control arrhythmias.

Supraventricular Tachycardia in Infants

The immediate treatment of supraventricular tachycardia in infancy depends on the severity of the clinical picture. In the acutely ill infant, DC cardioversion is the treatment of choice. This approach will terminate most re-entry tachycardias although some may restart and antiarrhythmic drug therapy may be necessary to suppress reinitiation. DC cardioversion will not be effective in patients exhibiting sinus tachycardia or junctional ectopic tachycardia (JET).

In less dire circumstances, both orthodromic reciprocating tachycardia and atrial flutter can be terminated by transesophageal pacing technique. This procedure has the further advantage of facilitating establishment of a definitive diagnosis by documenting the atrial and ventricular relationship and timing. If pacing facilities or expertise are not available, patients with orthodromic reciprocating tachycardia may be treated by vagal maneuvers (recalling that ocular compression is no longer considered safe) or parenteral administration of tensilon. Although use of parenteral verapamil in infants for acute termination of supraventricular tachycardia initially had many supporters, there have subsequently been reports of hemodynamic compromise with its use.[42] The latter has been a problem, particularly in infants with congestive heart failure or when verapamil was used in combination with other antiarrhythmic agents. Therefore, as a rule, verapamil should not be used in young infants, and particularly in the absence of a definitive tachycardia diagnosis.

Long-term prevention of recurrent orthodromic reciprocating tachycardia in infants has traditionally consisted of no treatment or the use of cardiac glycosides. The former is often effective in as much as many infants seem to "out grow" their tachycardia. In fact, the susceptibility to tachycardia probably remains but these infants manifest fewer initiating events (premature atrial or ventricular beats, sinus acceleration) over the first few months of life and consequently have fewer tachycardia episodes. However, tachycardia may recur later in life. Among patients treated with digoxin, on the other hand, tachycardia recurrences have been reported to be as frequent as in the untreated patient.[43]

Management of junctional ectopic tachycardia is critically dependent upon recognition and treatment of the underlying hemodynamic or metabolic problem. On occasion, rapid atrial pacing may be useful in order to achieve 2:1 AV block and thereby slow the ventricular rate. However, in many infants, AV nodal conduction is sufficiently rapid that this technique is ineffective. Pharmacological therapy addressing the tachycardia directly (such as use of beta-adrenergic blocking drugs or verapamil) may result in catastrophic hemodynamic deterioration. On occasion, procainamide has been effective as has the investigational antiarrhythmic agent propafenone. However, the negative inotropic effects and vasodilator capacity of antiarrhythmic drugs may result in exacerbation of an already tenuous hemodynamic state. Hypothermia has been noted to be useful adjunctive therapy in a few patients.

Summary

Supraventricular tachycardias comprise a wide range of arrhythmias, and for the most part, ECG findings alone are inadequate to provide a definitive diagnosis. Intracardiac electrophysiological studies have markedly increased our understanding of these arrhythmias and their treatment. Given the wide variety of treatment options now available, it is increasingly important to assess these arrhythmias fully before embarking upon long-term treatment programs. Consequently, familiarity with the differential diagnosis of supraventricular tachycardias and the clinical electrophysiological techniques available for their evaluation has important therapeutic implications.

Acknowledgment: The authors would like to express their appreciation to Barry L.S. Detloff and Barbara Borgwardt for technical assistance and Wendy Markuson for preparation of the manuscript.

References

1. Fisher JD: Role of electrophysiologic testing in the diagnosis and treatment of patients with known and suspected bradycardias and tachycardias. Prog Cardiovasc Dis 24:25, 1981.
2. Morady F, Scheinman MM: Paroxysmal supraventricular tachycardia. Mod Concepts Cardiovasc Dis 51:107, 1982.
3. Benditt DG, Benson DW Jr, Dunnigan A, Gornick CC, Anderson RW: Atrial flutter, atrial fibrillation, and other primary atrial tachycardias. Med Clin N Am 68:895, 1984.
4. Olshansky B, Waldo AL: Atrial fibrillation: update on mechanism, diagnosis, and management. Mod Concepts Cardiovasc Dis 56:23, 1987.
5. Gornick CC, Benson DW Jr: Electrocardiographic aspects of the preexcitation syndromes. In: Benditt DG, Benson DW Jr (eds), Cardiac Preexcitation Syndromes: Origins, Evaluation and Treatment. Boston, Martinus-Nijhoff, 1986, pp 43–73.
6. Anderson RH, Becker AE, Brechenmacher C, et al: Ventricular preexcitation: a proposed nomenclature for its substrates. Eur Heart J 3:27, 1975.
7. Allessie MA, Bonke FIM: Re-entry within the sinoatrial node as demonstrated by multiple micro-electrode recordings in the isolated rabbit heart. In: Bonke FIM (ed), The Sinus Node: Structure, Function and Clinical Relevance. The Hague, Martinus Nijhoff, 1978, pp 409–421.
8. Childers R, Arnsdorf M, De La Fuente D, et al: Sinus nodal echoes: clinical case report and canine studies. Am J Cardiol 31:220, 1973.
9. Narula OS: Sinus node re-entry: a mechanism for supraventricular tachycardia. Circulation 50:1114, 1974.
10. Weisfogel GM, Batsford WP, Paulay KL, et al: Sinus node re-entrant tachycardia in man. Am Heart J 90:295, 1975.
11. Curry PVL, Callowhill E, Krikler DM: Paroxysmal re-entry sinus tachycardia. Proceedings of the British Cardiac Society. (abstract) Br Heart J 38:311, 1976.
12. Wellens HJJ: Role of sinus re-entry in the genesis of sustained cardiac arrhythmias. In: Bonke FIM (ed), The Sinus Node: Structure, Function and Clinical Relevance. The Hague, Martinus Nijhoff, 1978, pp 422–427.
13. Strauss HC, Geer MR: Sinoatrial node re-entry. In: Kulbertus HE (ed), Reentrant Arrhythmias: Mechanisms and Treatment. Lancester, MTP Press, 1977, pp 39–62.
14. Gomes JA, Hariman RJ, Kang PS, et al: Sustained symptomatic sinus node reentrant tachycardia: incidence, clinical significance, electrophysiologic observations and the effects of antiarrhythmic agents. J Am Coll Cardiol 5:45, 1985.
15. Wellens HJJ: General conclusions. In: Bonke FIM (ed), The Sinus Node: Structure, Function and Clinical Relevance. The Hague, Martinus Nijhoff, 1978, pp 428.
16. Kirchhof CJHJ, Bonke FIM, Allessie MA: Sinus node reentry: fact of fiction.

In: Brugada P, Wellens HJJ. (ed), Cardiac Arrhythmias: Where to Go from Here? Mount Kisco, NY, Futura Publishing Company Inc., 1987. pp 53–65.
17. Dhingra RC, Wyndham C, Amat-y-Leon F, et al: Sinus nodal responses to atrial extrastimuli in patients without apparent sinus node disease. Am J Cardiol 36:445, 1975.
18. Dunnigan A, Pierpont ME, Smith S, et al: Cardiac and skeletal myopathy in patients with cardiac dysrhythmias. Am J Cardiol 53:731, 1984.
19. Gallagher JJ, et al: Multiple accessory pathways in patients with preexcitation syndrome. Circulation 54:571, 1976.
20. Gallagher JJ, Pritchett ELC, Sealy WC, et al: The preexcitation syndromes. Prog Cardiovasc Dis 20:285, 1978.
21. Klein GJ, Bashore TM, Sellers TD, et al: Ventricular fibrillation in the Wolff-Parkinson-White syndrome. N Engl J Med 301:1080, 1979.
22. Gallagher JJ: Role of nodoventricular and fasciculoventricular connections in tachyarrhythmias. In: Benditt DG, Benson DW Jr (eds), Cardiac Preexcitation Syndromes: Origins, Evaluation and Treatment. Boston, Martinus-Nijhoff, 1986, pp 201–232.
23. Benditt DG, Dunbar D, Almquist A, et al: AV node bypass tracts and enhanced AV conduction: relation to ventricular preexcitation. In: Benditt DG, Benson DW, Jr (eds), Cardiac Preexcitation Syndromes: Origins, Evaluation and Treatment. Boston, Martinus-Nijhoff, 1986, pp 507–526.
24. Benditt DG, Pritchett ELC, Smith WM, et al: Characteristics of atrioventricular conduction and spectrum of arrhythmias in Lown-Ganong-Levine syndrome. Circulation 57:454, 1978.
25. Benditt DG, Epstein ML, Arentzen CE, et al: Enhanced atrioventricular conduction in patients without preexcitation syndrome: relation to heart rate in paroxysmal reciprocating tachycardia. Circulation 65:1474, 1982.
26. Lown B, Ganong WF, Levine SA: The syndrome of short P-R interval, normal QRS complex and paroxysmal rapid heart action. Circulation 5:693, 1952.
27. Gettes L, Zipes DP, Gillet TC, et al: Personnel and equipment required for electrophysiologic testing: report of the Committee on Electrocardiography and Cardiac Electrophysiology, Council on Clinical Cardiology, American Heart Association. Circulation 69:1219, 1984.
28. Benditt DG, Pritchett ELC, Smith WM, et al: Ventriculoatrial intervals: diagnostic use in paroxysmal supraventricular tachycardia. Ann Intern Med 91:161, 1979.
29. Milstein S, Sharma AD, Guirandon GM, et al: An algorithm for the electrocardiographic localization of accessory pathways in the Wolff-Parkinson-White syndrome. PACE 10:555, 1987.
30. Benson DW Jr, Dunnigan A: Treatment of pediatric patients with preexcitation syndromes. In: Benditt DG, Benson DW Jr (eds), Cardiac Preexcitation Syndromes: Origins, Evaluation and Treatment. Boston, Martinus-Nijhoff, 1986, pp 465–480.
31. Benson DW Jr, Dunnigan A, Benditt DG, et al: Transesophageal cardiac pacing: history, application, technique. Clin Prog Pacing Electrophysiol 2:360, 1984.
32. Benson DW Jr, Dunnigan A, Benditt DG, et al: Transesophagel study of infant supraventricular tachycardia: electrophysiologic characteristics. Am J Cardiol 52:1002, 1983.

33. Garson A Jr, Gillette PC: Junctional ectopic tachycardia in children: electro-cardiography, electrophysiology, and pharmacologic response. Am J Cardiol 44:298, 1979.
34. Scheinman MM, Evans-Bell T, and the Executive Committee of the Percu-taneous Cardiac Mapping and Ablation Registry: Catheter ablation of the atrioventricular junction. Circulation 70:1024, 1984.
35. Ross DL, Johnson DC, Denniss AR, et al: Curative surgery for atrioven-tricular junctional (AV nodal) reentrant tachycardia. J Am Coll Cardiol 6:1383, 1985.
36. Cox JL, Holman WL, Cain ME: Cryosurgical treatment of atrioventricular node reentrant tachycardia. Circulation 76:1329, 1987.
37. Guirauden GM, Klein GJ, Sharma AD, et al: Closed-heart technique for Wolff-Parkinson-White syndrome: further experiences and potential limi-tations. Ann Thorac Surg 42:651, 1986.
38. Sealy WC, Hattler BG, Blumenshein SD, et al: Surgical treatment of Wolff-Parkinson-White syndrome. Ann Thorac Surg 8:1, 1969.
39. Cox JL, Gallagher JJ, Cain ME: Experience with 118 consecutive patients undergoing operation for the Wolff-Parkinson-White syndrome. J Thorac Cardiovasc Surg 90:490, 1985.
40. Scheinman MM: Catheter ablation for patients with ventricular preexcitation syndromes. In: Benditt DG, Benson DW Jr (eds), Cardiac Preexcitation Syn-dromes: Origins, Evaluation and Treatment. Boston, Martinus-Nijhoff, 1986, pp 493–506.
41. Jackman WM: New catheter techniques for recording accessory AV pathway activation. In: Benditt DG, Benson DW Jr (eds), Cardiac Preexcitation Syn-dromes: Origins, Evaluation and Treatment. Boston, Martinus-Nijhoff, 1986, pp 413–434.
42. Epstein ML, Kiel EA, Victorica BE: Cardiac decompensation following ver-apamil therapy in infants with supraventricular tachycardia. Pediatrics 75:737, 1985.
43. Benson DW Jr, Dunnigan A, Benditt DG, et al: Prediction of digoxin treat-ment failure in infant supraventricular tachycardia: role of transesophageal pacing. Pediatrics 75:288, 1985.

Chapter 7

Diagnosis and Management of Patients with Primary Atrial Arrhythmias

Ellison Berns and Gerald V. Naccarelli

Introduction

Primary atrial arrhythmias are those that require neither the conduction system (AV node, His-Purkinje) nor ventricular tissue for initiation or maintenance. Atrial fibrillation and flutter are the most commonly occurring primary atrial arrhythmias. Other include uniform and multiform ectopic atrial tachycardia and, less commonly, intra-atrial and sinus node re-entrant tachycardias. The purpose of this chapter is to provide an overview of the mechanism, natural history, and approach to diagnosis and management of the most common atrial arrhythmias.

Mechanism

The electrophysiological mechanisms of atrial arrhythmias in man remain unclear. Most theories are derived from cellular and animal models. Ectopic atrial arrhythmias appear to arise from disorders of impulse generation either by abnormal automaticity through enhancement of normal ionic mechanisms or by triggered activity during or following

From Naccarelli GV (ed): *Cardiac Arrhythmias: A Practical Approach.* Mount Kisco, NY, Futura Publishing Co., Inc., © 1991.

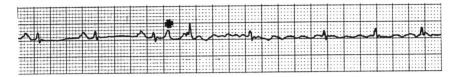

Figure 1. Lead 2 rhythm strip showing spontaneous initiation of atrial fibrillation by a premature atrial beat (asterisk). The ventricular response to the PAC is of right bundle branch block aberrancy typical of Ashman's phenomenon. The irregular baseline that follows the premature contraction is characteristic of atrial fibrillatory activity.

repolarization (afterdepolarizations).[1,2] This may explain why some of these arrhythmias occur with stress, exercise, or digitalis toxicity.

Re-entry is the most widely accepted mechanism used to explain atrial fibrillation and atrial flutter.[1,3] Anatomical or physiological conditions provide the necessary substrate to sustain re-entry within atrial tissue. In the case of atrial flutter, a single organized circuit usually propagates in a caudocranial direction at a particular cycle length, thereby determining the rate of tachycardia. On the other hand, multiple re-entrant wavelets with irregular and rapid propagation patterns are the most likely explanation for atrial fibrillation.[3] Premature atrial beats frequently act as a trigger to initiate the arrhythmia (Fig. 1). However, therapies directed toward reducing the frequency of these triggers may not prevent recurrences because supraventricular tachycardias such as AV nodal or orthodromic atrioventricular re-entrant tachycardias may precipitate or degenerate into an atrial arrhythmia (Fig. 2).[4,7]

Etiology and Natural History

Coronary artery disease, rheumatic and hypertensive heart diseases, and congestive heart failure from any cause are commonly associated with the development of atrial fibrillation and flutter. Table 1 lists other causes. Atrial fibrillation is more common than atrial flutter with the latter usually converting to sinus rhythm or degenerating into atrial fibrillation. A large left atrium predisposes toward the development of atrial fibrillation regardless of the type of underlying heart disease.[8] Patients with previous episodes of paroxysmal atrial fibrillation are at higher risk for recurrence and development of chronic atrial fibrillation.[9] Acute conversion and maintenance of sinus rhythm may depend more on the duration of atrial fibrillation than on left or right atrial

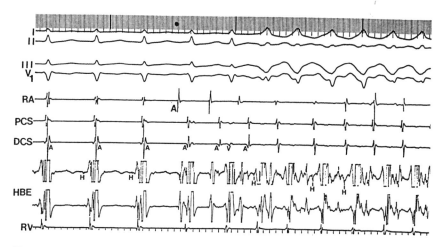

Figure 2. Intracardiac recording of AV nodal re-entrant supraventricular tachycardia with spontaneous development of atrial tachycardia. Following the third beat of tachycardia, an atrial tachycardia, labeled A on the RA channel, develops with 1:1 antidromic conduction at an average rate of 240 bpm. Surface recordings include limb leads 1–3 and precordial lead V_1. Intracardiac recordings are from the high right atrium (RA), proximal (PCS), and distal (DCS) coronary sinus, His bundle region (HBE), and right ventricular apex (RV).

Table 1
Etiologies of Atrial Fibrillations

Hypertensive cardiovascular disease
Coronary artery disease
Rheumatic mitral valve disease (mitral stenosis or regurgitation)
Cardiomyopathy (dilated or hypertrophic)
Congestive heart failure
Tachycardia-bradycardia (sick sinus) syndrome
Post-thoracotomy
Hyperthyroidism
Pericarditis
Congenital heart disease
Idiopathic
Wolff-Parkinson-White syndrome
Alcohol
Pulmonary embolism

---

size.[9–11] However, spontaneous or chemical conversion will more likely occur if there is a small rather than a large left atrium even if treatment is undertaken within a few days following the onset of atrial fibrillation.[9,14–17] Once established, atrial fibrillation more than doubles overall mortality, perhaps as a result of an increased thromboembolic risk from progressive left atrial enlargement, underlying cardiovascular disease and a generally older patient population in atrial fibrillation.[12,13,18,19] Patients without identifiable heart disease and "lone" or idiopathic atrial fibrillation have few complications and probably little change in mortality because of their arrhythmia.[18–21]

Patients with uniform ectopic atrial tachycardia generally have evidence of pulmonary or coronary artery disease. While frequently associated with an acute myocardial infarction, the most common cause is digitalis toxicity with or without hypokalemia.[9] Multiform ectopic atrial tachycardia (MAT) most commonly occurs in the setting of diabetes, decompensated pulmonary disease, or theophylline toxicity, but rarely as a manifestation of digitalis intoxication.[9]

Diagnosis and Electrocardiographic Features

Patients presenting with atrial arrhythmias may be asymptomatic or complain of palpitations, shortness of breath, or dizziness. Hypotension, syncope, and congestive heart failure are a function of ventricular rate, degree of underlying ventricular dysfunction, and dependence upon the atrial contribution for left ventricular filling and cardiac output. It is difficult to discern one atrial arrhythmia from another by physical examination. A jugular venous pulse pressure with discreet flutter waves suggests atrial flutter or tachycardia; fibrillatory waves associated with a variable intensity to S_1 during auscultation is consistent with atrial fibrillation.

Each atrial arrhythmia has distinctive electrocardiographic features.[2] Atrial fibrillation inscribes irregular baseline undulations or discrete atrial activity of variable amplitude at rates of 350–600 beats per minute. These atrial deflections are best seen in limb lead 2 or precordial lead V_1 (Fig. 3). In either case, the ventricular response is usually irregular (Fig. 3) ranging from 100 to 180 beats per minute in untreated patients. On the other hand, atrial flutter rates range from 250 to 350 beats per minute, with the usual being 300 beats per minute.

The P wave is usually negative in the inferior or precordial leads and there is no isoelectric segment between P waves. This results in the

V_1

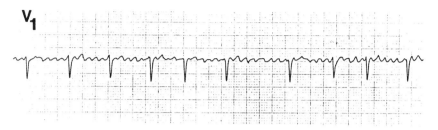

Figure 3. Lead V_1 rhythm strip demonstrating typical electrocardiographic features of atrial fibrillation. Note the irregular fibrillating undulations and the irregularly, irregular ventricular response.

characteristic sawtooth pattern. The ventricular response is usually regular and half the atrial rate, most commonly 150 beats per minute (Fig. 4).

Uniform ectopic atrial tachycardia inscribes a P wave that is morphologically distinct from the sinus P wave with rates of 150–280 beats per minute. Slower atrial rates with multiple P wave morphologies and variable P-P intervals differentiate multiform ectopic atrial tachycardia from the uniform variety (Fig. 5). In both instances, the P wave is separated from another by an isoelectric baseline. Table 2 summarizes the major ECG findings of each of the atrial arrhythmias. It should be noted that treated patients frequently have rates that are slower than those outlined for untreated arrhythmias.

Finally, patients with Wolff-Parkinson-White (WPW) syndrome who present with an atrial dysrhythmia associated with an antegrade conducting accessory pathway will have an ECG with a wide (>.12 sec) and bizarre-appearing QRS (Fig. 6). This can be confused with ventricular tachycardia when the atrial arrhythmia is associated with a regular ventricular response, as usually seen with atrial flutter or uniform ectopic atrial tachycardia. On the other hand, the highly irregular ven-

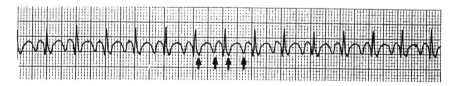

Figure 4. Lead 2 rhythm strip demonstrating typical atrial flutter with inscription of negative P waves (arrows) at a rate of 300 bpm. The ventricular response is one-half the atrial rate, or 150 bpm.

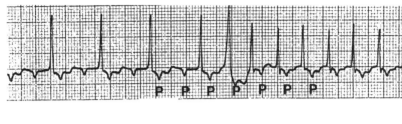

A

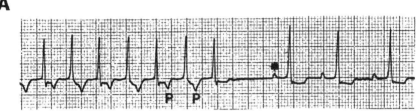

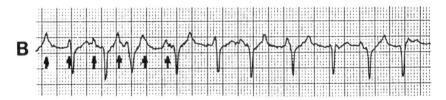

B

Figure 5. Different types of atrial tachycardias: (A) demonstrates uniform ectopic atrial tachycardia with 2:1 and 1:1 AV node conduction. Notice the P morphology of the tachycardia is different from sinus node activity (star). (B) shows the variable atrial rate and morphology characteristic of MAT. In both instances there is an isoelectric baseline between atrial deflections.

tricular response seen with other atrial arrhythmias makes the distinction from ventricular tachycardia easier because ventricular tachycardia is generally regular. In addition, grouping of narrow and then wide complexes with long pauses preceding the wide beats should also suggest conduction over an accessory pathway rather than ventricular tachycardia or aberrant conduction over the normal conducting system (Figs. 6 and 7). Aberrant conduction usually occurs when a short R-R interval follows a long R-R interval (Ashman's phenomenon) with the ensuing wide beats frequently assuming a right bundle branch block configuration (Figs. 1 and 8).

Table 2
ECG Features of Untreated Atrial Arrhythmias

	Atrial Activity	Ventricular Activity
Atrial fibrillation	No or irregular P waves, variable amplitude 350–600 bpm	Grossly irregular 100–160 bpm
Atrial flutter	Negative P waves, inferior levels, regular 250–350 bpm (usually 300)	Regular, ½ atrial rate usually 150 bpm
Uniform ectopic atrial tachycardia	Uniform, P waves distinct from sinus, gradual rate changes 100–280 bpm	Variable, can be same as atrial rate
Multiform atrial tachycardia	Three or more different P waves, irregular 100–220 bpm	Grossly irregular, same as atrial rate

Evaluation

History and physical examination may help diagnose an associated condition that is responsible for the arrhythmia. Echocardiography is useful to confirm the presence or absence of organic heart disease by demonstrating wall thickness and motion, chamber sizes, pericardial fluid, valvular abnormalities, and regurgitant jets. An echocardiographically determined left atrial size should not be solely used to determine if cardioversion should be attempted because there are no studies demonstrating an absolute atrial size which precludes restoration of sinus rhythm. Finally, echocardiographic detection of an atrial thrombus is technically difficult, making this test of little use for determining embolic risk.

Correlation of symptoms with the presence of arrhythmia is extremely important before treatment is undertaken to confirm the diagnosis and possibility to utilize symptoms as a guide to therapeutic efficacy.

Chronic arrhythmias are easily documented by ECG. Paroxysmal arrhythmias are more difficult to record. Continuous ECG monitoring (Holter monitoring) for 24–48 hours rarely captures infrequent, symp-

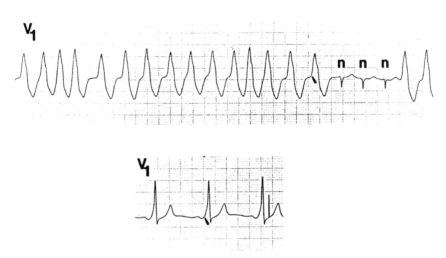

Figure 6. Top tracing demonstrates wide QRS irregular rhythm secondary to atrial fibrillation and antegrade conduction down an accessory pathway. Note several normal (n) conducting beats secondary to conduction down the AV node. Bottom tracing shows lead V₁ of same patient in sinus rhythm. Arrow marks delta wave. Note similarity in conduction of wide QRS beats to pre-excited beats in sinus rhythm.

tomatic episodes, but may record nonsustained asymptomatic runs that may represent an electrical instability and predisposition for a sustained event.[22] Holter recordings can also document concomitant ventricular arrhythmias and bradycardias that might influence therapy (Fig. 9). When a patient's history suggests exertion as a initiating factor, exercise treadmill testing may occasionally precipitate an episode of atrial fibrillation or uniform ectopic atrial tachycardia.[22–25] Finally, patient-activated transtelephonic event recorders can record the heart rhythm during symptoms and define the type of arrhythmia.[22]

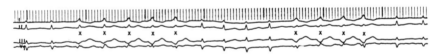

Figure 7. Recordings made during an electrophysiology study following induction of atrial fibrillation in a patient with WPW using surface recordings from limb leads 1–3 and precordial lead V₁. Notice the grouping of wide (labeled X) and narrow complexes, the irregularity of the wide beats, and the long pauses preceding the wide complexes. This pattern is most consistent with antidromic conduction over an accessory pathway.

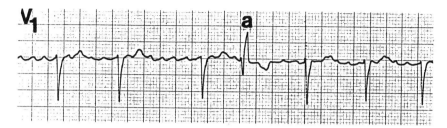

Figure 8. Lead V₁ rhythm strip demonstrating atrial fibrillation and a right bundle branch aberrant (a) beat secondary to Ashman's phenomena. Note that the aberrancy occurs when a short R-R interval follows a long R-R interval.

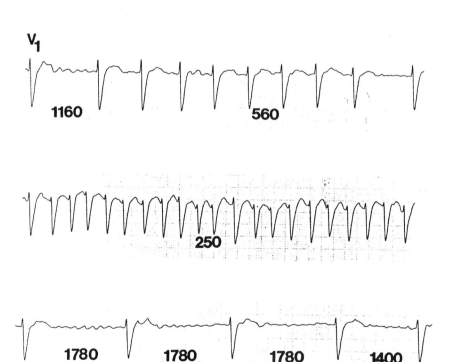

Figure 9. Holter lead V₁ of same patient, demonstrating relatively controlled ventricular response in top panel, rapid ventricular response averaging 240 bpm in middle panel, and a junctional escape rhythm at 34 bpm in bottom panel.

Once diagnosed, Holter monitoring or transtelephonic recordings may objectively confirm symptomatic recurrences and determine if the frequency of asymptomatic runs has been decreased by therapy. Patients with persistent atrial arrhythmias in whom the major therapeutic goal is to control the ventricular response under a variety of physiological conditions should have their heart rates recorded with Holter monitoring and possibly treadmill testing.

Treatment

There are two general acute and chronic treatment strategies for atrial arrhythmias: control of ventricular response or restoration and maintenance of sinus rhythm.[26] Except for the WPW syndrome, the ventricular response to an atrial arrhythmia is usually dependent upon propagation of impulses through the AV node. Table 3 outlines the most commonly used pharmacological agents that control the ventricular response to an atrial dysrhythmia. All of these agents that control heart rate act at the level of the AV node. The route of drug administration depends upon the urgency of the clinical situation. Intravenous beta- or calcium blocking agents are often more effective than digitalis for controlling the ventricular rate.[27,28]

When verapamil is administered over a 1–2 minute period, maximal effect on the AV node is achieved within 2–3 minutes with its total duration of action lasting about 30 minutes.[29] Verapamil should be used cautiously in patients with a history of left ventricular dysfunction, tachycardia-bradycardia syndrome, or concurrent use of beta-blockers. In addition, IV verapamil is a potent vasodilator and may produce profound hypotension, especially if the blood pressure is already low (<100 mm Hg).

Intravenous beta-blockers, such as propranolol, may also achieve significant AV node conduction slowing, especially when a rapid ventricular response is due to a heightened adrenergic state as frequently seen postoperatively. Esmolol is an IV beta-blocker with an acute onset of action similar to propranolol but a rapid half-life of 9 minutes.[30] Because of its short half-life, this medication may provide an added element of safety. Studies with esmolol, propranolol, and verapamil demonstrate that they are equally effective for controlling ventricular rates and have a similar incidence of drug-induced hypotension.[27,31,32] While hypotension is generally well tolerated, additional interventions besides discon-

Table 3
Pharmacological Therapies of Atrial Arrhythmias

Drug	Loading Dose	Maintenance Dose
Agents to Control Ventricular Response		
Digoxin	0.75–1.0 mg IV	0.125–0.25 mg QOD-QD
	0.75–1.5 mg PO	PO or IV
Propranolol	0.15–0.20 mg/kg IV	20–80 mg Q6H PO or IV
Esmolol	500 µg/kg/min IV	50–300 µg/kg/min IV
	loading doses	
Verapamil	5–10 mg IV	80–160 mg Q6–8 PO hr
		0.005 mg/kg/min IV
Agents to Restore and Maintain Sinus Rhythm		
Propranolol†	0.15–20 mg/kg IV	20–80 mg Q6H PO
Procainamide†	10–15 mg/kg IV	2–6 mg/min IV
		500–1000 mg Q4H PO
Quinidine†		200–600 mg Q6H PO
Disopyramide*†		100–200 mg Q6H PO
Flecainide*		100–200 mg BID PO
Encainide*		25–50 mg TID PO
Propafenone*		150–300 mg TID PO
Amiodarone*		200–800 mg QD PO

* Not FDA-approved for treatment of SVT.
† Sustained release formulations available.

tinuing the infusion are frequently required when agents other than esmolol are used.

Finally, patients who have severe hypotension, congestive heart failure, or angina associated with their arrhythmia should have immediate electrical cardioversion to sinus rhythm with a synchronized countershock. Atrial flutter is frequently terminated with as little as 10–20 joules. Other atrial arrhythmias, and atrial fibrillation in particular, generally require a minimum of 50–100 joules and up to 400 joules to restore sinus rhythm.[29] The need for temporary pacemaker support because of an inadequate sinus or junctional escape rhythm following conversion is unknown.[33] It is acceptable to insert a pacemaker prior to elective cardioversion in patients with known sinus or AV node dysfunction or documented episodes of bradycardia (tachycardia-bradycardia syndrome) or slow ventricular response to atrial fibrillation (<50 bpm) in the absence of drug therapy.

Overall it is more desirable to restore and maintain sinus rhythm than to control the ventricular response. Sinus rhythm frequently decreases embolic risk and improves symptoms and hemodynamics. Pharmacological agents of Vaughn-Williams classes IA, IC, and III often restore sinus rhythm (Table 3).

Digitalis and verapamil rarely terminate atrial arrhythmias.[15,16,27,31,34] On the other hand, propranolol and esmolol have been shown to terminate paroxysmal atrial fibrillation.[27,31] A type IA agent, such as quinidine or procainamide, will frequently terminate acute paroxysmal atrial fibrillation.[9,19] Excluding digitalis intoxication, uniform ectopic atrial tachycardia may be treated with type I agents.[2] On the other hand, MAT most frequently responds to removal of the offending agent, infrequently terminating with type IA agents, verapamil or metoprolol.[9,35,36] Atrial flutter is very resistent to pharmacological conversion and usually requires either pacing or direct current shock for restoration of sinus rhythm. The ability to acutely terminate and chronically maintain sinus rhythm may be enhanced when pharmacological therapy is instituted prior to pacing or electrical cardioversion and then continued after sinus rhythm is restored.[9,37]

While not approved by the FDA, flecainide, encainide, or propafenone are probably as effective as procainamide, quinidine, and disopyramide for acute termination of atrial fibrillation.[14,38–41] Even if a type IA agent has failed previously, one-half to two-thirds of patients treated with a type IC agent will be maintained in sinus rhythm with fewer side effects compared to patients taking the more conventional type IA agents.[14,40,41] Preliminary evidence suggests that flecainide and encainide are very effective for restoring and maintaining sinus rhythm in nearly all patients with uniform ectopic atrial tachycardia.[39,42,43] Amiodarone may be the most effective agent available for drug refractory, symptomatic, recurrent atrial fibrillation. Nearly two-thirds of patients treated remained in sinus rhythm for up to a year follow-up.[44,47] Frequent use of amiodarone for this and other atrial arrhythmias is limited by its potentially severe and life-threatening side-effects.

Special Considerations

Wolff-Parkinson-White Syndrome

Patients presenting with antegrade conduction over an accessory pathway during an atrial arrhythmia are frequently hemodynamically stable and may not require emergency electrical cardioversion. However, these patients represent the one subgroup with supraventricular tachyarrhythmias that may be at risk for sudden cardiac death if their ventricular response is rapid. These patients should not receive digitalis, beta- or calcium blocking agents because the ventricular rate is rarely slowed and frequently enhanced resulting in hypotension or precipitation of a ventricular tachyarrhythmia.[48,49] Acute IV administration of procainamide or disopyramide may slow conduction over the accessory pathway and terminate the atrial arrhythmia.[49,50] Lidocaine will not stop the atrial arrhythmia and may rarely enhance conduction over the accessory pathway.[49] In patients who are hemodynamically unstable, direct current cardioversion is the treatment of choice.

Individuals presenting with atrial arrhythmias and WPW should be stabilized and undergo electrophysiological evaluation to determine if pharmacological therapy with a type IA or IC agent to maintain sinus rhythm will also slow or prevent antegrade accessory pathway conduction should there be a recurrence. Surgical ablation of the accessory pathway may be advisable in young patients, in drug refractory individuals, or in those with short refractory periods determined at electrophysiology study.

Proarrhythmia

The definition of a drug-aggravated atrial arrhythmia is not clear. Because of its vagolytic effect and resultant rapid ventricular response, quinidine should not given without prior administration of agents to slow AV node conduction. Type IA and IC agents occasionally slow the atrial rate allowing for more impulses to be conducted resulting in faster ventricular rate (Fig. 10). This is commonly prevented or treated by the addition of agents that slow AV node conduction: digitalis, beta-blockers, calcium blockers. Occasionally, treatment of patients with the tachycardia-bradycardia syndrome worsens sinus node function resulting in symptomatic bradyarrhythmias that require pacemaker support.

Quinidine syncope is due to a drug-induced arrhythmia, torsades de pointes. This is a rapid, polymorphic ventricular tachycardia commonly associated with the use of type IA agents and frequently seen in patients with left ventricular dysfunction, hypokalemia, prolonged QTU interval, or atrial fibrillation. Patients in whom a trial of quinidine-like drugs is contemplated for restoration of sinus rhythm should have the agent initiated in hospital under telemetry monitoring for roughly 72–

REST

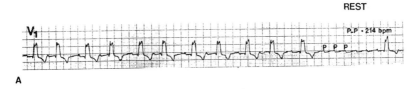

A

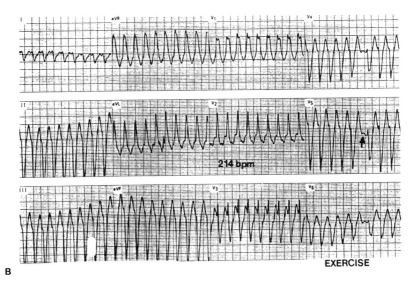

B

Figure 10. Rhythm strip of a patient taking flecainide (A) showing an atrial flutter rate of 214 bpm and a variable ventricular response with right bundle branch block aberrancy. With minimal exertion (B) there is 1:1 AV nodal conduction with a ventricular rate of 214 bpm. The arrow shows one non-conducted P wave.

96 hours, the usual time to see early proarrhythmic events with these drugs.[51] IC agents rarely precipitate serious ventricular arrhythmias except when patients have rapid dose escalations, coexistent, potentially lethal ventricular arrhythmias or left ventricular dysfunction.[40,52-56] These types of patients should also be monitored in hospital during drug titration to observe for unexpected proarrhythmic responses. Finally, the development of incessant atrial arrhythmias or atrial arrhythmias not previously documented is a rare but well-described atrial proarrhythmic response. These arrhythmias are frequently resistent to pharmacological and/or electrical cardioversion with spontaneous conversion

occurring after the drug is metabolized. Because it is difficult to predict the hemodynamic and ventricular responses to an incessant atrial proarrhythmia after the drug is discontinued, treatment is most safely done in hospital with telemetry monitoring.

Postoperative Arrhythmias

Postoperative atrial arrhythmias are most commonly seen following thoracic surgery, especially pneumonectomy and open heart surgery.[57,58]

Up to 20% of patients may develop an episode that is most often atrial fibrillation. There are few factors associated with the development of postoperative paroxysmal atrial fibrillation; but elderly patients and those in whom treatment with beta-blockers have recently been discontinued may be at higher risk. Acute treatment to restore sinus rhythm is often ineffective or associated with early recurrences. However, most patients who develop postoperative atrial fibrillation will have sinus rhythm restored either spontaneously or with pharmacological therapy within 1 week of surgery and will rarely require long-term treatment. Hemodynamic and embolic complications from postoperative paroxysmal atrial fibrillation are rare. Multiple studies have shown that prophylaxis with low-dose beta-blockers perioperatively frequently prevents the acute episodes. In randomized studies, 5–20 mg of propranolol q.i.d. preoperatively is effective prophylaxis against the development of postoperative paroxysmal atrial fibrillation. Randomized studies with digoxin are less conclusive. One 1.5 mg p.o. given 1–3 days preoperatively may be effective for prevention of postoperative paroxysmal atrial fibrillation.[57]

Anticoagulation

Many studies have demonstrated a 1–5% annual risk of peripheral embolic events in patients with atrial fibrillation, most commonly to arteries of the brain, mesentery, kidneys, heart, and large limbs. The risk of systemic embolism and ischemic stroke in patients with nonrheumatic, chronic atrial fibrillation is five to seven times higher compared to similar patients in sinus rhythm, particularly during the first year following onset.[9,19,59-61] Two recent trials have given us new information, suggesting that oral anticoagulation may be of benefit in reducing systemic embolization in patients with nonvalvular atrial fibrillation. The AFA-SAK study[62] demonstrated a statistical reduction of embolic strokes from 5.0% to 2.2% in nonvalvular, chronic atrial fibrillation patients treated with warfarin instead of aspirin or placebo. The SPAF study[63] showed a statistical reduction in embolic events form 8.3% per year in the placebo arm to 1.6% per year in the aspirin or warfarin arm (prothrombin times 1.3 to 1.8 time control) of the study in patients with paroxysmal or chronic atrial fibrillation. Aspirin was not beneficial in patients over 75 years of age. Based on the above studies, we would recommend low-dose warfarin or aspirin (in patients under 75 years of age) in an attempt to minimize the incidence of serious embolic phenomena in patients with nonvalvular atrial fibrillation. Although not as well controlled, patients with atrial fibrillation and hypertrophic or dilated cardiomyopathy appear to benefit from chronic anticoagulation.[59]

Episodes of paroxysmal atrial fibrillation, especially in patients under 40 years of age, may not carry the same risk of thromboembolism compared to patients with chronic atrial fibrillation. Patients with atrial flutter and fibrillation should be treated as if they have only atrial fibrillation.[64] Finally, patients with atrial arrhythmias other than atrial fibrillation are considered at low thromboembolic risk, and anticoagulation either for paroxysmal or chronic forms or prior to elective cardioversion is not generally required.[64]

Patients with atrial fibrillation and rheumatic valvular disease are at the highest risk for thromboembolic events and should be chronically anticoagulated even if sinus rhythm is restored.[64] Thus, it is recommended that patients with atrial fibrillation associated with rheumatic heart disease, hypertrophic or dilated cardiomyopathy be anticoagulated with warfarin to 1.2–1.5 times control.[59,64] Patients who have suffered an embolic event have a high rate of recurrence, particularly in the first month following the acute event, and should also be anticoagulated. Because the mortality rate associated with systemic embolism approaches 40%, especially with advancing age, it is recommended that patients with hypertension, coronary artery disease, and thyrotoxicosis who have chronic atrial fibrillation or frequent episodes of paroxysmal atrial fibrillation be anticoagulated with warfarin to 1.2–1.5 times control.[59,64] This must be weighed against the risk of major hemorrhagic complications that occur at a rate of up to 3% per year.[65] The risk of major bleeding increases with duration of therapy, prothrombin times more than 2.5 times control, and possibly in patients over age 70.[66]

The risk of thromboembolic events following cardioversion of atrial fibrillation ranges from 1 to 5% in nonanticoagulated patients to about

1% in those anticoagulated.[33,59,60] The rationale for the recommendations to anticoagulate prior to and following cardioversion are based largely on theory and have never been rigorously proven in controlled clinical trials. However, atrial fibrillation of long duration should be anticoagulated for 2–3 weeks prior to attempted cardioversion. Anticoagulation should then be maintained for roughly 4 weeks following cardioversion because mechanical atrial systole may not return for up to a month following restoration of sinus rhythm by ECG.[9,59,64,67,68] Thus, patients presenting with paroxysmal atrial fibrillation of less than 7 days' duration can undergo chemical and/or electrical cardioversion without delay so as to enhance the possibility of restoring sinus rhythm. Patients requiring emergency electrical cardioversion have rarely been in atrial fibrillation for a long period of time and should not have the procedure delayed to be anticoagulated. However, if they have been in atrial fibrillation for several days prior to cardioversion or are at high risk of recurrence of atrial fibrillation because of concurrent illness such as congestive heart failure, pneumonia, or untreated thyrotoxicosis, then anticoagulation following emergency cardioversion may be available.[64]

Nonpharmacological Therapies

There are many surgical and catheter ablative techniques for the treatment of atrial arrhythmias that are acceptable alternatives to drug therapy. As previously mentioned, surgical ablation of accessory pathways may be the most effective therapy for the WPW syndrome, frequently obviating the need for drug therapy and removing the stimulus for future episodes of paroxysmal atrial fibrillation.[69,70] Patients refractory to drug therapy, either because of inefficacy or adverse reactions, may be symptomatically improved by percutaneous catheter ablation of AV nodal structures which creates complete heart block.[74] In some cases, AV nodal conduction can be modified without the need for permanent pacing. Despite the need for a permanent pacemaker, quality of life and exercise tolerance are significantly improved.[72] Patients with infrequent episodes of paroxysmal atrial flutter, without the WPW syndrome, in whom medication is ineffective, not indicated, or not desirable may have acute episodes terminated by implantation of a permanent antitachycardia pacemaker.[73] Finally, resection or cryosurgical ablation of AV nodal structures in order to create complete heart block is indicated for drug refractory, rapid, and poorly tolerated atrial arrhythmias that have failed previous catheter ablative attempts.[74]

References

1. Braunwald E (ed): Heart Disease. Philadelphia, WB Saunders Co, 1984, pp 599–604.
2. Rinkenberger R: Cardiac rhythm in the critical care setting: pathophysiology and diagnosis. In: Dantzker DR (ed), Cardiopulmonary Critical Care. Orlando, Grune and Stratton, 1986, pp 403–479.
3. Allessie MA, Lemmers WJ, Rensma PL, et al: Flutter and fibrillation in experimental models: what has been learned that can be applied to humans? In: Brugada P, Wellens HJJ (eds), Cardiac Arrhythmias: Where Do We Go From Here. Mt. Kisco, Futura Publishing Inc, 1987, pp 67–82.
4. Hurwitz J, German L, Wharton JM, et al: Atrial fibrillation in atrioventricular nodal reentry tachycardia. PACE 12:684, 1989.
5. Roark SF, McCarthy EA, Lee KL, et al: Observations on the occurrence of atrial fibrillation and paroxysmal supraventricular tachycardia. Am J Cardiol 57:571, 1986.
6. Sharma AD, Klein GJ, Guiraudon GM, et al: Atrial fibrillation in patients with Wolff-Parkinson-White syndrome: incidence after surgical ablation of the accessory pathway. Circulation 72:161, 1985.
7. Klein GJ, Bashore TM, Sellers TD, et al: Ventricular fibrillation in the Wolff-Parkinson-White syndrome. N Engl J Med 301:1080, 1979.
8. Henry WL, Morganroth J, Pearlman AS, et al: Relation between echocardiographically determined left atrial size and atrial fibrillation. Circulation 52:273, 1976.
9. Braunwald E (ed): Heart Disease. Philadelphia, WB Saunders Co, 1984, pp 671–677.
10. Dittrich HG, Ericson JS, Schneiderman T, et al: Echocardiographic and clinical predictors for outcome of elective cardioversion of atrial fibrillation. Am J Cardiol 63:193, 1989.
11. Brodsky MA, Allen BJ, Capparelli EV, et al: Factors determining maintenance of sinus rhythm after chronic atrial fibrillation with left atrial dilatation. Am J Cardiol 63:1065, 1989.
12. Sanfilippo AJ, Abascal WM, Sheehan M, et al: Left atrial enlargement as a consequence of atrial fibrillation: a perspective echocardiographic study. J Am Coll Cardiol 13:206A, 1989.
13. Sosa-Suarez G, Lampert S, Grayboys TB, et al: Changes in left atrial size due to chronic atrial fibrillation. J Am Coll Cardiol 13:206A, 1989.
14. Borgeat A, Goy JJ, Maendly R, et al: Flecainide vs. quinidine for conversion of atrial fibrillation to sinus rhythm. Am J Cardiol 58:496, 1986.
15. Suttorp MJ, Kingma JH, Lie-a-huen L, et al: Intravenous flecainide vs. verapamil for acute conversion of paroxysmal atrial fibrillation or flutter to sinus rhythm. Am J Cardiol 63:693, 1989.
16. Wafa SS, Ward DE, Parker J, et al: Efficacy of flecainide acetate for atrial arrhythmias following coronary artery bypass grafting. Am J Cardiol 63:1058, 1989.
17. Goy JJ, Kaufmann U, Kappenberger L, et al: Restoration of sinus rhythm with flecainide in patients with atrial fibrillation. Am J Cardiol 62:38, 1988.

18. Kannel WB, Abbott RD, Savage DD, et al: Epidemiologic features of chronic atrial fibrillation. N Engl J Med 306:1018, 1982.
19. Alpert JS, Petersen P, Godtfredsen J: Atrial fibrillation: natural history, complications and management. Ann Rev Med 39:41, 1988.
20. Brand FN, Abbott RD, Kannel WB: Characteristics and prognosis of lone atrial fibrillation: 30 year follow-up on the Framingham study. JAMA 254:3449, 1985.
21. Kopecky SL, Jersh BJ, McGoon MD, et al: An actual history of lone atrial fibrillation: a population-based study over three decades. N Engl J Med 317:669, 1987.
22. Naccarelli GV, Dougherty AH, Berns E, et al: Assessment of antiarrhythmic drug efficacy in the treatment of supraventricular arrhythmias. Am J Cardiol 58:31C, 1986.
23. Strasberg B, Ashley WW, Wyndham CRC, et al: Treadmill exercise testing in the Wolff-Parkinson-White syndrome. Am J Cardiol 45:742, 1980.
24. Coelho E, Pailieo E, Ashley WW, et al: Tachyarrhythmias in young athletes. J Am Coll Cardiol 7:237, 1986.
25. Yeh SJ, Lin FC, Wu D: The mechanism of exercise provocation of supraventricular tachycardia. Am Heart J 117:1041, 1989.
26. Pritchett ELC, Anderson JL: Antiarrhythmic strategies for the chronic management of supraventricular tachycardias. Am J Cardiol 62:1D, 1988.
27. Platia EV, Waclawski SH, Pluth TA, et al: Management of acute-onset atrial fibrillation/flutter: esmolol vs. verapamil vs. digoxin vs. placebo. Circulation 76:IV-520, 1987.
28. Weiner P, Bassan MM, Jarchovsky J, et al: Clinical course of acute atrial fibrillation treated with rapid digitalization. Am Heart J 105:223, 1983.
29. Rinkenberger RL: Cardiac rhythm in the critical care setting: evaluation and treatment. In: Dantzker DR (ed): Cardiopulmonary Critical Care. Orlando, Grune and Stratton, 1986, pp 481–585.
30. Turlapaty P, Laddu A, Murthy VS, et al: Esmolol: short-acting intervenous beta-blocker for an acute critical care setting. Am Heart J 114:866–885, 1989.
31. Esmolol Multicenter Study Research Group: Efficacy and safety of esmolol vs. propranolol in the treatment of supraventricular tachyarrhythmias: a multicenter double-blind clinical trial. Am Heart J 110:913, 1985.
32. Platia EV, Michelson EL, Porterfield JK, et al: Esmolol vs. verapamil in the acute treatment of atrial fibrillation or atrial flutter. Am J Cardiol 63:925, 1989.
33. Mancini GBJ, Goldberger AL: Cardioversion of atrial fibrillation: consideration of embolization, anticoagulation, prophylactic pacemaker, and long-term success. Am Heart J 104:617, 1982.
34. Falk RH, Knowlton AA, Bernard SA, et al: Digoxin for converting recent-onset atrial fibrillation to sinus rhythm. Ann Int Med 106:503, 1987.
35. Levine JH, Michael JR, Guarnieri T: Treatment of multifocal atrial tachycardia with verapamil. N Engl J Med 312:21, 1985.
36. Arsura E, Lefkin AS, Scher DL, et al: A randomized, double-blind, placebo-controlled study of verapamil and metoprolol in treatment of multifocal atrial tachycardia. Am J Med 85:519, 1988.
37. Olshansky B, Okumura K, Hess PJ, et al: Use of procainamide with rapid

atrial pacing for successful conversion of atrial flutter to sinus rhythm. J Am Coll Cardiol 11:359, 1988.

38. Antman EM, Beamer AD, Cantillon C, et al: Long-term oral propafenone therapy for suppression of refractory symptomatic atrial fibrillation and atrial flutter. J Am Coll Cardiol 12:1005, 1988.
39. Connolly SJ, Hoffert DL: Usefulness of propafenone for recurrent paroxysmal atrial fibrillation. Am J Cardiol 63:817, 1989.
40. Anderson JL, Jolivette DM, Fredell PA: Summary of efficacy and safety of flecainide for supraventricular arrhythmias. Am J Cardiol 62:62D, 1988.
41. Makynen PJ, Koskimen PJ, Saaristo TE, et al: Comparison of encainide and quinidine for supraventricular tachyarrhythmias. Am J Cardiol 62:55L, 1988.
42. Berns E, Rinkenberger RL, Jeang MK, et al: Efficacy and safety of flecainide acetate for atrial tachycardia or fibrillation. Am J Cardiol 59:1337, 1987.
43. Kuck K-H, Kunze K-P, Schluter M, et al: Encainide vs. flecainide for chronic atrial and junctional ectopic tachycardia. Am J Cardiol 62:37L, 1988.
44. Horowitz LN, Spielman SR, Greenspan AM, et al: Use of amiodarone in the treatment of persistent and paroxysmal atrial fibrillation resistant to quinidine therapy. J Am Coll Cardiol 6:1402, 1985.
45. Gold RL, Haffajee CI, Charos G, et al: Amiodarone for refractory atrial fibrillation. Am J Cardiol 57:124, 1986.
46. Brodsky MA, Allen BJ, Walker CJ, et al: Amiodarone for maintenance of sinus rhythm after conversion of atrial fibrillation in the setting of a dilated left atrium. Am J Cardiol 60:572, 1987.
47. Kopelman HA, Horowitz LN: Efficacy and toxicity of amiodarone for the treatment of supraventricular tachyarrhythmias. Prog Cardiovas Dis 31:355, 1989.
48. McGovern B, Garan H, Ruskin JM: Precipitation of cardiac arrest by verapamil in patients with Wolff-Parkinson-White syndrome. Ann Intern Med 104:791, 1986.
49. Prystowsky EN: Diagnosis and management of the pre-excitation syndromes. Curr Prob Cardiol 13:231, 1988.
50. Fujimura O, Klein GS, Shamara AD, et al: Acute effect of disopyramide on atrial fibrillation in the Wolff-Parkinson-White syndrome. J Am Coll Cardiol 13:1133, 1989.
51. Jackman WM, Friday KJ, Anderson JL, et al: The long QR syndromes: a critical review, new clinical observations and a unifying hypothesis. Prog Cardiovasc Dis 31:115, 1988.
52. Morganroth J, Anderson JL, Gentzkow GD: Classification by type of ventricular arrhythmia predicts a frequency of adverse cardiac effects from flecainide. J Am Coll Cardiol 8:607, 1986.
53. Morganroth J, Horowitz LN: Flecainide: its proarrhythmic effect and expected changes on the surface electrocardiogram. Am J Cardiol 53:89B, 1984.
54. Morganroth J: Risk factors for the development of proarrhythmic events. Am J Cardiol 59:32E, 1987.
55. Soyka LF: Safety considerations and dosing guidelines for encainide in supraventricular arrhythmias. Am J Cardiol 62:63L, 1988.
56. Rinkenberger RL, Naccarelli GV, Berns E, et al: Efficacy and safety of class 1C antiarrhythmic agents for the treatment of coexisting supraventricular and ventricular tachycardia. Am J Cardiol 62:44D, 1988.

57. Krowka MJ, Pairolero PC, Trastek VF, et al: Cardiac dysrrhythmia following pneumonectomy. Chest 91:490, 1987.
58. Lauer MS, Eagle KA, Buckley MJ, et al: Atrial fibrillation following coronary artery bypass surgery. Prog Cardiovasc Dis 31:367, 1989.
59. Kadish SL, Lazar EJ, Frishman WH: Anticoagulation in patients with valvular heart disease, atrial fibrillation, or both. Cardiol Clin 5:591, 1987.
60. Roy D, Marchand E, Gagne P, et al: Usefulness of anticoagulant therapy in the prevention of embolic complications of atrial fibrillation. Am Heart J 112:1039, 1986.
61. Halperin JL, Hart RG: Atrial fibrillation and stroke: new ideas, persisting dilemmas. Stroke 19:937, 1988.
62. Petersen B, Boysen G, Godtfredsen J, et al: Placebo-controlled, randomized trial of warfarin and aspirin for prevention of thromboembolic complications of chronic atrial fibrillation. The Copenhagen AFASAK Study. Lancet 175–179, 1989.
63. Preliminary report of the stroke prevention in atrial fibrillation study. N Engl J Med 322:863, 1990.
64. Dunn M, Alexander J, DeSilva R, et al: Antithrombotic therapy in atrial fibrillation. Chest 89:68S, 1986.
65. Levine MN, Raskob G, Hersh J: Hemorrhagic complications of long-term anticoagulant therapy. Chest 89:16S, 1986.
66. Gurwitz JH, Goldberg RJ, Holden A, et al: AH-related risks of long-term oral anticoagulant therapy. Arch Intern Med 148:1733, 1988.
67. Shapiro EP, Effron MB, Lima S, et al: Transient atrial dysfunction after conversion of chronic atrial fibrillation to sinus rhythm. Am J Cardiol 62:1202, 1988.
68. Manning WJ, Leeman DE, Gotch PJ, et al: Pulsed Doppler evaluation of atrial mechanical function after electrical cardioversion of atrial fibrillation. J Am Coll Cardiol 13:617, 1989.
69. Sharma AD, Klein GJ, Guiraudon GM, et al: Atrial fibrillation in patients with Wolff-Parkinson-White syndrome: incidence after surgical ablation of the accessory pathway. Circulation 72:161, 1985.
70. Fischell TA, Stinson EB, Derby GC, et al: Long-term follow-up after surgical correction of Wolff-Parkinson-White syndrome. J Am Coll Cardiol 9:283, 1987.
71. Evans GT, Sheinman MM, Zipes DP, et al: The percutaneous cardiac mapping and ablation registry: final summary of results. PACE 11:1621, 1988.
72. Kay GN, Bubien RS, Epstein AE, et al: Effective catheter ablation of the atrioventricular junction on quality of life and exercise tolerance in paroxysmal atrial fibrillation. Am J Cardiol 62:741, 1988.
73. Barold SS, Wyndham CRC, Kappenberger LL, et al: Implanted atrial pacemakers for paroxysmal atrial flutter. Ann Intern Med 107:144, 1987.
74. Lowe JE, Sabiston DC: Surgical management of cardiac arrhythmia. J Appl Cardiol 1:1, 1986.

Chapter 8

Wolff-Parkinson-White Syndrome

Paul G. Colavita, John J. Gallagher,
Jay G. Selle, John M. Fedor,
Samuel H. Zimmern, and
Robert H. Svenson

Introduction

The Wolff-Parkinson-White (WPW) syndrome has fascinated electrocardiographers for many years. While the initial description of a case was in 1914,[1] it was not until 1930 that Wolff, Parkinson, and White reported a group of young healthy people with a short PR interval, bundle branch block and paroxysmal tachycardia.[2] Since this report, our understanding of the WPW syndrome has advanced tremendously. In this chapter, we will review the clinical and electrophysiological aspects of the WPW syndrome as we understand them today.

Recognition

The Wolff-Parkinson-White syndrome is characterized electrocardiographically by a short PR interval (less than 0.12 second), and a prolonged QRS complex characterized by a slurring of the initial QRS forces called a delta wave (Fig. 1). These result from ventricular pre-excitation or fusion of the cardiac impulse from the atria to the ventricles over the

From Naccarelli GV (ed): *Cardiac Arrhythmias: A Practical Approach*. Mount Kisco, NY, Futura Publishing Co., Inc., © 1991.

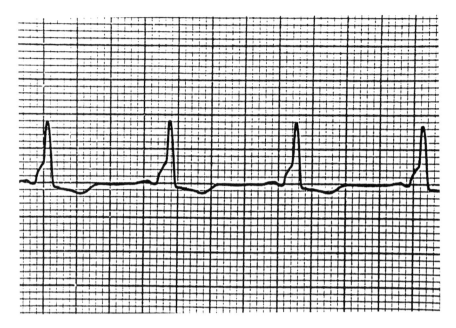

Figure 1. Lead I from an electrocardiogram of a patient with a right free wall accessory connection. Note the short PR interval and delta wave characteristic of patients with Wolff-Parkinson-White syndrome.

normal atrioventricular node and an accessory atrioventricular connection (Fig. 2). Multiple factors affect the degree of pre-excitation, including the location of the accessory connection, and conduction times through the atria, atrioventricular node, His-Purkinje system, and accessory connection. For example, a left lateral accessory connection may not be evident on a resting electrocardiogram if the activation reaches the ventricles via the atrioventricular node before it reaches the accessory connection. Although accessory atrioventricular connections most commonly function in both antegrade and retrograde directions, they can function in the antegrade or retrograde direction only. When antegrade conduction is present, pre-excitation is manifest with a shortened PR interval and a widened QRS complex. With connections that function only in the retrograde direction, pre-excitation is not present and the electrocardiogram is normal. These connections are therefore concealed.

The location of the accessory atrioventricular connection can also be identified electrocardiographically. There are two types of ventricular pre-excitation based on the morphology of the QRS complex in the pre-

NORMAL SINUS RHYTHM

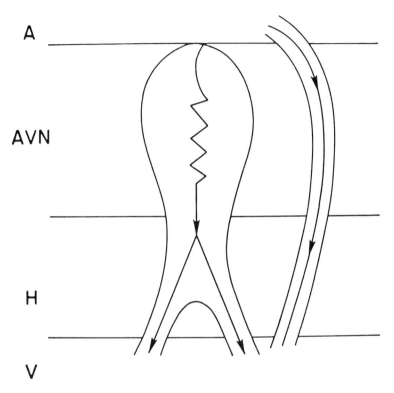

Figure 2. Schematic presentation of ventricular pre-excitation with ventricular activation via the atrioventricular node (AVN) and accessory connection.

cordial leads.[3] In type A, the R wave was the only dominant deflection in leads V_1 and V_2, and in type B, an S or QS deflection predominated in at least one of the right precordial leads. It was later hypothesized that type A was related to left posterior basal pre-excitation and type B was the result of right lateral pre-excitation. This classification was broad and failed to identify septal connections.

Localization was attempted by organizing the direction of the delta wave vector based on all 12 electrocardiographic leads.[4] Only maximally pre-excited beats were examined to minimize the influence of fusion with normal conduction. This resulted in the identification of 10 accessory connection sites although some overlap existed. Localization of the connection was confirmed by epicardial mapping and surgical ablation in that area. Only coexisting electrocardiographic abnormalities due to the presence of congenital or acquired cardiac disorders or the possible existence of multiple pathways limit this classification.

Arrhythmias

The spectrum of arrhythmias that can occur in association with the Wolff-Parkinson-White syndrome is broad. They can range from a mildly symptomatic reciprocating tachycardia to life-threatening ventricular fibrillation. The proportion of WPW patients with symptomatic arrhythmias varies from 4.3% to 90%, depending on the group studied.[5]

The most common type of arrhythmia in the WPW syndrome is orthodromic reciprocating tachycardia (Fig. 3). This arrhythmia utilizes a macro re-entrant circuit consisting of the atria, atrioventricular node, His-Purkinje system, ventricular myocardium, and the accessory pathway (Fig. 4). Antegrade conduction is via the atrioventricular node, therefore the QRS duration is usually normal, although bundle branch aberrancy may occur.

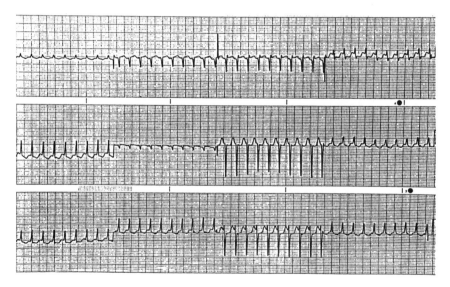

Figure 3. Twelve-lead electrocardiogram during orthodromic reciprocating tachycardia.

ORTHODROMIC RECIPROCATING
TACHYCARDIA

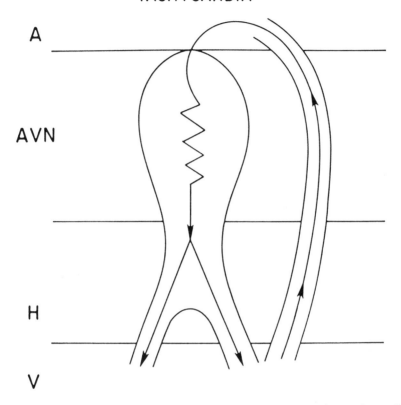

Figure 4. Schematic presentation of orthodromic reciprocating tachycardia with antegrade conduction over the atrioventricular node (AVN) and retrograde conduction via the accessory connection.

It is often difficult to determine the mechanism of a regular, narrow-complex supraventricular tachycardia on the basis of an electrocardiogram alone. The differential diagnosis could include an ectopic atrial tachycardia, atrial flutter, or atrioventricular node re-entrant tachycardia. Electrocardiographic features that may suggest participation of an accessory pathway include (1) fast heart rate (>200 bpm),[6,7] (2) QRS electrical alteration,[8] or (3) slowing of the tachycardia rate during bundle branch block.[9] Heart rate during AV node re-entry ranges from 115–214 bpm (mean 169 bpm) compared to 171–222 bpm (mean 194 bpm) for reciprocating tachycardia utilizing an accessory connection.[6] Faster heart rates, therefore, suggest reciprocating tachycardia although there is considerable overlap. The presence of electrical alternation in the QRS was felt to be highly specific for the participation of an accessory pathway. It has been recently shown, though, to be a rate-related phenomenon that depends on an abrupt increase to a critical rate.[10] Since the rate of reciprocating tachycardia is usually faster than atrioventricular node re-entry, electrical alternation has been noted more commonly during reciprocating tachycardia.

Bundle branch block aberration is most commonly rate-related and therefore occurs with fast heart rates. When the heart rate slows with bundle branch block during tachycardia, participation of an accessory connection is present. Tachycardia slowing occurs when the accessory connection is on the same side as the bundle branch block (i.e., left-sided accessory connection with left bundle branch block). The reason this occurs is that the re-entrant circuit is lengthened by transseptal activation time (e.g., instead of activating the left ventricle via the left bundle, the activation descends through the right bundle and right ventricle before activating the left ventricle via the intraventricular septum). With a free wall pathway, this usually adds ≥35 ms to the circuit and therefore slows the tachycardia accordingly. Failure to observe this phenomenon does not rule out participation of an accessory connection which may be septal or on the contralateral side to the block. Irrespective of changes in the tachycardia rate, the occurrence of left bundle branch block is suggestive of reciprocating tachycardia. Functional left bundle branch block has only rarely been associated with an ectopic atrial tachycardia or atrioventricular node re-entrant tachycardia.[7]

The location of the P wave is the most useful electrocardiographic feature to determine the mechanism of a narrow complex tachycardia.[11] Because retrograde conduction over the accessory connection is usually faster than antegrade conduction via the atrioventricular node during reciprocating tachycardia, the P wave is usually located shortly after the QRS complex (Fig. 5). Often the P waves are not recognizable either due to their small amplitude or to obscurement within the ST segment. In such cases, reciprocating tachycardia is indistinguishable from atrioventricular node re-entrant tachycardia. An esophageal lead has proven to be very helpful in identifying atrial activity and in differentiating atrioventricular node re-entrant tachycardia from reciprocating tachycardia.[12] A ventriculoatrial (VA) interval (measured from the onset of the QRS complex to the atrial deflection of the esophageal lead) of <70 ms rules out participation of an accessory connection and suggests atrioventricular node re-entrant tachycardia. A VA interval of >70 ms sug-

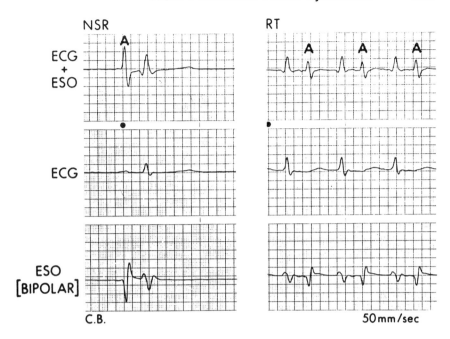

Figure 5. Left panel: Surface electrocardiogram (ECG) and esophageal electrogram (ESO) during normal sinus rhythm. Right panel: Surface electrocardiogram and esophageal electrogram during reciprocating tachycardia. The ventriculoatrial (VA) interval is about 160 ms, suggesting participation of an accessory connection.

gests reciprocating tachycardia, although there are some uncommon forms of supraventricular tachycardia that can also have a VA interval of >70 ms. A detailed electrophysiological study may be necessary to differentiate these.

Antidromic tachycardia is an uncommon arrhythmia seen in patients with WPW syndrome.[13] In this arrhythmia, the activation proceeds antegrade over the accessory connection and retrograde over the atrioventricular node, or more commonly, a second accessory connection (Fig. 6). This results in a wide maximally pre-excited QRS complex (Fig. 7). The rate of antidromic reciprocating tachycardia is usually 150–240 bpm. This rate, combined with the wide QRS complex, makes differentiation of this rhythm from ventricular tachycardia and atrial flutter with aberrancy difficult.

Atrial fibrillation and flutter are also common arrhythmias in patients with WPW syndrome. Atrial fibrillation is often initiated as the

ANTIDROMIC TACHYCARDIA

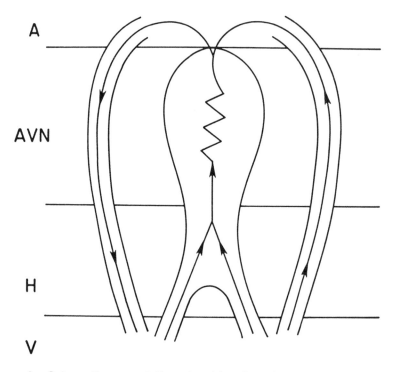

Figure 6. Schematic presentation of antidromic tachycardia with antegrade conduction over one accessory connection and retrograde conduction via the atrioventricular node (AVN) and/or a second accessory connection.

result of an episode of reciprocating tachycardia rather than as a primary arrhythmia.[14] Depending on the refractory periods and conduction properties of the atrioventricular node and accessory connection, the resultant QRS complexes may be narrow (via the atrioventricular node), wide due to bundle branch aberrancy, or wide secondary to ventricular pre-excitation. Frequently, all of these and QRS complexes with various degrees of fusion will be noted on an individual electrocardiogram (Fig. 8). Atrial fibrillation is identified by its irregularly irregular rhythm. The heart rate during atrial fibrillation may vary from 120 to 350 bpm.

Sudden cardiac death occurs in patients with the Wolff-Parkinson-White syndrome as a result of rapid atrial fibrillation leading to ventricular fibrillation (Fig. 9). Although most patients who experience ven-

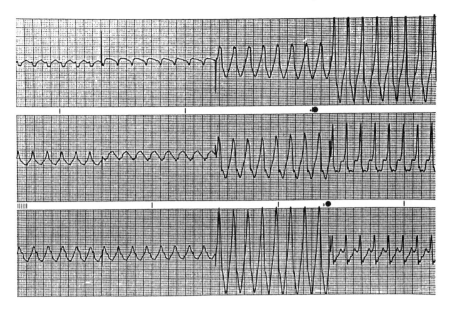

Figure 7. Twelve-lead electrocardiogram during antidromic tachycardia.

tricular fibrillation were previously symptomatic with atrial fibrillation and/or reciprocating tachycardia, ventricular fibrillation can be the initial presentation of the syndrome.

Patient Evaluation

The classic electrocardiographic pattern of Wolff-Parkinson-White syndrome has been noted to occur in 1–3 per 1,000 individuals.[4] The evaluation of a patient with Wolff-Parkinson-White syndrome will depend on the clinical presentation. Therapy for a patient with bothersome orthodromic reciprocating tachycardia will be different than for a patient with rapid atrial fibrillation, a potentially life-threatening arrhythmia.

The occasional occurrence of ventricular fibrillation as the initial manifestation of the Wolff-Parkinson-White syndrome has stimulated interest in the possibility of identifying asymptomatic patients who may be at risk for this complication. The shortest RR interval between two pre-excited beats during atrial fibrillation has been shown to be the most useful indicator of patients at risk of having ventricular fibrillation since all the patients with ventricular fibrillation had a shortest RR interval of

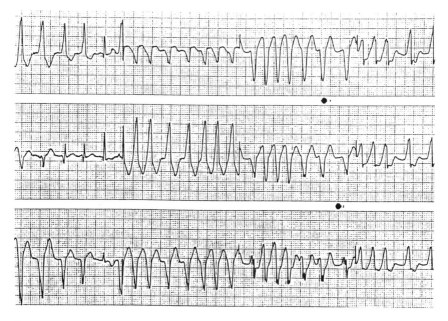

Figure 8. Twelve-lead electrocardiogram during atrial fibrillation. Considerable variation in QRS morphology reflects various degrees of preexcitation from nonpreexcited (5th complex) to maximally pre-excited (7th complex).

250 ms or less.[15] Patients with pathways that have a long antegrade refractory period (>270 ms) and slow ventricular rates during atrial fibrillation are not considered at risk for ventricular fibrillation.

The initial evaluation of an asymptomatic patient should include a thorough history and physical examination, as well as an echocardiogram to rule out associated cardiac anomalies, such as Ebstein's anomaly. The most important element of the initial evaluation, though, is to determine whether or not the connection is capable of rapid antegrade conduction.

Intermittent pre-excitation is defined as the abrupt loss of pre-ex-

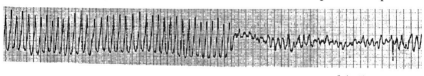

Figure 9. Rapid pre-excited ventricular response during atrial fibrillation results in ventricular fibrillation.

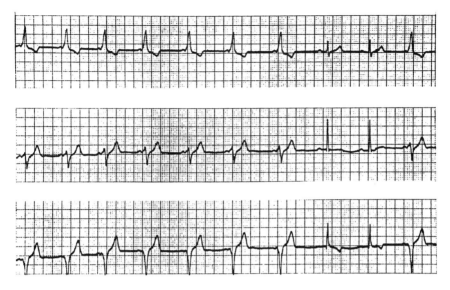

Figure 10. Intermittent pre-excitation. During normal sinus rhythm antegrade conduction block occurs over the accessory connection for two consecutive complexes (8th, 9th) with loss of pre-excitation.

citation during sinus rhythm in a manner resembling Mobitz II block (Fig. 10). This intermittent loss of the delta wave has been shown to occur in patients whose connection has a long antegrade refractory period and relatively slow rates during atrial fibrillation.[16] Loss of ventricular pre-excitation in this fashion may be observed on a Holter monitor or an exercise treadmill test. Loss of ventricular pre-excitation after administration of a type 1A antiarrhythmic agent has also been shown to occur more commonly in patients whose connection has a long antegrade refractory period, but false-positive and false-negative results have been obtained.[18,19] Induction of atrial fibrillation is still the best determinant of the conduction characteristics of the accessory connection. This can be accomplished invasively or noninvasively using an esophageal lead. An infusion of isoproterenol is also administered during this procedure. Isoproterenol increases the rate of conduction over the accessory connection during atrial fibrillation and allows a better assessment of the risk of excessively rapid rates occurring during atrial fibrillation.[20]

Natural history studies indicate the death rate of Wolff-Parkinson-White patients is quite low, yet the results of electrophysiological studies suggest the number of patients at risk according to this criterion to be about 17%.[21] The reason for this discrepancy is not clear, although a recent study suggests that accessory connections can lose their ability to conduct over time.[22]

Symptomatic patients should have a physical examination and a complete history should be taken. An assessment of the antegrade refractory period of the accessory connection and its ability to conduct during atrial fibrillation should also be performed. Further invasive evaluations are indicated for those patients with rapid antegrade conduction over the accessory connection and those patients whose conduction characteristics cannot be determined. Detailed invasive electrophysiological tests are indicated in patients being considered for surgical or electrical ablation of the accessory connection or for use of an anti-tachycardia pacemaker.[23] Patients being considered for surgical correction of either congenital or acquired cardiac disease in the presence of known ventricular pre-excitation should also undergo electrophysiological testing to determine the number, location, and characteristics of the accessory connection(s). Electrophysiological studies could also be considered to assess risk in athletes, airline pilots, or those who operate mass transportation vehicles.

Therapy

An electrocardiogram obtained during the symptomatic tachycardia is the most important piece of information necessary to plan therapy. Therapy is usually not prescribed unless this information is available.

Asymptomatic patients with a known long antegrade refractory period and slow ventricular response during atrial fibrillation are not at risk for sudden cardiac death and therapy is not indicated. The asymptomatic patient with a known short antegrade effective refractory period and rapid ventricular conduction during atrial fibrillation is more difficult to treat. Although such patients are known to have a sporadic risk of sudden death, the general prognosis is still good. No treatment can therefore be considered acceptable. Although insufficient data are available, medical therapy with antiarrhythmic medications to slow conduction over the accessory connection is our present recommendation until additional data are obtained.

Orthodromic reciprocating tachycardia is the most common tachycardia observed in patients with the WPW syndrome. Chronic prophylactic therapy is not always indicated in this intrinsically benign arrhythmia. Patients who have infrequent attacks may take no long-term therapy but instead deal with each attack when it occurs. Many attacks of orthodromc reciprocating tachycardia terminate spontaneously or can be terminated by vagal maneuvers, such as the Valsalva maneuver. In some patients, calcium channel blockers and/or beta-blockers can be taken at the onset of symptoms to terminate reciprocating tachycardia.[24] Occasionally, physician intervention is required for termination of reciprocating tachycardia. Again, if vagal maneuvers are unsuccessful, intravenous verapamil would be the drug of choice.[25] This should terminate almost 90% of reciprocating tachycardia.

Drugs that slow AV nodal conduction are excellent choices for long-term therapy of reciprocating tachycardia. Beta-blockers may be the best choice although calcium channel blockers, verapamil, and dilitazem as well as digitalis compounds are also useful. Caution should be exercised when using digitalis compounds in patients with ventricular pre-excitation since it may precipitate ventricular fibrillation in patients with atrial fibrillation.[26] It should therefore probably be used only for those patients with a slow ventricular response during atrial fibrillation or pathways that conduct only in the retrograde direction.

Type 1A antiarrhythmic agents such as quinidine, procainamide, or disopyramide are also excellent therapy for orthodromic reciprocating tachycardia. They act by preventing the premature atrial or ventricular beats that may initiate the tachycardia and by slowing conduction over the accessory connection. They are frequently used in combination with drugs that slow atrioventricular nodal conduction in difficult to manage patients and in patients with both reciprocating tachycardia and atrial fibrillation.

Atrial fibrillation or flutter as well as antidromic tachycardia is treated quite differently. In these arrhythmias, antegrade conduction is over the accessory pathway and can at times be quite rapid. The QRS complexes are usually wide and pre-excited. Initial therapy is DC cardioversion if the patient exhibits any hemodynamic compromise. Intravenous procainamide should be used when the patient is hemodynamically stable. Procainamide will not only slow conduction over the accessory connection but may also terminate the arrhythmia. Digitalis compounds and verapamil are contraindicated in patients with pre-excited atrial fibrillation. These drugs can accelerate the ventricular rate, causing hemodynamic compromise or ventricular fibrillation.[15,27] Lidocaine should probably also not be used to treat pre-excited atrial fibrillation or flutter since it can occasionally accelerate the ventricular response during atrial fibrillation and cause hemodynamic compromise.[28]

Chronic therapy for pre-excited atrial fibrillation should include a drug that slows conduction over the accessory connection. Quinidine, procainamide, disopyramide, encainide, flecainide, and amiodarone possess this effect. These drugs can also prevent atrial fibrillation and stabilize the ventricle to prevent ventricular fibrillation. Of these drugs, only quinidine, procainamide, and disopyramide are approved for the treatment of atrial fibrillation in the United States but studies of other compounds are presently ongoing.

Pharmacological therapy is successful in preventing symptomatic arrhythmias in a majority of patients with the Wolff-Parkinson-White syndrome. Surgical or other nonpharmacological therapy may be required for those patients with potentially life-threatening connections as well as those with medically refractory tachycardia and/or drug intolerance.

Nonpharmacological therapy includes antitachycardia pacemakers, catheter ablation of the accessory connection, or ablative surgery. Pacing techniques are usually employed to terminate episodes of reciprocating tachycardia but can also be used to prevent episodes of tachycardia.[29] Although studies have documented the efficacy of antitachycardia pacing, excessive limitations and adverse effects limit their applicability in Wolff-Parkinson-White patients. The major limitation is the development of atrial fibrillation, which can be quite hazardous to some patients with Wolff-Parkinson-White syndrome.

Surgical techniques are the most commonly used nonpharmacological therapy. Since the original description of the technique in 1968,[30] the procedure has evolved so that the overall success rate now approaches 100% with low mortality.[31,32] Because of the excellent success rate and low mortality, the indications for surgery have been liberalized and now include young healthy patients who no longer wish to be bothered with episodic tachycardia or who no longer wish to take daily antiarrhythmic therapy.

Catheter ablation of the accessory pathway is still considered experimental. There have been many reports of successful accessory connection ablation, especially when the connection is located in the posteroseptal position.[33,34] Left free wall ablation has been considered to be seldom effective and associated with an increased incidence of adverse effects including cardiac tamponade.[35] A recent report suggests improved success rates for accessory connections in diverse locations with a low complication rate.[36] These data, however, are still preliminary and need to be confirmed by other studies. Recently, catheter ablation of accessory pathways using radiofrequency current has reported success rates approaching surgery at several centers. In the future, the use of this technique may become more widespread if the safety and long-term efficacy prove similar to surgical procedures.

In summary, much has evolved since the original description of the WPW syndrome. We now understand the pathophysiology of the syndrome and have several successful methods of dealing with the problem.

References

1. Cohn AE, Fraser FR: Paroxysmal tachycardia and the effect of stimulation of the vagus nerves by pressure. Heart 4:93, 1913–1914.
2. Wolff L, Parkinson J, White PD: Bundle-branch block with short P-R interval in healthy young people prone to paroxysmal tachycardia. Am Heart J 5:685, 1930.
3. Rosenbaum FF, Hecht HH, Wilson FN, et al: The potential variations of the thorax and the esophagus in anomalous atrioventricular excitation. Am Heart J 29:281, 1945.
4. Gallagher JJ, Pritchett ELC, Sealy WC, et al: The preexcitation syndromes. Prog Cardiovasc Dis 20:285, 1978.
5. Chung KY, Walsh TJ, Massie E: Wolff-Parkinson-White syndrome. Am Heart J 69:116, 1965.
6. Wu D, Denes P, Amat-Y-Leon F, et al: Clinical, electrocardiographic and electrophysiologic observations in patients with paroxysmal supraventricular tachycardia. Am J Cardiol 41:1045, 1978.
7. Farshidi A, Josephson ME, Horowitz LN: Electrophysiologic characteristics of concealed bypass tracts: clinical and electrocardiographic correlates. Am J Cardiol 41:1052, 1978.
8. Green M, Heddle B, Dassen W, et al: Value of QRS alternation in determining the site of origin of narrow QRS supraventricular tachycardia. Circulation 68:368, 1983.
9. Kerr CR, Gallagher JJ, German LD: Changes in ventriculoatrial intervals with bundle branch block aberration during reciprocating tachycardia in patients with accessory atrioventricular pathways. Circulation 65:196, 1982.
10. Morady F, DiCarlo LA, Baerman JM, et al: Determinants of QRS alternans during narrow QRS tachycardia. J Am Coll Cardiol 9:489, 1987.
11. Kay GN, Pressley JC, Packer DL, et al: Value of the 12-lead electrocardiogram in discriminating atrioventricular nodal reciprocating tachycardia from circus movement atrioventricular tachycardia utilizing a retrograde accessory pathway. Am J Cardiol 59:296, 1987.
12. Gallagher JJ, Smith WM, Kasell J, et al: Use of the esophageal lead in the diagnosis of reciprocating supraventricular tachycardia. PACE 3:440, 1984.
13. Bardy GH, Packer DL, German LD, et al: Preexcited reciprocating tachycardia in patients with Wolff-Parkinson-White syndrome: incidence and mechanisms. Circulation 70:377, 1984.
14. Roark SF, McCarthy EA, Lee KL, et al: Observations on the occurrence of atrial fibrillation in paroxysmal supraventricular tachycardia. Am J Cardiol 57:571, 1986.

15. Klein GJ, Bashore TM, Sellers TD, et al: Ventricular fibrillation in the Wolff-Parkinson-White syndrome. N Engl J Med 301:1080, 1979.
16. Klein GJ, Gulamhusein SS: Intermittent preexcitation in the Wolff-Parkinson-White syndrome. Am J Cardiol 52:292, 1983.
17. Wellens HJJ, Braat S, Brugada P, et al: Use of procainamide in patients with the Wolff-Parkinson-White syndrome to disclose a short refractory period of the accessory pathway. Am J Cardiol 50:1087, 1982.
18. Critelli G, Grassi G, Perticone F, et al: Transesophageal pacing for prognostic evaluation of preexcitation syndrome and assessment of protective therapy. Am J Cardiol 51:513, 1983.
19. Fananapazir L, Packer DL, German LD, et al: Procainamide infusion test: inability to identify patients with Wolff-Parkinson-White syndrome who are potentially at risk of sudden death. Circulation 77:1291, 1988.
20. German LD, Gallagher JJ, Broughton A, et al: Effects of exercise and isoproterenol during atrial fibrillation in patients with Wolff-Parkinson-White syndrome. Am J Cardiol 57:1203, 1983.
21. Milstein S, Sharma AD, Klein GJ: Electrophysiologic profile of asymptomatic Wolff-Parkinson-White pattern. Am J Cardiol 57:1097, 1986.
22. Klein GJ, Yee R, Sharma AD: Longitudinal electrophysiologic assessment of asymptomatic patients with the Wolff-Parkinson-White electrocardiographic pattern. N Engl J Med 320:1229, 1989.
23. Waldo AL, Akhtar M, Benditt D, et al: Appropriate electrophysiologic study and treatment of patients with the Wolff-Parkinson-White syndrome. J Am Coll Cardiol 11:1124, 1988.
24. Yeh S-J, Lin F-C, Chou Y-Y, et al: Termination of paroxysmal supraventricular tachycardia with a single oral dose of diltiazem and propranolol. Circulation 71:104, 1985.
25. Waxman HL, Myerburg RJ, Appel R, et al: Verapamil for control of ventricular rate in paroxysmal supraventricular tachycardia and atrial fibrillation and flutter. Ann Intern Med 94:1, 1981.
26. Sellers TD, Bashore TM, Gallagher JJ: Digitalis in the pre-excitation syndrome: analysis during atrial fibrillation. Circulation 56:260, 1977.
27. Gulamhusein S, Ko P, Carruthers SG, et al: Acceleration of the ventricular response during atrial fibrillation in the Wolff-Parkinson-White syndrome after verapamil. Circulation 65:348, 1982.
28. Akhtar M, Gilbert CJ, Shenasa M: Effect of lidocaine on atrioventricular response via the accessory pathway in patients with Wolff-Parkinson-White syndrome. Circulation 63:435, 1981.
29. Osborn MJ, Holmes DR: Antitachycardia pacing. Clin Prog Electrophysiol Pacing 3:239, 1985.
30. Cobb FR, Blumenschein SD, Sealy WC, et al: Successful surgical interruption of the bundle of Kent in a patient with Wolff-Parkinson-White syndrome. Circulation 38:1018, 1968.
31. Gallagher JJ, Sealy WC, Cox JL, et al: Results of surgery for pre-excitation caused by accessory atrioventricular pathways in 267 consecutive cases. In: Josephson ME, Wellen HJJ (eds), Tachycardias, Mechanisms, Diagnosis and Treatment. Philadelphia, Lea and Febiger, 1984, pp 259–269.
32. Guiraudon GM, Klein GJ, Sharma AD, et al: Surgery for Wolff-Parkinson-

White syndrome: further experience with an epicardial approach. Circulation 74:525, 1986.
33. Bardy GH, Ivey TD, Coltorti F, et al: Developments, complications and limitations of catheter-mediated electrical ablation of posterior accessory atrioventricular pathways. Am J Cardiol 61:309, 1988.
34. Morady F, Scheinman MM, Kou WH, et al: Long-term results of catheter ablation of a posteroseptal accessory atrioventricular connection in 48 patients. Circulation 79:1160, 1989.
35. Fisher JD, Brodman R, Kim SG, et al: Attempted nonsurgical electrical ablation of accessory pathways via the coronary sinus in the Wolff-Parkinson-White syndrome. J Am Coll Cardiol 4:685, 1984.
36. Warin JF, Haissaguerre M: Fulguration of accessory pathways in any location: report of seventy cases. PACE 12:215, 1989.

General References

1. Prystowsky EN: Diagnosis and management of the preexcitation syndromes. Curr Probl Cardiol 13(4):225, 1988.
2. Benditt DG, Benson DW (eds): Cardiac Preexcitation Syndromes. Boston, Martinus Nijhoff, 1985.

Chapter 9

Wide QRS Tachycardias: Mechanism, Differential Diagnosis, and Acute Management

Patrick J. Tchou, Mohammad Jazayeri, Boaz Avitall, Paul J. Troup, and Masood Akhtar

Introduction

Accurate identification of the mechanism underlying a wide QRS tachycardia is important in guiding proper medical therapy. Since most of these tachycardias are paroxysmal in nature, patients usually present with these arrhythmias in an acute care or primary care setting. There is frequently a sense of urgency and concern when such a patient is seen since some of these arrhythmias can be life-threatening if not treated quickly and appropriately. This chapter will address the different mechanisms of ventricular activation that cause wide QRS complexes (>120 ms duration), the types of tachycardias, both supraventricular and ventricular in origin, which show wide QRS morphologies and an approach to the differential diagnosis and therapy of such tachycardias in the acute setting.

Why Are Some QRS Complexes Wide?

The QRS complex on the surface electrocardiogram represents transient voltage gradients created across the heart by propagation of a de-

From Naccarelli GV (ed): *Cardiac Arrhythmias: A Practical Approach.* Mount Kisco, NY, Futura Publishing Co., Inc., © 1991.

polarizing wave front as it spreads through the ventricular myocardium. Therefore, the QRS width, or its duration, approximates the time for an impulse to depolarize the entire ventricle. Synchronization of ventricular depolarization will result in a narrow QRS, while a factor that delays activation of any part of the ventricle will result in a wider QRS. Normal activation of the ventricles during supraventricular impulse propagation through the atrioventricular node will activate the myocardium through the His-Purkinje system. Activation of the His bundle and the bundle branches are not reflected in the surface QRS. Because of the branching network structure of the Purkinje system, a large portion of the ventricular endocardium is activated more or less synchronously. Such a branching network allows more synchronous activation of the entire endocardium from a supraventricular beat than from an impulse originating from the periphery of the Purkinje network or within the myocardium. Because of this synchronization, depolarization of the entire ventricle occurs more quickly during a supraventricular beat than during a ventricular beat, thus giving a narrower QRS appearance to the supraventricular beat. Given this understanding of how a normal supraventricular beat generates a narrow QRS, one can easily appreciate the various different mechanisms that generate a wide QRS tachycardia. Certainly, one mechanism would be ventricular tachycardia where the source of ventricular activation is in the myocardium. Activation of the ventricle via an accessory atrioventricular pathway would also manifest as a wide QRS since the ventricular myocardium is depolarized from the site of the accessory pathway and synchronization of endocardial activation is not present. A third type of wide QRS complex comes from activation of the ventricle via only one of the bundle branches. While relatively synchronized depolarization of the subendocardium occurs in the ventricle where bundle branch conduction is intact, the contralateral ventricle is activated via transeptal muscle conduction. Therefore, there is a delay in activating one of the ventricles and lack of synchronization of subendocardial activation in that ventricle leading to a wide QRS on the surface electrocardiogram.

Supraventricular Tachyarrhythmias with Wide QRS Morphologies

These are tachycardias that involve anterograde propagation of an electrical impulse over an accessory atrioventricular pathway or the atrioventricular node as an essential aspect of activating the ventricle. The exact mechanisms of the various forms of supraventricular tachycardias will not be discussed here as they are covered in a separate chapter. The discussion here will address issues relevant to how supraventricular tachyarrhythmias can present with wide QRS morphologies. Atrioventricular nodal re-entrant tachycardias, atrial tachycardias, or atrioventricular reciprocating tachycardias involving accessory pathways conducting in the retrograde direction can all manifest as wide QRS tachycardias if anterograde conduction through the normal pathway (atrioventricular node) encounters bundle branch block. This block can either be pathological, due to disease within the bundle branch system, or functional, due purely to normal conduction and refractory period properties of the bundle branches. If bundle branch block during tachycardia is pathological, it is also more likely that the patient will manifest a bundle branch block or other conduction abnormalities during normal sinus rhythm. With purely functional bundle branch blocks, the QRS during sinus rhythms is usually normal. It has also been an observation in our electrophysiology laboratory that functional bundle branch blocks tend to resolve spontaneously over several minutes. For this reason, while functional bundle branch blocks can be seen quite often at beginnings of tachycardias, especially ones induced by programmed stimulation in the laboratory, they are a much less likely source of wide QRS tachycardias in the primary care setting where a patient presenting with this tachycardia is usually having a sustained episode which had already lasted many minutes if not hours.

Some of the above-mentioned tachycardia mechanisms can also lead to wide QRS morphologies when the ventricles are predominantly or exclusively activated via an accessory pathway. Certainly, atrial tachycardias can conduct across an accessory pathway. In this respect, a major clinical concern is atrial fibrillation or atrial flutter with rapid conduction to the ventricle via the accessory pathway.[1,2] Some of these tachycardias may exhibit ventricular rates in the range of 300 beats per minute. Figures 1 and 2 show two examples of such rhythms. Aside from the hypotensive effect of such rates, there is a real potential for such rhythms to degenerate into ventricular fibrillation. Reports of sudden death in patients with the Wolff-Parkinson-White (WPW) syndrome are very likely due to this mechanism.[1,2]

With atrial or atrioventricular nodal re-entrant tachycardias that activate the ventricle through an accessory pathway, the width of the QRS will depend on competition between the accessory pathway and the normal atrioventricular nodal pathway for depolarization of the ventricles. In patients with the WPW syndrome, the width of the QRS may

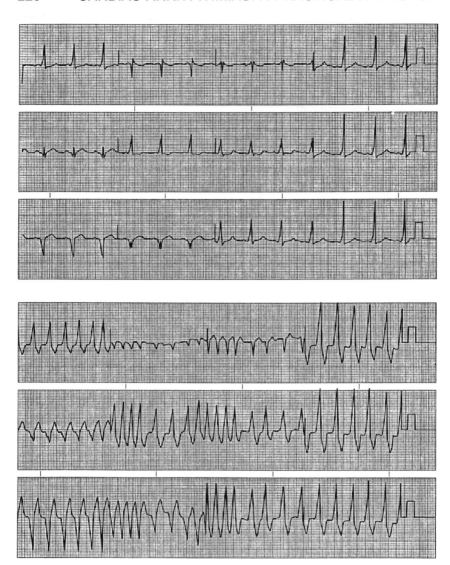

Figure 1. These two electrocardiograms are from a 28-year-old patient with the Wolff-Parkinson-White syndrome. The upper panel shows sinus rhythm with evidence of delta waves indicating ventricular pre-excitation. The lower panel shows atrial fibrillation with ventricular activation occurring almost exclusively over the accessory pathway giving a wide QRS appearance to the electrogram. Note that the shortest RR interval has a coupling of 210 ms (285 bpm).

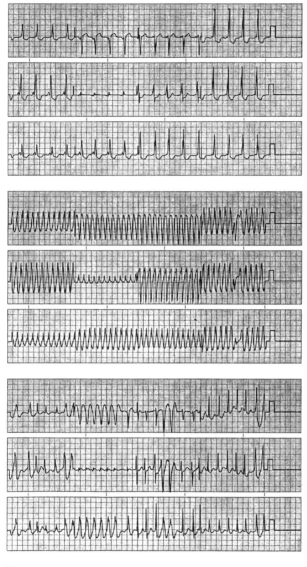

Figure 2. These three electrocardiograms are from a patient taken over a period of 2½ hours. The top panel shows sinus rhythm with ventricular pre-excitation demonstrated by delta waves. The second panel represents atrial flutter with 1:1 atrioventricular conduction over the accessory pathway resulting in a ventricular rate of 300 beats per minute. The third panel, taken 20 minutes later, shows the effect of intravenous procainamide. Ventricular rate has slowed considerably, averaging around 170 beats per minute, and conduction over the accessory pathway occurs only intermittently.

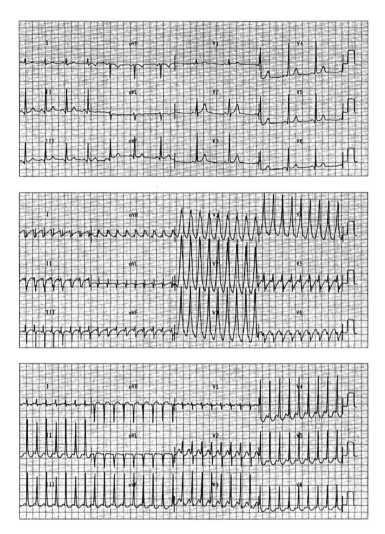

Figure 3. These three electrocardiograms are recorded from a 32-year-old male with recurrent episodes of palpitations. The upper panel show sinus rhythm. The amount of pre-excitation is quite subtle and can best be appreciated in lead V_2 where a delta wave can be seen. The absence of an S wave in lead V_1 also suggests ventricular pre-excitation. The S wave in lead V_1 is normally generated by late depolarization of the posterior left free wall. Its absence in this case suggests earlier activation of this portion of the left ventricle. The middle panel was obtained during right atrial pacing at a rapid rate. The QRS is now considerably wider with ventricular activation occurring mostly over the accessory pathway. This panel illustrates the ability of an atrial tachycardia to widen the QRS in patients with the WPW syndrome even

vary considerably from one supraventricular rhythm to another, depending on the extent of atrioventricular nodal conduction delay. For example, QRS widening during sinus rhythm can be minimal with only a subtle delta wave visible. With an atrial tachycardia, however, the QRS can become quite wide due to slowing of conduction in the node or quicker access of the ectopic atrial impulses to the accessory pathway than the node. An example of such differences is illustrated in Figure 3.

Another mechanism of wide QRS tachycardia that should be mentioned is the so-called antidromic tachycardia. The re-entrant circuit of this tachycardia involves anterograde atrioventricular conduction over an accessory pathway and retrograde ventriculoatrial conduction over the node or another accessory pathway. The former is sometimes referred to as "true antidromic" tachycardia. Figure 4 shows an example of a true antidromic tachycardia. True antidromic tachycardias are uncommon clinical entities in part due to the stringent electrophysiological requirements associated with initiation and sustenance of impulse propagation within the re-entrant circuit.[3]

Another infrequent mechanism of wide QRS supraventricular tachycardia is that associated with the so-called "Mahaim" fiber.[4,5] Recent reports have suggested that these tachycardias are more likely due to atriofascicular (right bundle branch) accessory pathways having node-like conduction properties rather than true nodoventricular pathways.[6,7] Because antegrade activation of the right bundle and ultimately the right ventricle during tachycardia occurs via this accessory pathway, the QRS morphology has a typical left bundle branch block pattern. An example of such a tachycardia is shown in Figure 5.

Mechanisms of Ventricular Tachycardias

The most common etiology of monomorphic wide QRS tachycardia seen in our institution as well as in others is ventricular tachycardia.[8–10] This is probably true at most institutions in the United States. It is

---

when delta waves are virtually unseen during sinus rhythm. The bottom panel shows orthodromic atrioventricular re-entrant tachycardia in the same patient. Because ventricular activation occurs exclusively via the atrioventricular node during this tachycardia, there is no pre-excitation at all. The presence of S waves in V_1 and V_2 confirms the fact that their absence during sinus rhythm (top panel) is due to ventricular pre-excitation.

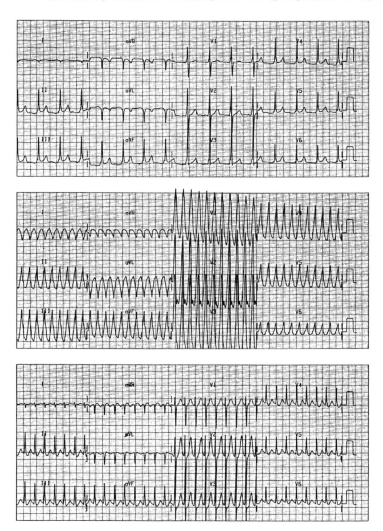

Figure 4. These three electrocardiograms are from a 14-year-old male who had recurrent episodes of palpitations. The top panel shows his normal atrial rhythm. The P wave axis is somewhat unusual ($-30°$) and may represent an ectopic atrial rhythm. Delta waves can be clearly seen preceding each QRS. The middle panel shows wide QRS tachycardia which was verified to be true antidromic tachycardia during electrophysiology study and intraoperative mapping. During tachycardia, atrioventricular conduction occurred via a left free wall accessory pathway while ventriculoatrial conduction propagated over the atrioventricular node. This tachycardia was quite rapid with a rate 250 beats per minute. The lower panel demonstrates that the patient is also capable of having a narrow QRS orthodromic atrioventricular re-entrant

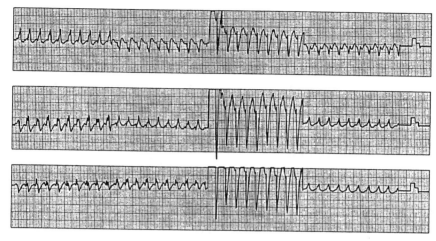

Figure 5. An example of supraventricular tachycardia is shown here in which the mechanism of re-entry involves an atriofascicular fiber with node-like slow conduction properties. Antegrade conduction during the re-entrant tachycardia occurs over the accessory pathway which connects from the anterior right atrium to the right bundle branch and, therefore, activates the ventricles preferentially over the right bundle branch giving the QRS a left bundle branch block appearance.

most commonly (80–90%) associated with coronary artery disease and a previous myocardial infarction. It is now generally accepted that the mechanism of monomorphic sustained ventricular tachycardia in patients with chronic myocardial infarctions is re-entry in the border zone between the scar and normal muscle.[11–15] The infarcted zones usually have subendocardial and subepicardial layers of surviving myocardial cell which are infiltrated with connective tissue resulting from the ischemic insult. Some types of scars, especially those involving the inferior wall, may have transmural islands of surviving muscle cells interspersed within the scar. Propagation of an electrical impulse within this scarred region may be quite slow even though the entrapped myocardial cells may have relatively normal action potentials. Slowed propagation cre-

tachycardia, which is the most common mechanism of tachycardia in patients with the Wolff-Parkinson-White syndrome. The re-entrant pathway of this tachycardia is the reverse of that described above involving antegrade conduction via the atrioventricular node and retrograde conduction over the accessory pathway.

ates the potential substrate for a re-entrant circuit leading to ventricular tachycardia in the presence of a triggering stimulus which initiates re-entry.

The next most common structural heart diseases associated with sustained monomorphic ventricular tachycardia are the dilated cardiomyopathies. These pathological entities also create scarring within the ventricles, although more on a microscopic scale compared to the large and better demarcated scarring present in healed myocardial infarctions. The pathological process, being more diffuse in nature, can involve the His-Purkinje system as well. These patients frequently have conduction abnormalities as reflected in abnormalities of the surface QRS complex during sinus rhythm. Such conduction abnormalities within the His-Purkinje system may play an important role in the mechanism of tachycardia in patients with dilated cardiomyopathies. Up to 30% or 40% of patients with dilated cardiomyopathies who have sustained monomorphic ventricular tachycardias may have so-called macro re-entry, or bundle branch re-entry, as the mechanism of ventricular tachycardia.[16,17]

There are several clinical characteristics that may help to identify a patient who is likely to have this mechanism as the cause of sustained monomorphic ventricular tachycardia.[16,17] These patients usually have a dilated cardiomyopathy with global hypokinesis of their ventricles even if they do have concomitant coronary artery disease and old myocardial infarcts. The PR interval on the surface 12-lead electrocardiogram is usually borderline or prolonged, reflecting increased conduction time within the His-Purkinje system. The 12-lead electrocardiogram commonly shows a nonspecific widening of the QRS, again reflecting conduction disturbances within the Purkinje system. When a 12-lead electrocardiogram of the tachycardia is available, the QRS morphology has a typical bundle branch block appearance, usually left bundle branch block. Examples of 12-lead electrocardiograms from a patient during sinus rhythm and during bundle branch re-entrant tachycardia are shown in Figure 6. Presence of these characteristics in a patient should prompt the physician to consider bundle branch re-entry as a cause of tachycardia. Diagnostic as well as therapeutic intervention should then be pursued with this mechanism in mind. Recognition of this mechanism in a patient has particular importance in deciding the approach to chronic therapy. Electrical transcatheter ablation of the right bundle branch is a very effective therapy which can usually be accomplished with very little morbidity and extremely low risk of mortality.[18,19] Ventricular tachycardias in patients with dilated cardiomyopathies unrelated to bundle branch re-entry could be related to intramural re-entry within

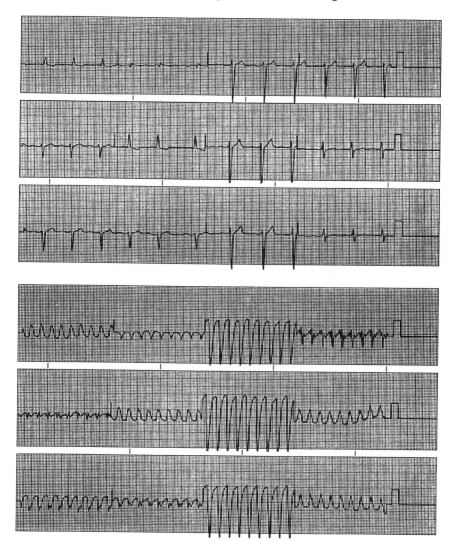

Figure 6. These two electrocardiograms were recorded from a man with a dilated cardiomyopathy superimposed on coronary artery disease. He had multiple clinical episodes of sustained monomorphic ventricular tachycardia which were associated with syncope. The top panel shows a 12-lead electrocardiogram during sinus rhythm. Note that the QRS has a nonspecific conduction delay with a duration of 116 ms and that the PR interval is prolonged. Electrophysiology study demonstrated an inducible bundle branch re-entrant ventricular tachycardia (lower panel) which was identical to the clinical tachycardia. A 12-lead electrocardiogram of this tachycardia revealed a left bundle branch block QRS morphology with left axis deviation. Catheter ablation of the right bundle branch abolished inducibility of this tachycardia and eliminated clinical recurrences.

the myocardium or due to automatic mechanisms. Definitive evidence, however, for either mechanism has not been reported in the literature.

While discussing ventricular tachycardias associated with cardio-myopathies, one should also include the syndrome of arrhythmogenic right ventricular dysplasia. This syndrome was first described in 1977,[20] and is characterized by a dysplastic right ventricle which is dilated, hy-pocontractile, and infiltrated by fatty deposits.[21,22] Because the source of ventricular tachycardia is from the right ventricle, the QRS morphology has a left bundle branch block appearance. However, the pathological process may not be limited to the right ventricle since left ventricular involvement has been reported on occasions.[23-25] Patients usually present at a young age and sometimes in the middle ages (before 50 years of age) with recurrent episodes of ventricular tachycardia, and on occasions, ventricular fibrillation. Long-term follow-up of 8 to 16 years have shown up to 20% mortality which is mostly due to sudden death and the causes are presumably arrhythmic in nature. The progressive nature of the disease may make efficacy assessment of both medical[21,25,26] and surgical therapies[27-29] difficult.

Recently, a syndrome has been described in the literature in which patients experience recurrent episodes of ventricular tachycardia having a right bundle branch block QRS morphology with a superior axis, yet they do not have any detectable structural heart disease.[30-39] Patients are generally young with ages ranging mostly from the teens to the thirties, although a few were in the 40- to 60-year-old range. An example of such a tachycardia is shown in Figure 7. This type of tachycardia seems to involve myocardial tissues within the left ventricle that have calcium-dependent slow conduction properties. The tachycardias can be facilitated or accelerated by catecholamines and suppressed with verapamil. Left ventricular endocardial mapping of these tachycardias indicates that they originate near the apex of the left ventricle.[35] While some reports in the literature suggest that triggered automaticity can be an explanation of the mechanism in these tachycardias,[32,39] more recent electrophysiological data are most consistent with a re-entrant phenomenon, with excitation of the myocardium during tachycardia occurring via the fascicular Purkinje network. It is, therefore, quite possible that the re-entrant pathway in these tachycardias involves the Purkinje network and a slowly conducting, calcium-dependent tissue as part of the circuit.

Exercised-induced ventricular tachycardia originating from the right ventricular outflow tract in patients with apparently normal hearts is another syndrome that was recently described in the literature.[40-46] This

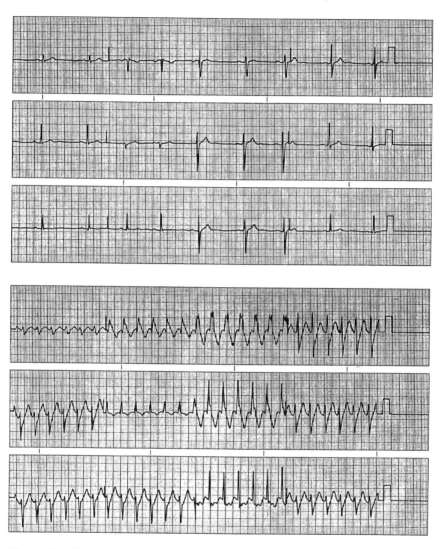

Figure 7. These two electrocardiograms are from an 18-year-old male with recurrent episodes of wide QRS tachycardia. Ventricular function was normal. The upper panel shows normal sinus rhythm. The lower panel reveals a wide QRS tachycardia initiated during electrophysiology study which was identical to his clinical arrhythmia. The tachycardia slowed initially and then became totally suppressed with verapamil infusion. The tachycardia QRS morphology suggests that the arrhythmic focus is located near the left ventricular apex.

type of arrhythmia is usually not inducible with programmed stimulation or is inducible only after infusion of isoproterenol. Because of their responsiveness to adrenergic stimulation and the difficulty in inducing these arrhythmias with programmed stimulation, it has been suggested that triggered automaticity related to delayed afterdepolarization of the myocardial action potential may be the underlying mechanism of this tachycardia.[42,43] This type of arrhythmia may respond to a variety of antiarrhythmic medications including type I and type III antiarrhythmics and beta-blockers. However, some patients do not have adequate control with any of these medication combinations and require surgical therapy.[45]

The ventricular tachycardia mechanisms discussed so far all manifest as monomorphic tachycardia. That is, the QRS complex maintains the same morphology from beat to beat. Some ventricular tachycardias, however, have polymorphic appearances. For physiological, pathological, as well as therapeutic reasons, it is important to clinically distinguish these tachycardias from the monomorphic variety. These tachycardias show beat to beat changes in their QRS morphologies which can sometimes be difficult to appreciate without multiple electrocardiographic leads. Nonsustained polymorphic ventricular tachycardias, when seen clinically, are a particularly alarming sign of impending cardiac arrest. Sustained versions of these tachycardias frequently degenerate into ventricular flutter or fibrillation with resultant cardiac arrest. These arrhythmias can be classified into two categories: those associated with lengthening of the QT interval and those associated with normal QT intervals. When this type of arrhythmia is associated with QT prolongation, it is labeled "torsades de pointes," which alludes to the twisting of the QRS axis in a continuous manner. Polymorphic ventricular tachycardias associated with prolonged QT can be further divided into those that are congenital versus those that are acquired secondary to drug therapy, electrolyte imbalances, or bradycardia. This division may be somewhat artificial since the acquired variety may represent a milder form, or a "subclinical" version of the disease which becomes manifest only when provoked by conditions that delay repolarization. A thorough review of the congenital syndrome is beyond the scope of this chapter.

Suffice it to say that these patients are at risk for multiple episodes of syncope as well as sudden death associated with polymorphic ventricular tachycardia. More commonly, patients presenting with polymorphic ventricular tachycardia and QT prolongation have electrolyte disturbances associated with diuretic therapy or secondary to gastrointestinal tract losses or are being treated with a drug that prolongs the

QT interval. Antiarrhythmic medications, especially the type Ia varieties (quinidine, procainamide, Norpace), are usually the culprits.[52-54] However, other medications that can affect the QT interval can also trigger this arrhythmia. Tricyclic antidepressants,[55] neuroleptic agents,[56,57] and even erythromycin[58] have been described to cause "torsades-like" arrhythmias. An example of torsades de pointes is shown in Figure 8. The mechanism of this tachyarrhythmia is not clearly delineated in the literature. Epicardial activation maps of polymorphic ventricular tachycardia in canine models indicate a shifting focus of earliest activation in the myocardium accounting for the changing electrocardiographic morphology.[59,60] At the membrane level, the mechanism may well be related to early afterdepolarizations seen during phase 3 of the cardiac action potential under certain pathological conditions.[61] Bradycardia and prolongation of repolarization appear to enhance early afterdepolarization similar to their effects on promoting torsades.

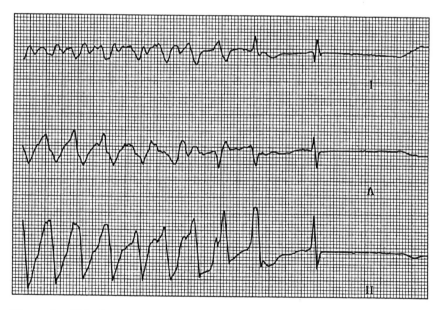

Figure 8. This three-lead electrocardiogram shows the initiation of torsades de pointes in a patient treated with quinidine. Note the markedly prolonged QT interval (>720 ms) just preceding initiation of polymorphic ventricular tachycardia. There is gradual beat-to-beat change in the QRS morphology which can be best appreciated in the "V" lead of this electrocardiographic monitor printout.

Polymorphic ventricular tachycardia not associated with QT prolongation appears to have a strong correlation with critical coronary disease. We recently examined the occurrence of polymorphic ventricular tachycardia unassociated with QT prolongation in a hospitalized patient population.[62] The most commonly associated cardiac disease in this population was high-grade coronary obstructions in vessels supplying viable myocardium. The tachyarrhythmias were usually very rapid. The polymorphic nature of these tachycardias is sometimes not evident on a single lead but can easily be appreciated when multiple leads are recorded (see Fig. 9). These tachycardias do not respond well to conventional antiarrhythmic medications. Acutely, they respond to beta-blocker therapy. However, because of their association with high-grade coronary stenosis, urgent myocardial revascularization surgery or angioplasty should be the therapy of choice. Long-term therapy with medications appears to have a poor outcome. If medical therapy is the only option, beta-blockers with perhaps the addition of amiodarone may have some effectiveness.

Acute Diagnosis and Treatment of Wide QRS Tachycardia

The most important distinction to be made prior to treatment of a wide QRS tachycardia in the acute setting is to determine whether the QRS morphology is monomorphic or polymorphic. The approach to therapy is quite different for these two entities. Appropriate therapy for monomorphic ventricular tachycardia could be disastrous if employed for the polymorphic types. Sustained polymorphic ventricular tachycardias are almost always hemodynamically unstable. Patients with this tachycardia would usually present in a cardiac arrest situation. However, these patients frequently have warning arrhythmias occurring as bursts of nonsustained polymorphic tachycardias. Treatment of these tachycardias with the usual antiarrhythmic agents should be avoided for they are either ineffective or may actually worsen the arrhythmia. The presence of QT prolongation may be difficult to detect. The T wave may not be prominent on a single lead and QT prolongation may only be visible after a long RR interval such as ones immediately following a premature beat. When polymorphic ventricular tachycardia is associated with QT prolongation, initial therapy should include intravenous magnesium sulfate (1 to 2 grams over 10–15 minutes) and isoproterenol to accelerate ventricular rate to 90 or 100 beats per minute. This approach

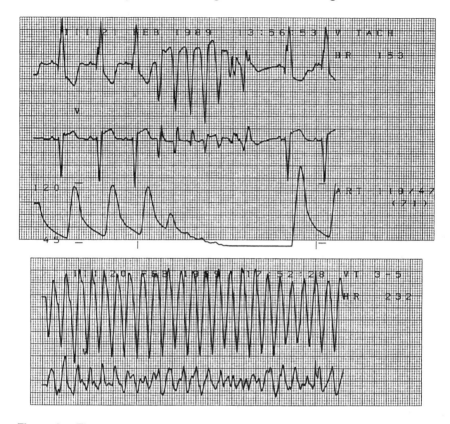

Figure 9. These two panels demonstrate the type of polymorphic ventricular tachycardia not associated with QT prolongation. This patient presented with syncope, and cardiac catheterization revealed high-grade obstruction of multiple coronary arteries supplying viable myocardium. The upper panel shows a nonsustained run of rapid tachycardia which is clearly polymorphic but the QT intervals of sinus beats are not prolonged. The arterial pressure tracing shows absence of ventricular ejection during the burst of tachycardia. The lower panel shows one of several sustained episodes in the same patient. Note the rather monomorphic appearance of the tachycardia in lead III (the upper lead). However, the "V" lead (lower) clearly shows beat-to-beat changes in QRS morphology.

would acutely stabilize the arrhythmia and allow insertion of a temporary pacemaker to replace isoproterenol as a means of accelerating heart rate. Any offending drug should be stopped immediately and serum electrolyte abnormalities, including K^+, Mg^{++}, and Ca^{++} deficiencies should be quickly corrected.

Polymorphic ventricular tachycardias unassociated with prolongation of QT interval or electrolyte abnormalities should raise the suspicion that there is high-grade ischemia within a large segment of myocardium. Beta-blockers appear to be most effective in acutely controlling the rhythm. Urgent definition of coronary anatomy should be pursued followed by appropriate revascularization of ischemic myocardium. It is important to emphasize the need to distinguish polymorphic ventricular tachycardias due to ischemia versus torsades de pointes. While beta-blocker therapy is contraindicated in many instances of torsades, it appears to be the most effective in ischemia-related polymorphic ventricular tachycardias. On the other hand, isoproterenol, which is probably the acute therapy of choice in torsades, could be disastrous if used in situations where there is ongoing myocardial ischemia.

Acute therapeutic approaches to monomorphic ventricular tachycardias are quite different from the polymorphic varieties. Identification of the origins of these tachycardias in the acute setting remains a clinical problem. Based on available literature, there appears to be a significant tendency by physicians to label a monomorphic wide QRS tachycardia as supraventricular in origin with aberrant ventricular conduction when the mechanism in the vast majority of cases is ventricular tachycardia.[8,9,63,64] Treatment of these tachycardias as supraventricular in origin, especially with intravenous verapamil, often results in acute hemodynamic decompensation.[65] Therefore, verapamil should be avoided in the acute therapy of wide QRS tachycardias unless one is certain that the tachycardia involves anterograde conduction over the atrioventricular node. The reason for misdiagnosis of ventricular tachycardia as supraventricular tachycardia appears to be in part related to a prevalent misconception that ventricular tachycardia is necessarily hemodynamically unstable.[65] While ventricular tachycardias in general may be more unstable than supraventricular tachycardias, one must consider the self-selection process that occurs with patients who present to a primary care setting with ventricular tachycardia. If unstable, they probably would present with a cardiac arrest. These rapid, hemodynamically unstable forms of ventricular tachycardias may degenerate quickly to ventricular fibrillation before cardiac monitoring can be initiated. Those who present with sustained ventricular tachycardia are those who remain hemodynamically stable, at least until they are treated with verapamil. Therefore, the decision to treat a wide QRS tachycardia as supraventricular in origin should not be made without conclusive evidence.

There are many previously reported clinical criteria that can be useful in making a bedside diagnosis of the underlying mechanism of a monomorphic wide QRS tachycardia. A patient's medical history can be quite useful. The presence of structural heart disease such as previous myocardial infarction or a dilated cardiomyopathy would indicate that the wide QRS tachycardia is highly likely to be ventricular tachycardia.[8,9] Physical examination can be helpful at times. Intermittent cannon waves in the jugular veins suggest atrioventricular dissociation that would be diagnostic of ventricular tachycardia. Wide variation in the intensity of S_1 on cardiac auscultation also suggests varying atrioventricular asynchrony consistent with ventricular tachycardia. The absence of these findings, however, does not exclude ventricular tachycardia.

A 12-lead electrocardiogram can also provide useful information in differentiating ventricular from supraventricular origins of a tachycardia. The presence of atrioventricular dissociation on the electrocardiogram is the most reliable evidence for ventricular origination of the tachycardia.[9] However, this criterion can be discerned from the surface electrocardiograms in only one-quarter of patients with ventricular tachycardia. On the other hand, one-to-one atrioventricular correspondence does not exclude ventricular tachycardia as approximately 25% of patients with ventricular tachycardia will have one-to-one retrograde conduction through the atrioventricular node.[9] The QRS morphology and its duration can also help differentiate supraventricular tachycardia with aberrancy from ventricular tachycardia.[9,66] Whenever QRS duration is greater than 140 ms, the physician should be suspicious that the tachycardia is ventricular in origin. The QRS axis may also be helpful. An extreme left axis, between $-90°$ and $-180°$, indicates ventricular tachycardia. The combination of left bundle branch block and right axis deviation is also highly suggestive of ventricular tachycardia.[9] The only QRS morphology that has good predictive value in identifying supraventricular tachycardia with aberrancy is the presence of a typical right bundle branch block QRS pattern in leads V_1 and V_6.[66] In V_1, this should be a rsR' pattern with a very distinct notch for the S wave. In lead V_6, the QRS pattern should be a QR complex with a terminal S wave that is slurred, a pattern that is typical of right bundle branch block.

In patients with bundle branch block during sinus rhythm, comparing a 12-lead electrocardiogram during sinus rhythm with the 12-lead electrocardiogram during wide QRS tachycardia could quite reliably distinguish between ventricular tachycardia and supraventricular tachycardia with aberrancy.[69] If lead by lead comparisons demonstrate identical QRS morphologies between the two electrocardiograms, then it is highly likely that the wide QRS tachycardia is supraventricular in origin.

If there are significant differences in any one lead, it is probable that the tachycardia is ventricular in origin.

In selecting acute therapy of a wide QRS tachycardia, it is wise to follow the old medical maxim "first do no harm." There are two potential problems in treating a ventricular tachycardia as supraventricular in origin. First, the use of drugs that have vasodilating properties such as verapamil can cause acute hemodynamic decompensation which can unnecessarily jeopardize the patient. Second, fortuitous termination of tachycardia following drug administration can mislead the physician to conclude that the tachycardia was supraventricular in origin and thus neglect further appropriate diagnostic and therapeutic interventions. While a particular ventricular tachycardia may be hemodynamically stable for a patient, the underlying substrate that generated that tachycardia may be capable of generating other less stable tachycardias. For example, a patient with a previous myocardial infarction may be capable of multiple ventricular tachycardias, some hemodynamically stable, while others could be quite unstable. Such patients should be thoroughly evaluated so that appropriate chronic therapies can be instituted.

Even when the origin of a wide QRS tachycardia is supraventricular, there are still circumstances where verapamil may cause hemodynamic deterioration. Atrial fibrillation or flutter with conduction across an accessory pathway can generate rapid ventricular responses. These accessory pathways do not usually respond to calcium channel blockade. However, the vasodilation caused by these drugs can further drop a patient's blood pressure and increase sympathetic tone. The increased sympathetic tone can, in turn, induce more rapid conduction across the accessory pathway leading to further blood pressure drop or production of ventricular fibrillation.[68] With all these potential pitfalls, it would seem wise to avoid use of verapamil altogether in the acute treatment of wide QRS tachycardias.

Drug therapy of a monomorphic wide QRS tachycardia should always be approached cautiously with continuous monitoring of the patient's cardiac rhythm. A defibrillator should be at bedside and ready to be used because heart rate and hemodynamic stability of these patients can change rapidly. While under close monitoring, one or two bolus doses of intravenous lidocaine, 1 mg/kg, can be used as an initial treatment of a wide QRS tachycardia without significant concern that it may harm the patient. Many tachycardias, however, will not respond to this medication. The next drug of choice available currently in the United States is intravenous procainamide. This drug should be infused at a rate no greater then 50 mg/min up to 10 mg/kg total dose. The patient's blood pressure should be checked after every 50 mg since this medication has the potential to lower blood pressure. The electrophysiological effect of procainamide should cause slowing if not termination of tachycardia whether the origin of the tachycardia is supraventricular or ventricular. In places where drugs such as ajmaline, adenosine, and even intravenous amiodarone are available, they can also be used in the acute setting. Adenosine may be particularly attractive since it is an extremely short-acting drug that markedly slows anterograde atrioventricular nodal conduction. Should the patient not respond to therapy or if the hemodynamic status deteriorates, one should terminate the tachycardia quickly with direct current cardioversion. Since response to therapy is not useful in identifying the origin of a tachycardia, a thorough diagnostic work-up should be pursued in all of these patients following acute termination of their tachycardia.

As this chapter has hopefully demonstrated, the differential diagnosis and therapeutic approach to a patient who presents with a wide QRS tachycardia can be quite complex. What may be appropriate under one set of circumstances may be disastrous in a different situation. In approaching the acute therapy of such tachycardias, one should always be cognizant of the possible underlying pathologies and avoid the pitfalls that could endanger a patient's well-being.

References

1. Dreifus L, Haiat R, Watanabe Y, et al: Ventricular fibrillation: a possible mechanism of sudden death in patients with Wolff-Parkinson-White syndrome. Circulation 63:520, 1971.
2. Klein G, Bashore T, Sellers TD, et al: Ventricular fibrillation in the Wolff-Parkinson-White syndrome. N Engl J Med 301:1080, 1979.
3. Lehmann MH, Tchou P, Mahmud R, et al: Electrophysiological determinants of antidromic reentry induced during atrial extrastimulation: insights from a pacing model of Wolff-Parkinson-White syndrome. Circulation Research 65:295, 1989.
4. Gallagher JJ, Smith WM, Kasell JH, et al: Role of Mahaim fibers in cardiac arrhythmias in man. Circulation 64:176, 1981.
5. Bardy GH, German LD, Packer DL, et al: Mechanism of tachycardia using a nodofasicular Mahaim fiber. Am J Cardiol 54:1140, 1984.
6. Tchou P, Lehmann M, Jazayeri M, et al: Atriofascicular connection or a nodoventricular Mahaim fiber? Electrophysiologic elucidation of the pathway and associated reentrant circuit. Circulation 77:837, 1988.
7. Klein GJ, Guiraudon GM, Kerr CR, et al: "Nodoventricular" accessory pathway: evidence for a distinct accessory pathway with atrioventricular node-like properties. J Am Coll Cardiol 11:1035, 1988.

8. Tchou P, Young P, Mahmud R, et al: Useful clinical criteria for the diagnosis of ventricular tachycardia. Am J Med 84:53, 1988.
9. Akhtar M, Shenasa M, Jazayeri M, et al: Wide QRS complex tachycardia: reappraisal of a common clinical problem. Ann Intern Med 109:905, 1988.
10. Steinman RT, Herrera C, Schuger CD, et al: Wide QRS tachycardia in the conscious adult: ventricular tachycardia is the most frequent cause. JAMA 261:1013, 1989.
11. Wellens HJJ, Duren DR, Lie KI: Observation on mechanism of ventricular tachycardia in man. Circulation 54:237, 1976.
12. Josephson ME, Horowitz LN, Farshidi A, et al: Recurrent sustained ventricular tachycardia. I. Mechanisms. Circulation 57:431, 1978.
13. Josephson ME, Horowitz LN, Farshidi A: Continuous local electrical activity: a mechanism of recurrent ventricular tachycardia. Circulation 57:659, 1978.
14. Josephson ME, Buxton AE, Marcchlinski FR, et al: Sustained ventricular tachycardia in coronary artery disease: evidence for reentrant mechanism. In: Zipes DP, Jalife J (eds), Cardiac Electrophysiology and Arrhythmia. Orlando, FL, Grune and Stratton, p 409, 1985.
15. DeBakker JMT, VanCapelle FJL, Janse MJ, et al: Reentry as a cause of ventricular tachycardia in patients with chronic ischemic heart disease: electrophysiologic and anatomic correlation. Circulation 77:589, 1988.
16. Caceres J, Jazayeri M, McKinnie J, et al: Sustained bundle branch reentry as a mechanism of clinical tachycardia. Circulation 79:256, 1989.
17. Tchou P, Blanck Z, McKinnie JJ, et al: Mechanism of inducible ventricular tachycardia in patients with idiopathic dilated cardiomyopathy. JACC 13:2, 174A, 1989.
18. Tchou P, Jazayeri M, Denker S, et al: Transcatheter electrical ablation of right bundle branch. Circulation 78:246, 1988.
19. Langberg JJ, Desai J, Dullet N, et al: Treatment of macroreentrant ventricular tachycardia with radiofrequency ablation of the right bundle branch. Am J Cardiol 63:1010, 1989.
20. Fontaine G, Guiraudon G, Frank R, et al: Stimulation studies and epicardial mapping in ventricular tachycardia: study of mechanism and selection for surgery. In: Kulbertus H (ed), Reentrant Arrhythmias, Mechanism and Treatment. Lancaster, MTP Publishing, 1977, p 334.
21. Marcus FI, Fontaine G, Guiraudon G, et al: Right ventricular dysplasia: a report of 24 adult cases. Circulation 65:384, 1982.
22. Frank R, Fontaine G, Guiraudon G, et al: Dysplasic ventriculaire droite arytmogene et maladie de Uhl. Arch Mal Coeur 75:361, 1982.
23. Manyari DE, Klein GJ, Gulamhusein S, et al: Arrhythmogenic right ventricular dysplasia: a generalized cardiomyopathy? Circulation 68:251, 1983.
24. Webb JG, Kerr CR, Huckell VF, et al: Left ventricular abnormalities in arrhythmogenic right ventricular dysplasia. Am J Cardiol 58:568, 1986.
25. Blomstrom-Lundqvist C, Sabel KG, Bertil Olsson S: A long-term follow-up of 15 patients with arrhythmogenic right ventricular dysplasia. Br Heart J 58:477, 1987.
26. Rossi P, Massumi A, Gillette P, et al: Arrhythmogenic right ventricular dysplasia: clinical features, diagnostic techniques, and current management. Am Heart J 103:415, 1982.

27. Guiraudon G, Fontaine G, Frank R, et al: Surgical treatment of ventricular tachycardia guided by ventricular mapping in 23 patients without coronary artery disease. Ann Thorac Surg 32:439, 1981.
28. Fontaine G, Guiraudon G, Frank R, et al: Surgical management of ventricular tachycardia unrelated to myocardial ischemia or infarction. Am J Cardiol 49:397, 1982.
29. Guiraudon GM, Klein GJ, Gulamhusein S, et al: Total disconnection of the right ventricular free wall: surgical treatment of right ventricular tachycardia associated with right ventricular dysplasia. Circulation 67:463, 1983.
30. Strasberg B, Kusniec J, Lewin R, et al: An unusual ventricular tachycardia responsive to verapamil. Am Heart J 111:190, 1986.
31. Sethi K, Manoharan S, Mohan J, et al: Verapamil in idiopathic ventricular tachycardia of right bundle branch block morphology: observations during electrophysiologic and exercise testing. PACE 9:8, 1986.
32. Lerman B, Belardinelli L, West GA, et al: Adenosine-sensitive ventricular tachycardia: evidence suggesting cyclic AMP-mediated triggered activity. Circulation 74:270, 1986.
33. Maisuls E, Maor N, Lorber A: Idiopathic recurrent sustained parasystolic ventricular tachycardia responsive to verapamil in a 15-year-old patient. Int J Cardiol 15:116, 1987.
34. Chiale PA, Sicouri SJ, Elizari MV, et al: Chronic idiopathic idioventricular tachycardia caused by slow response automaticity. PACE 10:1371, 1987.
35. Ohe T, Shimomura K, Aihara N, et al: Idiopathic sustained left ventricular tachycardia: clinical and electrophysiologic characteristics. Circulation 77:560, 1988.
36. Belhassen B, Rotmensch HH, Laniado S: Response of recurrent sustained ventricular tachycardia to verapamil. Br Heart J 46:679, 1981.
37. Lin FC, Finely CD, Rahimtoola SH, et al: Idiopathic paroxysmal ventricular tachycardia with QRS pattern of right bundle branch properties. Am J Cardiol 52:95, 1983.
38. German LD, Packer DL, Bardy GH, et al: Ventricular tachycardia induced by atrial stimulation in patients without symptomatic cardiac disease. Am J Cardiol 52:1202, 1983.
39. Zipes DP, Foster PR, Troup PJ, et al: Atrial induction of ventricular tachycardia: reentry versus triggered automaticity. Am J Cardiol 44:1, 1979.
40. Pietras RJ, Lam W, Bauernfeind R, et al: Chronic recurrent right ventricular tachycardia in patients without ischemic heart disease: clinical haemodynamic and angiographic findings. Am Heart J 105:357, 1983.
41. Mokotoff DM, Quinones MA, Miller RR: Exercise-induced ventricular tachycardia. Chest 77:10, 1980.
42. Sung RJ, Shen EN, Morady F, et al: Electrophysiologic mechanism of exercise-induced sustained ventricular tachycardia. Am J Cardiol 51:525, 1983.
43. Wu D, Lou HC, Hung JS: Exercise-triggered paroxysmal ventricular tachycardia: a repetitive rhythmic activity possibly related to after-depolarization. Ann Intern Med 95:410, 1981.
44. Palileo EV, Ashley WW, Swiryin S, et al: Exercise provocable right ventricular outflow tract tachycardia. Am Heart J 104:185, 1982.

45. Holt PM, Wainwright RJ, Curry PVL: Right ventricular outflow tract tachycardias in patients without apparent structural heart disease. Int J Cardiol 10:99, 1986.
46. Woelfel A, Foster JR, McAllister RG, et al: Efficacy of verapamil in exercise-induced ventricular tachycardia. Am J Cardiol 56:292, 1985.
47. Dessertenne F: La tachycardie ventriculaire a deux foyers opposes variable. Arch Mal Coeur 59:263, 1966.
48. Moss AJ, Schwartz PJ: Delayed repolarization (QT or QTU prolongation) and malignant ventricular arrhythmias. Mod Concepts Cardiovasc Med 51:85, 1982.
49. Schwartz PJ: The long Q-T syndrome. In: Kulbertus HE, Wellens HJJ (eds), Sudden Death. The Hague, Martinus Nijhoff, pp 358–378, 1980.
50. Schwartz PJ, Moss AJ: Q-T interval prolongation as predictor of sudden death in patients with myocardial infarction. Circulation 57:1074, 1978.
51. Schwartz PJ, Periti M, Malliani A: The long Q-T syndrome. Am Heart J 89:378, 1975.
52. Keren A, Tzivoni D, Gavish D, et al: Etiology, warning signs and therapy of torsades de pointes. Circulation 64:1167, 1981.
53. Kay GN, Plumb VJ, Arciniegas JG, et al: Torsades de pointes: the long-short initiating sequence and other clinical features. Observations in 32 patients. JACC 2:806, 1983.
54. Smith WM, Gallagher JJ: "Les torsades de pointes": An unusual ventricular arrhythmia. Ann Intern Med 93:578, 1980.
55. Fowler NO, McCall D, Chou TC, et al: Electrocardiographic changes and cardiac arrhythmias in patients receiving psychotropic drugs. Am J Cardiol 37:223, 1976.
56. Tri T, Combs DT: Phenothiazine-induced ventricular tachycardia. West J Med 123:412, 1975.
57. Hollister LE, Kosek JC: Sudden death during treatment with phenothiazine derivatives. JAMA 192:93, 1965.
58. McComb JM, Campbell N, Cleland J: Recurrent ventricular tachycardia associated with QT prolongation after mitral valve replacement and its association with intravenous administration of erythromycin. Am J Cardiol 54:922, 1984.
59. Bardy GH, Ungerleider RM, Smith WM, et al: A mechanism of torsades de pointes in a canine model. Circulation 67:52, 1983.
60. Inoue H, Murakawa Y, Toda I, et al: Epicardial activation patterns of torsades de pointes in canine hearts with quinidine-induced long QT interval but without myocardial infarction. Am Heart J 111:1080, 1986.
61. Brachmann J, Scherlag BJ, Rosenshtraukh LV, et al: Bradycardia-dependent triggered activity: relevance to drug-induced multiform ventricular tachycardia. Circulation 68:846, 1983.
62. Tchou P, Atassi K, Jazayeri M, et al: Etiology of polymorphic ventricular tachycardia in the absence of prolonged QT. JACC 13:2, 21A, 1989.
63. Stewart RB, Bardy GH, Greene HL: Wide complex tachycardia: misdiagnosis and outcome after emergent therapy. Ann Intern Med 104:766, 1986.
64. Dancy M, Camm AJ, Ward D: Misdiagnosis of chronic recurrent ventricular tachycardia. Lancet II:320, 1985.

65. Morady F, Baerman JM, DiCarlo LA Jr, et al: A prevalent misconception regarding wide complex tachycardias. JAMA 254:2790, 1985.
66. Wellens HJJ, Bar FW, Lie KI: The value of the electrocardiogram in the differential diagnosis of a tachycardia with a widened QRS complex. Am J Med 64:27, 1978.
67. Dongas J, Lehmann MH, Mahmud R, et al: Value of preexisting bundle branch block in the electrocardiographic differentiation of supraventricular from ventricular origin of wide QRS tachycardia. Am J Cardiol 55:717, 1985.
68. McGovern B, Garan H, Ruskin JN: Precipitation of cardiac arrest by verapamil in patients with Wolff-Parkinson-White syndrome. Ann Intern Med 104:791, 1986.

Chapter 10

Sinus Nodal Dysfunction and Atrioventricular Conduction Disturbances

William M. Miles and Lawrence S. Klein

Introduction

The purpose of this chapter is to discuss several entities that, in their extreme, result in bradycardia and often necessitate cardiac pacing. These entities include sinus nodal dysfunction (or sick sinus syndrome) and atrioventricular conduction delay or block located either in the AV node or in the His-Purkinje system.

Sinus Nodal Dysfunction

Sinus nodal dysfunction refers to a heterogeneous group of disorders that are often referred to as "sick sinus syndrome."[1,2] There are several abnormalities included in the sick sinus syndrome. These include *persistent spontaneous sinus bradycardia* not due to reversible factors such as drug therapy and which is inappropriate for the physiological conditions. *Sinus arrest* refers to sudden unexpected failure of arterial activity

From Naccarelli GV (ed): *Cardiac Arrhythmias: A Practical Approach.* Mount Kisco, NY, Futura Publishing Co., Inc., © 1991.

Supported in part by the Herman C. Krannert Fund, by grants HL-06308 and HL-07182 from the National Heart, Lung, and Blood Institute of the National Institutes of Health, U.S. Public Health Service, the American Heart Association, Indiana Affiliate, Inc., by the Attorney General of Indiana Public Health Trust and by the Roudebush Veterans Administration Medical Center, Indianapolis.

without a distinct pattern (see below) to suggest exit block. When sinus arrest occurs, asystole may result or an ectopic atrial or junctional escape rhythm. *Sinus exit block* is defined by sudden unexpected absence of a P wave in a distinct pattern, suggesting that the sinus node has discharged but the impulse has failed to exit from the perinodal tissue; examples would be exact doubling of the P-P interval (Fig. 1), or a pattern of P-P intervals suggestive of Wenckebach block within the perinodal tissue between the sinus pacemaker cells and the atrial myocardium (for example, a repetitive pattern of P-P intervals where the longest P-P interval is followed by the next longest P-P interval followed by decreasing P-P intervals until the longest interval occurs again, and the longest interval is less than twice the shortest; see the discussion of typical Wenckebach conduction below). *Combinations of sinoatrial and AV conduction abnormalities* exist in many patients, implying that the disease process causing sinus nodal dysfunction may be diffuse and may involve more than just the atrial or sinus nodal tissue. *Tachycardia-bradycardia syndrome* refers to alternation of paroxysmal atrial tachycardia or atrial fibrillation with marked sinus bradycardia or sinus arrest (Fig. 2). Some patients with this syndrome will demonstrate abnormal AV conduction

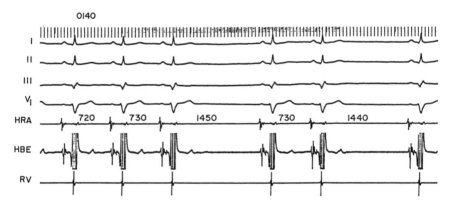

Figure 1. Sinus exit block. The format and abbreviations used here are employed for all of the subsequent intracardiac tracings in this chapter unless specified otherwise. Surface leads I, II, III, and VI are displayed with high right atrial (HRA), His bundle electrogram (HBE), and right ventricular (RV) electrograms. The patient has sinus rhythm interrupted by the sudden absence of a P wave after the third and fifth complexes. The cycle length of the pauses is approximately twice that of the predominant sinus rate, indicating that the sinus activation is occurring regularly but intermittently fails to conduct out of the perinodal tissues to the atrium.

234146

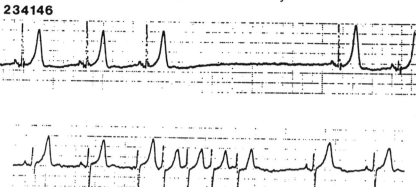

Figure 2. Electrocardiogram of a patient with tachycardia-bradycardia syndrome. This monitor strip illustrates sinus arrest (top panel) co-existing with short runs of atrial tachycardia (bottom panel).

with slow ventricular response during periods of atrial fibrillation. Many patients with the tachycardia-bradycardia syndrome will demonstrate marked suppression of sinus nodal activity immediately after termination of supraventricular tachycardia, resulting in a prolonged and often symptomatic sinus pause. Another manifestation of diffuse cardiac electrical involvement distal to the sinus node in this syndrome is the phenomenon of overdrive suppression of subsidiary pacemakers in addition to the sinus node, resulting in extremely slow ventricular rates in some patients once the sinus node fails. More than one manifestation of the sick sinus syndrome may be present in any one patient.

In summary, the sick sinus syndrome encompasses a variety of manifestations of sinus nodal dysfunction plus impaired AV conduction, atrial tachyarrhythmias, and suppression of subsidiary pacemakers. In its early stages, sick sinus syndrome may present as persistent inappropriate sinus bradycardia, paroxysmal atrial fibrillation, prolonged sinus pauses after spontaneous conversion or cardioversion of atrial fibrillation, an inappropriate sinus rate for physiological circumstances (for example, lack of rate acceleration with exercise), or shifting atrial pacemakers.

Etiology of Sinus Nodal Dysfunction

Sinus nodal dysfunction can be either intrinsic (i.e., an electrophysiological abnormality of the sinoatrial node or perinodal tissues) or autonomic (i.e., either an exaggerated response to autonomic influences or excessive autonomic influences on the sinus node and other subsidiary pacemakers). Reversible causes of sinus nodal dysfunction include excessive vagal tone, hyperkalemia, hypercarbia, hypothermia, increased intracranial pressure, and sepsis. Pharmacological agents that can depress sinus nodal function include beta-blocking drugs, calcium channel blockers, sympatholytic agents such as methyldopa or clonidine, type I and type III antiarrhythmic agents such as quinidine or amiodarone, cimetidine, lithium, amitriptyline, and chlorpromazine. Patients with sick sinus syndrome have been reported to be particularly sensitive to the effects of digitalis. Therefore, patients with known sinus nodal dysfunction should be closely observed upon initiation of digitalis therapy. These factors may cause reversible sinus nodal dysfunction in intrinsically normal sinus nodes or may unmask mild, latent sinus nodal dysfunction. Well-trained athletes with markedly increased vagal tone can occasionally develop such marked sinus nodal and AV nodal slowing that symptoms may occur from sinus bradycardia or AV block despite otherwise normal hearts.[3] These patients may benefit from moderate deconditioning to prevent these arrhythmias.

Intrinsic sinus nodal dysfunction can occur in patients with ischemic heart disease, rheumatic heart disease or other inflammatory myocardial disease, pericarditis, cardiomyopathy (especially amyloidosis), collagen vascular diseases, surgical injury, Friederich's progressive muscular dystrophy, Duchenne's and myotonic muscular dystrophy, metastatic disease, hemochromatosis, and other autoimmune diseases. Since many of these disorders tend to occur in older patients, sinus nodal dysfunction is most frequent in the older age groups. The most common cause of sinus nodal dysfunction appears to be idiopathic degenerative fibrosis of the sinus node.

In children, sinus nodal dysfunction occurs most commonly after surgical correction of congenital heart disease, especially the Mustard procedure for correction of transposition of the great arteries,[4] but it has been reported after correction of other congenital defects. The cause is probably surgical trauma to the sinus node during atriotomy or superior vena cava cannulation. Occasionally, children with unoperated congenital heart disease may develop sinus nodal dysfunction, or it may be familial or idiopathic and associated with no known cardiac abnormality.

Anatomy and Physiology of Sinus Nodal Dysfunction

The sinus node is located just beneath the epicardium near the junction of the right atrium and superior vena cava. The blood supply to the sinus node is usually from the sinus nodal artery that arises from the proximal right coronary artery in approximately 60% of patients and the proximal circumflex artery in the remainder. The sinus node has a collagenous framework and two types of specialized cells. The P cells are small round cells in grape-like clusters located mainly within the central portion of the sinus node and are probably the site of impulse formation. The transitional cells are elongated, interweaving fibers that probably function to conduct impulses toward the atrium. The sinus nodal area is richly innervated with autonomic nerves and ganglia. With increasing age, the collagen and other connective tissues increase.

Apparent sinus nodal dysfunction can be caused by either abnormal impulse formation within the sinus node or abnormal conduction of the sinus nodal impulse through the perinodal tissues. Sinus nodal cells have low resting membrane potentials and action potential contours similar to those of AV nodal cells, whereas the perinodal fibers have normal resting potentials and upstroke velocities but have longer refractory periods than sinus nodal pacemaker cells or the contiguous atrial cells. Therefore, this physiological substrate may prevent a sinus nodal impulse from reaching the atrial tissue should disease be present in the perinodal areas.

Several different pathological patterns have been reported in patients with the sick sinus syndrome,[5–7] emphasizing the heterogeneity of this condition. There may be total or subtotal destruction of the sinus node, or there may be areas where there is discontinuity between the nodal and the atrial tissue. Inflammatory or degenerative changes may also be seen in the nerves or ganglia surrounding the node, although changes in the arterial blood supply are infrequent. There may be fibrosis and fatty infiltration in the region of the sinus node, or changes in the adjacent atrial wall may occur. A sclerodegenerative process may involve the AV node and the His-Purkinje system as well as the sinus node. In some patients, a marked loss of nodal cells may occur beyond that normally expected for a particular age. Occasionally, no detectable morphologic abnormality in the sinus node can be found.

Symptoms

The symptoms from sinus nodal dysfunction and its associated conduction system abnormalities are often intermittent and unpredictable. Sinus nodal dysfunction is often benign, and marked sinus bradycardia and prolonged sinus pauses can be normal in apparently healthy young adults, especially at night.[8] It is critical to correlate the electrocardio-graphic abnormality suggesting sinus nodal dysfunction and the patient's symptoms because of the frequent occurrence of many of these electrocardiographic phenomena in asymptomatic people. The most common symptoms related to excessive bradycardia are presyncope and syncope. When these symptoms occur and are well-documented to be due to bradyarrhythmia, therapy is indicated. Some patients present with symptoms due to tachyarrhythmias as well as bradyarrhythmias. A classic presentation includes paroxysmal atrial fibrillation in a patient symptomatic with palpitations or dizziness, and upon termination of the tachyarrhythmia, a long asystolic pause may cause syncope. Some patients may have more nonspecific and less episodic manifestations such as fatigue, congestive heart failure, or angina related to low cardiac output due to chronic bradycardia. Systemic embolism may occur, especially in patients with the tachycardia-bradycardia syndrome.

Evaluation of the Patient with Suspected Sinus Nodal Dysfunction

Evaluation of the patient with sick sinus syndrome is most definitive when symptoms can be correlated with electrocardiographic abnormalities. This usually cannot be accomplished with a simple 12-lead electrocardiogram or short ECG rhythm strip and usually requires prolonged electrocardiographic monitoring. It is reasonable to start with a routine 24-hour Holter recording to identify frequently occurring arrhythmias, but in most patients symptomatic episodes are so infrequent that they cannot be reliably identified with only 24 or 48 hours of monitoring. In this situation, an event recorder that the patient can use for a month or more may be extremely useful. When the patient's symptoms occur, he can press the event marker and an electrocardiographic recording is stored, consisting of several seconds or minutes prior to (using a memory loop) and after the event. These long-term event monitors are the single most useful way of documenting symptoms from sinus nodal dysfunction but have the following drawbacks: (1) the patient must either remain conscious long enough to activate the monitor, remember to activate it immediately upon awakening from an event, or have a friend or spouse activate the monitor should an event occur; (2) it may not be advisable in some patients to allow another potentially serious event to occur in order to obtain the recording; and (3) the event must occur at least once over a several-month period in order to record it. Often a frank syncopal episode is not necessary to make the diagnosis; a relatively prolonged episode of bradycardia or tachycardia with dizziness may be sufficient.

One must remember that sinus bradycardia can be a normal phenomenon. It is most likely to be pathological when it is severe (less than 40 beats per minute), persistent over a long period of time, and inappropriate for the clinical situation, i.e., the heart rate not increasing with exercise. Likewise, sinus arrhythmia may be prominent in many normal people, and pauses of up to 2 seconds may occur commonly, especially at night. This emphasizes the difficulty in establishing a diagnosis of true sinus nodal dysfunction without correlation of electrocardiographic abnormalities with symptoms. When assessing the patient with suspected sinus nodal dysfunction, it is very important to exclude reversible causes, especially drug-related causes. Increased vagal tone, even though reversible acutely by vagolytic drugs such as IV atropine or transcutaneous scopolamine, is not always reversible chronically, and if symptomatic, more definitive therapy such as pacing may be required.

Because of the difficulty in establishing a diagnosis, several provocative tests may be useful in the evaluation of sinus nodal dysfunction. All provocative tests are limited by the occurrence of false positive and false negative results, and are not as desirable as documenting spontaneous arrhythmias with symptoms. Exercise testing may reveal a lack of the normal increase in sinus nodal rate with exercise[9] (remembering that well-trained athletes may also not increase their heart rate with exercise as much as the average person). An abnormal response to carotid sinus massage (arbitrarily defined as a pause greater than 3 seconds, using up to 5 seconds of carotid pressure) may be suggestive of sinus nodal dysfunction (Fig. 3), but this hypersensitive carotid sinus reflex may occur in many asymptomatic patients, especially the elderly.[10] The hypersensitive carotid sinus syndrome may coexist with the sick sinus syndrome. Care must be taken in applying carotid sinus pressure in the older age group because of the possibility of carotid disease and subsequent cerebrovascular accident.

Pharmacological testing of the sinus node by giving atropine or isoproterenol to increase or propranolol to decrease the sinus rate may be useful in some patients.[11] However, the criteria for normal versus abnormal responses are not well established, and the sensitivity and specificity of this pharmacological testing at detecting clinically significant sinus nodal dysfunction is not clear, re-emphasizing the need for correlation with clinical symptoms. The intrinsic heart rate after complete autonomic blockade (propranolol 0.2 mg per kg and atropine 0.04

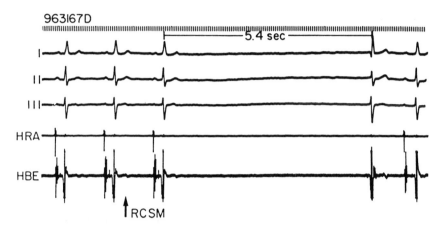

Figure 3. Abnormal sinus nodal slowing with carotid sinus massage. During sinus rhythm, right carotid sinus massage (RCSM, arrow) was applied and the patient had a prolonged asystolic pause (5.4 seconds) closed by a junctional escape prior to resumption of sinus rhythm. This exaggeration of the normal response of the sinus node to carotid sinus massage represents a hypersensitive carotid sinus reflex but may not always be responsible for symptoms.

mg per kg) represents the sinus nodal function devoid of autonomic influences. The normal intrinsic heart rate was defined in one study as $118.1 - (0.57 \times age)$ beats per minute and the 95% confidence limit, suggesting sinus nodal dysfunction, was ± 16 beats per minute or an intrinsic heart rate 15% or more below predicted.[12] Again, the determination of an abnormal intrinsic heart rate does not define whether this abnormality is responsible for symptoms in a given patient.

The two most widely used tests at electrophysiological study for evaluation of sinus nodal function are the sinus nodal recovery time and the sinoatrial conduction time.[13] The sinus nodal recovery time[14] is used to assess the automaticity of the sinus node by measuring the time that it takes for the sinus node to recover after atrial pacing (overdrive suppression of sinus nodal automaticity). The normal sinus node demonstrates mild to moderate overdrive suppression, but in patients with sinus nodal dysfunction, this property may be markedly exaggerated (Fig. 4). The specific pacing protocol to determine the sinus nodal recovery time varies from laboratory to laboratory. In general, the right atrium is paced for 30 seconds at several different cycle lengths (in our laboratory we use pacing cycle lengths 700 to 350 ms in 50 ms decre-

922486F

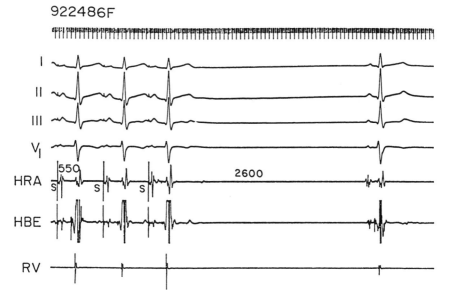

Figure 4. Abnormal sinus nodal recovery time. The high right atrium is paced (S) for 30 seconds at a cycle length of 550 ms. The last three complexes of atrial pacing prior to sudden cessation of pacing are illustrated. Subsequently, a pause of 2600 ms occurs before sinus activity resumes. This is an exaggeration of the normal phenomenon of overdrive suppression of sinus nodal automaticity. When corrected for the spontaneous sinus rate (800 ms in this patient), the corrected sinus nodal recovery time is 1800 ms (markedly prolonged).

ments). The sinus nodal recovery time is defined as the interval between the last paced atrial electrogram and the first spontaneous sinus depolarization. The sinus nodal recovery time is dependent upon the preexisting spontaneous sinus rate, and therefore it is generally corrected by subtracting the spontaneous sinus cycle length from the sinus nodal recovery time. A corrected sinus nodal recovery time less than 540 ms is considered normal in our laboratory. Occasionally, the sinus nodal recovery time itself is normal but a secondary pause occurs; that is, an abnormal prolongation of any sinus cycle after the first post-pacing cycle.[15] This appears to be especially common in patients with sinoatrial exit block (Fig. 5).

Sinoatrial conduction time is usually measured indirectly.[16] In this

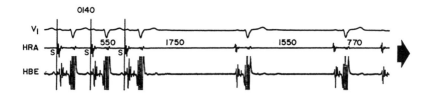

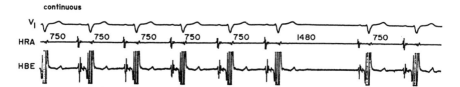

Figure 5. Abnormal sinus nodal recovery time with secondary pauses in a patient with sinoatrial exit block. The last three atrial paced complexes (S) of a 30-second pacing train at a cycle length of 550 ms are illustrated (top panel). With sudden cessation of pacing, sinus intervals of 1750 and 1550 ms occur followed by sudden acceleration to 770 and 750 ms. There is also a sudden doubling of the cycle length in the bottom panel. The first two prolonged sinus intervals after atrial pacing and the prolonged interval on the bottom strip probably represent 2:1 sinoatrial exit block induced by the atrial pacing. In addition, there is mild overdrive suppression of the sinus nodal pacemaker itself since the first two pauses are slightly greater than twice the subsequent sinus cycle length.

method (Fig. 6), premature atrial stimuli (A_2) are introduced progressively earlier during sinus rhythm (A_1), starting in late diastole, until atrial refractoriness is encountered. The late diastolic atrial extrastimuli collide with the impulse exiting the sinus node, and the return cycle (A_2A_3) is fully compensatory ($A_1A_3 = 2 \times A_1A_1$; zone of interference). However, as the atrial extrastimulus is introduced earlier in diastole,

Figure 6. Sinoatrial conduction time. The determination of a normal sinoatrial conduction time is illustrated. Surface lead V_1 and high right atrial (HRA) and His bundle (HBE) electrograms are shown. The ladder diagram illustrates impulse formation at the level of the sinus node (SN), conduction through the perinodal tissues (slanted lines), and activation of the atria (A). In panel A, sinus rhythm is present with a cycle length of 710 ms. An atrial premature stimulus (S) produces atrial activation with an A_1A_2 interval of 540 ms. This premature atrial impulse is late enough that it collides with the already generated sinus nodal impulse within the perinodal tissue and a completely compensatory pause of 880 ms results ($540 + 880 = 710 + 710$; zone of interference).

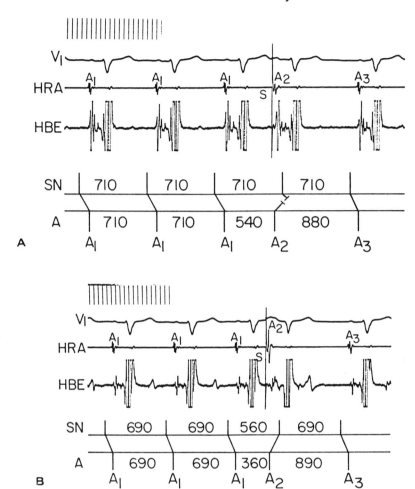

In panel B, the sinus cycle length is 690 ms and the A_1A_2 interval 360 ms (shorter than in panel A). The atrial extrasystole is now early enough that it can conduct retrogradely through the perinodal tissue and depolarize the sinus nodal pacemaker prematurely, before the latter has depolarized spontaneously. The sinus pacemaker is reset and theoretically discharges again 690 ms later, giving rise to A_3 and a less than compensatory pause after the atrial premature ($360 + 890 < 690 + 690$; zone of reset). Note that the difference between A_2A_3 and the presumed sinus nodal cycle length after reset ($890 - 690 = 200$ ms) should represent the time that it takes for the atrial premature impulse to travel retrogradely into the sinus node plus the time for the subsequent sinus nodal impulse to travel out of the sinus node. If these two conduction times were equal, then half of this value would be the sinoatrial conduction time.

the zone of reset is encountered; that is, the atrial premature beat enters the sinus node, resets it, and the subsequent return cycle (A_2A_3) is less than fully compensatory ($A_1A_3 < 2 \times A_1A_1$). Theoretically, when this occurs, the difference between the sinus cycle length (A_1A_1) and the return cycle length (A_2A_3) is the time that it takes for the atrial paced impulse to travel into the sinus node and the subsequent sinus impulse to extent the sinus node. Therefore, when the zone of reset is identified, the difference between the spontaneous cycle length (A_1A_1) and the return cycle length (A_2A_3) should represent twice the sinoatrial conduction time. Obviously this is an indirect measurement and involves several assumptions that may not be fully applicable, including (1) the premature atrial contraction does not alter the sinus rate by overdrive suppression; (2) conduction into and out of the sinus node are equal; (3) the premature atrial contraction does not cause a shift in the pacemaker site within the sinus node; and (4) the occurrence of a noncompensatory rather than compensatory pause always represents reset of the sinus node. Direct techniques for recording sinoatrial conduction time have been developed, but they cannot be obtained reliably in all patients.[17]

Like the other provocative tests, the occurrence of an abnormal sinus nodal recovery time or sinoatrial conduction time does not necessarily indicate that sinus nodal dysfunction is the cause of symptoms. The sensitivity of the corrected sinus nodal recovery time for sinus nodal dysfunction is approximately 54% and that of the sinoatrial conduction time 51%; when combined, the sensitivity increases to 64%.[18] In patients with symptomatic sinus nodal dysfunction and patients with sinoatrial exit block, this sensitivity increases. The specificity of the two tests taken together is about 88%.[18] It appears that the sinus nodal recovery time is probably the more reliable of the two tests, although these tests should be considered as only supporting evidence rather than diagnostic of sinus nodal dysfunction. Markedly prolonged uncorrected sinus nodal recovery times (greater than 2 to 3 seconds) are more likely of clinical significance than mildly prolonged values.[19]

Electrophysiological study should not be performed in patients whose symptoms are clearly documented to be due to bradyarrhythmias from sinus nodal dysfunction. It should also not be done in asymptomatic patients with sinus bradyarrhythmia or pauses at night during sleep. However, electrophysiological study is indicated in patients who are symptomatic with syncope or presyncope in whom sinus nodal dysfunction is suspected as the etiology of symptoms but the relationship between arrhythmia and symptoms cannot be established by noninvasive means. In addition, selected patients with known sinus nodal dysfunction may require electrophysiological study to determine anterograde or retrograde AV conduction properties to help select the type of pacemaker to be implanted, to determine the severity of sinus nodal dysfunction and response to drug interventions, or to exclude other arrhythmias contributing to symptoms such as ventricular tachycardia.[18]

Therapy

The patient should be withdrawn from drugs that may exacerbate sinus nodal dysfunction if possible. However, in many patients, drug therapy such as that for atrial or ventricular tachyarrhythmias cannot be safely withdrawn, and permanent pacing may be necessary if such drug therapy exacerbates bradycardia. Even though vagolytic or adrenergic therapy (atropine or isoproterenol) may temporarily increase the sinus rate, chronic drug therapy is usually associated with intolerable side effects and is unacceptable for long-term management. Therefore, the treatment of choice for most patients is permanent cardiac pacing once the relationship between symptoms and bradyarrhythmias has been established. Aminophylline therapy may benefit some young patients with vagally mediated sinus nodal dysfunction.[20]

The prognosis of patients with sinus nodal dysfunction is related more to underlying heart disease in older patients than to the sinus nodal dysfunction itself. Pacemaker implantation relieves symptoms in properly selected patients, although pacemakers have not been demonstrated to improve overall survival in some studies.[21]

Because of the risk of systemic embolization, patients with the tachycardia-bradycardia syndrome should be considered for chronic anticoagulation with warfarin if no contraindications exist. The development of permanent atrial fibrillation in patients with tachycardia-bradycardia syndrome may "cure" symptoms by preventing episodes of asystole due to sinus arrest at the termination of atrial fibrillation.

Permanent pacing is usually the preferred therapy, with adjunctive drug therapy necessary in patients with tachyarrhythmias. Ventricular pacing may be sufficient in many patients, but some patients may benefit from dual chamber pacing to preserve atrial synchrony; however, the sinus nodal function should not be relied upon to increase heart rate with exercise. Patients with intermittent atrial tachyarrhythmias may not benefit from dual chamber pacing if the pacemaker tracks the rapid atrial rate. Atrial pacing is usually not sufficient because of the commonly associated AV conduction abnormalities, which, if not apparent at the time of diagnosis, may subsequently develop as the conduction disease progresses.

Atrioventricular Conduction Disturbances

Anatomy of the AV Junction

After the sinus impulse activates the atria, the electrical impulse travels to the AV junction via working atrial myocardial cells. Although atrial cells that are oriented in a certain direction conduct more rapidly in that direction than in other directions, it is now widely believed that a specialized internodal conduction system does not exist. The first portion of the AV junction consists of a transitional cell zone forming the atrial approaches to the AV node. The second section, the compact portion or the AV node itself, is located superficially beneath the right atrial endocardium above the insertion of the septal leaflet of the tricuspid valve and anterior to the ostium of the coronary sinus. The third portion of the AV junction is termed the penetrating part of the AV bundle (bundle of His). This portion penetrates the central fibrous body and continues into the annulus fibrosis and the membranous septum. The more proximal cells of the penetrating portion resemble those of the compact node and the more distal cells resemble the Purkinje cells typical of the bundle branches. The penetrating portion is enclosed in connective tissue and bifurcates into the two major bundle branches distally in the membranous septum at the superior margin of the muscular septum. The left bundle branch distributes over the left septum and subsequently the entire left ventricle. It sometimes divides into separate anterosuperior and posteroinferior fascicles, but sometimes this distinct division is not present anatomically, although the concept of left anterior and left posterior fascicular blocks (hemiblocks) is still useful clinically. The right bundle branch travels (without any further branching) along the right septum to the base of the anterior papillary muscle. Both bundle branches continue as an arborizing network of Purkinje fibers that eventually terminate at ventricular myocardial cells. This extensive His-Purkinje system allows nearly simultaneous activation of multiple areas of the right and left ventricles and results in the relatively narrow QRS complex of normal ventricular activation.

Normal Atrioventricular Conduction

The time between the onset of the P wave and the onset of the QRS complex is termed the PR interval and for most normal heart rates in adults is ≤0.20 seconds. With the advent of His bundle recording, one can divide the PR interval into its component parts.[22] To record His bundle activation, a multipolar electrode catheter is positioned just across the septal leaflet of the tricuspid valve. Using bipolar recording techniques with filter settings of 30–500 Hz, one can record low right atrial activity near the entrance into the AV node, a sharp His bundle potential generated by rapid conduction of the electrical impulse down the His bundle after traversing the AV node, and local right ventricular activation (Fig. 7). Note that direct recording of the slow conduction through the AV node cannot be accomplished using the usual techniques. If the catheter is advanced slightly from the His bundle recording position, a potential from the right bundle branch can be recorded.

The PA interval is the interval from the onset of the P wave on the surface ECG tracings to the low right atrial electrogram recorded from the His bundle catheter. This interval represents the intra-atrial conduction time between the sinus nodal area and the approaches to the AV node. The AH interval is the interval between the low right atrial electrogram and the onset of the His bundle electrogram; since the low right atrial electrogram records atrial activity near the approach to the AV node and the His bundle electrogram represents activity exiting the AV node, the AH interval is a good estimate of AV nodal conduction time. The inclusion of AV nodal tissue in this interval is proven by an increase in the AH interval by manipulations that should prolong AV nodal conduction (for example, vagal stimulation or after premature atrial contractions).[23] The normal values for the AH interval vary widely and are markedly influenced by autonomic tone; however, the usual range in adults is 45 to 140 ms.[24] The interval between the onset of the His bundle deflection and the earliest ventricular activation recorded in any surface electrocardiographic or intracardiac lead is termed the HV interval and represents conduction time through the His-Purkinje system. The normal values in adults for HV intervals are relatively narrow and reproducible, ranging from 30 to 55 ms. Recording of the His bundle electrogram can be useful in selected patients to determine the site of atrioventricular conduction disturbances;[25] conduction delay or block in the AV node occurs with different disease processes and has different therapeutic and prognostic implications than that in the His-Purkinje system.

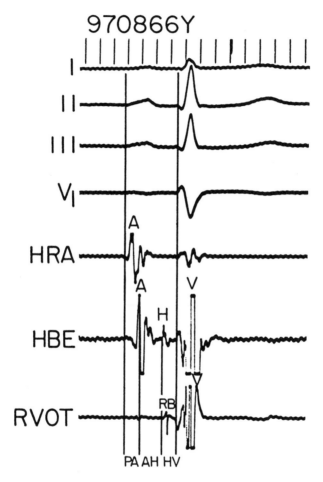

Figure 7. Normal intervals measured with intracardiac techniques. Surface leads I, II, III, and V_1 are displayed along with high right atrial (HRA) and His bundle electrograms (HBE). A catheter is placed in the right ventricular outflow tract (RVOT) in such a location that a right bundle branch potential can be recorded. The PA, AH, and HV intervals are determined as described in the text. A = atrial activation, H = His bundle activation, RB = right bundle branch activation, and V = ventricular activation. Note that the His bundle activation occurs prior to the right bundle branch activation.

Atrioventricular Block

Atrioventricular block refers to delay or nonconduction of an electrical impulse at a time when the AV junction should not be physiologically refractory. It must be distinguished from interference, which is a normal phenomenon whereby conduction delay or block occurs because of physiological refractoriness of the AV junction due to a previous impulse (for example, a sinus P wave following a preventricular contraction (PVC) is commonly not conducted to the ventricle; this is not due to AV block, but occurs because the preceding PVC depolarized the AV junction retrogradely, thus leaving it refractory to the subsequent sinus impulse).[26]

The most common causes of AV block in adults are drug toxicity, ischemic heart disease, and various degenerative processes. Drugs can cause AV block either in the AV node (for example, digitalis, beta-blockers, and calcium blockers) or in the His-Purkinje system (quinidine, procainamide, and other membrane-active antiarrhythmic drugs). AV nodal block may be due to excessive vagal activity in some young adults, especially highly trained athletes.[27] Chronic ischemic heart disease and degenerative processes involve primarily the His-Purkinje system. Lesions that involve the AV conduction system in the absence of associated myocardial disease include Lenegre's and Lev's diseases. Lenegre's disease is a sclerodegenerative process involving only the conduction system and is a common cause of bundle branch block and fascicular block in older people. Lev's disease[28] represents involvement of the conduction system by calcification or fibrosis extending from adjacent structures, an example being AV block in patients with calcific aortic stenosis. Atrioventricular block in acute myocardial infarction may be located either within the AV node or within the His-Purkinje system, as discussed below. Other more unusual causes of heart block include rheumatic fever, myocarditis, hypoxia and electrolyte disturbances, surgical trauma, Chagas' disease, myxedema, polymyositis, infiltrative processes such as amyloidosis or sarcoidosis, sclerodema, Reiter's disease, tumors, Hodgkin's disease, multiple myeloma, and progressive muscular dystrophy.

In children, AV block is usually congenital, approximately half of whom have no associated structural heart disease and half have some form of congenital heart disease. Pathology usually shows disruption of the atrial approaches to the conduction system or of the connection between the AV node and the more distal conduction system. Congenital heart block may have an immunologic etiology in some cases since it is more common in children whose mothers have connective tissue diseases and/or antibodies to ribonucleoprotein.[29]

First Degree AV Block

First degree AV block refers to delay in AV conduction, but every P wave is followed by a subsequent QRS complex. First degree AV block is usually defined in adults as a PR interval greater than 0.20 seconds. The PR interval can be very long (as long as 1.0 second) on rare occasions, and occasionally the PR interval may be longer than the P-P interval creating a "skipped" P wave, i.e., a P wave that conducts not to the immediately following QRS but to the subsequent QRS complex. First degree AV block may be due to delay in either the AV node or the His-Purkinje system (Fig. 8) but is more common in the AV node because of the node's unique ability to maintain slow conduction. First degree AV block with narrow QRS complexes is almost always located in the AV node, although it can occasionally be within the His bundle itself above the bifurcation into the bundle branches. First degree AV block with a bundle branch block QRS morphology can be located in either the AV node or the His-Purkinje system, and the differential diagnosis may not be made definitely without His bundle recordings.

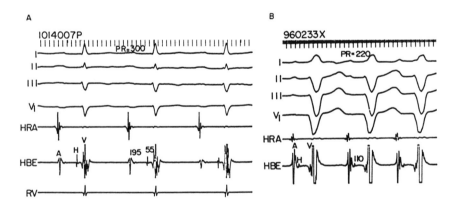

Figure 8. First degree AV block due to delay in the AV node (panel A) and the His-Purkinje system (panel B). In panel A, the PR interval is 300 ms, accounted for predominantly by the prolonged AH interval of 195 ms representing conduction delay within the AV node. In panel B, the PR interval is 220 ms with an HV interval of 110 ms, representing conduction delay in the His-Purkinje system. Note the wide QRS complexes of left bundle branch block in panel B but normal QRS complexes in panel A.

Second Degree AV Block

Second degree AV block is defined as failure of selected sinus impulses to conduct to the ventricles at a time when the AV junction should not be physiologically refractory. Using surface electrocardiographic criteria, second degree AV block is divided into type I and type II. Type I (Wenckebach) block is characterized by progressive prolongation of the PR interval prior to the nonconducted P wave (Fig. 9). In type II second degree AV block, there is sudden loss of AV conduction without prior prolongation of the PR interval (Fig. 10). One should emphasize that these are electrocardiographic patterns of second degree atrioventricular block, and although they are helpful in localizing the site of AV block (see below), the terms type I and type II are not synonymous with AV nodal or His-Purkinje sites of block. In general, Wenckebach periodicity

Schematic of 4:3 Wenckebach Cycle

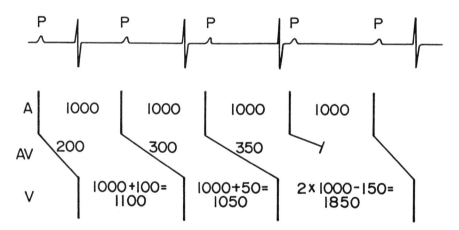

Figure 9. Schematic of typical Wenckebach periodicity. The top panel shows a schematic electrocardiogram of a 4:3 Wenckebach cycle with prolonging PR intervals until the fourth P wave fails to conduct to the ventricle. On the bottom is a diagram illustrating the atrial (A), AV junctional (AV), and ventricular (V) levels. Note that there is increasing conduction delay with each PR interval, but the amount of increase in conduction delay with each subsequent PR interval decreases. Therefore, the longest RR interval at the right of the figure is less than twice as long as the shortest RR interval immediately preceding it (see text for discussion).

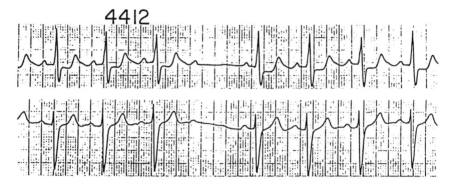

Figure 10. Electrocardiogram of type II second degree AV block. This electrocardiogram was obtained from a Holter recording of a patient with syncope. It shows constant RR and PR intervals until the fourth P wave suddenly fails to conduct to the ventricle. Note that bundle branch block is present.

is characteristic of block in AV nodal (slow-channel) tissue, whereas sudden type II (all-or-none) block is characteristic of His-Purkinje (fast-channel-dependent) tissue. However, diseased His-Purkinje tissue may demonstrate conduction prolongation prior to block (i.e., type I) in some patients.

A "typical" pattern of type I Wenckebach block has been described (Fig. 9), although it actually occurs in less than 50% of examples of type I AV block. However, the concept of typical Wenckebach periodicity is useful, especially when PR intervals are not available for analysis (for example, in sinoatrial exit block or exit block from a ventricular tachycardia or junctional focus). In typical Wenckebach AV block, the largest increment in AV delay (PR interval) occurs in the second beat after the pause, and even though the PR interval increases in each beat thereafter, the increment of PR prolongation decreases. Therefore, the following pattern emerges: (1) the duration between successive RR intervals after the pause progressively decreases; (2) the duration of the pause is less than twice the preceding RR interval; and (3) the duration of the RR interval following the pause is longer than the RR interval preceding the pause. Many examples of Wenckebach AV nodal conduction are not "typical," the most frequent example being a particularly prolonged PR interval just prior to AV block, possibly because of either tenuous conduction of this last conducted QRS complex or dual AV nodal pathways.

The two types of second degree AV block often occur in very different clinical circumstances and have different prognoses. Type II block often occurs in the presence of structural heart disease, prior to episodes of complete heart block and Stokes-Adams attacks (sudden transient loss of consciousness without warning). Type I block with a normal QRS duration frequently occurs in individuals without structural heart disease and usually has a benign prognosis. However, an occasional elderly patient can have a progressive form of type I block with narrow QRS complexes that may lead to Stokes-Adams attacks.[30] The mechanism and prognosis of these two types of AV block during an acute myocardial infarction are different. Type I block is common with inferior myocardial infarctions, tends to be transient, and usually does not require temporary or permanent pacing. On the other hand, type II block occurs more commonly with anterior myocardial infarction and is often related to the extent of myocardial damage. Pacing, both temporary and possibly permanent, are indicated for type II block associated with an acute myocardial infarction. Further, there is a high mortality due not so much to AV block but to the consequences of severe left ventricular dysfunction (heart failure or malignant ventricular arrhythmias).

First degree and type I second degree AV block may be normal in healthy young children.[31] In addition, these findings may be normal in well-trained athletes and are probably due to increased vagal tone. Occasionally, a highly trained athlete may develop symptomatic bradyarrhythmias that are only eliminated after deconditioning.

Localization of the Site of Block

Although the localization of second degree AV block to the AV node or the His-Purkinje system can be obtained with a His bundle recording at electrophysiological study (Figs. 11 and 12), this invasive technique is usually not required to determine the presumptive site of block (Table 1).[32] Type I block with a narrow QRS is almost always within the AV node; the exception is the rare occurrence of type I block within the His bundle itself above its bifurcation into the bundle branches, resulting in a narrow QRS complex. Type II block, especially if the QRS is wide, is usually within the His-Purkinje system. Type I block with a bundle branch block is more likely to be within the AV node than the His-Purkinje system but could be localized in either (one instance where the His bundle recording may be clinically relevant) (Fig. 13). The unusual situation of type II block with a narrow QRS could be localized within the His bundle on rare occasions, but a more likely cause would be type I block with very small increments in AV conduction that are not easily

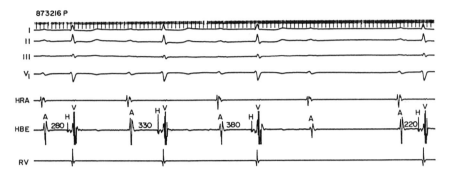

Figure 11. Intracardiac tracing of second degree AV block type I located within the AV node. Sinus rhythm is present and the AH interval gradually prolongs from 280 to 380 ms; subsequently, the fourth atrial depolarization fails to conduct to the ventricle and no His bundle potential follows atrial depolarization, demonstrating that the site of AV block is within the AV node. The subsequent sinus atrial depolarization conducts to the ventricle with a shorter AH interval.

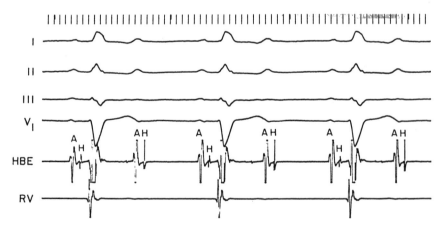

Figure 12. Intracardiac tracing of 2:1 second degree AV block located in the His-Purkinje system. Sinus rhythm with left bundle branch block is present. The AH intervals are constant but every other atrial complex fails to activate the ventricle even though each atrial depolarization is followed by a His bundle deflection. This demonstrates that the site of AV block is within the His-Purkinje system.

Table 1
Site of Second Degree Atrioventricular Block

Type of Block	Normal QRS	BBB
Type I	AVN > > > > HPS	AVN > HPS
Type II	HPS > AVN	HPS > > > > AVN
Fixed 2:1 or greater	AVN > HPS	HPS > > AVN

BBB = bundle branch block; AVN = atrioventricular node; HPS = His-Purkinje system. Arrows (>) indicte relative frequency of second degree AV block at different sites. Adapted from Zipes DP.[32]

detected on the electrocardiogram. This may happen if a rhythm strip contains only the last few complexes of a very long Wenckebach cycle where the increments of PR prolongation with each beat are very small.

Fixed 2:1 AV block (without ever recording its onset) could be located either in the AV node or His-Purkinje system and cannot be classified as either type I or type II; a narrow QRS complex would indicate that the site of block is probably in the AV node.

The AV node is rich with autonomic nerves and its conduction is accelerated with sympathetic stimulation and slowed with vagal stim-

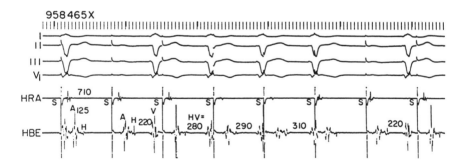

Figure 13. Type I second degree AV block located within the His-Purkinje system. The atrium is paced (S) at a constant cycle length of 710 ms. The AH interval is constant throughout the illustration. The first paced atrial impulse fails to conduct to the ventricle even though the His bundle (H) is activated. The HV interval following the second paced atrial depolarization is 220 ms and subsequent HV intervals increase gradually up to 310 ms prior to block of the sixth atrial paced depolarization below the recorded His bundle potential. This illustrates that Wenckebach AV block can occur within the His-Purkinje system.

ulation. The His-Purkinje system demonstrates much less response to sympathetic stimulation and little or no response to vagal stimulation. An abrupt alteration in autonomic tone may cause sudden changes in both AV nodal conduction and sinus rate. For example, a burst of vagal tone may result in sudden heart block with no change for the preceding PR interval to prolong (Fig. 14). This should be evident by observing an increase in the P-P interval simultaneously with the heart block. Massive sudden vagal discharges may cause block of several sequential P waves and this should not be interpreted as type II or "poor-prognosis" heart block.

One would expect that atropine might improve AV conduction in patients with AV nodal block but worsen conduction in patients with His-Purkinje block due to the increase in sinus rate (Fig. 15). Likewise, carotid sinus stimulation might worsen AV conduction in patients with AV nodal block but improve conduction in patients with His-Purkinje block due to sinus node slowing. However, the effect of any given intervention on the AV node may be weaker than that on the sinus node; thus, using these drugs to localize the site of AV block may be confusing in some patients. For example, a patient with AV nodal block who receives atropine may have improvement in AV nodal conduction, but if the sinus rate accelerates excessively, a higher percentage of P waves may paradoxically not conduct to the ventricle.

CSM

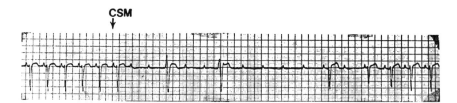

Figure 14. Carotid sinus massage causing high-grade AV block. This patient has sinus tachycardia with a rate of approximately 110 beats per minute. When carotid sinus massage is applied, sudden AV block occurs without preceding prolongation of the PR interval, resulting in 10 P waves without AV conduction (two slow ventricular escapes are present). Carotid sinus massage activates the vagus and results in AV block at the level of the AV node. In addition to AV block, the P-P interval prolongs such that the sinus rate is less than 100 before AV conduction resumes toward the right of the strip. This electrocardiogram illustrates that a sudden surge of vagal tone can create high-grade heart block that may mimic type II, although the subsequent prolongation of the P-P interval should alert one that vagal stimulation has occurred and is responsible for the AV block.

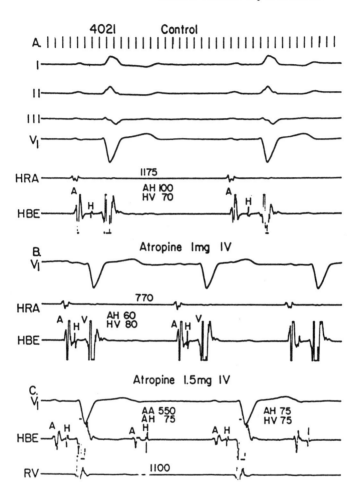

Figure 15. His-Purkinje AV block after an atropine-induced increase in sinus rate. Panel A shows sinus rhythm at a cycle length of 1175 ms with 1:1 AV conduction. Left bundle branch block is present, the AH interval is 100 ms, and the HV interval is prolonged (70 ms). In panel B, after atropine 1 mg IV, the sinus rate decreases to 770 ms and the HV increases to 80 ms but 1:1 AV conduction is still present. The AH interval shortens to 60 ms despite the faster sinus rate due to the direct effect of atropine to shorten AV nodal conduction time. In panel C, after atropine 1.5 mg, the sinus cycle length decreases to 550 ms and 2:1 AV block occurs below the recorded His bundle potential. Atropine worsens AV conduction in this patient not by a direct drug effect but because the atropine-induced increase in sinus rate stresses the already abnormal His-Purkinje system.

Complete AV Block

In complete AV block there is no conduction between the atria and the ventricles and both chambers are controlled by separate independent pacemakers. Ventricular escape foci that are closer to the AV node tend to be more stable, have a faster escape rate, and are under more autonomic influence than those located more distal to the AV node in the bundle branches. The ventricular escape rhythm is usually regular, and this feature can help distinguish complete from incomplete AV block. It should be noted that AV block and AV dissociation are distinct entities (see below) and that AV block is only one cause of AV dissociation. AV block can be located either within the AV node, the His bundle, or the bundle branches. If complete AV block is permanent and not caused by transient processes (such as drugs), block within the AV node is often congenital and results in a normal-appearing QRS escape morphology with rates of between 40 and 60 per minute. This escape focus usually increases its rate in response to atropine, isoproterenol, or exercise. Some patients with congenital AV block may have block localized to the bundle of His at electrophysiological study, but the prognosis of patients with congenital heart block does not seem to be predicted by the precise site of block.[33] Permanent AV block within the His-Purkinje system is usually acquired, the result of a diffuse disease process affecting all of the His-Purkinje system including both bundle branches. The ventricular escape QRS complex is wide with a rate of between 20 and 40 per minute. It is not as reliable as that in patients with congenital complete AV block and these patients are often symptomatic with syncope or presyncope.

His bundle electrograms in patients with congenital complete AV block show independent atrial and ventricular activity (Fig. 16). No His bundle potential is recorded after atrial depolarizations but a His bundle potential followed by a normal HV interval is recorded before each ventricular depolarization, localizing the site of AV block to the AV node. In patients with acquired complete AV block, a His bundle potential is recorded after each atrial depolarization (representing normal AV nodal conduction) but no His bundle potential is noted preceding the ventricular depolarization, indicating that the site of block is below the AV node (Fig. 17 and 18).

Patients with acquired complete AV block without any identifiable reversible cause require permanent ventricular pacing. Some children with congenital heart block may become symptomatic from bradycardia in the neonatal period, but most children are asymptomatic through

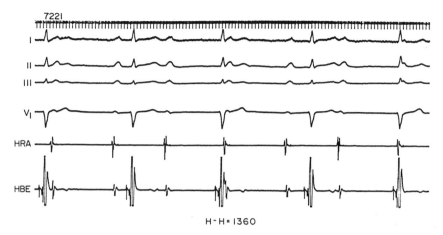

Figure 16. Congenital complete heart block located within the AV node. Sinus arrhythmia with a cycle length of approximately 860 ms is completely dissociated from a regular junctional escape rhythm with a cycle length of 1360 ms. There is no relationship between atrial and ventricular depolarizations. There is no His bundle deflection after any atrial depolarization. A His bundle electrogram with a normal HV interval precedes each junctional escape complex in the His bundle lead. Therefore, the site of AV block is within the AV node. Note the normal (narrow) morphology of the junctional escape QRS complexes.

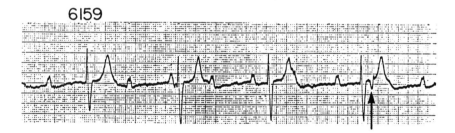

Figure 17. Electrocardiogram of acquired complete AV block. The P wave cycle length is 840 ms and is independent of the regular wide QRS escape mechanism at 1800 ms (less than 40 per minute). There is no relationship between the P waves and the QRS complexes at any time during the recording until the next to the last P wave (arrow), where there is early retrograde atrial activation representing ventriculoatrial conduction despite the fact that there is complete anterograde AV block. Therefore, in some patients, retrograde conduction may be intact even though anterograde conduction is not, or vice versa.

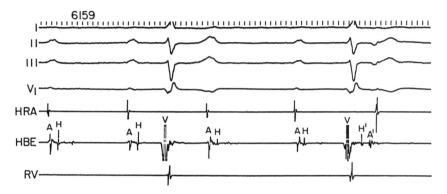

Figure 18. Acquired complete heart block located in the His-Purkinje system (same patient as in Fig. 16). The atrial cycle length is approximately 800 ms. There is AV dissociation, as demonstrated in the previous electrocardiogram, with ventricular escapes resembling right bundle branch block morphology. Each atrial complex (A) is followed by a His bundle electrogram (H), demonstrating that AV nodal conduction is intact. No ventricular escape complex is preceded by a His bundle electrogram, documenting their ventricular origin. Thus the site of block is located within the His-Purkinje system. Note that the very last ventricular escape complex results in retrograde His bundle (H') and atrial (A') activation, correlating with the intact retrograde conduction seen in the previous figure.

childhood. However, symptoms may appear as the child enters adulthood. If symptoms such as presyncope or syncope occur that are definitely attributable to bradycardia, then permanent pacing is indicated. A persistent escape rate less than 50 beats per minute throughout the day may be a sign that the junctional pacemaker will not remain adequate and is common in patients who subsequently develop syncope.[33,34] Other proposed predictors of subsequent symptoms are junctional escape exit block, lack of an increase in junctional escape rate with exercise, and frequent ventricular ectopy.[34] Short runs of ventricular tachycardia can suppress the junctional pacemaker and result in a long asystolic pause that may be symptomatic. Some authors have proposed that measurement of the junctional recovery time, similar to the sinus nodal recovery time described above, may be useful in identifying unreliable junctional escape pacemakers (Fig. 19).[35] The ventricle is paced for 30 seconds at progressively faster rates, and the time for the junctional escape to resume activity after abrupt cessation of pacing is measured. The normal values are not well established, but long junctional recovery times, especially if not improved by atropine, may indicate a poor junctional escape mechanism.

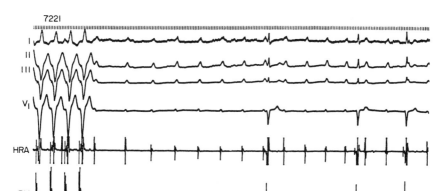

Figure 19. Junctional recovery time in a patient with congenital complete heart block (same patient as in Fig. 16). The ventricle is paced for 30 seconds at a cycle length of 450 ms (S). Sudden termination of the pacing results in a long pause (greater than 4 seconds) before the junctional rhythm resumes, at which time it gradually accelerates back to its original rate. The patient became dizzy during these pacing-induced pauses.

Many authors use the term advanced or high-grade AV block. This term is not defined uniformly; it often refers to instances where multiple consecutive P waves are blocked but complete AV block is not present, but some authors also include type II second degree AV block and/or complete infra-His block.

Symptoms and Signs of AV Block

Patients who have symptomatic second or third degree AV block usually present with syncope or dizziness. Some patients complain of palpitations or "missed heart beats." In addition, they may have other manifestations of inadequate cardiac output such as fatigue, angina, or congestive heart failure. If bradycardia is not severe and the heart is able to compensate by increasing its stroke volume, the patient may have no symptoms.

Clinical information regarding age, underlying heart disease, and cardiac medications may be helpful in some patients in identifying the site of AV block.

Physical examination may reveal the manifestations of the underlying cardiac disease. Furthermore, complete heart block results in jugular venous A waves that have variable amplitude and are not related to the ventricular contractions; the very large jugular A waves occurring when the atria contract intermittently against a closed mitral valve are referred to as cannon A waves. In addition, the variation in the degree of mitral valve opening at the onset of ventricular systole due to the AV dissociation results in a varying intensity of the first heart sound.

AV Dissociation

AV dissociation is defined as independent activation of the atria and ventricles. As mentioned above, AV block is only one example of AV dissociation. AV dissociation is not a diagnosis in itself but requires further examination of the ECG to define the underlying cause, which may be one of three possibilities, either alone or in combination: (1) slowing of the dominant (usually sinus) pacemaker allowing escape of a subsidiary pacemaker. An example would be the patient with inferior myocardial infarction and marked sinus bradycardia with junctional escape, leading to AV dissociation but not AV block. In this situation, the P wave may intermittently capture the ventricle if it occurs at a time when the AV junction is not physiologically refractory. (2) Acceleration of a subsidiary pacemaker that usurps control of the heart from the dominant pacemaker. An example of this would be accelerated (nonparoxysmal) junctional tachycardia in a patient with digitalis toxicity. (3) Atrioventricular block. Transient interruption of AV dissociation with intermittent AV or ventriculoatrial conduction is termed incomplete AV dissociation.

Electrophysiological Study in Acquired AV Block

Electrophysiological study is not indicated in those patients who have AV block on electrocardiographic recording that is well correlated with symptoms of syncope or presyncope. In addition, asymptomatic patients who have transient AV block associated with sinus slowing (the typical situation being type I second degree AV block at night) should not have an electrophysiological study. Electrophysiological study should be performed in patients in whom AV block is suspected but cannot be documented as the cause of symptoms (syncope or presyncope) by noninvasive means. In addition, an occasional patient with known episodes of AV block may have symptoms from another cause (for example, ventricular tachycardia) and may benefit from electrophysiological study.[18]

Selected patients may benefit from electrophysiological study when the site of AV block is not evident from surface electrocardiographic tracings and if the site of AV block would determine whether a pacemaker should be implanted. Examples would include an asymptomatic patient with type I second degree (Wenckebach) AV block and bundle branch block, fixed 2:1 AV block and bundle branch block, or apparent type II block with a normal QRS complex (i.e., suspected intra-His AV block). In addition, electrophysiological study may be useful in an occasional patient suspected of having concealed junctional extrasystoles as a cause of apparent type I or type II AV block (i.e., pseudo AV block) (Fig. 20).[36]

At electrophysiological study, in addition to measuring the AH and HV intervals, the atria are paced and the minimal atrial pacing cycle length maintaining 1:1 AV conduction within the AV node or the His-Purkinje system is determined. Many patients have relatively prolonged AV nodal conduction times, and improvement of conduction in response to atropine may determine whether the AV node is intrinsically diseased or under the influence of excess vagal tone. AV block below the recorded His bundle electrogram during decremental atrial pacing is considered abnormal, especially if it occurs at slower pacing rates. If His-Purkinje block does not occur during decremental atrial pacing, procainamide or disopyramide may be infused to facilitate block in a patient who is predisposed to His-Purkinje block (Fig. 21).[37] Some patients who have documented paroxysmal His-Purkinje block have apparently normal His-Purkinje function at the time of electrophysiological study. The reason for this is unclear; however, acute reversible ischemia may play a role.

Chronic Intraventricular Conduction Delay

The prognosis in patients with chronic bundle branch block depends predominantly upon the severity of underlying structural cardiac disease. Progression to complete AV block is infrequent and no clinical or physical exam or electrocardiographic finding is predictive of those patients who will develop complete AV block. Even patients with chronic bifascicular block (right bundle branch block plus left anterior or left posterior fascicular block) do not subsequently develop complete AV block frequently enough to warrant prophylactic permanent pacing.

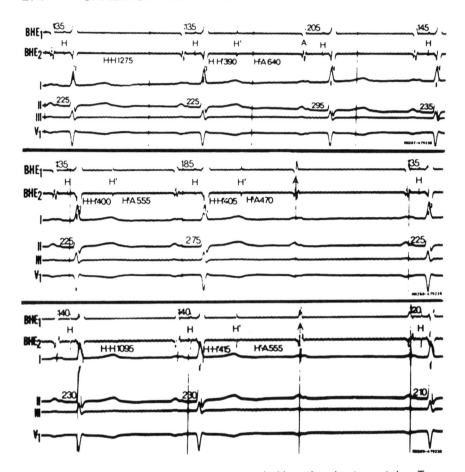

Figure 20. Pseudo AV block due to concealed junctional extrasystoles. Two bipolar His recordings (BHE₁ and BHE₂) are illustrated along with surface leads I, II, III, and V₁. In the top panel, the AH interval is 135 ms and the PR interval is 225 ms. A concealed junctional extrasystole (H′) conducts neither to the atria nor to the ventricles; however, it must have penetrated into the AV node because of the prolongation of the subsequent AH interval to 205 ms and the PR interval to 295 ms (concealed conduction). Thus, sudden unexpected first degree AV block is due to the concealed junctional extrasystole.

The middle panel represents pseudo-Wenckebach AV block due to concealed junctional extrasystoles. On the left, the AH interval is 135 ms and PR interval 225 ms. The first junctional extrasystole (H′) fails to conduct to the atria or ventricles but penetrates into the AV node as evidenced by prolongation of the subsequent AH interval to 185 ms and PR interval to 275 ms. Subsequently, another concealed junctional extrasystole (H′) causes the subsequent atrial depolarization to block completely in the AV node.

The bottom panel illustrates pseudo-type II second degree AV block due

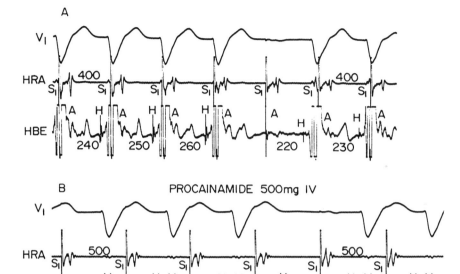

Figure 21. Development of His-Purkinje block after IV infusion of procainamide. Panel A illustrates atrial pacing at a cycle length of 400 ms prior to procainamide infusion in this patient with a left bundle branch block but normal HV interval. The AH interval increases gradually from 240 to 260 ms before the fourth paced atrial complex does not conduct to the ventricle because of Wenckebach block in the AV node. This is normal function of the AV conduction system. However, in panel B after procainamide infusion, atrial pacing at a cycle length of 500 ms results in abnormal AV block located below the recorded His bundle potential. Thus, in patients with suspected His-Purkinje block, provocative testing with intravenous drugs may unmask His-Purkinje abnormalities.

---

to a concealed junctional extrasystole. The AH interval on the left is 140 ms and the PR interval is 230 ms. The concealed junctional extrasystole (H′) conducts neither to the atria nor to the ventricle but penetrates retrogradely into the AV node and causes the subsequent atrial impulse to suddenly not conduct to the ventricle without any preceding PR or AH prolongation. On the surface tracing, this would mimic type II AV block. The diagnosis of pseudo AV block due to concealed junctional extrasystoles cannot be made definitively from surface ECG tracings; however, if unexpected AV block is noted in a patient who also has multiple *manifest* premature junctional extrasystoles (i.e., that conduct to the ventricle), then *concealed* junctional extrasystoles should be suspected as the cause of AV block. Reprinted with permission from Bonner AJ and Zipes DP.[36]

However, the percentage of patients who eventually progress to complete AV block increases if the HV interval is prolonged (4.5% if the HV is prolonged versus 0.6% with a normal HV)[38] and the percent progressing to AV block increases if the HV interval is markedly prolonged.[38,39] The dividing line is controversial, but many authors recommend prophylactic permanent pacing in patients with bifascicular block if the HV interval is greater than 90–100 ms.

The sensitivity of decremental atrial pacing for producing block distal to the His recording is relatively low, but if it occurs, the risk of development of complete AV block is high.[40,41] It should be noted that functional block distal to the His recording due to *abrupt* shortening of the pacing coupling intervals is not abnormal (Ashman's phenomenon). In addition, abnormalities other than AV block may commonly be the cause of syncope or presyncope in many patients with bifascicular block, and therefore electrophysiological study in these patients should also include evaluation of sinus nodal function and programmed atrial and ventricular stimulation.

Electrophysiological study should not be performed in asymptomatic patients with intraventricular conduction delay, even bifascicular block. However, patients who have symptoms (syncope or near syncope) and bundle branch block may be candidates for electrophysiological study in order to determine (1) the severity of conduction delay (i.e., HV interval and response to atrial pacing) and its response to drugs in order to help define prognosis and plan therapy; and (2) whether ventricular arrhythmias or sinus nodal dysfunction may be a cause for the symptoms.[18]

Therapy for Bradyarrhythmias Caused by Sinus Nodal Dysfunction or AV Block

Pharmacological therapy can be used transiently (minutes or hours) for treatment of symptomatic bradyarrhythmias due to sinus nodal dysfunction or AV block, but patients who require therapy for longer periods should be managed with temporary or permanent cardiac pacing. Pharmacological therapy causes side effects and is not as reliable as pacing. Atropine can be used for disorders of the sinus node or AV node. Isoproterenol will increase the sinus nodal rate and accelerate conduction through both the AV node and the His-Purkinje system;[42] however, it increases myocardial oxygen demand and may precipitate or exacerbate ventricular arrhythmias.

Temporary Pacing

Pacemaker therapy may be either temporary or permanent. Temporary pacemakers are used when reversible causes for bradycardia are suspected or as a temporary measure prior to implantation of a permanent pacemaker. Temporary pacing is indicated when a symptomatic bradycardia is either present or likely to occur. Such situations include post-cardiac surgery, right heart catheterization in patients with left bundle branch block (where the right heart catheter may traumatize the right bundle branch and result in transient complete AV block), and in the presence of drugs that slow the heart rate (either therapeutic or toxic effects).

Temporary Pacing in Patients with Acute Myocardial Infarction

Table 2 lists the indications for a temporary pacemaker in patients with acute myocardial infarction. Any patient with an acute infarction and a symptomatic bradyarrhythmia unresponsive to or recurrent during drug therapy requires temporary pacing. However, temporary pacing may be indicated in selected patients with myocardial infarctions as prophylaxis in case of sudden complete AV block.

Type I second degree AV block commonly occurs with acute inferior myocardial infarctions and is probably due to transient AV nodal ischemia or increased vagal tone. It is usually transient (24–48 hours), localized to the AV node, is not symptomatic, and usually does not require pacing unless the resultant bradycardia causes hypotension, angina, or congestive heart failure. On the other hand, type II AV block is usually associated with a large acute anterior myocardial infarction, is located in the His-Purkinje system, is often preceded by new bundle branch or fascicular block, progresses to complete heart block in a high percentage of cases, and requires temporary (and probably permanent) pacing. Even though these generalizations are usually valid, an occasional patient with inferior myocardial infarction may develop AV block that is not transient and requires pacing. Patients with first degree AV block or asymptomatic type I second degree AV block with a normal QRS duration do not require pacing.

In patients with acute anterior myocardial infarction and complete AV block, mortality is influenced mostly by the degree of myocardial damage. However, abrupt deaths occur due to the AV block itself, and

Table 2
Indications for a Temporary Pacemaker in Acute
Myocardial Infarction

ECG Abnormality	Indication for Pacemaker
PR prolongation	−
Second degree AV block type I	−
Second degree AV block type II	+
Complete AV block	usually +
AV dissociation without complete AV block	−
Alternating BBB RBBB + LAFB RBBB + LPFB LBBB + PR prolongation } new	+
RBBB + nl axis LBBB + nl PR } new	+/−
LBBB RBBB ± axis deviation } old	−

RBBB = right bundle branch block, LBBB = left bundle branch block, LAFB = left anterior fascicular block, LPFB = left posterior fascicular block.

therefore it is reasonable to provide these patients with temporary pacing support if necessary. It is important in some patients with an inferior myocardial infarction not to confuse AV dissociation due to marked sinus bradycardia and junctional escape with complete heart block; the former does not require pacing unless symptomatic.

Prophylactic temporary ventricular pacing is advised for patients with acute myocardial infarction who have a new bifascicular block manifested by alternating right and left bundle branch block, right bundle branch block with left or right axis deviation, and possibly left bundle branch block with an increased PR interval; these patients have an approximately 45% chance of progressing to complete heart block.[43] The indications for pacing are not so clear for patients with new right bundle branch block with normal axis or new left bundle branch block with normal PR intervals, although some authors have reported up to 43% of patients with new right bundle branch block progressing to complete heart block. Pacing is not generally indicated for patients with new left anterior fascicular block. Patients with pre-existing left bundle branch block or right bundle branch block with or without axis deviation are not candidates for pacing during an acute myocardial infarction because their risk of progressing to complete AV block is low. With the advent of transthoracic pacemakers that deliver high-energy, wide-pulse width impulses for external pacing through special large skin patches (for example, the Zoll external pacemaker,[44] one can be somewhat more conservative than in the past with these patients since they can be paced quickly if complete AV block occurs.

Indications for Permanent Pacing

Symptomatic bradycardia from any cause that is apparently permanent or may recur is an induction for permanent pacing (Table 3).

Table 3
Indications for Permanent Pacemaker (Bradycardia)

I. *Symptomatic Permanent Bradycardias:*
Fixed or intermittent acquired third degree AV block
Sick sinus syndrome:
  sinus arrest or exit block
  severe sinus bradycardia
  tachycardia-bradycardia syndrome
  exacerbation of bradycardia by drugs necessary for tachycardia
    therapy
  atrial fibrillation with slow ventricular response
  asystole at the termination of supraventricular tachycardia
  hypersensitive carotid sinus syndrome
II. *Prophylaxis:*

ECG	Indication for Pacemaker
Asymptomatic third degree AV block:	
acquired	+
congenital	−
Asymptomatic second degree AV block type I	−
Asymptomatic second degree AV block type II	+
Chronic BBB ± axis deviation	−
± PR	−
Survivors of acute myocardial infarction complicated by BBB and transient high-grade AV block	probably +

Bradycardia caused by nonessential drug therapy or associated with an acute myocardial infarction should be excluded. The two most common indications for permanent pacemaker implantation are fixed or intermittent third degree AV block and the sick sinus syndrome.

In addition to symptomatic bradycardias, there are certain conditions in which permanent pacing is indicated for prophylaxis against possible future AV block. This includes patients with asymptomatic acquired third degree AV block, but patients with asymptomatic congenital AV block are not paced unless symptoms occur or they have criteria for instability of the junctional escape as described above.[34] Patients with asymptomatic type I second degree AV block do not require pacing, but patients with asymptomatic second degree type II AV block are at high risk of sudden complete AV block and should receive prophylactic permanent pacemakers. Patients with chronic bundle branch block with or without axis deviation or long PR intervals are at low risk of developing complete AV block and should not receive permanent pacemakers. Some studies have suggested that survivors of acute myocardial infarction complicated by bundle branch block and transient high-grade AV block (here defined as type II second degree AV block, or third degree AV block which is preceded by type II block or which develops suddenly) have a better long-term prognosis if they receive a permanent pacemaker.[45,46]

References

1. Surawicz B, Reddy CP: Tachycardia-bradycardia syndrome. In: Surawicz B, et al (eds), Tachycardias. Boston, Martinus Nijhoff, 1984, p 199.
2. Crossen KJ, Cain ME: Assessment and management of sinus node dysfunction. Mod Concepts Cardiovasc Dis 55:43, 1986.
3. Abdon NJ, Landin K, Johansson BW: Athlete's bradycardia as an embolising disorder? Symptomatic arrhythmias in patients aged less than 50 years. Br Heart J 52:660, 1984.
4. Duster MC, Bink-Boelkens MT, Wampler D, et al: Long-term follow-up of dysrhythmias following the Mustard procedure. Am Heart J 109:1323, 1985.
5. Bharati S, Nordenberg A, Bauernfeind R, et al: The anatomic substrate for the sick sinus syndrome in adolescents. Am J Cardiol 46:163, 1980.
6. Rossi L: The pathologic basis of cardiac arrhythmias. Cardiol Clin 1:13, 1983.
7. Davies MJ, Anderson RH, Becker AE: Pathology of atrial arrhythmias. In: The Conduction System of the Heart. Butterworth Scientific Publication, London, 1983.
8. Brodsky M, Wu D, Denes P, et al: Arrhythmias documented by 24-hour continuous electrocardiographic monitoring in 50 male medical students without apparent heart disease. Am J Cardiol 39:390, 1977.

9. Holden, W, McAnulty JH, Rahimtoola SH: Characterization of heart rate response to exercise in the sick sinus syndrome. Br Heart J 40:923, 1978.
10. Peretz DI, Abdulla A: Management of cardioinhibitory hypersensitive carotid sinus syncope with permanent cardiac pacing: a seventeen year prospective study. Can J Cardiol 1:86, 1985.
11. Desae JM, Scheinman MM, Strauss HC: Electrophysiologic effects of combined autonomic blockade in patients with sinus node disease. Circulation 63:953, 1981.
12. Jose AD, Collison D: The normal range and determinants of the intrinsic heart rate in man. Cardiovasc Res 4:160, 1970.
13. Reiffel JA: Electrophysiologic evaluation of sinus node function. Cardiol Clin 4:401, 1986.
14. Mandel W, Hayakawa H, Danzig R, et al: Evaluation of sino-atrial node function in man by overdrive suppression. Circulation 44:59, 1971.
15. Benditt DG, Strauss HC, Scheinman MM, et al: Analysis of secondary pauses following termination of rapid atrial pacing in man. Circulation 54:436, 1976.
16. Strauss HC, Saroff AL, Bigger JT Jr, et al: Premature atrial stimulation as a key to the understanding of sinoatrial conduction in man: presentation of data and critical review of the literature. Circulation 47:86, 1973.
17. Gomes JAC, Kang PS, El-Sherif N: The sinus node electrogram in patients with and without sick sinus syndrome: techniques and correlation between directly measured and indirectly estimated sinoatrial conduction time. Circulation 66:864, 1982.
18. A report of the American College of Cardiology/American Heart Association Task Force on assessment of diagnostic and therapeutic cardiovascular procedures (Subcommittee to assess clinical intracardiac electrophysiologic studies): Guidelines for clinical intracardiac electrophysiologic studies. Circulation 80:1925, 1989.
19. Morady F: The evaluation of syncope with electrophysiologic studies. Cardiol Clin 4:515, 1986.
20. Benditt DG, Benson DW Jr, Kreitt J, et al: Electrophysiologic effects of theophylline in young patients with recurrent symptomatic bradyarrhythmias. Am J Cardiol 52:1223, 1983.
21. Shaw DB, Holman RR, Gowers JI: Survival in sinoatrial disorder (sick-sinus syndrome). Br Med J 1:139, 1980.
22. Scherlag BJ, Lau SH, Helfant RH, et al: Catheter technique for recording His bundle activity in man. Circulation 39:13, 1969.
23. Damato AN, Lau SH, Helfant RH, et al: Study of atrioventricular conduction in man using electrode catheter recordings of His bundle activity. Circulation 39:287, 1969.
24. Josephson ME, Seides SF: Clinical Cardiac Electrophysiology: Techniques and Interpretations. Philadelphia, Lea & Febiger, 1979.
25. Damato AN, Lau SH, Helfant R, et al: A study of heart block in man using His bundle recordings. Circulation 39:297, 1969.
26. Fisch C: Electrocardiography of Arrhythmias. Philadelphia, Lea & Febiger, 1990.
27. Zeppilli P, Fenici R, Sassara M, et al: Wenckebach second degree AV block in top ranking athletes: an old problem revisited. Am Heart J 100:281, 1980.
28. Lev M: Anatomic basis for atrioventricular block. Am J Med 37:742, 1964.

29. Scott JS, Maddison PJ, Taylor PV, et al: Connective-tissue disease, antibodies to ribonucleoprotein, and congenital heart block. N Engl J Med 309:209, 1983.
30. Shaw DB, Kekwick CA, Veale D, et al: Survival in second degree atrioventricular block. Br Heart J 53:587, 1985.
31. Southall DP, Johnston F, Shinebourne EA, et al: 24-hour electrocardiograph study of heart rate and rhythm patterns in a population of healthy children. Br Heart J 45:281, 1981.
32. Zipes DP: Second-degree atrioventricular block. Circulation 60:465, 1979.
33. Karpawich PP, Gillette PC, Garson A Jr, et al: Congenital complete atrioventricular block: clinical and electrophysiologic predictors of need for pacemaker insertion. Am J Cardiol 48:1098, 1981.
34. Dewey RC, Capeless MA, Levy AM: Use of ambulatory electrocardiographic monitoring to identify high-risk patients with congenital complete heart block. New Engl J Med 316:835, 1987.
35. Narula OS, Narula JT: Junctional pacemakers in man: response to overdrive suppression with and without parasympathetic blockade. Circulation 57:880, 1978.
36. Bonner AJ, Zipes DP: Lidocaine and His bundle extrasystoles: His bundle discharge conducted normally, conducted with functional right or left bundle branch block or blocked entirely (concealed). Arch Intern Med 136:700, 1976.
37. Bergfeldt L, Rosenqvist M, Vallin H, et al: Disopyramide-induced second and third degree atrioventricular block in patients with bifascicular block: an acute stress test to predict atrioventricular block progression. Br Heart J 53:328, 1985.
38. Dhingra R, Palileo E, Strasberg B, et al: Significance of the HV interval in 517 patients with chronic bifascicular block. Ciculation 64:1265, 1981.
39. Scheinman MM, Peters RW, Modin G, et al: Prognostic value of infranodal conduction time in patients with chronic bundle branch block. Circulation 56:240, 1977.
40. Dhingra RC, Wyndham C, Bauernfeind R, et al: Significance of block distal to the His bundle induced by atrial pacing in patients with chronic bifascicular block. Circulation 60:1455, 1979.
41. Fujimura O, Yee R, Klein GJ, et al: The diagnostic sensitivity of electrophysiologic testing in patients with syncope caused by transient bradycardia. N Engl J Med 321:1703, 1989.
42. Dhingra RC, Winslow E, Pouget JM, et al: The effect of isoproterenol on atrioventricular and intraventricular conduction. Am J Cardiol 32:629, 1973.
43. Mullins CB, Atkins JM: Prognosis and management of ventricular conduction blocks in acute myocardial infarction. Med Concepts Cardiovasc Dis 45:129, 1976.
44. Zoll PM, Zoll RH, Falk RH, et al: External noninvasive temporary cardiac pacing: clinical trials. Circulation 71:937, 1985.
45. Hindman MC, Wagner GS, JaRo M, et al: The clinical significance of bundle branch block complicating acute myocardial infarction. 1. Clinical characteristics, hospital mortality, and one year follow-up. Circulation 58:679, 1978.
46. Hindman MC, Wagner GS, JaRo M, et al: The clinical significance of bundle branch block complicating acute myocardial infarction. 2. Indications for temporary and permanent pacemaker insertion. Circulation 58:689, 1978.

Chapter 11

Management of Peri-infarctional Ventricular Arrhythmias and Conduction Disturbances

Anil K. Bhandari and Philip T. Sager

Introduction

Ventricular arrhythmias and conduction disturbances are common in the peri-infarction period and their early recognition and treatment is of paramount importance.[1–5] In the first 48 hours after acute myocardial infarction (MI), ventricular arrhythmias are almost invariably present.[6–27] While some forms of ventricular arrhythmias are considered benign, others need to be treated because they may be the harbingers of ventricular fibrillation.[28–40] At times, prompt treatment is indicated because of the hemodynamic compromise related directly to the presence of ventricular arrhythmias.[41,42] In the late hospital phase, although the ventricular arrhythmias decrease in their frequency and complexity, their presence correlates with an increased risk of sudden and total cardiac mortality during the first year after discharge from the hospital.[53–59] However, there is no universal consensus on the issue of whether asymptomatic ventricular arrhythmias should be treated or not. More recent data suggest that programmed ventricular stimulation (PVS) and signal-averaged ECG may have a potential role in more accurately identifying patients at an increased risk for sudden death.[60–71]

From Naccarelli GV (ed): *Cardiac Arrhythmias: A Practical Approach.* Mount Kisco, NY, Futura Publishing Co., Inc., © 1991.

The purpose of this chapter is to review the clinical significance and the management of the ventricular arrhythmias and the conduction disturbances that occur soon after and in the first few weeks after acute MI.

Ventricular Arrhythmias

In the peri-infarction period, the mechanisms of ventricular arrhythmias are varied and complex and much of the current knowledge is based on the experimental data.[6-11] After acute experimental MI, ventricular arrhythmias occur in three distinct phases.[8] *Early phase* arrhythmias occur in the first 30 to 60 minutes after acute coronary artery occlusion and include rapid ventricular tachycardias and fibrillation. Immediately after coronary occlusion, there is an accumulation of anaerobic metabolites, an abnormal alteration in the intracellular and extracellular ionic concentrations, and a dysfunction of the autonomic nervous system. The resultant cellular electrophysiological abnormalities produce a milieu for ventricular arrhythmias that appear to be predominantly re-entrant in mechanism.[9,10]

After an electrical quiescence of 1 to 5 hours, the *delayed phase* of arrhythmias sets in and lasts for approximately 6 to 10 hours. This phase is characterized by the appearance of relatively slow (60 to 120 bpm) ventricular tachycardia (VT) that appears to be automatic in mechanism since it can neither be induced or terminated by PVS. *The late phase* of arrhythmias occurs at 3 to 10 days after experimental MI and includes relatively rapid nonsustained and sustained VT. They appear to be re-entrant in mechanism because of their reproducible initiation and termination by PVS.

These experimental findings should perhaps not be extrapolated to the survivors of acute MI but the broad similarities exist in the patterns of the experimental arrhythmias and the peri-infarctional arrhythmias in man. *The early phase* arrhythmias appear to correspond with the prehospital phase in man where the predominant arrhythmias are rapid polymorphic VT or ventricular fibrillation (VF). The *delayed phase* appears to correspond with the accelerated idioventricular rhythms which are frequently observed in the coronary care unit phase of acute MI in man. *The late phase* arrhythmias are probably analogous to those seen during the first 1 to 2 weeks after MI in man. Also, PVS performed just prior to discharge in the survivors of acute MI induce sustained VT or VF in

17–46% of the patients and the incidence is remarkably similar to that observed during PVS after experimental MI.[60–71]

Pre-hospital Phase Ventricular Arrhythmias

Pre-hospital phase usually refers to the period of the first 4 hours (or less) after the onset of acute MI before the patient arrives in the hospital. Using continuous oscilloscopic monitoring in 294 patients, Pantridge et al. found premature ventricular complexes (PVC) in 58% of the patients in the first hour and in 93% of the patients by 4 hours after acute MI.[12] Primary VF represents the most serious arrhythmia in this phase and occurs in an average of 10% of the patients (range 4% to 36%) with a vast majority occurring in the first 2 hours after the infarction.[12–14] At least half of all deaths from MI take place during this period and are predominantly due to VF. Although significant bradyarrhythmias occur in about 8% to 38% of the patients, the deaths during the pre-hospital phase are only rarely due to severe bradyarrhythmias or asystole.

Coronary Care Unit Phase

The incidence of ventricular arrhythmias ranges from 34% to 100% during the coronary care unit phase of the acute MI.[1–4,15] The varying incidence reflects probably the differences in the techniques of electrocardiographic monitoring, in the time elapsed between onset of symptoms and admission to the hospital and in the proportion of patients with complicated infarctions. In general, the ventricular arrhythmias tend to occur more often in patients with larger infarct size, congestive heart failure, and conduction disturbances. While some arrhythmias may be benign and need no treatment, others may be harbingers of the sustained life-threatening ventricular arrhythmias and need to be promptly treated.

Ventricular arrhythmias in the coronary care unit phase may be divided into four categories: (1) warning arrhythmias, (2) VF, (3) paroxysmal VT, and (4) accelerated idioventricular rhythms (AIVR). The incidence and the prognostic significance of these arrhythmias will be discussed in the following section.

Warning Arrhythmias

It is well accepted that there is a vulnerable period for induction of VF when a ventricular stimulus was delivered in the late systole or early diastole after acute MI.[9] Earlier experience in the coronary care unit appeared to confirm this concept as several investigators demonstrated a precipitation of primary VF by early cycle PVC.[6,7,15] In the subsequent years, other forms of ventricular arrhythmias were also identified that predisposed the patients with acute MI to the development of VF. These include ventricular arrhythmias with the following characteristics: PVC frequency of ≥5 beats per minute, R-on-T phenomenon PVC with a prematurity index (as defined by the ratio of the coupling interval of PVC and the QT interval of preceding sinus beat) of less than 0.85, multiform PVC, and PVC occurring in pairs or runs.[15]

The concept of warning arrhythmias has not withstood the test of time. The R-on-T phenomenon PVC appeared to be no more malignant than the late cycle PVC as the latter precipitated primary VF in less than half of the episodes and R-on-T PVCs were noted in approximately half of the patients who never developed primary VF. Thus, the warning arrhythmias are neither sensitive nor specific precursors of primary VF and should not be used as a sole guide to antiarrhythmic therapy in patients with acute MI. Moreover, the detection of warning arrhythmias is highly dependent upon the capability of the electrocardiographic monitoring system and on the level of training of the nursing staff and, thus, is subject to significant interobserver variability.

Ventricular Fibrillation

VF may occur as a primary or secondary event in patients with acute MI. Primary VF is defined as the fibrillation that occurs unexpectedly within the first 48 hours after acute MI and is not preceded by advanced heart failure, hypotension, or cardiogenic shock. Secondary, VF, on the other hand, develops as a terminal complication of the above clinical situations. The distinction of the two forms of VF is of clinical importance since the resuscitation rate is very high (95–100%) and the subsequent prognosis is favorable in patients with primary VF. Conversely, in patients with secondary fibrillation, the resuscitation rate is low (40–50%) and the subsequent prognosis is poor.[18–20]

Primary VF has been reported to occur in 1–10% of the hospitalized patients with acute MI.[1–5] The incidence is highest in the first hour after

MI and declines rapidly in the ensuing hours. In a recent review of the temporal course of primary VF in patients experiencing it as a complication of an acute MI,[20] the vast majority of episodes occurred in patients within the first 4 to 12 hours. In no patient did the primary VF occur more than 48 hours after the infarction. Primary VF was usually preceded by the appearance of warning ventricular arrhythmias in approximately half of the patients, but in others, it may be the first manifestation of the underlying electrical instability.[16,17]

Although the exact electrophysiological mechanism of primary VF is not known, it appears to be an isolated electric event and bears no significant relation to the size and location of the infarct or to presence or absence of left ventricular dysfunction.[18-20] Controversy exists as to the short-term prognostic implication of the primary VF. Although earlier studies[18-20] suggested no adverse effects of this arrhythmia, two recent large studies have demonstrated a significantly higher in-hospital mortality in patients with primary VF than in those without this arrhythmia.[21,22] The long-term prognosis, however, was not adversely affected by primary VF.

Accelerated Idioventricular Rhythms

Accelerated idioventricular rhythm (AIVR) is defined as a ventricular rhythm with rates ranging from 55 to 120 beats per minute. This is a common arrhythmia in the first 24 hours of acute MI and occurs at a frequency ranging from 8% to 46%.[1-4,23,25] AIVR may emerge as an escape rhythm in the setting of a slow sinus rhythm. More often, this arrhythmia is initiated by a PVC and the QRS morphological pattern of the AIVR is often similar to that of the PVC (Fig. 1). Frequently, AIVR shows a variable rate at the onset (warm-up phenomenon) and termination of the arrhythmia. It is equally common in patients with anterior and inferior MI and the frequency is not affected by the size of the infarction or the extent of left ventricular dysfunction. The presence of AIVR is not associated with a higher in-hospital mortality and it is not considered to be a precursor of VF.[24,25] However, there are several documented instances where the relatively slow AIVR progressed to faster sustained VT and the rate of the faster VT was exactly double that of the slower rhythm, and the QRS morphology (in the monitored rhythm strips) appeared to be identical.[24] Such a progression is, however, quite rare and may reflect the presence of a variable exit block of the automatic AIVR focus in the myocardium. In recent years, there has been a re-

12 HOURS POST MI

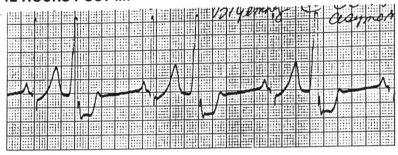

20 HOURS POST MI

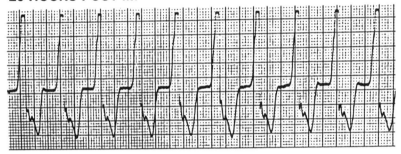

36 HOURS POST MI

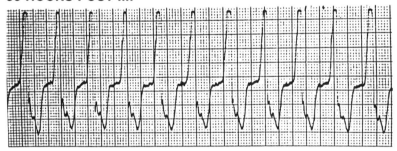

Figure 1. Rhythm strips of a patient with an acute anterior wall myocardial infarction showing premature ventricular complexes (PVC) in bigeminy (top strip) accelerated idioventricular rhythm (AIVR) at a rate of 105 beats per minute (middle strip) and AIVR at a rate of 118 beats per minute (bottom strip). Note that the PVC resembles in morphology the QRS configuration during AIVR. The AIVR resolved spontaneously and required no treatment.

newed interest in AIVR as a manifestation of reperfusion arrhythmia. This will be dealt with separately under the section entitled *Reperfusion Arrhythmias.*

Ventricular Tachycardia

VT is defined as three or more consecutive QRS complexes of ventricular origin at a rate of more than 120 beats per minute. The tachycardia is considered nonsustained when it lasts less than 30 seconds in duration and terminates spontaneously without symptoms of hemodynamic compromise. Sustained VT, on the other hand, is defined as tachycardia that lasts 30 seconds or longer in duration or tachycardia that causes immediate hemodynamic compromise requiring termination in less than 30 seconds.

VT has been reported to occur in 6–40% of patients with acute MI, with an average frequency of 10%.[1–4] The vast majority of the episodes are nonsustained, lasting up to a few seconds in duration, and do not produce any significant hemodynamic compromise. The VT occurs equally frequently in patients with anterior or inferior infarctions and its presence in the first 48 hours after acute MI does not adversely affect the long-term prognosis.

Sustained VT is relatively infrequent in the first 48 hours after acute MI.[2–4,15] It occurs generally in the setting of an extensive infarction and congestive heart failure. The in-hospital mortality is high and reflects probably the severity of underlying left ventricular dysfunction. It is traditionally thought that the sustained ventricular arrhythmias in the first 48 hours after acute MI are peculiar to the acute stage of the infarction and their presence does not adversely affect the long-term prognosis.[4,15–20] However, this viewpoint is based on the results of few studies that had small numbers of patients and the vast majority of the included patients had either primary VF or AIVR as the underlying sustained arrhythmia. The authors have had the opportunity of witnessing several patients with sustained monomorphic VT in the first 48 hours of acute MI in whom the arrhythmia recurred during follow-up and was difficult to manage with antiarrhythmic drugs (Fig. 2).

Recently, attention has also been drawn to the polymorphic sustained VT in the setting of acute MI which is not associated with marked QT prolongation and does not occur in association with other known predisposing factors of torsades de pointes[26] (Fig. 3). The exact mechanism of this arrhythmia is not known. In some patients, it appeared

SINUS RHYTHM

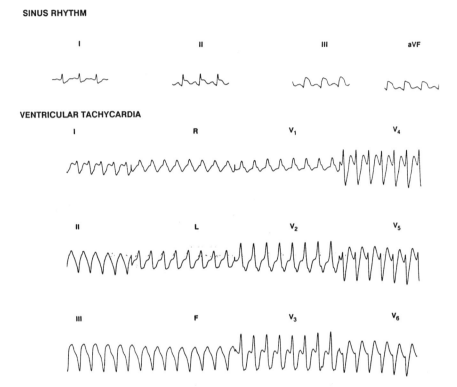

VENTRICULAR TACHYCARDIA

Figure 2. Sustained ventricular tachycardia in a patient with 1-day-old inferior myocardial infarction. During sinus rhythm (top panel), the ST segment shows a 3–5 mm elevation in leads II, III, and AVF. The patient developed a rapid sustained ventricular tachycardia at a rate of 200 beats per minute (12-lead ECG shown) from which he had to be cardioverted with a 50-joule shock. The VT recurred on the 10th hospital day and was inducible during programmed ventricular stimulation was well. The control of arrhythmias required treatment with amiodarone.

to be related to the presence of severe myocardial ischemia and was suppressed by anti-ischemic therapy consisting of intravenous beta-blockers, intra-aortic balloon pump, or emergent coronary artery bypass surgery.[27] In one report of nine such patients, the arrhythmia was resistant to multiple antiarrhythmic drugs and overdrive pacing, but intravenous verapamil was effective in three of the four patients in whom it was administered.[26] The in-hospital mortality and the long-term prognosis is poor in these patients.

ON ADMISSION

I III aVF

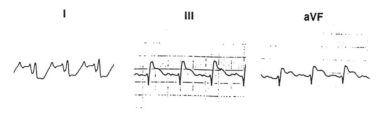

6 HOURS LATER

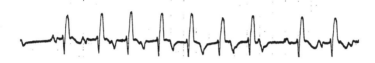

7 HOURS LATER

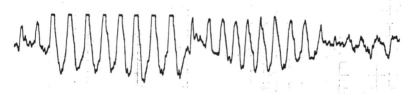

7 1/2 HOURS LATER

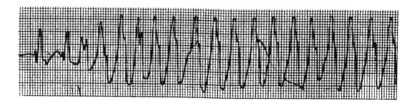

Figure 3. Polymorphous ventricular tachycardia in a patient with an acute inferior myocardial infarction. The three ECG leads obtained on admission show ST segment elevation in leads III and F. Six hours later, the rhythm strip shows a short paroxysm of atrial tachycardia. Note that the QT interval is not prolonged. Shortly thereafter, the patient developed multiple runs of polymorphous ventricular tachycardia (third and bottom strip) some of which required cardioversion. The treatment with intravenous lidocaine, procainamide, and bretylium was ineffective and the control of arrhythmia required administration of intravenous amiodarone.

Reperfusion Arrhythmias

Since the advent of thrombolytic therapy, there has been increased interest in the prevalence, pathophysiology, and the significance of the reperfusion arrhythmias.[28–30] The arrhythmias occur in over 80% of the patients who have successful restoration of the antegrade coronary flow. The AIVR is the most common ventricular arrhythmia and some have characterized this arrhythmia to be a useful noninvasive marker of the coronary recanalization, especially if it occurs in close proximity to the administration of the thrombolytic agents.[28,29] AIVR is a benign arrhythmia and only rarely degenerates to VF. At times, reperfusion may be associated with sinus bradycardia and high-grade atrioventricular blocks. These bradyarrhythmias are generally transient in nature and rarely require treatment with intravenous atropine or temporary cardiac pacing.

Management of Arrhythmias

With the advent of coronary care units and a prompt recognition and treatment of the ventricular arrhythmias, there has been a significant reduction in the incidence of primary arrhythmic deaths during the first 72 hours after acute MI.[2–8] The vast majority of in-hospital deaths now are due to cardiogenic shock or cardiac rupture and only rarely does a patient succumb to the refractory incessant ventricular arrhythmias.

General Measures

In approaching ventricular arrhythmias, the patient should undergo a comprehensive evaluation of the underlying medical condition. One ought to identify and correct the reversible predisposing factors that may contribute to the genesis and perpetuation of the ventricular arrhythmias. These factors include myocardial ischemia, arterial hypoxemia, electrolyte imbalance, congestive heart failure, systemic hypotension or hypertension, acid base abnormalities, and the proarrhythmic effects of antiarrhythmic agents.

Warning Arrhythmia and Lidocaine Prophylaxis

It is generally agreed upon that the warning arrhythmias in the first 48 hours after acute MI should be treated. The treatment is based upon the premise that warning arrhythmias indicate an increased propensity of the ventricles to fibrillate and that their suppression will lead to protection against primary VF.[15] Others have argued for giving antiarrhythmic prophylaxis to all survivors of acute MI, regardless of the presence or absence of warning arrhythmias.[31-33] The latter viewpoint is supported by the fact that the warning arrhythmias are neither a sensitive nor a specific marker for primary VF and at least half of the patients who develop primary VF after acute MI do not demonstrate preceding warning arrhythmias.

Intravenous lidocaine is the drug of choice for warning arrhythmias as well as for routine antiarrhythmic prophylaxis. Several studies have documented the efficacy of lidocaine in suppressing PVC and in reducing the frequency of primary VF.[33] Intravenous lidocaine suppresses PVC is in 70–80% of the patients in the first few hours after acute MI and in 80–90% of the patients thereafter. The available data support the use of prophylactic lidocaine in the survivors of acute MI who are hemodynamically stable and are under the age of 70 years. In patients older than 70 years or in those with heart failure, prophylactic lidocaine is likely to be of benefit, but its efficacy has not been systematically evaluated. However, the side effects are likely to be more frequent in these patients and the plasma levels of lidocaine ought to be closely monitored. Furthermore, it needs to be recognized that the low-dose lidocaine regimens have not been shown to reduce the incidence of primary VF.[33] The recommended loading dose includes an initial bolus of 1.5 mg/kg body weight (usually 100 mg) followed by two repeat boluses of half of the initial dose at intervals of 8 minutes each.[34] The maintenance infusion is 2 to 4 mg/minute administered over the next 36 to 48 hours. The administration of the repeat boluses is important because of the rapid half-life of lidocaine in the initial redistribution phase. Alternatively, the loading dose of lidocaine may also be infused at 5 mg/kg body weight over 20 to 30 minutes followed by a maintenance infusion. The loading and maintenance doses of lidocaine should be decreased by half in patients with significant heart failure or hepatic dysfunction.

The prophylactic use of other antiarrhythmic agents (such as procainamide, disopyramide, phenytoin, quinidine, aprindine, etc.) has not been shown to be beneficial.[4] However, early use of intravenous betablockers may be accompanied by a reduction in the incidence of sustained ventricular arrhythmias. In a double-blind trial of 1395 patients with acute MI, intravenous metoprolol 15 mg given soon after admission reduced significantly the incidence of in-hospital VF although the total in-hospital mortality was not different between the treated group and the placebo group.[35] Another large trial of intravenous and oral atenolol given soon after acute MI showed a significant reduction of ventricular arrhythmias in the treated group.[36] The use of intravenous beta-blockers, thus, may be of benefit in the first several hours after acute MI when the hyperadrenergic activity may contribute to the genesis of the ventricular arrhythmias. As noted previously, intravenous thrombolytic agents have not been shown to reduce the incidence of primary VF.[21] When asymptomatic ventricular arrhythmias are not suppressed by lidocaine, or if they show a breakthrough after an initial suppression, it does not constitute an indication to change the antiarrhythmic drug. The beneficial effect of lidocaine for primary VF appears to be more related to its ability in raising the fibrillation threshold rather than in suppressing PVC.[31] In patients with symptomatic of hemodynamically significant ventricular arrhythmias that fail to respond to lidocaine, intravenous procainamide is the next drug of choice. The loading dose of 15 mg/kg body weight (usually 1000 mg) is infused slowly over 20 minutes at a rate of 50 mg/minute followed by a maintenance infusion of 2–4 mg/minute.

Lidocaine Prophylaxis in the Pre-hospital Phase

Because 50–60% of all deaths due to acute MI occur before the patient arrives in the hospital and because the majority of the deaths are due to VF, there is need to have a safe and effective drug, which when given prophylactically, can reduce the mortality in the pre-hospital phase. A single intramuscular injection of lidocaine (in the deltoid muscle) at a dose of 300 mg has been recommended but the available data are conflicting.[37,38] At present, the prophylactic use of intramuscular lidocaine is not routinely recommended in the pre-hospital phase of patients with documented or suspected acute MI.

Accelerated Idioventricular Rhythms

AIVR is generally considered a benign arrhythmia and does not need to be routinely treated with an antiarrhythmic agent. However, occasionally, this arrhythmia may be associated with a significant hemodynamic compromise, probably due to the loss of atrioventricular synchrony. It may then be suppressed by accelerating the underlying sinus rhythm by intravenous atropine or by atrial overdrive pacing.[24,25] Rarely when the AIVR shows a sudden jump to the faster rate, its treatment is similar to that of sustained ventricular arrhythmias.

Sustained Ventricular Tachycardia

When sustained VT is associated with a significant hemodynamic decompensation or collapse, or if the rate of VT is more than 160 beats per minute, the treatment of choice is an immediate direct current synchronized cardioversion.[39] The recommended energy for the first shock is 50 joules. If the first shock is ineffective, the energy of subsequent shocks may be increased to 100 and then 200 joules. A precordial thump is only rarely effective in terminating sustained VT and its routine use is not recommended.

If the patient is hemodynamically stable, and the ventricular rate is less than 160 beats per minute, treatment with intravenous lidocaine or procainamide may sometimes be effective.[39] The dosage schedules have been described above. The use of bretylium tosylate is reserved for patients who have recurrent sustained VT refractory to lidocaine and procainamide.[40] Bretylium is administered as a loading dose of 5 to 10 mg/kg (usually 300 mg) over 5 minutes followed by a maintenance infusion of 1 to 2 mg per minute. Hypotension is the main side effect of the drug, and may require withdrawal of the drug in up to one-third of the patients. Infrequently, when a patient continues to have frequent episodes of otherwise well-tolerated sustained VT, a temporary ventricular pacemaker may be inserted to perform overdrive pacing or deliver timed premature stimuli in order to pace terminate the tachycardia. Intravenous amiodarone remains an investigational agent and its use is reserved for patients who fail to respond to the above antiarrhythmic agents.[41] Amiodarone is administered as a bolus of 300 mg (5 mg/kg body weight) over 5 to 10 minutes followed by a maintenance infusion of 1 mg/minute. If the VT recurs, half of the initial bolus may be repeated at 30-minute intervals.

Polymorphic VT (torsades de pointes) is a rare complication of acute MI and often fails to respond to conventional therapy. The control of arrhythmia may require the use of intravenous beta-blockers (provided the patient has no congestive heart failure), intravenous amiodarone, overdrive ventricular pacing, intra-aortic balloon pump, or rarely map guided infractectomy.[26,27,42]

Ventricular Fibrillation

Immediate defibrillation with 200 joules direct current counter shock is the recommended treatment of choice.[39] If VF persists, the energy of subsequent shocks may be increased to 300 and 360 joules. Appropriate cardiopulmonary resuscitation and a correction of the metabolic and electrolyte disturbances is of crucial importance. For patients with recurrent VF, intravenous bretylium is the drug of choice since it raises the threshold for VF. The resuscitation rate is excellent (>95%) for patients with primary VF, but is low (40–50%) for patients with secondary VF. As noted above, the latter patients, even if successfully resuscitated have a high in-hospital mortality rate of 50–75%.[18]

Late In-hospital Phase

After the first 48 to 72 hours in the coronary care unit, the frequency of ventricular arrhythmia declines for the next 3 to 4 days and then begins to increase again, reaching its peak probably around 6 to 12 weeks after the MI. In most previous studies,[43–50] the prevalence of ventricular arrhythmias has been studied between 1 and 3 weeks after the infarction. An interest in this time period stems from the fact that the survivors of acute MI face an increased risk of sudden death after discharge from the hospital and the risk of sudden death is highest in the first 6 months after the discharge.

Table 1 summarizes the prevalence of ventricular arrhythmias during the late in-hospital phase. Frequent PVCs (as defined by ≥10/hour) occur in about 15–30%, multiform PVCs in 18–30%, ventricular couplets in 10–20%, and nonsustained VT in 6–10%. The runs of VT are generally brief (three to five beats) and the vast majority do not experience more than one or two episodes a day. In general, the ventricular arrhythmias occur more frequently in patients with left ventricular dysfunction and wall motion abnormalities. However, it should be recognized that the ventricular arrhythmias in the late in-hospital phase bear no relationship to those observed in the coronary care unit.[44]

Prognostic Significance of Ventricular Arrhythmias

Almost every study that examined the prognostic significance of ventricular arrhythmias in the late in-hospital phase of acute MI has

Table 1
Prevalence of Ventricular Arrhythmias in the Late Hospital Phase of Acute MI

Study	No. of Pts.	Time from AMI	Hours of ECG	Ventricular Arrhythmias				
				Any PVC	Freq. PVC	Pairs	VT	Multi.
Moss et al.[43]	100	21 days	6	72%	20%	18%	4%	20%
Vismara et al.[44]	64	11 days	10	76%	34%	34%	6%	—
Ruberman et al.[45]	1739	2 wks–3 yrs	1	51%	26%	26.6%	26.6%	
Moss et al.[46]	940	Predischarge	6	50%	—	3%	1%	13%
Mukharji et al.[47]	533	10 days	24	84%	15%			66%
Bigger et al.[48]	819	—	24	86%	15%	26%	11%	64%
Kostis et al.[49]	1640	2–21 days	24	84%	13%	20%	20%	32%

Frequent PVC >10/hour, Pts = patients, AMI = acute myocrdial infarction, VT = ventricular tachycardia, Multi = multiform.

shown a relationship between the arrhythmia and the subsequent sudden cardiac mortality.[43-50] The mortality is lowest in patients without PVC and increases by two to threefold in patients with ventricular arrhythmias depending upon the frequency and complexity of the arrhythmia. In most studies, the presence of frequent PVC ($\geq$10 per hour) has been the most significant predictor of subsequent cardiac mortality, although in one study the mortality risk reached the maximum at a frequency as low as 3 PVC per hour.[48] The repetitive PVC (as defined by ventricular couplets or nonsustained VT) have consistently been found to increase the risk of sudden and total cardiac mortality. Some studies have reported a threefold or higher mortality in patients with nonsustained VT than in those without this arrhythmia.[48-50] However, this arrhythmia is encountered in only a small percentage (5 to 10%) of the survivors of acute MI and its sensitivity in predicting sudden death is too low to be of clinical utility (Table 2).

It should be emphasized that the mortality in post infarction patients is best predicted by the presence of left ventricular dysfunction. This relationship has been shown to be consistent in all reported studies. Because the prevalence of ventricular arrhythmias bears a strong relationship with the severity of left ventricular dysfunction, many have argued whether the ventricular arrhythmias contribute to the increased cardiac mortality independent of the underlying left ventricular dysfunction. Shortly after an MI (within 2 weeks), ventricular arrhythmias are uncommon with an ejection fraction of >40% and occur in more than half of the patients with an ejection fraction of <40%. Sudden deaths during a short-term follow-up of 7 months occurred almost exclusively among the patients with complex arrhythmias and depressed left ventricular ejection fraction. A significant association has been demonstrated between ventricular arrhythmias and cardiac mortality, after an adjustment was made for the left ventricular ejection fraction. However, the results of five large studies have convincingly demonstrated an association between ventricular arrhythmias and cardiac mortality independent of the left ventricular dysfunction (Table 3). The risk of sudden death is synergistically increased when frequent PVCs coexist with depressed ejection fraction. In the MILIS study,[47] patients with left ventricular ejection fraction <40% and PVC $\geq$10 per hour had a 2-year sudden mortality rate of 18%. In contrast, the incidence of sudden death was only 2% in patients with ejection fraction >40% and a mean PVC frequency of <10 per hour (Table 3).

Although the presence of the asymptomatic ventricular arrhythmia is an established risk factor for sudden death in the survivors of acute

Table 2
Prognostic Significance of Ventricular Arrhythmias in Survivors of Acute MI

Study	No. of Pts.	F/U Mo.	Method of LV Function	PVC Independent	Odds Ratio for Increased Sudden Deaths			
					Freq. PVC	Rep. PVC	Freq. PVC	Rep. PVC
Ruberman et al.[45]	1739	36	Clinical	Yes	—	3.33	—	2.13
Moss et al.[46]	940	48	Clinical	Yes	—	—	—	—
Mukharji et al.[47]	533	18	RNEF	Yes	3.4	2.4	4.0	2.2
Bigger et al.[48]	766	24	RNEF	Yes	4.0	3.6	3.0	3.2
Kostis et al.[49]	1640	25	Clinical	Yes	1.80	1.30	2.20	1.5

F/U = Follow-up, Mo = month, PVC = premature ventricular complex, Rep = repetitive, Freq = frequent.
* Complex PVC: Pairs, bigeminy, multiform, or R-on-T.
** Frequent PVCs defined as >10/hour.
RNEF = radionuclide ejection fraction.

Table 3

Mortality in Survivors of Acute MI in MILIS* Study: Interaction of PVC and LVEF

Group	No. of Pts.	Total Deaths	Sudden Death	Relative Risk Sudden Death
EF >40% PVC <10/HR	314	16 (5%)	5 (2%)	1
EF <0.40%, PVC <10/HR	141	27 (19%)	14 (10%)	6
EF >40%, PVC >10/HR	38	7 (20%)	3 (8%)	5
EF <0.40%, PVC >10/HR	40	16 (40%)	7 (18%)	11

EF = Left ventricular ejection fraction; PVC = premature ventricular complex.
* Mukharji JT, et al: The MILIS study group.
Risk factors for sudden death after acute myocardial infarction: two-year follow-up. Am J Cardiol 54:31, 1984.

MI, it should be emphasized that its sensitivity in predicting sudden deaths has been disappointingly low and ranges from 15% to 45%, depending upon the definition of abnormal end-points for ventricular arrhythmias[49] (Table 4). In general, with an increasing complexity of ventricular arrhythmias, there is a decline in the sensitivity, although the specificity tends to be higher.

Table 4

The Sensitivity and the Specificity of Ventricular Arrhythmias in Predicting Sudden and Total Cardiac Mortality in Post-Infarction Patients in the BHAT Study*

Characteristic	Sudden Death		Total Deaths	
	Sensitivity %	Specificity %	Sensitivity %	Specificity %
>10/hour	25	87	26	88
Repetitive	34	80	33	82
Either	43	75	44	76
Both	16	94	14	94

* Kostis JB, Byington R, Friedman LM, et al: Prognostic significance of ventricular ectopic activity in survivors of acute myocardial infarction. J Am Coll Crdiol 10:231, 1987.

Management of Asymptomatic Ventricular Arrhythmias

The question of whether the post-MI patient with asymptomatic ventricular arrhythmias should be treated with antiarrhythmic drugs represents a difficult problem. Although these patients represent an easily identifiable high-risk subset, the benefit of antiarrhythmic therapy has not been convincingly shown in any of the randomized trials. In a recent review of the results of six randomized studies of antiarrhythmic drugs in the survivors of acute MI involving a total of 1620 patients and using diphenylhydantoin, tocainide, or aprindine, there was no significant reduction in mortality in the treated versus the placebo group.[53] These studies however, had significant drawbacks. The number of patients enrolled was relatively small, the patient risk stratification was not performed, only one antiarrhythmic drug was used in each study, and the suppression of PVC was not documented. Some of these drawbacks were corrected in two relatively recent studies. In 1984, the International Mexiletine and Placebo antiarrhythmic coronary trial (IMPACT) reported its findings in the 630 patients with recent acute MI.[54] These patients underwent a baseline Holter monitoring prior to treatment and then at 1, 4, and 12 months after the infarction. Although mexiletine-treated patients had a lower prevalence of ventricular arrhythmias at 1 and 4 months, there was a trend toward higher mortality in the mexiletine group (7.6%) than in the placebo group (4.8%). In 1987, Gotlieb et al.[55] studied 143 high-risk survivors of acute MI who had ventricular arrhythmias of Lown grade 3 or higher, left ventricular ejection fraction <40%, or both. There was no significant difference in the 1-year mortality between the aprindine group (17%) and the placebo group (22%).

Because of the serious design problems and the relatively small number of patients in the above-mentioned studies, the National Heart, Lung and Blood Institute initiated the Cardiac Arrhythmia Pilot Study (CAPS) in 1983[56] and the Cardiac Arrhythmia Suppression Trial (CAST) in 1987.[57] The CAPS was a feasibility study in which 502 patients with recent MI were randomized to therapy with encainide, flecainide, moricizine, imipramine, or placebo. Except for imipramine, which had a low efficacy and a high incidence of intolerable side effects, the other three drugs were highly effective in suppressing PVC and were well tolerated. Based on these findings, the CAST study sought to determine the effects on survival of flecainide, encainide, or moricizine in 1727 survivors of acute MI. Prior to randomization, all patients had shown an 80% or greater reduction in PVC and a 90% or greater reduction of repetitive

PVC by one of the study drugs. During an average of 10 months of follow-up, the total cardiac mortality was 2.5-fold higher in 730 patients treated with encainide or flecainide (7.7%) than in 725 patients on placebo (3.0%). The incidence of sudden cardiac death and nonfatal cardiac arrest was also significantly higher in the flecainide or encainide group (4.5%) compared with the placebo group (1.2%). Although the exact reasons remain to be determined, the increased mortality from encainide or flecainide could not be attributed to the baseline differences in the patient populations since the clinical and laboratory characteristics appeared to be similar to the two groups.

Thus, a careful review of the available data provides no meaningful support for using antiarrhythmic drugs in the treatment of asymptomatic ventricular arrhythmias. The CAST has shown that both flecainide and encainide ought not to be used in these patients since their use is associated with a two- to threefold higher risk of mortality. Furthermore, the failure of class I antiarrhythmic agents needs to be contrasted against a consistently beneficial effect of the prophylactic beta-blocker therapy in reducing sudden and total cardiac mortality.[58] This beneficial effect may be mediated by an anti-ischemic action or a direct antiarrhythmic action of the beta-blockers. Although beta-blockers reduce the mortality risk in all subsets of patients, the benefit appears to be greater in those who had experienced an electrical or mechanical complication during their hospitalization for acute MI.[59]

Role of Programmed Ventricular Stimulation

In recent years, PVS has been used widely in the management of recurrent sustained VT or VF. In these patients, the clinical VT can be reproducibly induced and terminated by PVS, providing a reliable endpoint for selection of antiarrhythmic therapy. Because the mechanism of sudden death in the vast majority of post-infarct patients is sustained VT or VF, one may expect that the technique of PVS may be useful in identifying those who are at an increased risk of subsequent sudden cardiac death.

Several investigators have examined the prognostic significance of electrically inducible ventricular arrhythmias in post-MI patients and the results have been controversial.[60–69] Whereas some failed to show the benefit of this technique,[60–62,64,65] others[63,66–69] have reported favorable results. In the reported studies, the number of patients has been relatively small and major differences existed in the patient populations studied, the stimulation protocols used and the definitions of abnormal responses to PVS. Therefore, caution needs to be exercised before extrapolating these data to the routine management of patients with recent MI.

Table 5 summarizes the available data regarding the use of PVS in post-infarct patients. The incidence of inducibility ranged from 17% to 40%, depending on the vigor of the stimulation protocol. Patients with inducible arrhythmias, in general, had more severe left ventricular wall motion abnormalities, a higher prevalence of congestive heart failure and left ventricular aneurysms, and a lower left ventricular ejection fraction. In almost every study, patients with inducible arrhythmias tended to fare worse than those without inducible arrhythmias, but the difference in the outcome reached statistical significance only in studies that included high-risk patients with a post-infarction course complicated by the development of congestive heart failure, unstable angina, and/or nonsustained VT. The morphological configuration of the induced arrhythmia appears to be of prognostic significance as well. Although rapid polymorphic VT or VF is induced in approximately 10% of the patients, its inducibility does not correlate with the development of subsequent arrhythmic events.[61,66,69] On the other hand, monomorphic sustained VT with a relatively slow cycle length (>240 ms) appears to be a specific and reproducible response to PVS and its inducibility appears to predict the risk of subsequent arrhythmic events.

It should be emphasized that PVS remains an investigational technique in the survivors of acute MI. In patients with uncomplicated MI, the risk of recurrent arrhythmic events is low and the inducible ventricular arrhythmia has too low a sensitivity and positive predictive accuracy to be of clinical utility.[60–62] On the other hand, this technique appears to be promising in patients with complicated MI but it remains to be determined whether the inducible arrhythmia provides prognostic information independent of other simple clinical variables and whether an antiarrhythmic therapy based on the results of PVS may help in reducing mortality in these patients. More data are also needed on the day-to-day reproducibility of the induced response,[70] the long-term time course of evolution of inducible arrhythmia,[71] and the effects of thrombolysis on the inducibility of ventricular arrhythmias.[72] Finally, recent studies[64,66,73] have shown the technique of signal-averaged ECG to be useful in predicting the likelihood of subsequent arrhythmic events. Thus, this technique along with the other high-risk clinical variables may help in better selection of patients in whom the results of PVS are likely to be of more benefit. Until the answers to many of these questions

Table 5

Prognostic Significance of Induced Ventricular Arrhythmias in Survivors of Acute Myocardial Infarction

Study	No. of Pts.	Complicated MI	Induced Response		Arrhythmic Events in		MO
			NEG(%)	VT/VF(%)	NEG(%)	VT/VF(%)	
Roy et al.[60]	150	No	77	23	1	5	12
Bhandari et al.[61]	75	No	56	44	5	15	18
Santarelli et al.[62]	50	No	54	46	0	0	11
Richards et al.[63]	165	–	77	23	3	33*	12
Breithardt et al.[64]	132	–	54	46	4	16	15
Marchliuski et al.[65]	46	–	78	22	9	17	18
Denniss et al.[66]	403	–	66	34	4	12*	12
Hamer et al.[67]	70	Yes	83	17	9	42*	12
Waspe et al.[68]	50	Yes	66	34	0	41*	23
Bhandari et al.[69]	53	Yes	66	33	6	37*	10

* $p < 0.05$

Pts. = patients; MI = myocardial infarction.

NEG = negative.

become available, signal-averaged ECG and PVS remain investigational tools in survivors of acute MI and their routine clinical use is not recommended.

Late In-hospital Sustained Ventricular Tachyarrhythmias

Sustained VT or VF that develops 48 hours after the infarct represents a serious but rare complication of acute MI.[74,75] This arrhythmia develops in less than 1% of the patients and is more likely to occur in patients with larger infarcts, left ventricular aneurysms, depressed left ventricular ejection fraction, and intraventricular conduction delay. In patients with anteroseptal MI complicated by bundle branch block, approximately one-third develop late in-hospital VF during a monitored period of 6 weeks,[76] and patients with sustained VT or VF continue to be at high risk after discharge for recurrent arrhythmic events. Empiric antiarrhythmic therapy or coronary artery bypass surgery alone does not appear to significantly improve the course of these patients and the recurrent arrhythmic events develop in 30% to 50% of the patients during a short follow-up of 1 to 2 years. Recent data suggest that antiarrhythmic therapy guided by PVS may improve the outcome of these patients.[74,75] Using this approach, the clinical arrhythmia can be induced in 80% to 90% of these patients and the inducibility provides a reliable end-point for determining the efficacy of different antiarrhythmic agents. Approximately one-third of the patients may respond to therapy with one or more of the antiarrhythmic agents and they have a low incidence of recurrent arrhythmic events during follow-up. Patients in whom the drugs fail to suppress VT have a poor long-term prognosis. In these patients, the options include amiodarone, implantation of automatic implantable cardioverter defibrillators, and intraoperative map-guided subendocardial resection with or without left ventricular aneurysmectomy.[77]

At times the occurrence of sustained VT or VF may be directly related to the presence of severe myocardial ischemia. Typically these arrhythmias are preceded by the symptoms of myocardial ischemia or silent ST segment depression and the coronary angiography almost always demonstrates the presence of severely stenotic or ulcerated lesions in one or more of the coronary arteries. PVS only rarely induces ventricular arrhythmias and these patients may not need to be treated with antiarrhythmic agents. Instead, the relief of myocardial ischemia by percutaneous transluminal coronary angioplasty or coronary artery bypass grafting may be the most reasonable approach.

Bradyarrhythmias and Conduction Defects During Acute Myocardial Infarction

Bradyarrhythmias and conduction abnormalities are relatively common during acute myocardial infarction. Sinus node dysfunction occurs in up to 40% of patients, conduction abnormalities occur in 6% to 18% of patients, and complete heart block develops in approximately 5% of patients. These abnormalities of impulse formation or conduction can be secondary to ischemia or infarction, increased autonomic tone, or mediated by chemical metabolites.

Most conduction abnormalities that occur during myocardial infarction can be predicted based upon anatomical considerations. The sinus node receives its blood supply via the sinus node artery, which is the only major atrial artery in most patients. In 55% of hearts, it originates from the right coronary artery (RCA) and in 45%, it originates from the left circumflex coronary artery. Sinus node ischemia or infarction is almost always due to an occlusion of a major coronary vessel proximal to the take off of the sinus node artery.[78,79]

The AV node and the bundle of His receive their blood supply primarily from the AV node artery which originates from the RCA in 85–90% of patients and from the left circumflex artery in the remaining patients. In addition, most patients appear to have significant collateral circulation to the AV node and the bundle of His from septal perforators of the left anterior descending coronary artery (LAD). While conduction block within the AV node is most commonly associated with inferior wall myocardial infarction, it is very rarely associated with actual necrosis of the AV node,[78] presumably secondary to the dual circulation of the structure. In fact, AV block is most common in inferior wall infarction when there is coexistent significant proximal disease of the LAD.[80]

The bundle of His gives rise to the right and left bundle branches which initially travel together as a common bundle. The first fibers to branch off are those of the posterior division of the left bundle.[78] The dual blood supply from the LAD and the posterior descending artery, and the fact that the left posterior fascicle is a shorter and thicker structure than the other two fascicles, render it much less vulnerable to ischemic injury. It transverses inferiorly and posteriorly, inserting into the posterior papillary muscle. The anterior fascicle travels to the base of the anterior papillary muscle and its blood supply is from the septal perforators of the LAD. The proximal third of the right bundle is usually perfused by the AV nodal artery. However, once the fascicle exits the membranous septum and enters the muscular septum, blood supply is provided by the LAD.[78,79] Thus, proximal occlusion of the LAD often damages the right bundle branch and the left anterior fascicle but does not significantly affect the AV node or the left posterior fascicle. Meanwhile, a relatively small inferior wall infarction can result in proximal damage to the right bundle branch and cause block within the AV node.

Bradyarrhythmias

The most common bradyarrhythmia during myocardial infarction is sinus bradycardia which occurs in 25–40% of patients during the first 4 hours of myocardial infarction[78] and in 15–20% of patients after this time interval.[81] Sinus bradycardia is more commonly associated with inferior wall than anterior or lateral wall infarction despite the fact that the sinus node artery originates from the RCA in only slightly more than 50% of patients. Reflex vagotonia is probably the most common etiology of sinus bradycardia during myocardial infarction.[78,81] The lower posterior aspect of the intra-atrial septum and the inferior posterior wall of the left ventricle are richly supplied by receptors with cholinergic afferent pathways.[82] It is hypothesized that ischemia during inferior wall infarction causes stimulation of these receptors with subsequent increased activity of vagal efferents intervating the sinus node, AV node, and peripheral vasculature.[78,82] Experimental stimulation of this area results in the Bezold-Jarisch reflex, characterized by atropine-sensitive bradycardia and hypotension.[78,82] Morphine or severe pain can also exacerbate this reflex.[83] It has also been suggested that the release of metabolites from neighboring ischemic or infarcted tissue may result in negative chronotropic effects. The prognosis of patients with sinus bradycardia during myocardial infarction does not appear to be worse than patients without this arrhythmia.

Sinus arrest or sinus exit block (failure of a sinus beat to exit the SA node and depolarize the surrounding tissue) are observed much less frequently during acute infarction than during sinus bradycardia. Sinus arrest is characterized by a lack of sinus node activity; an atrial pause which is a noninteger multiple of the sinus cycle length is observed. The pause associated with sinus exit block is a multiple of the sinus cycle length. While these phenomenon can be secondary to increased vagotonia, either ischemia or infarction of the SA node are also common.

Therapy

Therapy is directed towards the symptomatic patient with hypotension, congestive heart failure, or arrhythmias. In most patients, careful observation is all that is required for the patient with sinus bradycardia or sinus pauses. In patients with severe sinus bradycardia (heart rate of less than 40 bpm) or hemodynamic symptoms, intravenous atropine (0.5–0.6 mg) is usually effective in increasing the sinus rate and correcting hypotension. This may be followed by small (0.3–0.4 mg, up to 2.5 mg over 2½ hours) doses of atropine if an adequate response was not initially achieved. One must be prudent in administering this agent as sinus tachycardia can result in increased ischemia, infarct extension, and possibly malignant ventricular arrhythmias. Other secondary therapeutic approaches to the patient with bradyarrhythmias include isopoterenol administration (initially at a dose of 0.5 µg/min titrated against the chronotropic response) or temporary cardiac pacing. Isopoterenol should only be a temporary approach since its positive inotropic effects can increase oxygen consumption, exacerbate ischemia, and its vasodilatory effects can provoke hypotension.

Sinus node dysfunction from vagotonia is most common during the first 4 to 6 hours of myocardial infarction.[78,81,83] After this time period, atropine appears to be less effective in correcting bradyarrhythmias and the hypotensive patient may require tranvenous cardiac pacing. Consideration should be given to AV sequential pacing in tenuous patients who would benefit from the contribution of atrial systole. An external pacemaker can be successfully utilized in some patients,[84] and is a reasonable option in patients in whom pacing may be needed only for a short time period and in whom this device functions appropriately and is well tolerated.

AV Block

The site of AV block can be intranodal (i.e., in the AV node or in the proximal portions of the bundle of His) or infranodal (in the bundle branches themselves or possibly in the distal aspect of the bundle of His). The location of block is important since intranodal block usually develops gradually and when complete, is commonly associated with a narrow complex escape rhythm located in the AV node or His bundle, has a rate of more than 40–60 bpm, is reliable, and is hemodynamically well tolerated (Fig. 4). The escape rhythm associated with infranodal

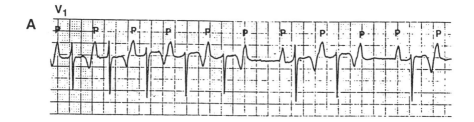

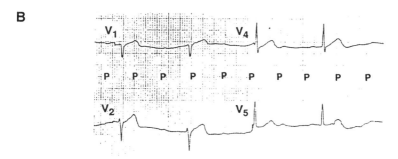

Figure 4. Two patients with inferior wall MI and AV block. (A) A patient with AV Wenckebach characterized by increasing PR intervals, a nonconducted P wave, and a shorter PR interval of the first conducted beat in each series. (B) Complete heart block with a narrow complex escape rhythm at a rate of 50 bpm. P = P wave.

block (located in the bundle branches or ventricle) is often unreliable, slow (less than 40 bpm), associated with hypotension, and up to 80% of such patients develop asystole (Fig. 5).

First Degree AV Block

This conduction defect exists when the PR interval is greater than 200 ms and occurs in 4–15% of patients with acute myocardial infarction.[78,80] Because 1:1 AV conduction is intact, this conduction defect does not result in bradycardia or hemodynamic instability. The site of block is within the AV node in the great majority of patients. Therapeutic interventions are not necessary but the patient should be carefully monitored for progression to higher forms of AV block. The administration of pharmacological agents that impair AV conduction (e.g., beta-blockers, calcium blockers, digoxin) should be administered judiciously in these patients.

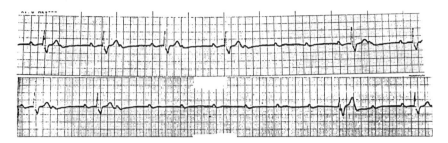

Figure 5. Anterior wall MI with Mobitz II AV block progressing to high-grade AV block in the lower tracing.

Second and Third Degree AV Block

Mobitz I second degree AV block occurs in 3–12%[85,86] of patients with myocardial infarction and is characterized by progressive increases in the PR interval with eventual failure of an atrial depolarization to conduct to the ventricle. Electrophysiological studies have demonstrated that this conduction abnormality is located within the AV node.[87] Type II second degree AV block is much less common than type I second degree AV block, occurring in less than 1% of patients of myocardial infarction, and is characterized by failure of atrial impulses to conduct to the ventricle without progressive changes in the PR interval. The site of block is in the His-Purkinje system.[88] In a patient with 2:1 AV block, a prolonged PR interval and a narrow QRS complex favor type I block while a normal PR interval and a wide QRS complex are usually found in patients with type II block. The diagnosis of complete heart block is made when AV dissociation is not present. During inferior wall myocardial infarction, AV block is most commonly localized in the AV node while in anterior wall infarction, AV block almost always occurs in the distal His-Purkinje system.[87,88]

Inferior Wall Myocardial Infarction

When patients with inferior wall infarction develop second degree AV block, it is almost exclusively type I block.[86–89] Of patients who developed complete heart block, it may be preceded by the development of first or second degree AV block in nearly one-half to three-quarters of the patients.[86,89] In one series, 39% of patients with first degree AV block and 48% of patients with type I second degree AV block progressed to complete heart block.[89] In almost all patients with advanced AV nodal block and inferior wall infarction, the block resolves.[86,87] HIgh-grade AV block can be divided into two time frames. Patients who develop block within the first 6 hours usually develop their block suddenly and respond well to atropine with increased AV conduction,[85] suggesting that vagotonia plays a major etiologic role in these patients' heart block. The second group of patients developed block more than 6 hours (range 6 hours to 8 days) after the onset of infarction, and AV block was characterized by gradually increasing AV block (i.e., first degree, then second degree, then complete AV block), did not respond to atropine, and it lasted considerably longer (more than 3 days versus several hours) than in patients with early block. Thus, late block may be secondary to ischemia, atrial infarction, edema, or metabolic alterations but probably not to vagotonia.[86–89]

Patients with inferior wall infarctions who develop second degree or complete AV block have a greater short-term mortality (15–30% compared to 5–10% without AV block), even when the block is transient.[90,91] The increased mortality in these studies appears to have been secondary to an increased incidence of cardiogenic shock. Patients with AV block tend to have lower left ventricular ejection fractions and lower right ventricular ejection fractions than patients without AV block.[91] The in-hospital mortality of patients with inferior wall infarction and complete heart block has been demonstrated to be significantly greater than that of patients without complete heart block. The early increased mortality in this study was secondary to increased congestive heart failure and cardiogenic shock.

The Indications for Therapy

The indications for therapy of AV block during acute inferior wall myocardial infarction are similar as those for bradyarrhythmias. The early form of AV block usually responds to atropine while the late form is commonly unresponsive to sympathetic agents. In almost all patients, the AV block resolves, but in some patients this may require several weeks,[85,86] and patient rehabilitation may be facilitated in selected temporary pacemaker-dependent patients by early permanent pacing.[83] The majority of patients who develop complete heart block with inferior wall infarction are hemodynamically stable and when hypotension is present, it is usually mild. Thus, temporary cardiac pacing is frequently not necessary in the patient with inferior wall infarction who develops complete heart block because of the stability of the escape rhythm and the lack of associated hemodynamic symptoms. However, patients with hemodynamic symptoms in whom the escape rhythm is a wide complex rhythm or who have severe bradycardia (pulse less than 40 bpm) should receive temporary cardiac pacing.

Anterior Wall Myocardial Infarction

Complete heart block occurs in approximately 5% of patients with anterior wall myocardial infarction, and while Mobitz II second degree AV block occurs much less frequently, it is almost completely confined to patients with anterior wall infarctions.[89] Such blocks are almost always infranodal and are caused by ischemia or infarction of the bundle branches. In complete heart block, the site of the escape rhythm is located distal to the site of block, either in a fascicle of the conduction system or in the ventricle itself. Advanced AV block with anterior wall infarction often occurs suddenly without warning, is associated in many patients with the prior development of intraventricular conduction defects, and is associated with a high incidence of asystole. Complete heart block is associated with a large infarction and the mortality rate is as high as 70–85%.[89,91] The cause of death in these patients is usually cardiogenic shock.

Intraventricular Conduction Blocks

Intraventricular conduction blocks (left anterior fascicular block (LAFB), left posterior fascicular block (LPFB), right bundle branch block (RBBB), left bundle branch block (LBBB), or combinations of these blocks) are observed in 8–15% of patients with acute myocardial infarctions.[89,92–96] In approximately half of patients, the conduction defect predates the acute infarction.[92–94] These defects are caused by ischemia or infarction of the bundle branches, and as would be expected from the anatomy of the conduction system and its blood supply, bundle branch blocks are significantly more common in anterior than inferior infarctions. While some pathological series have found infarction of the bundle branches[91] in patients who developed acute conduction defects, other studies have demonstrated a low incidence of infarction and have instead found ischemic changes within the cells comprising the bundle branches.[97] That bundle branch block in some patients may be mediated by ischemia and not only secondary to infarction of the His-Purkinje system would explain why they often resolve during the post-infarction period. Recently, Wilber et al.[98] described two patients with anterior wall infarctions and complete heart block who underwent angioplasty of their total LAD lesions more than 40 hours after infarction. Both patients had abrupt return of AV conduction with restoration of LAD patency. The major clinical importance of intraventricular conduction defects during infarction is their propensity to progress to complete heart block and the associated high mortality rate.

Left anterior fascicular block occurs in approximately 4% of patients and left posterior fascicular block in less than 1% of patients with acute infarctions[92–96,99,100] (Table 6). When these fascicular blocks are observed alone, they rarely progress to complete heart block. However, LPFB occurs almost exclusively in patients with large anterior wall infarctions and is associated with a mortality incidence as high as 40%.[92,94] The mortality occurrence with LAFB is approximately 20%. RBBB occurs in both inferior and anterior infarctions while left bundle branch block occurs most commonly in patients with anterior infarctions. The incidence of developing right bundle branch block is 2% and left bundle branch block is 4% and approximately 13% with either conduction defect develop complete heart block.[92,94–96] Overall mortality associated with either bundle branch block is about 23%.

The likelihood of progressing to complete heart block and of hospital

Table 6
Conduction Defects During Acute MI

Type of Conduction Defect	Incidence	Progression to CHB	Hospital Mortality
None		4%	12%
LAHB	4%	2%	20%
LPHB	1%	1%	40%
RBBB	2%	13%	23%
RBBB + LAHB	5%	27%	28%
RBBB + LPHB	1%	29%	45%
LBBB	4%	13%	23%
ABBB	1%	45%	45%

CHB = complete heart block; LAHB = left anterior hemiblock; LPHB = left posterior hemiblock; LBBB = left bundle branch block; RBBB = right bundle branch block; ABBB = alternating bundle branch block.

mortality is greatest in patients with bilateral bundle branch block (i.e., RBBB/LAFB or RBBB/LPFB).[92,96,100] While several studies[97] have suggested that the mortality is as high in patients who develop LBBB as in patients with bilateral bundle branch block, the majority of studies have found lower mortality rates, similar to those of patients with RBBB.[92,96,100] The risk of progression to complete heart block appears to be about twice as great if the conduction defect is new or of indeterminate age compared to patients in whom the defect is known to be old.[93,100]

Patients with alternating bundle branch block have trifascicular block and thus have a very high rate of progression to complete heart block (approximately 45%).[93] Similarly, patients with PR interval prolongation and bilateral bundle branch block, especially LBBB, have a significantly increased incidence of progressing to high-grade AV block compared to patients who have normal PR intervals.[93,95] This is because first degree AV block in many of these patients represents disease in the third fascicle instead of in the AV node. In one study,[93] the association of first degree AV block with a new RBBB or LBBB increased the likelihood of developing high-grade AV block from 11% to 19%, while in another study, patients with first degree AV block and LBBB or RBBB/LAFB had a 35% incidence of progression compared to 11% in patients with normal PR intervals.[95]

Indications for Prophylactic Temporary Cardiac Pacing

Prophylactic temporary transvenous cardiac pacing is considered in patients who are at high risk of developing complete heart block. Complete heart block can result in asystole, hypotension, shock, or congestive heart failure. Multiple studies have shown, however, that the mortality associated with the development of high-grade AV block (Mobitz II second degree AV block or complete heart block) is largely secondary to pump failure and cardiogenic shock.[89,93–95] Indeed, a statistical benefit from prophylactic pacing has not been demonstrated in any study. However, we and other authors believe that high-risk patients should be prophylactically paced as it can prevent the complications associated with complete heart block in individual patients, despite the lack of evidence of statistically improved survival.[89,95,99] Given that the mortality is so high in these patients, it would require a very large study population to demonstrate a significantly improved outcome in patients who are prophylactically paced. Many studies have also demonstrated that prophylactic pacing can be of benefit in individual patients.[89,93,95,99,101] Patients who developed high-grade AV block in the *absence* of pulmonary edema or shock have a significantly higher mortality than similar patients who did not develop advanced AV block.[92] In almost all of these patients without shock, death was due to the abrupt development of AV block, and thus it might be expected that survival would have been improved with prophylactic pacing.

Based on the above discussion, prophylactic pacing should be performed (Table 7) in patients with (probable) new trifascicular block (alternating bundle branch block, bilateral bundle branch block with first degree AV block, or Mobitz II AV block) or in patients with new bilateral bundle branch block. Patients with old bilateral bundle branch block (even with PR prolongation) or unifascicular blocks do not require prophylactic pacing while consideration should be given to pacing patients with an anterior infarction and documented new LBBB. There is a simple electrocardiographic system that may be used to predict the occurrence of complete heart block.[101] One point was assigned for the presence of each of the following risk factors: first degree AV block, second degree AV block, LAFB, LPFB, LBBB, or RBBB. A score equaling the sum of each patient's risk factors was correlated with the risk of developing complete heart block (CHB): a score of 0, 1.2% developed CHB; a score of 1, 7.8% developed CHB; a score of 2, 25% developed CHB; and a score of more than or equal to 3, 36.4% developed CHB. This scoring system appears to be a useful guide to patient management. Patients with high scores (more than or equal to 2), particularly with anterior wall infarctions, should be considered for temporary cardiac pacing. As discussed earlier, many patients with inferior wall infarctions might receive the most benefit from watchful waiting or use of an external cardiac pacemaker. One limitation of this approach is that the scoring system does not take into account whether the conduction abnormality was old, which carries an approximately 50% lower risk of advancing to complete heart block.[92,100] This must be considered when using this system.

In making the decision to utilize temporary pacing, the risks of this procedure need to be considered.[102] Complications have included ventricular arrhythmias in 2–4%, perforation in 2–3%, sepsis in 2%, and new cardiac friction rubs (which do not necessarily indicate perforation) in 5%. In these studies, femoral, internal jugular, and subclavian venous approaches have been associated with a lower incidence of complications and pacemaker malfunction than the brachial approach.[102] Consideration should be given to using a #4-French catheter in patients with inferior wall infarctions with right ventricular involvement who

Table 7
Indications for Cardiac Pacing

Temporary Pacing	*Indicated*
SA + AV Blocks	
Sinus node dysfunction without Sx ± medications	No
Sinus node dysfunction with hemodynamic Sx despite medical Rx	Yes
First degree AV block	No
Mobitz I without Sx	No
Mobitz I with Sx without adequate response to pharmacologic agents	Yes
Mobitz II	Yes
Complete heart block, AWMI	Yes
Complete heart block, IWMI with narrow escape rhythm without Sx	No
Complete heart block, IWMI with hemodynamic Sx or new wide complex escape rhythm	Yes
Bundle Branch Blocks	
New unifascicular block or isolated RBBB	No
New LBBB	Possible
New first degree AV block and RBBB or LBBB	Possible
New bilateral BBB	Yes
Alternating BBB	Yes
Old bilateral BBB, RBBB, LBBB	No
Permanent Pacing	
Old bundle branch block, bifascicular, or trifascicular block	No
New first degree AV block or bundle branch block	No
New bilateral bundle branch block	Possible
New first degree AV block and new bundle branch block	Probable
Alternating bundle branch block	Yes
New bundle branch block and transient high grade AV block*	Yes
Persistent high grade AV block*	Yes

* Mobitz II AV block or complete heart block.
BBB = bundle branch block; RBBB = right bundle branch block; LBBB = left bundle branch block; SX = symptoms; AW = anterior wall; IW = inferior wall.

require temporary pacing, since the flexibility of the catheter is much less likely to perforate the infarcted right ventricle.

Patients at intermediate risk of developing complete heart block may benefit from prophylactic use of the external cardiac pacemaker.[84] This device can be utilized in the standby mode and placement of a temporary transvenous pacemaker can be deferred unless the patient develops high-grade heart block. Patients should be considered for this approach only after it is demonstrated that the device paces the individual patient appropriately and that it is sufficiently well tolerated.

Indications for Permanent Pacing

Permanent cardiac pacing after myocardial infarction is controversial.[93-96] Three retrospective nonrandomized studies have demonstrated that patients with bundle branch block during infarction and transient high-grade or complete heart block have an improved long-term survival if they are permanently paced.[93,96,103] Patients receiving permanent pacemakers died less frequently during follow-up than patients who were not paced.[93] The issue of permanent cardiac pacing after infarction is compounded by the fact that many of the late deaths in high-risk patients are secondary to malignant ventricular arrhythmias and not complete heart block.[104] While electrophysiological studies to measure the HV interval (and possibly stress the AV conduction system) might help determine whether certain individual patients might benefit from permanent pacing, this approach has not been critically evaluated.

We recommend permanent pacing (Table 7) for patients with persistent advanced AV block (Mobitz II or complete heart block), patients with new bundle branch blocks who have had transient high-grade AV block during their infarction, or patients with alternating bundle branch block. Consideration should also be given to patients with first degree AV block and new persistent bundle branch blocks or bilateral bundle branch blocks.[105] Patients with only first degree block, new bundle branch block, new bilateral bundle branch block, or patients with inferior infarctions and transient advanced AV block without associated conduction abnormalities should not routinely be paced.

References

1. Julian DG, Valentine PA, Miller GG: Disturbances of rate, rhythm and conduction in acute myocardial infarction: a prospective study of 100 con-

secutive unselected patients with the aid of electrocardiographic monitoring Am J Med 37:915, 1964.

2. Meltzer LE, Kitchell JR: The incidence of arrhythmias associated with acute myocardial infarction. Prog Cardiovasc Dis 9:50, 1966.
3. Lawrie DM, Greenwood TW, Goddard M, et al: A coronary care unit in the management of acute myocardial infarction. Lancet 2:109, 1967.
4. Bigger JT, Dresdale RJ, Heissenbuttel RH, et al: Ventricular arrhythmias in ischemic heart disease: mechanism, prevalence, significance and management. Prog Cardiovasc Dis 19:255, 1977.
5. Dhurandhar RW, MacMillan RL, Brown KWG: Primary ventricular fibrillation complicating acute myocardial infarction. Am J Cardiol 27:347, 1971.
6. Jewitt D: The genesis of cardiac arrhythmias in acute myocardial infarction. Prog Cardiol 1:61, 1972.
7. Naito M, Michelson EL, Kaplinsky E, et al: Role of early cycle ventricular extasystoles in initiation of ventricular tachycardia and fibrillation: evaluation of the R-on-T phenomenon in myocardial infarction. Am J Cardiol 49:317, 1982.
8. Harris AS: Delayed development of ventricular ectopic rhythms following experimental coronary occlusion. Circulation 1:1318, 1950.
9. Wiggers CJ, Wegria R: Ventricular fibrillation due to single localized induction and condenser shocks applied during the vulnerable phase of ventricular systole. Am J Physiol 128:500, 1940.
10. Scherlag BJ, El-Sherif N, Hope R, et al: Characterization and localization of ventricular arrhythmias resulting from myocardial ischemia and infarction. Circ Res 35:372, 1974.
11. Wit AL, Bigger JT: Possible electrophysiologic mechanisms for lethal ventricular arrhythmias accompanying myocardial ischemia and infarction. Circulation 52(Suppl)3:96, 1975.
12. Pantridge JF, Adgey AAJ, Geddes JS, et al: The Acute Coronary Attack. New York, Grune & Stratton, 1975, pp 26–42.
13. Lewis RP, Warren JV: Factors determining mortality in the prehospital phase of acute myocardial infarction. Am J Cardiol 33:152, 1974.
14. Moss AJ, Goldstein S, Green W, et al: Prehospital precursors of ventricular arrhythmias in acute myocardial infarction. Arch Intern Med 129:756, 1972.
15. Lown B, Kosowsky BD, Klein MD: Pathogenesis, prevention and treatment of arrhythmias in myocardial infarction. Circulation 40(Suppl)4:261, 1969.
16. El-Sherif N, Myerburg RJ, Scherlag BJ, et al: Electrocardiographic antecedents of primary ventricular fibrillation: value of the R-on-T phenomenon in myocardial infarction. Br Heart J 38:415, 1976.
17. Lie KI, Wellens HJJ, Downar E, et al: Observations on patients with primary ventricular fibrillation complicating acute myocardial infarction. Circulation 52:755, 1975.
18. Stannard M, Sloman G: Ventricular fibrillation in acute myocardial infarction: prognosis following successful resuscitation. Am Heart J 77:573, 1969.
19. Conley MJ, McNeer JF, Lie KL, et al: Cardiac arrest complicating acute myocardial infarction: predictability and prognosis. Am J Cardiol 39:7, 1977.
20. Lawrie DM: Long-term survival after ventricular fibrillation complicating acute myocardial infarction. Lancet 2:1085, 1969.
21. Volpi A, Maggioni A, Franzosi MG, et al: In-hospital prognosis of patients

with acute myocardial infarction complicated by primary ventricular fibrillation. N Engl J Med 317:257, 1987.

22. Goldberg RJ, Gore JM, Haffajec CCI, et al: Outcome of the cardiac arrest during acute myocardial infarction. Am J Cardiol 59:251, 1987.

23. Lichstein E, Ribas-Meneclier C, Gupta PK, et al: Incidence and description of accelerated ventricular rhythm complicating acute myocardial infarction. Am J Med 58:192, 1975.

24. DeSoyza N, Bisset JK, Kane JJ, et al: Association of accelerated idioventricular rhythm and paroxysmal ventricular tachycardia in acute myocardial infarction. Am J Cardiol 34:667, 1974.

25. Norris RM, Mercer CJ: Significance of idioventricular rhythms in acute myocardial infarction. Prog Cardiovasc Dis 16:455, 1974.

26. Grenadier E, Alpan G, Maor N, et al: Polymorphous ventricular tachycardia in acute myocardial infarction. Am J Cardiol 53:1280, 1984.

27. Hanson EC, Levine FH, Kay HR, et al: Control of postinfarction ventricular irritability with the intraaortic balloon pump. Circulation 62(Suppl 1):I-130, 1980.

28. Cercek B, Lew AS, Laramee, et al: Time course and characteristics of ventricular arrhythmias after reperfusion in acute myocardial infarction. Am J Cardiol 60:214, 1987.

29. Gorgels APM, Vos MA, Letsch IS, et al: Usefulness of the accelerated idioventricular rhythm as a marker for myocardial necrosis and reperfusion during thrombolytic therapy in acute myocardial infarction. Am J Cardiol 61:231, 1988.

30. Pogwizd SM, Corr PB: Electrophysiologic mechanisms underlying arrhythmias due to reperfusion of ischemic myocardium. Circulation 75:404, 1987.

31. Lie KL, Wellens HJ, Capelle F, et al: Lidocaine in the prevention of primary ventricular fibrillation: a double-blind randomized study of 212 consecutive patients. N Engl J Med 291:1324, 1974.

32. Wyman MG, Hammersmith L: Comprehensive treatment plan for the prevention of primary ventricular fibrillation in acute myocardial infarction. Am J Cardiol 33:661, 1974.

33. DeSilva RA, Hennekens CH, Lown B, et al: Lignocaine prophylaxis in acute myocardial infarction: an evaluation of randomised trials. Lancet 2:855, 1981.

34. Wyman MG, Lalka D, Hammersmith L, et al: Multiple bolus technique for lidocaine administration during the first hours of an acute myocardial infarction. Am J Cardiol 41:313, 1978.

35. Ryden L, Ariniego R, Arnman K, et al: A double-blind trial of metoprolol in acute myocardial infarction: effects on ventricular tachyarrhythmias. N Engl J Med 308:614, 1983.

36. Yusuf S, Sleight P, Rossi P, et al: Reduction in infarct size, arrhythmias and chest pain by early intravenous beta-blockade in suspected acute myocardial infarction. Circulation 67(6:part 2):I-32, 1983.

37. Valentine PA, Frew JL, Mashford ML, et al: Lidocaine in the prevention of sudden death in the pre-hospital phase of acute infarction: a double-blind study. N Engl J Med 291:1327, 1974.

38. Lie KI, Liem KL, Louridtz WJ, et al. Efficacy of lidocaine in preventing primary ventricular fibrillation within 1 hour after a 300-mg intramuscular

injection: a double-blind randomized study of 300 hospitalized patients with acute myocardial infarction. Am J Cardiol 42:486, 1978.

39. Thirteenth Bethesda Conference: Emergency cardiac care. Am J Cardiol 50:345, 1982.

40. Heissenbuttel RH, Bigger JT Jr: Bretylium tosylate: a nearly available antiarrhythmic drug for ventricular arrhythmias. Ann Intern Med 91:229, 1979.

41. Morady F, Scheinman MM, Shen E, et al: Intravenous amiodarone in the acute treatment of recurrent symptomatic ventricular tachycardia. Am J Cardiol 51:156, 1983.

42. Garan H, Ruskin JM, DiMarco JP, et al: Refractory ventricular tachycardia complicating recovery from acute myocardial infarction: treatment with map-guided infarctectomy. Am Heart J 107:571, 1984.

43. Moss A, Schnitzler R, Green R, et al: Ventricular arrhythmias 3 weeks after acute myocardial infarction. Ann Intern Med 75:837, 1975.

44. Vismara LA, Anderson EA, Mason DT: Relation of ventricular arrhythmias in the late-hospital phase of acute myocardial infarction to sudden death after hospital discharge. Am J Med 59:6, 1975.

45. Ruberman W, Weinblatt E, Goldberg JD, et al: Ventricular premature beats and mortality after acute myocardial infarction. N Engl J Med 297:750, 1977.

46. Moss AJ, Davis HT, DeCamilla J, Bayer LW: Ventricular ectopic beats and their relation to sudden and nonsudden cardiac death after myocardial infarction. Circulation 60:998, 1979.

47. Mukharji J, Rude RE, Poole WK, et al: The MILIS study group. Risk factors for sudden death after acute myocardial infarction: two-year follow-up. Am J Cardiol 54:31, 1984.

48. Bigger JT, Fleiss JL, Kleiger K, et al: The multicenter post-infarction research group. The relationship between ventricular arrhythmias, left ventricular dysfunction and mortality in the two years of myocardial infarction. Circulation 69:250, 1984.

49. Kostis JB, Byington R, Friedman LM, et al: Prognostic significance of ventricular ectopic activity in survivors of acute myocardial infarction. J Am Coll Cardiol 10:231, 1987.

50. Schulze RA Jr, Strauss HW, Pitt B: Sudden death in the year following myocardial infarction relation to ventricular premature contractions in the late hospital phase and left ventricular ejection fraction. Am J Med 62:192, 1977.

51. Califf M, Burks JM, Behar VS, et al: Relationships among ventricular arrhythmias, coronary artery disease and angiographic indications of myocardial fibrosis. Circulation 57:725, 1978.

52. Calvert A, Lown B, Gorlin R: Ventricular premature beats and anatomically defined coronary artery disease. Am J Cardiol 39:627, 1977.

53. Furberg CD: Effect of antiarrhythmic drugs on mortality after myocardial infarction. Am J Cardiol 52:32C, 1983.

54. IMPACT Research Group: International mexiletine and placebo antiarrhythmic coronary trial: report on arrhythmia and other findings. J Am Coll Cardiol 6:1148, 1984.

55. Gotlieb SM, Achuff SC, Mellits ED, et al: Prophylactic antiarrhythmic ther-

apy of high-risk survivors of myocardial infarction: lower mortality at 1 month but not at 1 year. Circulation 75:792, 1987.

56. The Cardial Arrhythmia Pilot Study (CAPS) Investigators: Effects of encainide, flecainide, imipramine and moricizine on ventricular arrhythmias during the year after acute myocardial infarction: the CAPS. Am J Cardiol 61:501, 1988.

57. The Cardiac Arrhythmia Suppression Trial (CAST) Investigators Preliminary report: Effect of encainide and flecainide on mortality in a randomized trial of arrhythmia suppression after myocardial infarction. N Engl J Med 321:406, 1989.

58. Frishman WH, Furberg CD, Friedewald WTB: Adrenergic blockade for survivors of acute myocardial infarction. N Engl J Med 310:830, 1984.

59. Furberg CD, Hawkins M, Lichstein E, et al: Effect of propranolol in postinfarction patients with mechanical or electrical complications. Circulation 69:761, 1984.

60. Roy D, Marchand E, Theroux P, et al: Programmed ventricular stimulation in survivors of an acute myocardial infarction. Circulation 72:487, 1985.

61. Bhandari AK, Hong R, Kotlewski A, et al: Prognostic significance of programmed ventricular stimulation in survivors of acute myocardial infarction. Br Heart J 61:410, 1989.

62. Santarelli P, Bellocci F, Loperfido F, et al: Ventricular arrhythmia induced by programmed ventricular stimulation after acute myocardial infarction. Am J Cardiol 55:391, 1985.

63. Richards DA, Cody DV, Dennis AR, et al: Ventricular electrical instability: a predictor of death after myocardial infarction. Am J Cardiol 50:223, 1982.

64. Breithardt G, Borggrefe M, Haerten K: Role of programmed ventricular stimulation and noninvasive recording of ventricular late potentials for the identification of patients at risk of ventricular tachyarrhythmias after acute myocardial infarction. In: Zipes DP, Jalife J (eds), Cardiac Electophysiology and Arrhythmias. New York, Grune and Stratton, 553, 1985.

65. Marchlinski FE, Buxton AE, Waxman HL, et al: Identifying patients at risk of sudden death after myocardial infarction: value of the response to programmed stimulation, degree of ventricular ectopic activity and severity of left ventricular dysfunction. Am J Cardiol 52:1190, 1983.

66. Denniss AR, Richards DA, Cody DV, et al: Prognostic significance of ventricular tachycardia and fibrillation induced at programmed stimulation and delayed potentials detected on the signal-averaged electrocardiograms of survivors of acute myocardial infarction. Circulation 74:731, 1986.

67. Hamer A, Vohra J, Hunt D, Sloman G: Prediction of sudden death by electrophysiologic studies in high risk patients surviving acute myocardial infarction. Am J Cardiol 50:223, 1982.

68. Waspe LE, Seinfeld D, Ferrick A, et al: Prediction of sudden death and spontaneous ventricular tachycardia in survivors of complicated myocardial infarction: value of the response to programmed stimulation using a maximum of three ventricular extrastimuli. J Am Coll Cardiol 5:1292, 1985.

69. Bhandari A, Hong R, Kotlewski A, et al: Prognostic significance of programmed stimulation in high-risk patients surviving acute myocardial infarction (Abstract). J Am Coll Cardiol 11:6A, 1988.

70. Bhandari A, Hong R, Kulick D, et al: Day to day reproducibility of response

to programmed ventricular stimulation in patients with recent myocardial infarction. J Am Coll Cardiol (in press).

71. Bhandari AK, Au PK, Rose JS, et al: Decline in inducibility of sustained ventricular tachycardia from two to twenty weeks after acute myocardial infarction. Am J Cardiol 59:284, 1987.

72. Sager PT, Perlmutter RA, Rosenfeld LE, et al: The electrophysiologic effects of thrombolytic therapy in patients with a transmural anterior wall myocardial infarction complicated by left ventricular aneurysm formation. J Am Coll Cardiol 12:19, 1988.

73. Gomes JA, Winters SL, Stewart D, et al: A new noninvasive index to predict sustained ventricular tachycardia and sudden death in the first year after myocardial infarction: based on signal-averaged electrocardiogram, radionuclide ejection fraction and Holter monitoring. J Am Coll Cardiol 10:349, 1987.

74. Marchlinski FE, Waxman HL, Buxton AE, et al: Sustained ventricular tachyarrhythmias during the early post-infarction period: electrophysiologic findings and prognosis for survival. J Am Coll Cardiol 2:240, 1983.

75. DiMarco JP, Lerman BB, Kron IL, et al: Sustained ventricular tachyarrhythmias within 2 months of acute myocardial infarction: results of medical and surgical therapy in patients resuscitated from the initial episode. J Am Coll Cardiol 6:759, 1985.

76. Lie KI, Liem KL, Schuilenburg RM, et al: Early identification of patients developing late in-hospital ventricular fibrillation after discharge from the coronary care unit: a 5½ year retrospective and prospective study of 1897 patients. Am J Cardiol 41:674, 1978.

77. Miller JM, Machlinski FE, Harken AH, et al: Subendocardial resection for sustained ventricular tachycardia in the early post-acute infarction period. Am J Cardiol 55:980, 1985.

78. James TN: The coronary circulation and conduction system in acute myocardial infarction. Prog Cardiovasc Dis 10:410, 1968.

79. Kennel AJ, Titus JL: The vasculature of the human atrioventricular conduction system. Mayo Clin Proc 47:562, 1972.

80. Bassan R, Maia IG, Bozza A: Atrioventricular block in acute inferior wall myocardial infarction: harbinger of associated obstruction of the left anterior descending coronary artery. J Am Coll Cardiol 8:773, 1986.

81. Adgey AAJ, Geodes JS, Mulholland HC, et al: Incidence, significance and management of early bradyarrhythmias complicating acute myocardial infarction. Lancet 2:1097, 1968.

82. Mark AL: The Bezold-Jarisch reflex revisited: clinical implications of inhibitory reflexes originating in the heart. J Am Coll Cardiol 1:90, 1983.

83. Rosenfeld LE: Bradyarrhythmias, abnormalities of conduction, and indications for pacing in acute myocardial infarction. Cardiol Clin 6:49, 1988.

84. Zoll PM, Zoll RH, Falk RH, et al: External noninvasive temporary cardiac pacing: clinical trials. Circulation 71:937, 1985.

85. Feigl D, Ashkenazy J, Kishon Y: Early and late atrioventricular block in acute inferior myocardial infarction. J Am Coll Cardiol 4:35, 1984.

86. Tans AC, Lie KI, Durrer D: Clinical setting and prognostic significance of

high degree atrioventricular block in acute inferior myocardial infarction: a study of 144 patients. Am Heart J 99:4, 1980.

87. Narula OS, Scherlag BJ, Samet P, et al: Atrioventricular block: location and classification by His bundle recordings. Am J Med 50:146, 1971.

88. Rosen KM, Loeb HS, Chuquimia R, et al: Site of heart block in acute myocardial infarction. Circulation 42:925, 1970.

89. Norris RM, Mercer CJ: Significance of idioventricular rhythms in acute myocardial infarction. Prog Cardiovasc Dis 16:455, 1974.

90. Nicod P, Gilpin E, Dittrich H, et al: Long-term outcome in patients with inferior myocardial infarction and complete atrioventricular block. J Am Coll Cardiol 12:589, 1988.

91. Strasberg B, Pinchas A, Arditti A, et al: Left and right ventricular function in inferior acute myocardial infarction and significance of advanced atrioventricular block. Am J Cardiol 54:985, 1984.

92. Hindman MC, Wagner GS, JaRo M, et al: The clinical significance of bundle branch block complicating acute myocardial infarction. 1. Clinical characteristics, hospital mortality, and one-year follow-up. Circulation 58:679, 1978.

93. Hindman MC, Wagner GS, JaRo M, et al: The clinical significance of bundle branch block complicating acute myocardial infarction. 2. Indication for temporary and permanent pacemaker insertion. Circulation 58:689, 1978.

94. Klein RC, Vera Z, Mason DT: Intraventricular conduction defects in acute myocardial infarction: incidence, prognosis, and therapy. Am Heart J 108:1007, 1984.

95. Waugh RA, Wagner GS, Haney TL, et al: Immediate and remote prognostic significance of fascicular block during acute myocardial infarction. Circulation 47:765, 1973.

96. Atkins JM, Leshin SJ, Blomqvist G, et al: Ventricular conduction blocks and sudden death in acute myocardial infarction: potential indications for pacing. N Engl J Med 288:281, 1973.

97. Becker AE, Lie KI, Anderson RH: Bundle-branch block in the setting of acute anteroseptal myocardial infarction: clinicopathological correlation. Br Heart J 40:773, 1978.

98. Wilber D, Walton J, O'Neill W, et al: Effects of reperfusion on complete heart block complicating anterior myocardial infarction. J Am Coll Cardiol 4:1315, 1984.

99. Hollander G, Nadiminti V, Lichstein E, et al: Bundle branch block in acute myocardial infarction. Am Heart J 105:738, 1983.

100. Gann D, Balachandran PK, Sherif NE, et al: Prognostic significance of chronic versus acute bundle branch block in acute myocardial infarction. Chest 67:298, 1975.

101. Hynes JK, Holmes DR Jr, Harrison CE: Five-year experience with temporary pacemaker therapy in the coronary care unit. Mayo Clin Proc 58:122, 1983.

102. Lamas GA, Muller JE, Turi ZG, et al: A simplified method to predict occurrence of complete heart block during acute myocardial infarction. Am J Cardiol 57:15, 1986.

103. Ritter WS, Atkins JM, Blomqvist CG, et al: Permanent pacing in patients

with new transient trifasicular block during acute myocardial infarction. Am J Cardiol 38:205, 1976.

104. Sager PT, Batsford WP: Ventricular arrhythmias: medical therapy, device treatment and indications for electrophysiologic study. Cardiol Clin 6:37, 1988.

105. Frye RL, Collins JJ, DeSanctis RW, et al: Guidelines for permanent cardiac pacemaker implantation. J Am Coll Cardiol 4:2, 1984.

Chapter 12

Management of Arrhythmias and Conduction Disturbances in the Perioperative Setting

Brian Olshansky, Bruce Kleinman, and David J. Wilber

Introduction

It is difficult to give an exact definition of the perioperative period. For our purposes, we will say that the perioperative period begins prior to the onset of surgical anesthesia (with the administration of preoperative medications) and ends 1 to 2 weeks later. While cardiac rhythm disturbances are frequently diagnosed during this interval, scant data and few contemporary reports help clinicians effectively manage patients. Controlled trials are scarce. The extent, type, and severity of arrhythmias that occur during this characteristically unstable period pose a challenge to the surgeon, anesthesiologist, and medical consultant. Rhythm disturbances during this period are usually benign and self-limited, and are only rarely associated with a poor outcome. Serious rhythm abnormalities are associated with the extent and severity of underlying heart disease. Many rhythm "abnormalities" come to the attention of the managing physician only because the heart is placed under closer scrutiny during this period. However, it is clear that surgery,

From Naccarelli GV (ed): *Cardiac Arrhythmias: A Practical Approach*. Mount Kisco, NY, Futura Publishing Co., Inc., © 1991.

particularly cardiac surgery, can result in an assortment of de novo rhythm disturbances. In addition, virtually any pre-existing cardiac arrhythmia may become more pronounced during or just following surgery. This chapter focuses on the unique arrhythmia management problems during both the intraoperative and the postoperative periods.

Intraoperative Arrhythmias: Physiology

The pathophysiology of most intraoperative rhythm disturbances is multifactorial. Abrupt changes in autonomic tone play an important role in both the initiation and tolerance of arrhythmias.[1] Endotracheal intubation, peritoneal irritation, urologic manipulation, and neck dissection, for example, can trigger a vagal response.[2] Blood loss, hypotension, pain, and inadequate or excess anesthesia can trigger a sympathetic response. Rarely, autonomic manipulations lead to asystole or ventricular tachycardia.

Anesthetic drugs may result in transient rhythm abnormalities largely by effects on autonomic tone.[3–6] Spinal anesthesia can result in sympathetic blockade or indirectly provoke vagal discharge.[7] Local anesthetics used for spinal anesthesia can theoretically have other neurogenically mediated cardiovascular effects as well.[8] Bupivacaine and procaine infused into the lateral ventricle of cats creates a potent stimulus for malignant ventricular arrhythmias.[9] Nevertheless, a definite relationship between the incidence of serious intraoperative arrhythmias and the anesthetic drug used has yet to be demonstrated.

Halogenated inhalational anesthetics, such as halothane, can sensitize the myocardium to sympathetic stimulation thus triggering atrial and even sustained ventricular tachycardia in susceptible patients.[4] Isoflurane causes less sensitization and enflurane causes the least sensitization of the major inhalational anesthetics.[10] The mechanism of sensitization is not fully known. Presently it is thought to be multifactorial.[11] Increased automaticity plays a role as well as re-entry.[12,13] Therefore, in the face of increased sympathetic tone (such as related to exogenous catecholamines), halothane can induce automatic rhythms. However, because halothane has also been shown to depress intraventricular conduction, a condition for re-entrant rhythms also exists.[14] In addition, these anesthetics may also inhibit the baroreflex. Halothane is the most inhibitory;[15] enflurane and isoflurane are less so.[16,17] The importance of this clinically is that the expected reflex sinus tachycardia normally seen with hypotension may not be seen during an anesthetic with these inhalational drugs. These drugs can also directly depress sinus node automaticity.[4] Nitrous oxide generally has not been felt to have arrhythmogenic effects aside from its ability to rarely cause a sympathetic response. However, it has been implicated in the genesis of junctional rhythms.[18] Ketamine can cause tachycardia by a sympathetic effect.[14] Barbiturates can accentuate vagal tone and directly prolong the AV nodal conduction time.[14] Morphine and fentanyl can cause central vagal stimulation or can directly effect AV nodal conduction time.[14] Sufentanil is associated with bradycardias.[19] Alfentanil has shown little effect on heart rate.[20] Although usually well tolerated, succinylcholine can provoke bradycardia or ventricular ectopy.[14] Pancuronium can increase sinus rate and enhance AV conduction by a vagolytic effect.[14] Vercuronium has been associated with sinus bradycardia.[21,22] Atracurium, generally, has little effect on sinus rates.[22]

Pre-existing rhythm abnormalities, such as supraventricular tachycardia in patients with accessory atrioventricular connections, may be exacerbated by surgery.[23] Droperidol at moderate and large doses lengthened significantly the antegrade and retrograde effective refractory periods of the accessory pathways. Other anesthetic drugs such as thiopental, nitrous oxide, and fentanyl had no significant effect on the accessory pathway. This was also true of the muscle relaxant pancuronium. Various anesthetic combinations, especially nitrous oxide and narcotic combinations, have been advocated for these susceptible patients based on little data.[25,26]

Metabolic alterations including acidosis, hypoxemia, hypercarbia, and, possibly, electrolyte disturbances can initiate arrhythmias which are generally benign.[1,4] Ventricular ectopy during surgery may simply indicate that one or more of these metabolic abnormalities are present. Despite cautionary opinions by some investigators,[27] available data suggest that hypokalemia is not a significant cause of serious intraoperative rhythm disturbances.[28] In one study of patients with preoperative serum values between 2.6 and 3.4 mEq/L, one-third had intraoperative arrhythmias including benign arrhythmias not requiring therapy (sinus tachycardia, junctional rhythm atrial ectopy, or ventricular ectopy).[28] In patients with normal preoperative serum potassium, arrhythmias occurred in nearly half. There was no evidence that preoperative hypokalemia increased the frequency of serious or even benign intraoperative rhythm disturbances. An examination of the relationship between preoperative hypokalemia and frequency of Holter monitor confirmed intraoperative arrhythmias in patients undergoing major cardiac or vascular operations indicating that more than half were normokalemic, one-third were hypokalemic (3.1–3.5 mEq/L), and severe hypokalemia (<3.0 mEq/L) prior to surgery occurred infrequently. Hypokalemia did not increase the incidence or severity of ventricular or atrial arrhythmias, even in patients with underlying heart disease. Hypokalemia alone rarely causes intraoperative cardiac arrest. This is so even though it may exacerbate ventricular arrhythmias (including torsades de pointes) in the setting of impaired ventricular function or when a type I antiarrhythmic agent or digitalis is being used. Postponing elective surgery to correct preoperative potassium abnormalities may not be indicated. Finally, although hypomagnesemia is common in the postoperative patient, the preoperative incidence of this abnormality in these patients and its potential contribution to perioperative arrhythmias is unknown.[30]

Intraoperative changes in blood pressure, ventricular filling pressure, blood volume, and body temperature can trigger arrhythmias by various mechanisms, including a reflex sympathetic response, myocardial stretch, myocardial ischemia, or myocardial infarction. Direct intraoperative trauma to the heart during cardiac surgery can also lead to ventricular or atrial arrhythmias, AV block, and sinus bradycardia. These are frequently transient.[31] Cardioplegic solution, cooling the heart, as well as cardiopulmonary bypass may only partially protect the myocardium allowing for ischemic injury. The pathophysiology of arrhythmias during cardiac surgery will be discussed in a later section of this chapter.

Intraoperative Arrhythmias: Noncardiac Surgery

Nearly 80% of individuals undergoing surgery demonstrate some form of arrhythmia immediately following anesthesia induction and during intubation. The majority are benign and include sinus bradycardia, sinus tachycardia, and ventricular ectopic beats (a frequent cause for intraoperative medical/cardiac consultation). Life-threatening and hemodynamically intolerable arrhythmias including sinus arrest, asystole, and ventricular fibrillation occur rarely. Some investigations have failed to distinguish between serious and trivial arrhythmias, making the clinical significance of their findings questionable. Moreover, the influence of antiarrhythmic therapy on this incidence is rarely considered.

In a review of surgical patients, a 21% incidence of arrhythmias during intubation was noted. During anesthetic maintenance, the incidence was only 13%. The total incidence of all forms of arrhythmias (serious and benign) was about 50%. Premature ventricular beats were seen in 12.5% of patients, half of whom had preoperative ventricular ectopy. Arrhythmias were diagnosed more frequently in patients with cardiac disease than in those without. The type of anesthesia used (including spinal anesthesia) did not influence the incidence. The most common rhythm abnormalities were slow supraventricular rhythms and ventricular ectopy. Less than 1% of patients had serious rhythm disturbances and these occurred predominantly in patients with a preoperative diagnosis of heart disease.

These previous observations are limited by inadequate monitoring techniques. When Holter monitors are used to more carefully assess the frequency of intraoperative arrhythmias, the total incidence of arrhythmias was 61.7%. The incidence was greater in intubated patients than in those not intubated. These arrhythmias included: wandering atrial pacemaker, isorhythmic AV dissociation, junctional rhythm, sinus bradycardia, premature atrial beats, supraventricular tachycardia, and ventricular tachycardia. Most rhythm disturbances were transient. No apparent relationship existed between the preoperative cardiac (or arrhythmic) diagnosis and the presence of arrhythmias intraoperatively. However, the type of arrhythmia, its clinical importance, and severity were not considered when analyzing the data. Arrhythmias were more commonly noted in patients undergoing neurosurgical and thoracic procedures and, not surprisingly, in patients undergoing more prolonged procedures (>3 hours) who had prolonged monitoring. The type or severity of arrhythmia was not correlated with outcome.

Serious intraoperative rhythm disturbances are rare.[1,33] The postoperative risk of death and serious rhythm abnormalities increases with the extent and severity of the underlying cardiac disease.[31] However, intraoperative fatalities due to rhythm disturbances are highly uncommon. In one series, atrial and ventricular ectopy predicted a poor surgical outcome.[33] Ventricular ectopy was not correlated with the risk for development of more malignant ventricular arrhythmias, but was correlated with the severity of the underlying cardiac disease. Death in those with atrial ectopy occurred in elderly and in medically or surgically unstable patients. There is no evidence that preoperative suppression of complex ventricular ectopy or asymptomatic nonsustained ventricular tachycardia influence the risk of developing intraoperative arrhythmias or operative mortality.

Patients with serious, sustained, hemodynamically intolerable tachycardia who are adequately treated preoperatively can generally undergo surgery safely as long as medical therapy is continued.[33] An attempt to control such tachycardias with medication prior to elective surgery is preferable and, if necessary, by serial electrophysiological testing. Even though risk of death due to an intraoperative arrhythmia is rare in these patients, hemodynamic deterioration related to a sustained tachycardia will certainly complicate management. For serious arrhythmias, type I antiarrhythmic drugs, as well as beta-blockers, can be continued safely during and following surgery. Esmolol may be infused intraoperatively because it has a short half-life, making it relatively safe during the entire perioperative period.[34]

If drugs are being used for control of ventricular or supraventricular arrhythmias, it is prudent to continue these agents.[35] Prophylactic antiarrhythmic therapy in patients without hemodynamically compromising arrhythmias is potentially dangerous. It has not been shown to decrease serious intraoperative arrhythmias. Admittedly, controversy exists concerning use of prophylactic digoxin for cardiac surgery (discussed below). The suppression of new-onset, hemodynamically well-tolerated, ventricular ectopy in the intraoperative period is probably not necessary and may be dangerous since antiarrhythmic drugs may exacerbate intraoperative bradyarrhythmias and sustained ventricular tachyarrhythmias as well as interact poorly with some anesthetic agents.[36] When this occurs in an otherwise healthy patient, hypoxia, hypercarbia, hyperthermia, and "light" anesthesia should be considered causative. New-onset ventricular ectopy may signify ischemia due to coronary artery disease. For this, lidocaine is often administered acutely. Lidocaine, compared with other antiarrhythmic agents, rarely has serious proarrhythmic effects in this setting, but it is uncertain whether lidocaine administration will improve the outcome. Therefore, a firm recommendation for its use cannot be made. If sustained or hemodynamically compromising tachycardia occurs during surgery (serious arrhythmias), DC shock or antiarrhythmic therapy are indicated. Lidocaine and procainamide are first-line antiarrhythmic agents for the treatment of sustained and hemodynamically intolerable ventricular arrhythmias. Bretylium may be more dangerous.[37] Intravenous digoxin, verapamil, and beta-blockers are useful for atrial arrhythmias (type IA antiarrhythmic agents are occasionally useful as well for supraventricular tachycardias).

Intraoperative Conduction Disturbances: Noncardiac Surgery

Complete heart block may not directly increase the mortality of an operation but it can lead to deleterious hemodynamic instability during the perioperative period. Complete heart block and Mobitz II AV block has been less of a concern recently, as such patients, especially if symptomatic, are appropriately identified and treated with a permanent pacer prior to surgery. The concern has been more for those who *may develop* heart block during surgery. Bifascicular block (right bundle branch block with left anterior or posterior hemiblock, or left bundle branch block) especially in the presence of a long PR interval was suspected previously as being a frequent precursor of complete heart block. Combined data on 138 patients with bifascicular block, including 25 patients with bifascicular block and prolonged PR interval and 7 patients with bifascicular block and rhythms other than sinus underwent surgery without developing complete heart block.[33] These data are not surprising because the long-term risk of developing complete heart block in patients with chronic bifascicular block is small.[40] A temporary pacer is not required intraoperatively in patients with bifascicular block unless complete heart block has been documented. Intraoperative complications from a temporary pacemaker (and for that matter, a centrally placed large bore cannula) may actually outweigh its benefits.[41] It has been suggested, however, that prior to surgery, patients with chronic bundle branch block (of all types) have a large bore central cannula placed if a temporary pacer is required during or after surgery. Type I antiarrhythmic agents should be used with caution in these patients since these agents may interfere even further with His-Purkinje conduction and provoke complete heart block.

Intraoperative Arrhythmias: Cardiac Surgery

Intraoperative rhythm abnormalities, including sustained and hemodynamically unstable ventricular tachyarrhythmias, have been noted since the inception of cardiac surgery.[43] The development of arrhythmias during cardiac surgery has been related to the type of operation, the length of cardiopulmonary bypass, the severity of the underlying cardiac disease, the hemodynamic stability of the patient, and the preoperative diagnosis. Fortunately, unexpected cardiac arrest during cardiac surgery is rare. It has been suggested that, during cardiopulmonary bypass, ventricular fibrillation in the presence of ventricular hypertrophy might increase mortality by inducing subendocardial ischemia.

The cause for spontaneous intraoperative ventricular fibrillation immediately following institution of cardiopulmonary bypass, prior to aortic cross-clamping and cardioplegic arrest,[46] has been assessed in patients with ventricular fibrillation compared to controls. Ventricular fibrillation was more common during urgent coronary bypass graft surgery or when unstable angina was diagnosed prior to surgery. Mortality was much higher in the ventricular fibrillation group as was the incidence of perioperative myocardial infarction. It was unclear if ventricular fibrillation worsened the prognosis or was just a marker for a deleterious outcome. Although not directly comparable, ventricular fibrillation is frequently induced in the operating room in patients off cardiopulmonary bypass following cardiac surgery to test internal defibrillator patches. These patients have not been reported to have a high postoperative mortality, suggesting that intraoperative ventricular fibrillation alone is not the cause for a poor prognosis. Ultimately, during cardiac surgery, most tachyarrhythmias are transient and, if hemodynamically intolerable, easily controlled with an internal DC shock.

Intraoperative Conduction Disturbances and Bradycardia: Cardiac Surgery

Following discontinuation of cardiopulmonary bypass, bradyarrhythmias, including sinus arrest, sinus bradycardia, junctional rhythm, and AV block and bundle branch block are often noted. When bradyarrhythmias occur, they tend to be transient and are often improved or reversed by intravenous atropine. A temporary pacemaker is useful if the episode persists. The incidence of intraoperative bundle branch varies from 4% to 34%.[47] Cold cardioplegia has been implicated as a cause for transient bundle branch block. In one study of patients undergoing coronary artery bypass grafting, 34% receiving cardioplegia developed transient bundle branch block which resolved within 12 hours following surgery; three developed new permanent bundle branch block but there was no higher incidence of perioperative myocardial infarction in those developing bundle branch block.[48] In contrast, using cold cardioplegia, fewer patients developed new bundle branch block, of which 50% were transient in case study.[47] The risk of death was seven times higher when bundle branch block developed in this study. The incidence of myocardial infarction assessed by CK-MB fraction was four times higher in patients with new bundle branch block. In patients undergoing core hypothermia and induced ventricular fibrillation, fascicular conduction abnormalities occurred in 20% (39/200) of patients; the abnormality was transient in 12/39.[49] Persistent bundle branch block was associated with a higher incidence of new myocardial infarction and sudden death during long-term follow-up.

A few large studies have examined the cause for intraoperative fascicular conduction abnormalities in detail. The incidence of new fascicular conduction disturbances was evaluated in 200 consecutive patients undergoing coronary artery bypass grafting.[50] Forty-five patients (22.5%) developed fascicular conduction blocks of which six were transient. Right bundle branch block was the most commonly seen and represented 47% of all conduction disturbances. There was a correlation between fascicular conduction disturbances and left main coronary artery disease, chronic hypertension, preoperative digitalis use, and patient age. No correlation existed between the number of bypass grafts implanted, the ejection fraction, or the presence of perioperative infarction. New fascicular conduction disturbances were not associated with a poor prognosis. In another study of fascicular conduction defects following coronary revascularization procedures involving 227 patients, 24 had preoperative and 52 developed intraoperative fascicular block. Hemiblocks and right bundle branch blocks were transient. When left bundle branch block or an intraventricular conduction delay developed, it was permanent in 62% of such patients and was associated with a much higher 1-year mortality rate (38% vs. 4%). This higher mortality appeared to be related to the degree of myocardial dysfunction and was not caused by a bradyarrhythmia or complete heart block. A poorer survival rate is not uniformly seen in all studies evaluating patients with new onset bundle branch blocks; a new left bundle branch block does not even indicate a poor prognosis in all studies.[52]

Surgery for correction of valvular heart disease may also lead to bundle branch block. Conduction defects following aortic valve replacement have been reported in 5.3% to 29% of patients, most being transient. Left bundle branch block is the most common fascicular conduction disturbance following aortic valve replacement. When it occurs, it tends to persist.[53] Following aortic valve replacement and mitral valve replacement,[54] transient complete heart block is common, but there was a very low incidence of late heart block over a 4-year follow-up. Intraoperative heart block did not predict the need for permanent pacing. Prophylactic permanent pacer implantation was unnecessary.

The time course of conduction defects following coronary revascularization has also been investigated.[55] In 42 of 93 patients, new fascicular block or bundle branch block developed; four patients had third degree AV block. Their operative technique included cold, hyperkalemic cardioplegia. Conduction defects resolved partially or completely in 54%

and were associated with longer cardiopulmonary bypass time (as well as more cold cardioplegia), longer aortic cross-clamp times and more vessels bypassed. All patients with third degree heart block had eventual resolution of heart block even though three of four of them had been discharged in complete heart block with a permanent pacemaker. The investigators concluded that the most likely mechanism for conduction defects in their patients was ischemic injury to the cardiac conduction system. Temporary epicardial pacer leads appear to be helpful and should be used until there is resolution of AV block. If complete AV block or hemodynamically unstable second degree AV block persists near the time of hospital discharge, a permanent pacemaker is often considered and implanted even though the data do not suggest that a pacemaker will always be required in the future.

Intraoperative bundle branch block and AV block may be caused by ischemia or infarction.[50,55] Animal models have been used to assess the mechanism of His-Purkinje damage following cardiac surgery. Myocardial hypothermia lengthened the Wenckebach cycle length and the AH interval but high potassium cardioplegic arrest did not impair AV nodal conduction. The HV interval remained unchanged. This suggests that potassium cardioplegic arrest is not deleterious to the AV conduction system. In an evaluation of spontaneous cardiac electrical activity in dogs undergoing hyperkalemic, hypothermic arrest utilizing 25 intramural cardiac plunge electrodes per animal, atrial electrical activity returned first at the His atrial electrode, suggesting the presence of incomplete atrial (and especially His-Purkinje) protection. Therefore, cardioplegic arrest does not prevent all cardiac activity and ischemic conduction system damage may occur. Hypothermic cardioplegia appears to be more difficult to maintain in the atria compared to the ventricles as confirmed experimentally by lower cardioplegic solution flow and more rapid return of electrical activity to the atrial septum.[58] During cardioplegia, electrical activity was adequately inhibited in the ventricle but it persisted in the atrium especially in the AV nodal/His bundle region. Persistent electrical activity was correlated with the development of "ischemic" heart block and junctional rhythm. These data suggest that inadequate protection of conduction tissue with subsequent ischemic injury is a major determinant of intraoperative conduction disturbances, although the type of cardioplegic solution has also been implicated.[60] Despite contradictory data, hyperkalemia, by an unknown mechanism, and hypothermia appear capable of causing transient complete heart block.

Atrioventricular block, conduction abnormalities, and sinus node dysfunction may follow various types of cardiac surgery due to direct surgical trauma. Reparative operations for valvular heart disease, particularly aortic valve disease, may cause fascicular blocks, or second or third degree heart block. This may be due to (1) direct surgical manipulation or trauma of normal structures, (2) traumatic disruption of an already diseased His-Purkinje system, or (3) an aberrant suture in the cardiac conduction system.[61] Similarly, repair of various forms of congenital heart disease including ventricular septal defects, tetralogy of Fallot, and AV canal defects can cause bundle branch block (especially right bundle branch block), which rarely progresses to complete heart block.[62,63] The Senning and Mustard (as well as the Blalock) procedures may lead to various arrhythmias including complete heart block.[64] Atrial septal defect repair can cause sinus node dysfunction (sinus bradycardia, sinus arrest) secondary to direct sinus node damage. Despite damage that occurs during surgery, the conduction system is remarkably resilient so that intraoperative heart block and bradyarrhythmias are usually transient and almost always disappear in the late postoperative period over days to weeks.

Special Intraoperative Problems: Pacemakers and Automatic Internal Cardioverter Defibrillators

Intraoperative management becomes more complicated when a patient has an implanted mechanical device to control the heart rhythm.[65,66] Transient pacemaker dysfunction may occur during electrocautery especially if the pacemaker is unipolar and electrocautery is used near the pacemaker or the heart. Electrocautery may be sensed as atrial or ventricular activity and inhibit the pacemaker; temporary asystole may ensue.[67] Alternatively, the ventricular lead of a DDD pacemaker may track electrocautery as apparent atrial activity and ventricular pacing may occur at the upper rate limit. Electrocautery, as well as DC shock, can temporarily cause pacemaker exit block by interfering with the lead-myocardial interface. Electrocautery may cause pacemaker reprogramming or loss of pacemaker "identity."[68–70] Many of the new model pacemakers automatically convert to the asynchronous mode or perform ventricular "safety" pacing (asynchronous ventricular pacing in a DDD pacemaker when the ventricular electrode senses abnormal signals following the atrial electrogram) when "noise" (signals not considered intracardiac activity, such as electrocautery) is sensed or filter out "noise" altogether. Bipolar pacemakers are not immune to the above problems. Pacemakers whose rate is determined by myopotential activity (rate responsive pacemakers) will accelerate with increased myopotential activity. Electrocautery may generate myopotential activity near the pacemaker and therefore accelerate the pacing rate.

A pacemaker-dependent patient, in whom electrocautery is to be used during surgery, especially if the pacer is unipolar and the electrocautery is to be used close to the pacemaker or the heart, should have the pacemaker reprogrammed to the asynchronous mode. The same can be accomplished by placing a magnet, for most pacemakers, over the unit during the entirety of operation. Occasionally, a magnet can alter the permanent multiprogrammable pacemaker settings. It may be wise to monitor the arterial pulse tracing in pacemaker patients undergoing electrocautery as the electrocardiogram may be temporarily obliterated making rhythm interpretation even more difficult. Proper electrocautery grounding and avoidance of strong electrocautery signals, such as those generated by electrocautery cutting, may also prevent pacemaker inhibition.[71]

With a DDD pacemaker, intraoperative atrial fibrillation may precipitate rapid ventricular pacing rates. Intraoperative changes in autonomic tone may facilitate ventriculo-atrial conduction allowing for pacemaker-mediated tachycardia to develop even if this was not a prior problem. During pacemaker-mediated tachycardia, the ventricular rate occurs at the upper rate limit. Many new model DDD pacemakers sense persistent upper rate limit pacing activity and automatically attempt to abort it by failing to pace in the ventricle after a fixed number of paced beats.

Automated internal cardioverter defibrillators (AICD) are increasingly being implanted in patients who have had cardiac arrest secondary to ventricular fibrillation or have had sustained ventricular tachycardia not responsive to other measures.[72–75] Such patients (now numbering well over 6000) are at high risk for a malignant ventricular arrhythmia during surgery. Electrocautery can be sensed by the AICD as a rapid ventricular rate and commit the device to shock the patient even in sinus rhythm; approximately 4–7 seconds of a rapid rate sensed above the rate cut-off of the AICD is all that is required to commit the AICD to deliver a shock. Implantable defibrillators that allow programming of the sensing interval will soon be widely available but the problem remains. The presence of an activated AICD is a two-edged sword: it may appropriately convert the patient from a malignant sustained ventricular arrhythmia but it may also inappropriately shock the patient in sinus rhythm. Also, a rapid ventricular rhythm (secondary to a malignant ventricular arrhythmia or to a supraventricular arrhythmia) occurs during surgery, the device may unexpectedly deliver a shock jarring the patient to the consternation of the surgeon. In selected patients, such as those undergoing delicate surgery or in whom electrocautery is to be used, it is more acceptable to deactivate the AICD device during surgery. The patient can be externally defibrillated, if necessary. Application of adhesive defibrillator pads directly to the chest attached to an external defibrillator is recommended during the procedure for such patients. As internal defibrillator patches could theoretically shield the heart from external defibrillator shocks, it has been recommended that the external shocks be delivered in an anterior-posterior fashion. However, as placement of the internal patches may vary, the location for delivery of the optimal external shock is unpredictable.

Postoperative Arrhythmias: Noncardiac Surgery

Few studies assess postoperative rhythm disturbances following noncardiac surgery. Patients undergoing noncardiac surgery with a stable or controlled pre-existing rhythm abnormality are at low risk for arrhythmias, especially of the life-threatening type, in the postoperative period.[33,76] In a series of 1001 patients, 39 developed supraventricular tachycardia in the operating room and postoperatively. This included atrial fibrillation, atrial flutter, multifocal atrial tachycardia, "paroxysmal atrial tachycardia," and supraventricular tachycardia of unclear type. New supraventricular tachycardias occurred in 10% of those over age 70, in 13% of those with symptomatic congestive heart failure, and in 9% of those with chronic obstructive pulmonary disease. Twelve of these 39 patients were taking digoxin before the onset of supraventricular tachycardia. There were no reported cases of ventricular tachycardia.

Not all operations, however, have the same risk for postoperative arrhythmias. The risk of arrhythmias following thoracic surgery, for example, is high. In one review of 100 patients undergoing thoracic surgery, 34 developed arrhythmias, 16 patients developed atrial fibrillation, 2 developed atrial flutter, 8 demonstrated frequent atrial ectopy, and 12 developed frequent ventricular ectopy.[77]

Postoperative Arrhythmias: Cardiac Surgery

Cardiovascular surgery, particularly coronary revascularization procedures, has increased over the past decade. The number of patients undergoing coronary artery bypass graft procedures has escalated from 114,000 in 1979 to over 228,000 in 1986 in the United States despite a decline in incidence of new coronary artery disease.[78] Many of these are second cardiac operations for revascularization and, with the advent of angioplasty, often represent more complex cases. Cardiac arrhythmias are frequently seen and are considered a major complication of cardiac surgery. Knowledge of the types of arrhythmic complications that follow cardiac surgery, their clinical significance, and their management is increasingly important for consultants to help manage these patients adequately.

Contrary to the lack of data following noncardiac surgery, arrhythmias following cardiac surgery have been more extensively evaluated. This is of little surprise as postoperative supraventricular tachycardias following cardiac surgery may occur in as many as 72%[79] or even 100% of patients depending on the definition of "arrhythmia" and depending on the monitoring technique.[80] While supraventricular tachycardias are the most frequent rhythm abnormality seen following cardiac surgery, various rhythm disturbances are common including ventricular arrhythmias, AV dissociation, junctional rhythm, accelerated junctional rhythm, and AV block (of various types). These all tend to be transient and usually resolve within 2 months following cardiac surgery.

In the 1970s, the incidence of arrhythmias following cardiac surgery was evaluated.[31] Forty-eight percent had "significant" arrhythmias detected by "clinical observation," not hard copy monitoring. In congenital heart disease patients, junctional rhythm was the most common postoperative arrhythmia. No patient in this group died due to an arrhythmia. Valvular heart disease was associated with a 58% incidence of postoperative atrial fibrillation. Ventricular ectopy was the most common arrhythmia in coronary artery disease patients.

In contrast to earlier investigations examining the incidence of postcardiac surgical arrhythmias,[31,81,82] recent studies demonstrate a relatively low incidence of ventricular arrhythmias and a high frequency of atrial arhythmias.[83-91] Nearly two-thirds of patients undergoing coronary artery bypass grafting had postoperative arrhythmias.[83] Atrial arrhythmias including atrial fibrillation, atrial flutter, supraventricular tachycardia, and premature atrial beats were as common as ventricular arrhythmias including premature ventricular contractions and nonsustained ventricular tachycardia (>3 beats). Postoperative arrhythmias were also frequently detected in patients undergoing valvular surgery, the most common arrhythmia being atrial fibrillation. There was no relationship between these arrhythmias and other complications. Others have reported a 21–37.5% incidence of atrial fibrillation or flutter following various cardiac surgical procedures.[53,84,87]

It is difficult to predict which patient undergoing cardiac surgery will develop postoperative arrhythmias, most of which are supraventricular, self-limited, and unlikely to alter the long-term prognosis. Following coronary artery bypass graft surgery, patients with supraventricular arrhythmias tend to be older, have more bypass graft implantations, and have longer aortic cross-clamp times.[86,87,89] Following aortic valve replacement for aortic stenosis, the preoperative predictors for postoperative atrial tachyarrhythmias include age (>70), preoperative atrial fibrillation, diabetes mellitus, and use of antiarrhythmic therapy.[87] Postoperative predictors in these patients included prolonged respirator therapy, use of catecholamine support, and vasodilators. There may also be an association between the presence of postoperative atrial fibrillation and the occurrence of new bundle branch block.[90]

Patients with a preoperative history of sustained supraventricular or ventricular tachycardia (hemodynamically unstable or lasting >30 seconds) who do not undergo a corrective ablative procedure or implantation of a device to control their arrhythmia at the time of cardiac surgery are at continued or even increased risk for recurrent tachycardia in the postoperative setting. Myocardial revascularization alone rarely corrects sustained monomorphic ventricular tachycardia even though it may decrease the frequency and severity of episodes.[92] Patients with sustained or symptomatic tachycardia, particularly if inadequately treated prior to elective cardiac surgery, deserve complete preoperative evaluation, including electrophysiological testing, if necessary, to (1) assess the hemodynamic risk of the sustained ventricular or supraventricular tachycardia, (2) determine if effective drug therapy can be prescribed, and (3) assess surgical therapeutic options.

Patients undergoing cardiac surgery with the "substrate" for malignant arrhythmias but who have not yet manifest a symptomatic episode are more difficult to assess. This includes patients with (1) left ventricular dysfunction and nonsustained ventricular tachycardia who are at risk for sudden death despite myocardial revascularization, (2) ventricular aneurysms requiring aneurysmectomy or revascularization who are at risk for sustained ventricular tachycardia, and (3) the pattern of Wolff-Parkinson-White syndrome on the surface electrocardiogram but no symptomatic tachycardia. While controlled studies have not been performed in these patient groups, it has been our experience that these patients may also be at risk to develop tachycardia(s) postoperatively. Hemodynamic problems related to development of a new rapid rhythm disturbance could be devastating. An appropriate management plan has yet to be developed for these situations.

Diagnostic Evaluation of Arrhythmias Following Cardiac Surgery

The diagnostic techniques available to evaluate and treat cardiac rhythm disturbances following cardiac surgery include routinely available methods of rhythm analysis and therapy as well as epicardial atrial and ventricular wire electrodes which serve multiple functions.[93] These wires may be placed on either the atria or the ventricles (or both) to (1) facilitate accurate rhythm diagnosis when an arrhythmia cannot be diagnosed from the surface ECG (atrial flutter vs. atrial fibrillation, or the cause for a wide QRS tachycardia, for example), (2) provide an effective method to terminate, presumably re-entrant, tachyarrhythmias such as atrial flutter, (3) provide backup pacing should AV block or a bradyarrhythmia occur, (4) suppress atrial or ventricular ectopy which may trigger a tachyarrhythmia, and (5) permit a noninvasive approach to perform electrophysiological testing.[94] It is never clear who should receive epicardial pacer wires during cardiac surgery, and on which cardiac chambers, until a rhythm problem develops that is otherwise difficult to diagnose or treat. Since the initial reports in the 1960s,[95,96] epicardial pacer wires are being used frequently. Atrial epicardial leads have been reported to be useful in over 60% of those cardiac surgery patients in whom they are placed.[93,97] As a diagnostic or therapeutic tool, the wires are rarely nonfunctional.[98] If lead placement is not properly performed or if the wires are not properly attended to, they may become rapidly dysfunctional. Epicardial pacer wires rarely caused a complication. Removal of epicardial pacer wires was not associated with any serious problems including infection even though many remained in place for many days or weeks. In pediatric cardiac patients, single lead electrocardiographic evaluation may be improved substantially with the use of epicardial atrial electrodes postoperatively.[99] This suggests a need for intracardiac recordings to help assure an accurate diagnosis in postoperative pediatric patients.

The common occurrence of transient cardiac arrhythmias, especially atrial fibrillation and atrial flutter, following cardiac surgery, invites a careful search for the etiology. Potential responsible factors include (1) trauma and inflammation due to surgical manipulation including the development of postoperative pericarditis,[100] (2) autonomic influences,

(3) ischemia or new myocardial injury, (4) effects of cardioplegia and cardiopulmonary bypass,[101] (5) postoperative hemodynamic changes, and (6) a subsequent effect of previously damaged myocardial tissue.[102]

Epicardial leads are invaluable to terminate atrial and ventricular tachycardias and provide backup pacing for transient AV block and sinus bradyarrhythmias. Hemodynamic deterioration is not infrequent following cardiac surgery due to the presence a junctional or a ventricular rhythm (i.e., a slow rhythm without AV synchrony). This can usually be corrected by pacing to provide a more rapid ventricular rate and/or to provide AV synchrony.[103] Additionally, the hemodynamic response may be influenced by the site of location of the epicardial pacer leads in the ventricle.[104]

Causes of Postoperative Arrhythmias

Intraoperative atrial ischemia due to poor myocardial protection during cardiopulmonary bypass may trigger supraventricular tachycardias. The return of atrial activity during cardiopulmonary bypass has been demonstrated in the animal laboratory and in humans.[57,105] Although persistent intraoperative atrial activity has been seen to correlate with postoperative atrial arrhythmias, this is not found in all studies.[101] One reason may be that the best method to assess persistent atrial activity is still uncertain. The relationship between postoperative bundle branch block and atrial arrhythmias, however, is not surprising.[90] Cardiopulmonary bypass time has been correlated with postoperative atrial fibrillation but the damage may have been caused by the exposure to cardioplegic solution (which could cause ischemic injury or have a direct toxic effect) or hypothermia.[57,101] A strong correlation has been demonstrated between length of cardioplegic arrest and the presence of postoperative supraventricular tachyarrhythmias. This correlation is more apparent when using hyperkalemic crystalloid cardioplegia with systemic hypothermia than it is with the use of blood cardioplegia.[101]

Autonomic tone can influence the development of postoperative arrhythmias but its effect is difficult to assess. Experimentally, vagal stimulation precipitates atrial fibrillation. However, high vagal tone is usually not present postoperatively. Catecholamine-initiated atrial fibrillation is rare outside the postoperative period and beta-blockade rarely prevents atrial fibrillation outside the postoperative period.[106,107] Nevertheless, a growing body of evidence implicates beta-blockade as a successful therapy to prevent and terminate various supraventricular tachycardias, including atrial fibrillation, in the postoperative period. These data suggest that a catecholamine excess or increased sensitivity to catecholamines following cardiac surgery may promote an environment that allows the initiation of unusual forms of common rhythm abnormalities, including atrial fibrillation and atrial flutter.

Norepinephrine release is triggered by hypoxia and presumably by ischemia in the isolated, perfused, animal heart.[108] Similarly, cardiopulmonary bypass can lead to a tenfold increase in epinephrine and twofold increase in norepinephrine levels, possibly due to provocation by myocardial ischemia.[109] Although results have varied between studies, catecholamine levels can remain elevated for at least 3 days.[110] Catecholamine excess may then interfere with adequate myocardial protection during cardiopulmonary bypass by increasing myocardial oxygen demand in nonquiescent tissue triggering a vicious cycle of myocardial ischemia. However, no relationship has been demonstrated between the peak catecholamine level and postoperative arrhythmias.

Atrial Arrhythmias Following Cardiac Surgery

Atrial flutter is often considered along with atrial fibrillation postoperatively. While it is true that the two rhythms often occur in the same patients, and one frequently changes to the other, the mechanisms responsible for atrial flutter may be different from those responsible for atrial fibrillation. Four types of atrial fibrillation and two types of atrial flutter have been characterized in patients during the postoperative period using fixed bipolar epicardial atrial electrodes.[111–113] Type I (classic) atrial flutter exhibits rates between 230 to 340 beats/min and type II atrial flutter has rates between 340 and 433 beat/min. Both types demonstrate uniform morphology, polarity, and amplitude of atrial electrograms separated by an equally spaced isoelectric interval.[111] The essential difference between the two types is that type I atrial flutter can be terminated or otherwise influenced by rapid atrial pacing, but type II cannot. Present data do not suggest that categorization of atrial fibrillation types provides insight into the mechanism or treatment of atrial fibrillation. Moreover, these "distinct" types of atrial fibrillation, which have been categorized by epicardial atrial electrogram recordings, can change from one to the other and various types may be present in any given patient at different atrial sites. All types of atrial fibrillation and atrial flutter type II cannot be terminated by rapid atrial pacing.

The concepts of transient entrainment, the details of which are beyond the scope of this chapter, were initially developed by observing changes in flutter wave morphology during rapid atrial pacing of atrial flutter. During transient entrainment of atrial flutter, the tissue involved in the tachycardia is accelerated to the pacing cycle length with resumption of the same atrial flutter immediately upon pacing termination.[113] Criteria for transient entrainment can be demonstrated for postoperative, type I atrial flutter (and some postoperative atrial tachycardias). Re-entry, with an "excitable gap" of tissue (to allow entrance of the pacing wave front of depolarization into the re-entry circuit), is the most likely cause for this phenomenon. The atrial flutter reentrant circuit appears to be macro re-entrant with a discrete area of slow conduction.[114,115] The postoperative conditions necessary to create the milieu for atrial flutter are uncertain.

A canine model of sterile pericarditis may provide an experimental counterpart to study postoperative atrial flutter. Re-entry, not requiring an anatomical barrier, has been shown to be the cause for this experimental atrial flutter. This model reflects the conditions of the usual postoperative patient who develops atrial flutter.[100] Some episodes of postoperative atrial flutter may instead be due to anatomical disruption of the atria (for which there are also experimental models of re-entry).

Are Arrhythmias Following Cardiac Surgery Preventable?

Pharmacological alteration in autonomic tone to control and to prevent postoperative supraventricular tachyarrhythmias, particularly atrial fibrillation and atrial flutter, is conceptually appealing. This is because of the presence of a postoperative hyperadrenergic state. Prophylactic beta-blockade appears to reduce the incidence of postoperative atrial arrhythmias.[80,84,90,116–122] This may be especially true for those patients taking beta-adrenergic blocking agents preoperatively. Using acebutolol administered early postoperatively (within 36 hours) to prevent postoperative atrial fibrillation or atrial flutter,[118] no atrial arrhythmias were reported in the treatment group but 40% of those in the placebo group developed supraventricular tachycardia. With prophylactic timolol in a double-blind, prospective manner,[80] there were fewer episodes of postoperative atrial fibrillation and flutter in the timolol group than in the placebo group (291 vs. 5). No patient enrolled had a low ejection fraction (<41%). Patients taking beta-adrenergic blocking drugs preoperatively appear especially likely to derive arrhythmia prevention with postoperative beta-blockade.[119,120] Postoperative beta-blockade also appears to be superior to digoxin alone in preventing atrial arrhythmias. In a comparison of digoxin to propranolol to placebo, it was found that only propranolol reduced the incidence of sustained (>30 seconds) atrial fibrillation (37.5% control, 32.6% digoxin, 16.2% propranolol) following cardiac surgery.[84] The utility of combining digoxin and propranolol was evaluated following coronary artery bypass graft surgery[121] and resulted in a marked reduction in postoperative supraventricular arrhythmias. There was no increase in ventricular arrhythmias or other side effects.

While the preponderance of evidence suggests a beneficial effect of beta-blockade in reducing the incidence of postoperative atrial arrhythmias, several important limitations must be recognized. In general, atrial fibrillation tends to be a benign and often self-limiting arrhythmia (particularly in patients with good ventricular function most amenable to prophylactic beta-adrenoreceptor blockade). Thus the need for prophylactic therapy is unclear.[122] In patients with severely compromised ventricular function who are at greatest risk of adverse hemodynamic effects with the onset of postoperative atrial arrhythmias, prophylactic beta-adrenergic blockade may compromise an already limited cardiac reserve. In addition, not all studies demonstrate benefit of beta-adrenergic blockade for the prevention of all types of supraventricular tachycardias.[123] In one study, the incidence of postoperative atrial arrhythmias was 16.1% with placebo and 13.2% with beta-blockade.[124] Thus from available data, a universal recommendation with regard to the use of prophylactic beta-blockade cannot be made. Patients who have been treated preoperatively with a beta-blocker are at particularly high risk for postoperative supraventricular tachycardia and for these patients, beta-blockade should be continued postoperatively.

The benefits of prophylactic digoxin are even less clear. A variable change in the incidence of postoperative supraventricular tachycardia has been reported using prophylactic digoxin.[126] It is the authors' practice to reserve the use of digoxin to those patients who have had spontaneous tachycardia that may respond to digoxin therapy both preoperatively and postoperatively.

Therapy for Atrial Arrhythmias Following Cardiac Surgery

Postoperative atrial flutter is generally transient and self-limiting. If atrial wires are present, an attempt to terminate atrial flutter (type I) with rapid atrial pacing is warranted.[129] Other methods of pacing, including use of an esophageal lead, may be useful. Normally, pacing begins at a rate 10 beats/minute faster than the atrial flutter rate for at least 15 seconds. If the atria have been captured but the tachycardia is not terminated, atrial flutter was most likely transiently entrained. Pacing is then accomplished at progressively faster rates (increment of 10 beats/minute) until atrial flutter is terminated or atrial fibrillation ensues. Atrial pacing faster than 400 beats/minute may be undesirable as atrial fibrillation may be precipitated (unless atrial fibrillation is desired). Often, transient atrial fibrillation (<24 hours) is induced before the return to sinus rhythm. Unfortunately, rapid atrial pacing does not reliably terminate atrial flutter with the return of sinus rhythm; atrial fibrillation may be induced. If atrial flutter cannot be terminated with rapid atrial pacing at rates up to 400 beats/minute, it may be useful to add an intravenous type I antiarrhythmic agent such as procainamide to help facilitate the termination of atrial flutter by pacing techniques.[130]

If one episode of atrial flutter occurs, without a preoperative history of atrial flutter, long-term antiarrhythmic therapy, including AV nodal blocking drugs is not necessary. Many such patients will not have a recurrence of atrial flutter. In patients with recurrent atrial flutter, pharmacological therapy (type I antiarrhythmic agents or AV nodal blocking drugs) may be helpful. Unfortunately, there have been no prospective data documenting the comparative efficacy or safety of any therapeutic regimen in postoperative patients with recurrent atrial flutter. Additionally, the pharmacokinetics of antiarrhythmic agents may vary markedly in the early perioperative period due to the presence of acute phase reactants such as α_1-acid glycoprotein. These acute phase reactants may alter the free (unbound) fractions of antiarrhythmic agents by over 200% making it difficult to manage effectively antiarrhythmic drug therapy in the postoperative period.[131] Nevertheless, patients with recurrent atrial flutter should be considered for medical therapy for at least 6 weeks following cardiac surgery. It has been our experience that patients with recurrent atrial flutter benefit from type I antiarrhythmic agents in the postoperative period in normal therapeutic dosages because these drugs probably help prevent recurrent postoperative atrial flutter. Verapamil and digoxin appear to work mainly by slowing conduction in the AV node without prevention atrial flutter.[132] These drugs may control the ventricular response rate at rest but changes in sympathetic tone, as may occur with standing or walking, may easily override this effect even with large doses. Electrical cardioversion should be reserved as the last therapeutic maneuver, unless it is late in the hospitalization or if the patient is hemodynamically unstable. This is so because atrial flutter or fibrillation often recurs early in the postoperative period despite cardioversion. If all else fails, in the early period following cardiac surgery atrial flutter may be treated with continuous rapid atrial pacing to maintain atrial fibrillation. This may help control the ventricular response rate and maintain improved hemodynamics.[133] Long-term medical management must be individually tailored to the patient's overall condition, the hemodynamic severity of the arrhythmia, and the response to AV nodal blocking drugs and type I (and occasionally, type III) antiarrhythmic drugs.[86,134]

The most frequent time for the first occurrence of atrial fibrillation following cardiac surgery is in the first 2–5 postoperative days but it may recur or persist for weeks before it finally remits.[89] Atrial fibrillation cannot be terminated with rapid atrial pacing. The initial treatment in the early postoperative period should be an AV nodal blocking drug such as digoxin or verapamil, or both (with care to avoid digitalis toxicity), infused to slow the ventricular response rate. It is rare that either of these drugs will terminate atrial fibrillation. Beta-blockers, including esmolol, may help terminate atrial fibrillation or at least control the ventricular response rate.[34] If the patient is hypotensive or in worsening congestive heart failure, DC cardioversion should be performed. Atrial pacing, at rates between 90–110 beats per minute after cardioversion to sinus rhythm, may help maintain sinus rhythm by suppressing atrial ectopy. If the patient is hemodynamically stable, cardioversion may be deferred until late in the hospital course, as atrial fibrillation frequently recurs. Type IA or occasionally type III (amiodarone) antiarrhythmic drugs may help maintain sinus rhythm following conversion from atrial fibrillation. The comparative utility of a type IA antiarrhythmic agent to a type IC drug or amiodarone has not been reported. However, considering the potential toxicities of the drugs involved, it is most reasonable to initiate therapy with a quinidine or procainamide preparation. All of these drugs may additionally help convert atrial fibrillation directly to sinus rhythm. Often these drugs are not required for more than a few weeks to maintain sinus rhythm. This is because atrial fibrillation is often transient after cardiac surgery. The use of these drugs in the perioperative period should be tempered with a fundamental understanding of their potential toxicity. Their use should be reserved for those patients who manifest persistent and hemodynamically intolerable arrhythmias.[135]

Anticoagulation

In the postoperative period, anticoagulants may be helpful to prevent thromboemboli. This is particularly true for patients with transient atrial fibrillation and those with poor left ventricular function. Unfortunately, anticoagulants may increase bleeding complications. No randomized trial of anticoagulants has been undertaken in postoperative patients with transient atrial fibrillation. While the risks of thromboemboli may be relatively high following cardiac surgery due to a transient hypercoagulable state, it is unusual for transient atrial fibrillation to precipitate a clinically important thromboembolic event in the early postoperative period. With persistent atrial fibrillation following surgery, especially in those who ultimately may require cardioversion to sinus rhythm, it may be worth considering anticoagulation.[122]

Ventricular Arrhythmias Following Cardiac Surgery

Ventricular arrhythmias may occur following various types of cardiac surgery. They occur both early and late in the postoperative period. They represent a spectrum of disorders ranging from the exacerbation of benign ventricular ectopy to new onset ventricular fibrillation or ventricular tachycardia.[31,136–144] Ventricular arrhythmias occurring in the first 48 hours following surgery may represent a transient phenomenon caused by inotropic support, hypoxia (myocardial ischemia), and cardiac trauma. Malignant, hemodynamically intolerable, ventricular tachyarrhythmias that occur during this period may resolve spontaneously. Following stabilization, long-term therapy may not be necessary.

Ventricular Ectopy Following Cardiovascular Surgery

Asymptomatic ventricular arrhythmias, including ventricular ectopy and nonsustained ventricular tachycardia, are often seen in the early postoperative period following cardiac surgery for coronary revascularization and valve replacement.[137,138] Patients with impaired left ventricular function postoperatively are most likely to experience an aggravation of ventricular ectopy but, if there is improvement in ventricular function due to surgery, the ectopy may decrease in frequency and severity. In a report of prospectively evaluated coronary artery bypass patients who had postoperative couplets, nonsustained ventricular tachycardia, and the "R-on-T" phenomenon, all had good left ventricular function (ejection fraction >0.55).[142] In the long term, complex ventricular arrhythmias were not associated with a higher incidence of sudden or cardiac death, syncope, or myocardial infarction. Patients with poor ventricular function may have a greater frequency of postoperative complex ventricular ectopy and nonsustained ventricular tachycardia,[143] but there appears to be no relationship between these arrhythmias and total mortality or sudden death. Following aortic valve surgery, there has been reported a small but significant late mortality of 3.6%/year.[140] This mortality has been related to ventricular hypertrophy and unoperated occluded lesions, not to asymptomatic ventricular ectopy. Thus, the prognostic value of asymptomatic arrhythmias, postoperatively, is unclear. The occurrence of these arrhythmias may be related to electrolyte disorders, worsening heart failure, and ischemia plus a hyperadrenergic state following cardiac surgery. Evidence for a hyperadrenergic state causing serious, postoperative ventricular arrhythmias is demonstrated by the presence of intraoperative myocardial "bombs" (high, local intra-axonal accumulations of catecholamines within cardiac tissue as determined by intraoperative right atrial biopsy) in patients who subsequently developed postoperative ventricular tachycardia and ventricular fibrillation as late as the second postoperative week.[145] Ischemia, however, does not appear to be a prime factor. This is because there appears to be little or no change in the presence of exercise-induced ventricular ectopy following coronary revascularization.[146] Some advocate empiric antiarrhythmic treatment for asymptomatic, nonsustained ventricular tachyarrhythmias. However, there is no evidence to demonstrate that postoperative ventricular ectopy is a predictor of long-term prognosis, or that arrhythmia suppression will alter prognosis. Arrhythmia suppression may, in fact, worsen the prognosis. Signal-averaging and electrophysiological testing to evaluate and guide therapy for asymptomatic or nonsustained arrhythmias are investigational.

Sustained Ventricular Arrhythmias Following Cardiac Surgery

Sustained ventricular tachyarrhythmias in the postoperative period often require aggressive medical (or surgical) treatment and extensive evaluation, especially those occurring late (>48 hours postoperatively). Electrophysiological guided antiarrhythmic testing, and hence the need for long-term therapy may be necessary. The actual incidence of new-onset sustained ventricular tachyarrhythmias following cardiac surgery is uncertain. Of those patients dying from ventricular fibrillation, in whom autopsy was performed, there was no evidence for vein graft occlusion or recent myocardial infarction. More recently, it has been suggested that vein graft occlusion may have caused new-onset malignant ventricular arrhythmias following coronary artery bypass surgery. However, it was not clear that the ventricular arrhythmias had anything to do with surgery as some first episodes occurred as late as 5 months following surgery.[139] In a retrospective report of patients who had undergone various cardiac operations, new sustained ventricular tachycardia or ventricular fibrillation rarely developed. Lidocaine, interestingly, was already being used to suppress ventricular ectopy in many of these patients. Moreover, two of five deaths were related to an adverse effect of antiarrhythmic therapy in these patients. Electrophysiological testing appeared to be useful to predict effective therapy. Two patients died who continued to have ventricular tachycardia inducible by electrophysiological testing, despite medical therapy. The overall early mortality in this patient group was high (44%) with a 1-year mortality of 56%. Refractory hypotension developed in three patients who were treated with bretylium and in one treated with procainamide. The time of the first episode of ventricular tachycardia or ventricular fibrillation was within 48 hours postoperatively in the majority of patients. Some developed their first episode of ventricular tachycardia as late as 6 weeks postoperatively. It appears that following cardiac surgery, the new onset of sustained ventricular tachycardia or ventricular fibrillation is difficult to treat and is associated with a poor short- and long-term prognosis. Electrophysiological testing should be considered for these patients as it may help guide effective antiarrhythmic therapy in some (but clearly not all) patients.

Urgent cardiac surgery of any type poses a higher risk to the patient with preoperative tachycardias or ventricular fibrillation. This is especially true when a recent history of acute myocardial infarction is present. The early post-myocardial infarction or unstable angina patient in whom urgent myocardial revascularization is required becomes a management problem if a preoperative ventricular tachyarrhythmia (including ventricular fibrillation) is diagnosed. Recurrent or refractory ventricular tachyarrhythmias may occur following surgery, but it is difficult to predict who will develop these arrhythmias. Considering the long-term risk of ventricular tachycardia, and the frequent lack of efficacy of antiarrhythmic drugs and their side effects, it is often prudent to consider implantation and testing of epicardial internal defibrillator patch electrodes at the time of cardiac surgery for such patients. Implantation of patch electrodes can apparently be undertaken without adding major operative risk.[147]

Summary

Cardiac arrhythmias are common following cardiac and noncardiac surgery. The conditions under which they occur and their clinical severity is dependent on the underlying cardiac disease and the type of rhythm disturbance. Most are transient and do not require therapy. Treatment must be directed at the serious, hemodynamically intolerable, tachy- and bradyarrhythmias. Treatment of asymptomatic nonsustained atrial or ventricular ectopy has not yet been shown to have benefit.

Acknowledgment: We appreciate the secretarial assistance of Darlene Cognati in the preparation of this manuscript.

References

1. Katz RL, Bigger JT Jr: Cardiac arrhythmias during anesthesia and operation. Anesthesiology 33:193, 1970.
2. Baxandall ML, Thron JL: The nasocardiac reflex. Anesthesia 43:480, 1988.
3. Vanik PE, Davis HS: Cardiac arrhythmias during halothane anesthesia. Anesth Analg 47:299, 1968.
4. Atlee JL: Anesthesia and cardiac electrophysiology. Eur J Anesth 2:215, 1985.
5. Kuner J, Enescu V, Fumihiku U, et al: Cardiac arrhythmias during anesthesia. Dis Chest 52:580, 1967.
6. Reinikainen M, Pöntinen P: On cardiac arrhythmias during anesthesia and surgery. Acta Med Scand 180(suppl):1, 1966.
7. Wetstone DL, Wong KL: Sinus bradycardia and asystole during spinal anesthesia. Anesthesiology 41:87, 1974.
8. Albright GA: Cardiac arrest following regional anesthesia with etidocaine or bupivacaine. Anesthesiology 51:285, 1979.
9. Heavner JM: Cardiac dysrhythmias induced by infusion of local anesthetics into the lateral cerebral ventricle of cats. Anesth Analg 65:133, 1986.
10. Johnston RR, Eger EI, Wilson C: A comparative interaction of epinephrine with enflurane, isoflurane and halothane in man. Anesth Analg 55:709, 1976.
11. Reynolds AK: On the mechanism of myocardial sensitization to catecholamine by hydrocarbon anesthetics. Can J Physiol Pharmacol 62:183, 1984.
12. Hashimoto K: The mechanism of sensitization of the ventricle to epinephrine by halothane. Am Heart J 83:652, 1972.
13. Hashimoto K, Endoh M, Kimura T, et al: Effects of halothane on auto-

maticity and contractile force of isolated blood-perfused canine ventricular tissue. Anesthesiology 42:15, 1975.

14. Pratila MG, Pralilas V: Anesthetic agents and cardiac electromechanical activity. Anesthesiology 49:338, 1978.
15. Duke PC, Fownes O, Wade JG: Halothane depresses baroreflex control of heart rate in man. Anesthesiology 46:184, 1977.
16. Morton M, Duke PC, Ong B: Baroreflex control of heart rate in man awake and during enflurane and enflurane-nitrous oxide anesthesia. Anesthesiology 52:221, 1980.
17. Kotrly K, Ebert TJ, Vucing E, et al: Baroreceptor reflex control of heart rate during isoflurane anesthesia in humans. Anesthesiology 60:173, 1984.
18. Roizen MR, Plummer GO, Lichtor L: Nitrous oxide and dysrhythmias. Anesthesiology 66:427, 1987.
19. Starr NJ, Sethna DH, Estafarious FG: Bradycardia and asystole following the rapid administration of sufentanil with vercuronium. Anesthesiology 64:521, 1986.
20. Nauta J, Koopman D, Spierdijk J, et al: Alfentanil, a new narcotic anesthetic induction agent. Anesth Analg 61:267, 1982.
21. Salmenpera M, Peltola K, Takkunen O, et al: Cardiovascular effects of pancuronium and vecuronium during high-dose fentanyl anesthesia. Anesth Analg 62:1059, 1983.
22. Heinonen J, Salmenpera M, Suomivuori M: Contribution of muscle relaxant to the hemodynamic course of high-dose fentanyl anesthesia: a comparison of pancuronium, vecuronium and atracurium. Can Anaesth Soc J 33:597, 1986.
23. Sadowski AR, Moyers JR: Anesthetic management of the Wolff-Parkinson-White syndrome. Anesthesiology 51:553, 1979.
24. Gomez-Arnau J, Marquez-Montes J, Avello F: Fentanyl and droperidol effects on the refractoriness of the accessory pathway in the Wolff-Parkinson-White syndrome. Anesthesiology 58:307, 1983.
25. Katz J, Kadis L: Anesthesia and Uncommon Disorders. Philadelphia, WB Saunders, 1973, pp 217–219.
26. Van der Starre PJA: Wolff-Parkinson-White syndrome during anesthesia. Anesthesiology 48:369, 1978.
27. McGovern B: Hypokalemia and cardiac arrhythmias. Anesthesiology 63:127, 1985.
28. Vitez TS, Soper LE, Wong KC, et al: Chronic hypokalemia and intraoperative dysrhythmias. Anesthesiology 63:130, 1985.
29. Hirsch IA, Tomlinson DL, Slogoff S, et al: The over-stated risk of preoperative hypokalemia. Anesth Analg 67:131, 1988.
30. Chernow B, Bamberger, Stolko M, et al: Hypomagnesemia in postoperative intensive care. Chest 95:391, 1989.
31. Angelini P, Feldman MI, Lufschanowski R, et al: Cardiac arrhythmias during and after heart surgery: Diagnosis and management. Prog Cardiovasc Dis 26:469, 1974.
32. Dodd RB, Sims WA, Bone DJ: Cardiac arrhythmias observed during anesthesia. Surgery 51:440, 1962.
33. Goldman L, Caldera DL, Southwick, FS, et al: Cardiac risk factors and complications in non-cardiac surgery. Medicine 57:357, 1978.

34. Gray RJ, Bateman TM, Czer LS, et al: Esmolol: a new ultrashort-acting beta-adrenergic blocking agent for rapid control of heart rate in postoperative supraventricular tachyarrhythmias. J Am Coll Cardiol 5:1451, 1985.
35. Wells PH, Kaplan JA: Optimal management of patients with ischemic heart disease for noncardiac surgery by complementary anesthesiologist and cardiologist interaction. Curr Cardiol 12:1029, 1981.
36. Gallagher J, Gessman LJ, Moreno P, et al: Electrophysiologic effects of halothane and quinidine on canine Purkinje fibres: evidence for a synergistic interaction. Anesthesiology 65:278, 1986.
37. Kron IL, Nolan SP: Severe hypotension due to the use of bretylium for postcardiotomy ventricular arrhythmias. Ann Thorac Surg 35:271, 1983.
38. Vandam LD, McLemore GA Jr: Circulatory arrest in patients with complete heart block during anesthesia and surgery. Am J Med 47:518, 1957.
39. Kunstadt D, Punja M, Cagin N, et al: Bifascicular block: a clinical and electrophysiologic study. Am Heart J 86:173, 1973.
40. McAnulty JH, Rahimtoola SH, Murphy, et al: Natural history of "high risk" bundle branch block. N Engl J Med 307:137, 1982.
41. Zaidan JR: Pacemakers. In: Cardiac Anesthesia. JA Kapkin (ed), New York, Grune and Stratton, 1979, pp 347–367.
42. McAnulty JH, Rahimtoola SH: Bundle branch block. Prog Cardiovasc Dis 26:333, 1983.
43. Jaruszewski FJ, Hellerstein HK, Feil H: Electrocardiographic studies during cardiac surgery. Circulation 7:175, 1953.
44. Spanos PK, Brown AL, McGoon DC: The significance of intraoperative ventricular fibrillation during aortic valve replacement. J Thorac Cardiovasc Surg 73:605, 1977.
45. Hottenrott CE, Towers B, Kurkji HJ, et al: The hazard of ventricular fibrillation in hypertrophied ventricles during cardiopulmonary bypass. J Thorac Cardiovasc Surg 66:742, 1973.
46. Salerno TA, Stefaniszyn HJ: Brief communications. Spontaneous ventricular fibrillation occurring immediately after institution of cardiopulmonary bypass: possible clinical implications. J Thorac Cardiovasc Surg 86:306, 1983.
47. Caspi J, Amar R, Elami A, et al: Frequency and significance of complete atrioventricular block after coronary artery bypass grafting. Am J Cardiol 63:526, 1989.
48. O'Connell JB, Wallis D, Johnson SA, et al: Transient bundle branch block following use of hypothermic cardioplegia in coronary artery bypass surgery: high incidence without perioperative myocardial infarction. Am Heart J 103:85, 1982.
49. Zeldis SM, Morganroth J, Horowitz LN, et al: Fascicular conduction disturbances after coronary bypass surgery. Am J Cardiol 41:860, 1978.
50. Wexelman W, Lichstein E, Cunningham JN, et al: Etiology and clinical significance of new fascicular conduction defects following coronary bypass surgery. Am Heart J 111:923, 1986.
51. Bateman TM, Weiss MH, Czer LS, et al: Fascicular conduction disturbances and ischemic heart disease: Adverse prognosis despite coronary revascularization. J Am Coll Cardiol 5:632, 1985.

52. Chu A, Califf RM, Pryor DB, et al: Prognostic effect of bundle branch block related to coronary artery bypass grafting. Am J Cardiol 59:798, 1987.
53. Høie J, Forfang K: Arrhythmias and conduction disturbances following aortic valve implantation. Scand J Thorac Cardiovasc Surg 14:177, 1980.
54. Keefe DL, Griffin JC, Harrison DC, et al: Atrioventricular conduction abnormalities in patients undergoing isolated aortic or mitral valve replacement. PACE 8:393, 1985.
55. Baerman JM, Kirsh MM, deBuitleir M, et al: Natural history and determinants of conduction defects following coronary artery bypass surgery. Ann Thorac Surg 44:150, 1987.
56. Silverman NA, DuBrow I, Kohler J, et al: Etiology of atrioventricular-conduction abnormalities following cardiac surgery. J Surg Res 36:198, 1984.
57. Ferguson TB, Smith PK, Buhrman WC, et al: Monitoring of the electrical status of the ventricle during cardioplegic arrest. Circulation 68:II27, 1983.
58. Smith PK, Buhrman WC, Ferguson TB, et al: Conduction block after cardioplegia arrest: prevention by augmented atrial hypothermia. Circulation 68:41, 1983.
59. Magilligan DJ, Vij D, Peper W, et al: Failure of standard cardioplegic techniques to protect the conducting system. Ann Thorac Surg 39:403, 1985.
60. Ellis RJ, Mavroudis C, Gardner C, et al: Relationship between atrioventricular arrhythmias and the concentration of K^+ ion in cardioplegic solution. J Thorac Cardiovasc Surg 80:517, 1980.
61. Thompson R, Mitchell A, Ahmed M, et al: Conduction defects in aortic valve disease. Am Heart J 98:3, 1979.
62. Rosenbaum MB, Corrado G, Oliveri R, et al: Right bundle branch block with left anterior hemiblock surgically induced in Tetrology of Fallot. Am J Cardiol 26:12, 1970.
63. Van Lier TA, Harinck E, Hitchcock JF: Complete right bundle branch block after surgical closure of perimembraneous ventricular septal defect. Eur Heart J 6:959, 1985.
64. Marquez-Montes J, O'Connor F, Burgos R, et al: Comparative electrophysiological evaluation of atrial activation and sinoatrial node function following Senning and Mustard procedures: an experimental study. Ann Thorac Surg 36:692, 1983.
65. Irnich W, Barold SS: Interference protection in cardiac pacemakers. In: Modern Cardiac Pacing. Barold SS (ed), Mt. Kisco, Futura Publishing Co., 1985, pp 839–856.
66. Hayes DL: Practical Considerations. In: A Practice of Cardiac Pacing. Furman S, Hayes DL, Holmes L (eds), Mt. Kisco, Futura Publishing Co., 1986, pp 451–462.
67. Sager DP: Current facts on pacemaker electromagnetic interference and their application to clinical care. Heart Lung 16:211, 1987.
68. Domino KB, Smith TC: Electrocautery-induced reprogramming of a pacemaker using a precordial magnet. Anesth Analg 62:609, 1983.
69. Belott PH, Sands S, Warren J: Resetting of DDD pacemakers due to EMI. PACE 7:169, 1984.
70. Bourke J, Gold RG, Adams PC, et al: Diathermy-induced loss of DDD pacemaker identity. Ann Thorac Surg 40:97, 1985.

71. Sebben JE: Electrosurgery and cardiac pacemakers. J Am Acad Dermatol 9:457, 1983.
72. Thomas AC, Moser SA, Smutka MC, et al: Implantable defibrillation: eight years clinical experience. PACE 11:2053, 1988.
73. Marchlinski F, Flores BT, Buxton, et al: The automatic implantable cardioverter defibrillator: efficacy complications and device failures. Ann Int Med 104:481, 1986.
74. Cannom OS, Winkle A: Implantation of the automatic implantable cardioverter defibrillator (AICD): practical aspects. PACE 9:793, 1986.
75. Troup PJ: Lessons learned from the automatic implantable cardioverter defibrillator: past, present and future. J Am Coll Cardiol 11:1287, 1988.
76. Rahimtoola SH: Management of patients with heart disease for noncardiac surgery. JAMA 246:1348, 1981.
77. Ghosh P, Pakrashi BC: Cardiac dysrhythmias after thoracotomy. Br Heart J 34:374, 1972.
78. Feinleib M, Havlik RJ, Gillum RF, et al: Coronary heart disease and related procedures: National Hospital Discharge Survey Data. Circulation 79:I-13, 1989.
79. Chee TP, Prakash S, Desser KB, et al: Postoperative supraventricular arrhythmias and the role of prophylactic digoxin in cardiac surgery. Am Heart J 104:974, 1982.
80. White HD, Antman EM, Glynn MA, et al: Efficacy and safety of timolol for prevention of supraventricular tachyarrhythmias after coronary artery bypass surgery. Circulation 70:479, 1984.
81. Thormann J, Schwarz F: Long-term observations of cardiac arrhythmias during and after surgery. I. Acquired heart disease. Scand J Thorac Surg 10:31, 1976.
82. Thormann JH, Schwarz F: Long-term observation of cardiac arrhythmias during and after cardiac surgery. II. Congenital heart disease. Scand J Thorac Surg 10:149, 1976.
83. Michelson EL, Morganroth J, MacVaugh H: Postoperative arrhythmias after coronary artery and cardiac valvular surgery detected by long-term electrocardiographic monitoring. Am Heart J 97:442, 1979.
84. Rubin DA, Nieminski KE, Reed GE, et al: Predictors, prevention, and long-term prognosis of atrial fibrillation after coronary artery bypass graft operations. J Thorac Cardiovasc Surg 94:331, 1987.
85. Parker FB, Greiner-Hayes C, Bove EL, et al: Supraventricular arrhythmias following coronary artery bypass. J Thorac Cardiovasc Surg 86:594, 1983.
86. Gavaghan TP, Feneley MP, Campbell TJ, et al: Atrial tachyarrhythmias after cardiac surgery: results of disopyramide therapy. Aust N Z J Med 15:27, 1985.
87. Douglas PS, Hirshfeld JW Jr, Edmunds LH Jr: Clinical correlates of atrial tachyarrhythmias after valve replacement for aortic stenosis. Circulation 72:II159, 1985.
88. Roffman JA, Fieldman A: Digoxin and propranolol in the prophylaxis of supraventricular tachydysrhythmias after coronary artery bypass surgery. Ann Thorac Surg 31:496, 1981.
89. Fuller JA, Adams GG, Buxton B: Atrial fibrillation after coronary artery

bypass grafting: Is it a disorder of the elderly? J Thorac Cardiovasc Surg 97:821, 1989.

90. Ormerod OJM, McGregor CGA, Stone DL, et al: Arrhythmias after coronary bypass surgery. Br Heart J 51:618, 1984.

91. Dixon FE, Genton E, Vacek JL, et al: Factors predisposing to supraventricular tachyarrhythmias after coronary artery bypass grafting. Am J Cardiol 58:476, 1986.

92. Wilber DJ, Olshansky B, Blakeman B, et al: Determinants of early implantable defibrillator discharges: role of coronary revascularization (abstract). Circulation (in press).

93. Waldo AL, MacLean WA, Cooper TA, et al: Use of temporarily placed epicardial atrial wire electrodes for the diagnosis and treatment of cardiac arrhythmias following open-heart surgery. J Thorac Cardiovasc Surg 76:500, 1978.

94. Dailey SM, Kay GN, Epstein AE, et al: Comparison of endocardial and epicardial programmed stimulation for the induction of ventricular tachycardia. J Am Coll Cardiol 13:1608, 1989.

95. Harris PD, Malm JR, Bowman FO Jr, et al: Epicardial pacing to control arrhythmias following cardiac surgery. Circulation 37:178, 1968.

96. Harris PD, Singer DH, Malen JR: Chronically implanted epicardial leads in man (abstract). Physiologist 9:199, 1966.

97. DeSanctis RW: Diagnostic and therapeutic uses of atrial pacing. Circulation 43:748, 1971.

98. Mills NL, Ochsner JL: Experience with atrial pacemaker wires implanted during cardiac operations. J Thorac Cardiovasc Surg 66:878, 1973.

99. Humes RA, Porter CJ, Puga FJ, et al: Utility of temporary atrial epicardial electrodes in postoperative pediatric cardiac patients. Mayo Clin Proc 64:516, 1989.

100. Pagé PL, Plumb VJ, Okumura K, et al: A new animal model of atrial flutter. J Am Coll Cardiol 8:872, 1986.

101. Mullen JC, Khan N, Weisel RD, et al: Atrial activity during cardioplegia and postoperative arrhythmias. J Thorac Cardiovasc Surg 94:558, 1987.

102. Lake CL, Sellers TD, Crosby IK, et al: Effects of coronary grafting technique upon reperfusion cardiac rhythm, ventricular function, and other variables. Am Surg 51:497, 1985.

103. Litwak RS, Kuhn LA, Gadboys HL, et al: Support of myocardial performance after open cardiac operations by rate augmentation. J Thorac Cardiovasc Surg 56:484, 1968.

104. Raichlen JS, Campbell FW, Edie RN, et al: The effect of the site of placement of temporary epicardial pacemakers on ventricular function in patients undergoing cardiac surgery. Circulation 70:118, 1984.

105. Tchervenkov CI, Wynands E, Symes JF, et al: Persistent atrial activity during cardioplegic arrest: a possible factor in the etiology of postoperative supraventricular tachyarrhythmias. Ann Thorac Surg 36:437, 1983.

106. Coumel P, Escoubet B, Attuel P: Beta-blocking therapy in atrial and ventricular tachyarrhythmias: experience with nadolol. Am Heart J 108:1098, 1984.

107. Harrison DC, Griffin JR, Fiene TJ: Effects of beta-adrenergic blockade with

propranolol in patients with atrial arrhythmias. N Engl J Med 273:410, 1965.

108. Wollenberger A, Shabab L: Anoxia-induced release of noradrenaline from isolated perfused heart. Nature 207:88, 1965.

109. Reves JG, Karp RB, Buttner EE, et al: Neuronal and adrenal catecholamine release in response to cardiopulmonary bypass in man. Circulation 66:49, 1982.

110. Engelman RM, Haag B, Lemeshow S, et al: Mechanism of plasma catecholamine increases during coronary artery bypass and valve procedures. J Thorac Cardiovasc Surg 86:608, 1983.

111. Wells JL, MacLean WAH, James TN, et al: Characterization of atrial flutter: studies in man after open heart surgery using fixed atrial electrodes. Circulation 60:665, 1979.

112. Waldo AL, Henthorn RW, Epstein AE, et al: Diagnosis and treatment of arrhythmias during and following open heart surgery. Med Clin N Am 68:1153, 1984.

113. Waldo AL, Henthorn RW, Plumb VJ: Atrial flutter and atrial fibrillation: drug therapy and recent observations. Ann NY Acad Sci 432:258, 1984.

114. Olshansky B, Okumura K, Henthorn RW, et al: Entrainment of human atrial flutter localizes the area of slow conduction in the inferior right atrium. J Am Coll Cardiol 7:128A, 1986.

115. Olshansky B, Okumura K, Henthorn W, et al: Atrial mapping of human atrial flutter demonstrates re-entry in the right atrium. J Am Coll Cardiol 7:194A, 1986.

116. Leone L, Silverman A, Siouffi S, et al: Efficacy of nadolol in preventing supraventricular tachycardia after coronary artery bypass grafting. Am J Cardiol 60:51D, 1987.

117. Silverman NA, Wright R, Lefitsky S: Efficacy of low-dose propranolol in preventing postoperative supraventricular tachyarrhythmias: a prospective, randomized study. Ann Surg 196:194, 1982.

118. Daudon P, Corcos T, Gandjbakhch I, et al: Prevention of atrial fibrillation or flutter by acebutolol after coronary bypass grafting. Am J Cardiol 58:933, 1986.

119. Oka Y, Frishman W, Becker RM, et al: Clinical pharmacology of the new beta-adrenergic blocking drugs. Part 10. Beta-adrenoceptor blockade and coronary artery surgery. Am Heart J 99:255, 1980.

120. Janssen J, Loomans L, Harink J, et al: Prevention and treatment of supraventricular tachycardia shortly after coronary artery bypass grafting: a randomized open trial. Angiology 37:601, 1986.

121. Mills SA, Poole GV, Breyer RH, et al: Digoxin and propranolol in the prophylaxis of dysrhythmias after coronary artery bypass grafting. Circulation 68:222, 1983.

122. Lauer MS, Eagle KA, Buckley MJ, et al: Atrial fibrillation following coronary artery bypass surgery. Prog Cardiovasc Dis 31:367, 1989.

123. Khuri SF, Okike ON, Josa M, et al: Efficacy of nadolol in preventing supraventricular tachycardia after coronary artery bypass grafting. Am J Cardiol 60:51D, 1987.

124. Ivey MF, Ivey TD, Bailey WW, et al: Influence of propranolol on supra-

ventricular tachycardia early after coronary artery revascularization: a randomized trial. J Thorac Cardiovasc Surg 85:214, 1983.

125. Parker F, Greiner-Hayes C, Bove EL, et al: Supraventricular arrhythmias following coronary artery bypass. J Thorac Cardiovasc Surg 86:594, 1983.
126. Tyras DH, Stothert JC, Kaiser GC, et al: Supraventricular tachyarrhythmias after myocardial revascularization: a randomized trial of prophylactic digitalization. J Thorac Cardiovasc Surg 77:310, 1979.
127. Csicsko JF, Schatzlein MH, King RD: Immediate postoperative digitalization in the prophylaxis of supraventricular arrhythmias following coronary artery bypass. J Thorac Cardiovasc Surg 81:419, 1981.
128. Rose MR, Glassman, Spencer FC: Arrhythmias following cardiac surgery: relation to serum digoxin levels. Am Heart J 89:288, 1975.
129. Cooper TB, Mac Lean WAH, Waldo A: Overdrive pacing for supraventricular tachycardia. PACE 1:196, 1978.
130. Olshansky B, Okumura K, Hess PG, et al: Use of procainamide with rapid atrial pacing for successful conversion of atrial flutter to sinus rhythm. J Am Coll Cardiol 11:359, 1988.
131. Davies RF, Dube LM, Mousseau N, et al: Perioperative variability of binding of lidocaine, quinidine, and propranolol after cardiac operations. J Thorac Cardiovasc Surg 96:634, 1988.
132. Waldo AL, Plumb VJ, Arciniegas JG, et al: Verapamil therapy in the treatment of supraventricular arrhythmias following open heart surgery. Angiology 34:755, 1983.
133. Waldo AL, MacLean WAH, Karp R, et al: Continuous rapid atrial pacing to control recurrent or sustained supraventricular tachycardias following open heart surgery. Circulation 54:245, 1976.
134. Campbell TJ, Morgan JJ: Treatment of atrial arrhythmias after cardiac surgery with intravenous disopyramide. Aust NZ J Med 10:644, 1980.
135. Stanton MS, Prystowsky EN, Fineberg NS, et al: Arrhythmogenic effects of antiarrhythmic drugs: a study of 506 patients treated for ventricular tachycardia or fibrillation. J Am Coll Cardiol 14:209, 1989.
136. Garson A, Randall DC, Gillette PC, et al: Prevention of sudden death after repair of tetralogy of Fallot: treatment of ventricular arrhythmias. J Am Coll Cardiol 6:221, 1985.
137. Olshausen KV, Amann E, Hofmann M, et al: Ventricular arrhythmias before and late after aortic valve replacement. Am J Cardiol 54:142, 1984.
138. DeSoyza N, Thenabada PN, Murphy ML, et al: Ventricular arrhythmias before and after coronary bypass surgery. Int J Cardiol 1:123, 1981.
139. Topol EJ, Lerman BB, Baughman KL, et al: De novo refractory ventricular tachyarrhythmias after coronary revascularization. Am J Cardiol 57:57, 1986.
140. Föppl M, Hoffmann A, Amann FW, et al: Sudden cardiac death after aortic valve surgery: incidence and concomitant factors. Clin Cardiol 12:202, 1989.
141. Gradman AH, Harbison MA, Berger HJ, et al: Ventricular arrhythmias late after aortic valve replacement and their relation to left ventricular performance. Am J Cardiol 48:824, 1981.
142. Rubin DA, Nieminski KE, Monteferrante JC, et al: Ventricular arrhythmias after coronary artery bypass graft surgery: incidence, risk factors and long-term prognosis. J Am Coll Cardiol 6:307, 1985.

143. Goenen M, Jacquemart JL, Gulvez, et al: Preoperative left ventricular dysfunction and operative risks in coronary bypass surgery. Chest 92:804, 1987.
144. Kron IL, DiMarco JP, Harman PK, et al: Unanticipated postoperative ventricular tachyarrhythmias. Ann Thorac Surg 38:317, 1984.
145. Kyosola AU, Mattila K, Harjula T, et al: Life-threatening complications of cardiac operations and occurrence of myocardial catecholamine bombs. J Thorac Cardiovasc Surg 95:334, 1988.
146. Huikuri HV, Korhonen VR, Takkanen JT: Ventricular arrhythmias induced by dynamic and static exercise. Am J Cardiol 55:948, 1985.
147. Manolis AS, Rastegar H, Estes NAM: Prophylactic automatic implantable cardioverter-defibrillator patches in patients at high risk for postoperative ventricular tachyarrhythmias. J Am Coll Cardiol 13:1367, 1989.

Chapter 13

What Physicians Who Treat Primarily Adults Need to Know About Managing Arrhythmias in the Pediatric Patient

James C. Perry and Arthur Garson, Jr.

Introduction

The point has been made by pediatricians that, in matters of health care, "children are not little adults." This is no less true in the realm of pediatric cardiac arrhythmias. Similarities do exist in the electrocardiographic appearance and acute therapy of many pediatric arrhythmias when compared to their adult counterparts. The physician who cares for adult patients has a "head start" with a fund of knowledge for decision-making when confronted with an infant, child, or adolescent with a cardiac arrhythmia. However, differences in the presumed substrate, clinical presentation, electrocardiographic appearance, and therapy of some pediatric arrhythmias are important. In addition, some teenagers and young adults, especially after repair of congenital heart defects, despite their "advanced age" are more similar to younger children. It is the purpose of this chapter to point out some of the differences that have direct bearing on age-appropriate management.

From Naccarelli GV (ed): *Cardiac Arrhythmias: A Practical Approach.* Mount Kisco, NY, Futura Publishing Co., Inc., © 1991.

Different ECG Morphologies and Mechanisms of Arrhythmias

The basic tenets of surface electrocardiographic arrhythmia diagnosis for adults apply to children as well. There are distinct age-related differences of both heart rate and the incidence of certain arrhythmias within the pediatric population. The first aspect, differences in heart rate, is relatively straightforward. The range of "normal" heart rates varies as a function of age, largely due to progressive maturation of cardiovascular control by the autonomic nervous system. The normal mean heart rate increases from 123/min at birth to 149/min by the end of the second month of life.[1] Heart rate then gradually declines to reach a mean of 119/min by 1–2 years and 85/min in early adolescence. The diagnosis of sinus bradycardia is therefore age-dependent (Table 1). For example, the newborn with a heart rate of 100/min may have sinus bradycardia, whereas this is sinus tachycardia for an adult. A rough guide for potentially significant bradycardia while awake is 60–70/min for an infant, 50–60/min for a child, and 40–50/min for an adolescent.

A slow ventricular rate in the newborn has many causes. Blocked premature atrial contractions (PACs)—atrial beats that do not conduct to the ventricles—are a relatively common occurrence in newborns (Fig. 1). Though they can serve as a trigger for arrhythmia in a patient with

Table 1
Range of Normal Heart Rates by Age

Age Group	Heart Rate	Mean
Less than 1 day	93–154	123
1–2 days	91–159	123
3–6 days	91–166	129
1–3 weeks	107–182	148
1–2 months	121–179	149
3–5 months	106–186	141
6–11 months	109–169	134
1–2 years	89–151	119
3–4 years	73–137	108
5–7 years	65–133	100
8–11 years	62–130	91
12–15 years	60–119	85

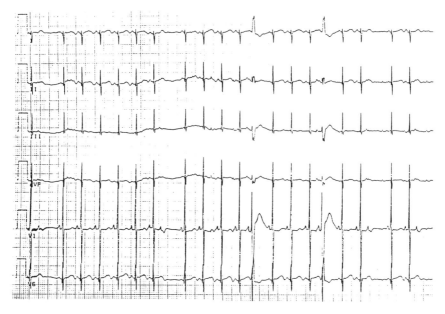

Figure 1. Premature atrial contractions in a newborn. This tracing shows both blocked PACs (at a P-P interval of 240 ms) and PACs conducted with aberrancy (P-P interval of 270 ms).

the proper substrate (e.g., a bypass tract) or result in somewhat slow ventricular rates, blocked PACs are benign. They generally disappear by 3 months of age and do not require therapy. Bradycardia in the newborn may also be due to congenital complete atrioventricular block (CCAVB). In nearly half of cases, there is clinical or laboratory evidence of a maternal collagen vascular disease, most often systemic lupus erythematosus.[2] Antibodies associated with this disorder, anti-Rho (SSA), may cross the placenta and react with the heart (primarily conduction tissue) in the fetus, resulting in abnormalities of AV conduction. Most newborns with CCAVB have an adequate junctional escape rate and do not have evidence of hemodynamic compromise. With an otherwise normal heart, a ventricular rate above 60 is usually well tolerated, while most of those below 50 have symptoms. Some patients, in fact, may not be discovered until several years of age, when a presumptive diagnosis of "congenital" complete AV block is made. Of note, infants with CCAVB are at a higher risk of having symptoms and sudden death if the corrected QT interval is also prolonged[3] (Fig. 2). This occurs in ap-

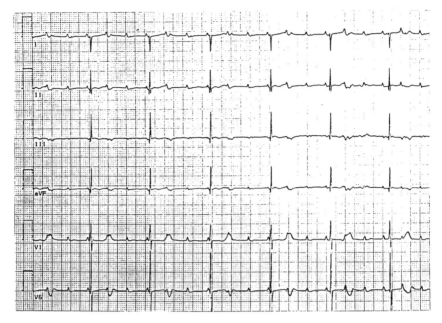

Figure 2. Congenital complete atrioventricular block with prolonged QTc. The ventricular rate is 48/min and the QTc is 0.46 seconds.

proximately 20% of these infants and is an indication for therapy, regardless of heart rate.

Junctional ectopic tachycardia (JET or nonparoxysmal junctional tachycardia) is occasionally seen in the adult following acute myocardial infarction.[4] This arrhythmia has a congenital form as well, although the underlying substrate is likely to differ. Congenital JET has rates of 140 to 300/min and is generally unresponsive to conventional medical therapy; amiodarone has been reported to be effective.[5] This arrhythmia carries a grave prognosis (37% mortality) and its prompt recognition (Fig. 3) is therefore of obvious importance. JET also occurs in children in the postoperative setting (ventricular septal defect, tetralogy of Fallot, Mustard operation, atrioventricular canal defect). It also occurs occasionally following the arterial switch procedure for d-transposition of the great arteries. JET in the postoperative patient can cause severe reduction of cardiac output and also is resistant to many standard medical interventions. We have found that an appropriate initial approach to postoperative JET consists of cooling the patient (by use of a cooling blanket) to 35–36°C. This usually slows the junctional rate adequately.

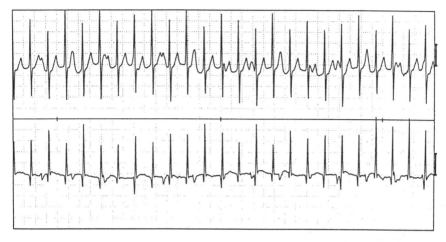

Figure 3. Congenital junctional ectopic tachycardia. The rate is 188/min and AV dissociation is evident.

At that time, atrioventricular sequential pacing at a reasonable rate is then possible, using epicardial wires placed at the time of surgery. Digoxin may slow the JET slightly but should improve contractility. We have reported the use of propafenone for this arrhythmia.[6] The drug causes significant hypotension, and volume loading is therefore a necessary part of its use.

A form of "chaotic atrial tachycardia" (CAT) occurs in infants (Fig. 4). An analogous arrhythmia in adult patients might be the atrial tachyarrhythmia seen in the face of hypoxic pulmonary disease. This arrhythmia manifests frequent shifts of P wave axis and morphology and has atrial rates ranging from 200 to 500/min. Brief runs of atrial flutter and atrial fibrillation may also be apparent on the ECG. High-grade AV block frequently co-exists with CAT, but ventricular rates can still be very fast and irregular. Some help in understanding the cellular basis of this arrhythmia may be derived from investigations of the development of atrial muscle action potentials and automaticity. Several studies[7–9] showing rapid atrial conduction velocities, short refractory periods, parasympathetic dominance, and developmental changes in potassium currents may play a role in the initiation and maintenance of this rapid atrial arrhythmia. It is likely that the mechanisms allowing triggering and maintenance of this arrhythmia incorporate many of the classic notions of automaticity, micro re-entry and macro re-entry.

The diagnosis of atrial flutter is based on the classic ECG "sawtooth"

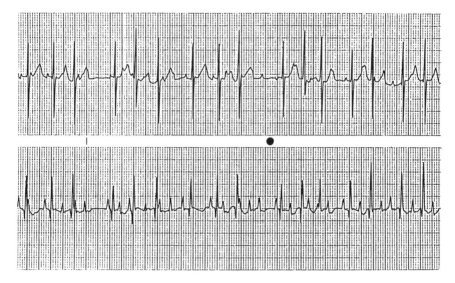

Figure 4. Chaotic atrial tachycardia in a newborn. The atrial rate varies from 136–375/min and the P wave morphology changes in the upper tracing.

pattern in the inferior and lateral leads. After the first year of life, atrial flutter is most commonly found in the child who has undergone atrial surgery for congenital heart disease. In these patients, probably due to the altered anatomy by scarring, atrial flutter is likely to consist of the surface ECG appearance of small, flat flutter waves with isoelectric periods, making diagnosis difficult (Fig. 5). In atrial flutter, atrial rates can range from 200 to 500/min, with variable AV conduction. One extremely important difference between adults and children is that in children and even in young adults, one-to-one conduction frequently occurs. As in adults, the atrial rate is slower in patients on antiarrhythmic agents (especially amiodarone). Atrial flutter may also occur in patients with cardiomyopathy, pericarditis, mitral valve prolapse, and rheumatic disease. It has been shown by intracardiac electrophysiology study[10] and operative mapping studies[11,12] that there are critical areas of very slow conduction in atrial muscle in patients following atrial surgery for congenital heart defects. Tachycardia may then be maintained by a re-entrant mechanism that incorporates these slow areas bordering the long suture lines inherent in the surgical procedure.

The permanent form of junctional reciprocating tachycardia (PJRT) occurs more frequently in children than in adults. The anatomical sub-

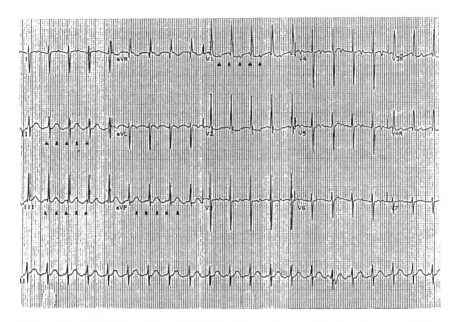

Figure 5. Atrial flutter in a child after Mustard operation for d-transposition of the great arteries. Note the low voltage flutter waves (arrowheads) and the intervening isoelectric period. The flutter cycle length is 310 ms and 2:1 AV conduction occurs.

strate of PJRT likely consists of antegrade conduction through the AV node and retrograde conduction through a slowly conducting pathway that may have decremental properties and enters the atrium at the mouth of the coronary sinus.[13,14] During tachycardia, rates of 120–250/ min can occur and a 1:1 AV relationship necessarily exists. Because of slow retrograde conduction, the retrograde P wave (P') appears closer to the QRS complex that follows than to the preceding QRS, resulting in a longer R-P' than P'-R during tachycardia (Fig. 6). The P' waves in tachycardia are deeply inverted in leads II, III, and AVF. Differential diagnosis (based on the ECG) includes low right atrial ectopic tachycardia, "fast-slow" AV node re-entry, atrial flutter with 2:1 AV conduction, His bundle re-entry, Ebstein's anomaly with accessory connection, and a decrementally conducting right-sided accessory connection. The diagnosis can usually be surmised from Holter monitoring, but can be easily demonstrated in the electrophysiology laboratory.

As the posterior septal area is densely populated with parasym-

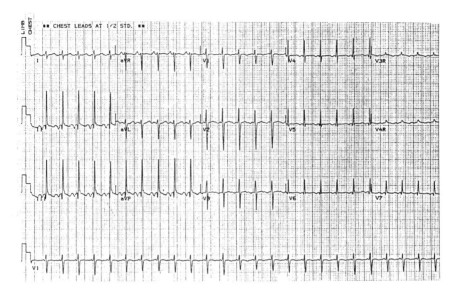

Figure 6. The permanent form of junctional reciprocating tachycardia. See text for explanation.

pathetic ganglia, it is conceivable that postganglionic fibers of these ganglia play either a primary or a secondary role in mediating PJRT. As autonomic influences change with age, it is possible that the substrate for PJRT no longer sustains tachycardia. The fact that PJRT is so rare in adults implies that the arrhythmia either resolves at some point during childhood or that patients with PJRT do not survive until adulthood.

Two forms of ventricular tachycardia (VT) in children deserve special mention: (1) incessant (present most of the day) VT associated with ventricular hamartomas in children under age 3 years and (2) VT occurring after repair of a congenital heart defect. Whereas VT in the adult typically occurs following myocardial infarction and is presumed to involve a re-entrant mechanism, the "mechanism" of these pediatric forms of VT is less clear.

Incessant infant VT may present as a relatively narrow QRS (0.06–0.11 sec), rapid tachycardia. There may be evidence of AV dissociation and the QRS has a different morphology from that seen in sinus rhythm. VT rates in infants are usually 250–300/min (Fig. 7), but can be as fast as 500/min.[15] Females outnumber males by 2:1. The typical presentation is cardiac arrest or severe congestive heart failure. In incessant VT, the etiology most often has been a myocardial hamartoma that is so small

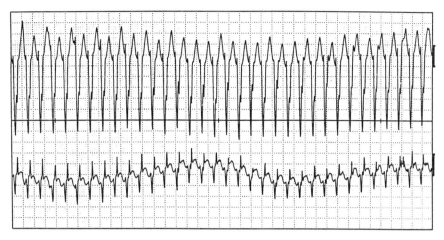

Figure 7. Ventricular tachycardia in an infant. Note the relatively narrow QRS complexes.

that it is detected only at surgery. Nearly half of these patients have a right bundle branch block with left axis deviation and tumors located in the left ventricular septum or apex. Occasionally, tumor is spread over the endocardial surface in a "candle wax" appearance. Some of these patients may have disruption of the electrical isolation of atrium and ventricle and have ECG manifestation of pre-excitation in sinus rhythm.

Microelectrode studies of excised hamartomatous tissue and surrounding ventricular myocardium have shown that the "tumor'" tissue itself is electrically silent.[16] VT probably occurs as a micro re-entrant circuit at the border of the tumor where myocardial cell anisotropy and discontinuity due to the tumor are evident.

Sudden death is a well-recognized risk in the patient who has undergone surgery for congenital heart defect, most notably tetralogy of Fallot. During electrophysiology study, as many as 33% of postoperative tetralogy patients will have inducible nonsustained VT[17,18] and 10% will have sustained VT. Recently, it has been recognized that 26% of postoperative transposition (atrial switch) patients will have nonsustained or sustained ventricular tachycardia (C. Marchal, personal communication). Many of these arrhythmias develop clinically several years following repair, leading to the hypothesis that extensive scarring in the region of the repair provides the substrate for arrhythmia. Additionally, partial cardiac autonomic denervation at the time of surgery and subsequent reinnervation may contribute to the late appearance of these arrhythmias. Adrenergic hypersensitivity in the border zones of myocardial infarction has been documented and is felt to play a part in the development of postinfarction VT.[19] A similar mechanism may be applicable after ventriculotomy.

Differences in Acute Arrhythmia Intervention

One of the more important facets of acute termination of pediatric arrhythmias and intervention for bradyarrhythmias is an appreciation of what a "sick" infant or young child looks like. An infant who is sick because of arrhythmia may show the following: poor feeding or frequent "rest periods" during feeding, lethargy, decreased muscle tone, poor capillary refill, and intercostal retractions. A gravely ill infant is extremely pale and/or mottled, diaphoretic, and has difficult-to-palpate peripheral pulses. The infant with a heart rate of 140/min, a respiratory rate of 30/min, and a blood pressure of 80/50 mm Hg may be perfectly normal, whereas these vital signs for an adult would be alarming.

Figure 8 shows the approach to acute management of supraventricular tachycardia (SVT) in children. Classic vagal maneuvers tend to be unsuccessful under the age of 4 years but may be extremely effective in the adolescent who has taught himself to stop tachycardia by gagging, using the Valsalva maneuver, or standing on his head. Use of the "diving reflex" is generally applied to infants. This maneuver consists of placing a plastic bag (or surgical glove) filled with ice water over the infant's face for 15–20 seconds. Apnea may play a role in the response. It is prudent to have intravenous access, as significant bradycardia may follow termination of tachycardia. Ocular pressure as a vagal stimulant should be avoided because of the risk of retinal detachment. Transesophageal overdrive pacing of SVT is readily accomplished in the infant and young child. Adolescents are less accepting of the nasogastric electrode tube and some even reject the pill electrode. Atrial electrograms can be recorded and atrial tissue paced from the esophagus using a pulse width of 10 milliseconds and an output of 10–20 milliamperes.[20,21] It is imperative to obtain a standard ECG following conversion to normal sinus rhythm. If the QRS morphology in sinus rhythm differs from that seen during tachycardia, then the tachycardia was most likely VT, as "SVT with aberrancy" is a rarity in pediatric patients.

A major point must be made regarding the use of intravenous verapamil for the conversion of SVT in children. Its use in patients under

Supraventricular tachycardia

1. Ice bag
2. Vagal maneuvers
3. Transesophageal pacing
4. Adenosine, ATP

Hemodynamic compromise?

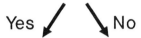

Yes / \ No

1. DC cardioversion (0.25-2.0 w-s/kg, Lidocaine if on digoxin)	1. IV verapamil (OK if >1 yo, no CHF and no beta-blockers)
2. Transvenous pacing	2. IV digoxin (D/C if WPW in NSR)
	3. IV procainamide

Figure 8. Acute management of SVT. WPW = Wolff-Parkinson-White syndrome; CHF = congestive heart failure; NSR = normal sinus rhythm.

1 year of age is contraindicated because of the significant hypotension and bradycardia that occur.[22] Verapamil should also be avoided in those patients on beta-adrenergic blocking agents or who have congestive heart failure.

The acute therapy for SVT, atrial flutter (Fig. 9), and VT (Fig. 10) are otherwise similar to that used in adults. Patients with atrial flutter who are likely to have underlying sinus node dysfunction (postop Mustard, Senning, Fontan) should have some provision made for back-up pacing prior to cardioversion. Patients with atrial ectopic tachycardia generally present with a long history of tachycardia that does not warrant acute therapy. When these patients become acutely ill, however, the tachycardia does not respond to cardioversion. The use of procainamide infusion (20–50 μg/kg/min) or constant atrial pacing at a rate sufficient to produce 2:1 atrioventricular block are potential temporizing measures while instituting chronic therapy.

Atrial flutter

Possible sick sinus syndrome?

 Yes   No \

Transesophageal/Transvenous   Overdrive pacing
pacing or DC cardioversion   or DC cardioversion
with back-up pacing ready

↓

If recurs immediately:
1. IV digoxin (if no WPW)
2. IV procainamide∗ if already on digoxin
3. IV propranolol∗

∗ Do not use with or in the presence of cardiac compromise

Figure 9. Acute management of atrial flutter. WPW = Wolff-Parkinson-White syndrome.

Acute atrioventricular block occurs most often in the postoperative setting. In surgical AV block, we wait 10–14 days prior to implanting a permanent pacing system. Conduction occasionally may return during this time.

Differences in Chronic Arrhythmia Therapy

A general review of antiarrhythmic drug dosing in children is beyond the scope of this chapter, but a few important points need to be covered. First, drug dosing in children is done on a dose per body weight or dose per body surface area method. For some agents, dose/body surface area has been found more predictive of subsequent drug serum level than dose/body weight.[23] Second, while drug pharmacodynamics may be similar to the adult patient, drug pharmacokinetics vary markedly with age. This is especially true of the infant under 6–12 months,

Ventricular tachycardia
Hemodynamic compromise?

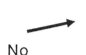

No

1. Lidocaine 1 mg/kg,
   infusion 10-50 mcg/kg/min
2. DC cardioversion 1-2 w-s/kg
3. continue as below

Correct underlying metabolic abnormality

Yes

1. Lidocaine bolus, then infusion
2. Procainamide 10 mg/kg over 30-60 min
3. Phenytoin 1-2 mg/kg q 15 min x 4
4. Propranolol 0.05-0.10 mg/kg in 3
   divided doses, 5 min apart
5. ?Amiodarone 10 mg/kg over 1 hour

Figure 10. Acute management of VT.

whose absorption, protein binding, liver metabolism, and excretion indices are generally less "mature" and require drug dosing adjustments. Children between 1 year and adolescence generally "hypermetabolize" and more frequent dosing may be necessary. Determination of drug serum levels for drugs such as quinidine, procainamide, flecainide, encainide, and propafenone therefore become important.

With the exception of age-specific heart rate as a diagnositic consideration, there are no significant differences in the approach to sinus bradycardia. Some postoperative patients (mentioned earlier) may have underlying sinus bradycardia as a manifestation of sinus node dysfunction. When these patients require sinus-suppressant antiarrhythmic agents for therapy of tachyarrhythmias (nearly every drug except digoxin and mexiletine), consideration must be given toward placement of a pacing system to prevent exacerbation of bradycardia and significant pauses. What is a "significant" pause is also age-related: 1.8 seconds for infants, 2.0 seconds for young children, and 3.0 seconds for adolescents.

As outlined in Figure 11, the approach to chronic management of the patient with congenital complete AV block is dependent on age, heart rate, and symptoms. The preschooler and elementary-school age child with untreated CCAVB may have very subtle early symptoms.

Atrioventricular block

Congenital (symptomatic):

Medical therapy: atropine
                          isoproterenol
                          dopamine for BP
Pacing for: 1) infants, vent rate ‹ 50
2) infants w/ CHD, rate ‹ 55
3) block below His
4) ventricular arrhythmias
5) irregular rate
6) temporary, if stressed infant
7) older child, rate ‹40
8) older child w/ syncope, CHF
9) older child w/ exer. intol.

Surgical: Wait 14 days (conduction may return)
temporary pacing in interim for support
Permanent pacing if no return of AV
conduction

Figure 11. Management issues in complete AV block.

These may consist of midday naps or irritability or excessive fatigue at the end of the day. Frank exercise intolerance is rare, but improvement is often noted after pacemaker implantation. Subtle "developmental delay" may also disappear when infants begin to run after pacing therapy. During sleep, escape rhythms may be erratic, leading to prolonged pauses. The resultant lack of cardiac output and cerebral anoxia may then be responsible for nightmares that occasionally occur. Endocardial dual-chambered pacing systems or single-chamber activity-related systems can be implanted in children who are as small as 10–15 kg. Therapy for the patient with CCAVB with co-existing long QT consists of pacing and beta-adrenergic blockade with propranolol (1–5 mg/kg/day).

Atrial flutter is considered one of the most dangerous arrhythmias in pediatrics. Adequate medical therapy is difficult to achieve and usually consists of trials of quinidine (15–60 mg/kg/day) or procainamide (15–60 mg/kg/day) in addition to digoxin. Amiodarone is one of the better drugs for flutter and sotalol may prove useful in children as well. While amiodarone is often effective, we are reluctant to use it on a long-term basis because of side effects, especially photosensitivity. For that reason, we are currently investigating the feasibility of direct surgical intervention for children with atrial flutter.[24] We do not favor AV node ablation for atrial arrhythmias since this leaves the child with 60–70 years of pacemaker dependence.

Antiarrhythmic therapy for most types of pediatric SVT is similar to that used in the adult population. Many arrhythmias in infancy will become quiescent by 1–2 years of age, including SVT secondary to Wolff-Parkinson-White (WPW) syndrome, CAT, and accelerated ventricular rhythms. With this in mind, antiarrhythmic therapy can either be discontinued or the patient can be allowed to "grow out" of his dose at this age. Close follow-up is obviously necessary to watch for recurrences. Our experience has been that in nearly one-third of patients with WPW and SVT in infancy, the arrhythmia disappears, then reappears at an average age of 7 years. The vast majority of SVT in patients over 5–7 years of age is persistent.

Another persistent arrhythmia is PJRT. This "permanent" tachyarrhythmia is generally resistant to traditional antiarrhythmic agents. Good chronic control of PJRT has been reported with both flecainide[23] and encainide.[25] Propafenone and sotalol may be useful in the future. Amiodarone is reserved for patients unresponsive to any of these agents.

Persistent tachyarrhythmias and the need for a long life of taking medicines frequently causes us to consider the possibility of surgical interventions.[26] This is especially true for the teenage population, where compliance with drugs may be low and recurrence of arrhythmia, need for medication, and side effects impinge on lifestyle. Recently, our success rate with WPW/SVT surgery has been 95%. Many life insurance companies will insure successfully operated patients at standard rates, while unoperated patients are either uninsurable or covered only at high premiums. Surgery for PJRT has been extremely successful (>95%), as the accessory connection can be frozen in the mouth of the coronary sinus, well away from the normal conduction tissue. Atrial ectopic tachycardia is also very amenable to surgical cryoablation. In children, right atrial ectopic tachycardias tend to have more than one focus, requiring placement of several cryoblative lesions, while left atrial foci tend to be single. The dilated "cardiomyopathy" that can occur secondary to chronic, inappropriate tachycardia has resolved in the majority of our patients postoperatively.

Surgical therapy for the infant with a "normal" heart and incessant ventricular tachycardia has been well-documented in the literature. The poor response to most antiarrhythmic agents (with the possible exception of flecainide) and the discovery that most of these patients have had clearly delineated and readily excisable ventricular "hamartomas" have made surgical intervention a practical and successful approach.[13] However, it is possible that this arrhythmia may disappear during later childhood. A child without development of dilated cardiomyopathy who has adequate medical control may then be able to be followed for disappearance of the arrhythmia. This has occurred only once in our experience in an 18-month-old with typical clinical and ECG features of "hamartoma" but who responded to flecainide. She is now 3 years old, off medication, and without cardiac dysfunction or arrhythmia.

Summary

The management of arrhythmias in the pediatric population frequently requires a different approach from comparable adult arrhythmias for many reasons. First, the natural history of pediatric arrhythmias may be dramatically different, especially for supraventricular tachycardia. This may allow long periods of arrhythmia- and medication-free management and may influence decision-making regarding surgical intervention. Second, the underlying substrate for the arrhythmias may not be similar in adults and children. This becomes important as we attempt to tailor antiarrhythmic therapy to presumed mechanisms of arrhythmia. Third, pediatric patients face a long life of antiarrhythmic therapy, thus necessitating a consideration of long-term drug effects, both organic and psychological. This becomes especially true in the area of pacing. Direct surgical elimination of arrhythmia, therefore, becomes appealing. Fourth, pharmacodynamics may be similar, but the variability of pharmacokinetics of antiarrhythmic agents in infants and children demands a thorough knowledge of their metabolism and disposition. These drug characteristics have direct bearing on choice of drug, efficacy, and side effects.

References

1. Davignon A, Rautaharju P, Boiselle E, et al: Normal ECG standards for infants and children. Pediatr Cardiol 1:123, 1979.

2. Reed BR, Lee LA, Harmon C, et al: Autoantibodies to SS-A/Ro in infants with congenital heart block. J Pediatr 103(6):889, 1983.
3. Esscher E, Michaelsson M: QT interval in congenital complete heart block. Pediatr Cardiol 4:121, 1983.
4. Koenecke LL, Knoebel SB: Nonparoxysmal junctional tachycardia complicating acute myocardial infarction. Circulation 45(2):367, 1972.
5. Villain E, Garson A Jr: Evolving concepts in the management of congenital junctional ectopic tachycardia: a multicenter study (abstract). J Am Coll Cardiol 11(2):155A, 1988.
6. Garson A Jr, Moak JP, Smith RT Jr, et al: Usefulness of intravenous propafenone for control of postoperative junctional ectopic tachycardia. Am J Cardiol 59(15):1422, 1987.
7. Escande D, Loisance D, Planche C, et al: Age-related changes of action potential plateau shape in isolated human atrial fibers. Am J Physiol (Heart Circ Physiol 18):H843, 1985.
8. Pickoff AS, Singh S, Flinn CJ, et al: Atrial vulnerability in the immature canine heart. Am J Cardiol 55:1402, 1985.
9. Toda N: Age-related changes in the transmembrane potential of isolated rabbit sino-atrial nodes and atria. Cardiovasc Res 14:58, 1980.
10. Vetter VL, Tanner CS, Horowitz LN: Electrophysiologic consequences of the Mustard repair of d-transposition of the great arteries. J Am Coll Cardiol 10:1265, 1987.
11. Hesslein PS, Finlay CD, Trusler G, et al: Atrial flutter after Mustard operation: evidence for a common reentry pathway (abstract). Am J Cardiol 62:510, 1988.
12. Wittig JH, de Leval MR, Stark J: Intraoperative mapping of atrial activation before, during and after Mustard operation. J Thorac Cardiovasc Surg 73:1, 1977.
13. Critelli G, Gallagher JJ, Manda V, et al: Anatomic and electrophysiologic substrate of the permanent form of junctional reciprocating tachycardia. J Am Coll Cardiol 4:601, 1984.
14. Gallagher JJ, Sealy WC: The permanent form of junctional reciprocating tachycardia: further elucidation of the underlying mechanism. Eur J Cardiol 8:413, 1978.
15. Garson A Jr, Smith RT, Jr, Moak JP, et al: Incessant ventricular tachycardia in infants: myocardial hamartomas and surgical cure. J Am Coll Cardiol 10:619, 1987.
16. Moak J, Ilkiw R, Hawkins E, et al: Cellular electrophysiology of ventricular tachycardia in human infants (abstract). Am J Cardiol 62:502, 1988.
17. Garson A Jr, Porter CJ, Gillette PC, et al: Induction of ventricular tachycardia during electrophysiology after repair of tetralogy of Fallot. J Am Coll Cardiol 1:1493, 1983.
18. Deal BJ, Scagliotti D, Miller SM, et al: Electrophysiologic drug testing in symptomatic ventricular arrhythmias after repair of teralogy of Fallot. Am J Cardiol 59:1380, 1987.
19. Kimura S, Bassett AL, Kohya T, et al: Automaticity, triggered activity and responses to adrenergic stimulation in cat subendocardial Purkinje fibers after healing of myocardial infarction. Circulation 75:651, 1987.
20. Pongiglione G, Saul JP, Dunnigan A, et al: Role of transesophageal pacing

in evaluation of palpitations in children and adolescents. Am J Cardiol 62(9):566, 1988.
21. Benson DW Jr: Transesophageal electrocardiography and cardiac pacing: state of the art. Circulation 75(4 Pt2):III-86, 1987.
22. Kirk CR, Gibbs JL, Thomas R, et al: Cardiovascular collapse after verapamil in supraventricular tachycardia. Arch Dis Child 62(12):1265, 1987.
23. Perry JC, McQuinn RL, Smith RT Jr, et al: Flecainide acetate for resistant arrhythmias in the young: efficacy and pharmacokinetics. J Am Coll Cardiol 14:185, 1989.
24. Klein GJ, Guiraudon GM, Sharma AD, Milstein S: Demonstration of macroreentry and feasibility of operative therapy in the common type of atrial flutter. Am J Cardiol 57:587, 1986.
25. Strasburger JF, Smith RT Jr, Moak JP, et al: Encainide for resistant supraventricular tachycardia in children: a follow-up report. Am J Cardiol 62(19):50L, 1988.
26. Garson A Jr, Moak JP, Friedman RA, et al: Surgical treatment of arrhythmias in children. Cardiol Clin 7(2):319, 1989.

Chapter 14

Syncope

John H. McAnulty

Introduction

Syncope is the sudden, complete loss of consciousness with full recovery within a few minutes. While easily put into words, it can be difficult to determine if syncope has occurred. When questioning the patient, particularly an elderly patient who may have had the event weeks or months earlier, it is often not so clear whether complete loss of consciousness occurred or not.

A diagnosis of syncope leads to a potentially extensive evaluation. Before going in that direction it can be useful to think through diagnostic possibilities (Fig. 1). Loss of consciousness is rarely caused by primary neurological abnormalities. It may be a transient neurological event, more specifically, a transient loss-of-consciousness event. Only three transient loss-of-consciousness syndromes are common: seizures, transient sleep, and syncope. Sleep will not be discussed here. It is important and often difficult to distinguish between syncope and seizures.

While seizures may be included within the differential diagnosis of syncope, an alternative approach is to consider it as a separate syndrome. By history, it may be difficult to distinguish between seizure and syncope (Table 1). The most useful is the *absence* of a post-ictal state. The presence of a post-ictal state does not allow differentiation between a seizure and syncope, but the clear absence of a post-ictal phase excludes, for the most part, a seizure as an explanation for a loss-of-consciousness episode.

Clonic or tonic motion has often been considered diagnostic of epi-

From Naccarelli GV (ed): *Cardiac Arrhythmias: A Practical Approach.* Mount Kisco, NY, Futura Publishing Co., Inc., © 1991.

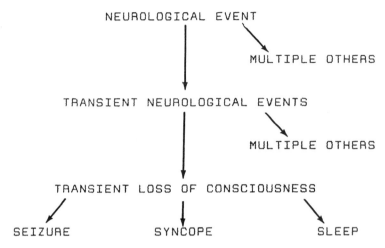

Figure 1. When a patient presents with a neurological event, it can be confusing because there are too many diagnostic possibilities. Thinking through the possibilities in the manner outlined in this figure can help our certainty in understanding which syndrome occurred before beginning a potentially expensive and dangerous evaluation.

lepsy. However, motions occur often in syncope and they may not be useful diagnostic observations. Subtle characteristics may distinguish the motions caused by a seizure from those caused by syncope, but most lay observers and most physicians would probably not be able to use these subtleties to make the diagnosis. What causes the abnormal motor

Table 1
Diagnostic Features of Seizures and Syncope

Diagnostic Features	Seizure*	Syncope
Prodrome	+ +	+ + +
Clonic-Tonic Motion	+ + +	+ +
Incontinence	+ +	+ +
Tongue Biting	+ +	+
Post-Ictal Phase	+ + +	±

* Seizure refers to grand mal epilepsy, the usual syndrome confused with syncope.

+ + + = occurs very frequently; + + = occurs frequently; + = usually occurs; ± = may or may not be observed.

function during syncope? Could a cause of syncope, for example an arrhythmia, be causing the clonic-tonic motion by causing a seizure? Possibly in some cases, but in a recent study,[1] electroencephalographic (EEG) monitoring performed during induction of ventricular fibrillation and tachycardia showed no focal seizure activity despite concurrent clonic-tonic motion. Thus, even these motor abnormalities, so typically related to epilepsy may be misleading. An example emphasizing these observations (Fig. 2) follows.

> A 41-year-old patient presented with transient loss of consciousness associated with repetitive extremity motion. Considering epilepsy a likely cause, he was studied with an ambulatory EEG. The EEG recording also had an electrocardiogram lead. The recordings show how we made the right diagnosis for the wrong reason. Expecting seizure activity, the monitor instead showed his primary problem was ventricular tachycardia. During the event he lost consciousness and had repetitive motor activity.
>
> The recordings are also interesting for other reasons: (1) With the arrhythmia, the EEG does not show seizure activity, but rather progressively finer CNS activity. (2) The prolonged polymorphic ventricular tachycardia and/or coarse ventricular fibrillation stopped spontaneously (after 118 seconds) and was followed by 18 seconds of asystole before a junctional and then a sinus rhythm returned. (3) With return of a rhythm, the activity seen on the EEG gradually returned to normal. The patient recovered completely and an antiarrhythmia drug was started.*

Syncope: Is It Common?

Practitioners are repeatedly forced to assess patients for loss of consciousness. It is estimated that 30–50% of the general population has had at least one syncopal episode, and even young Air Force recruits whose flying status is potentially compromised admit to a 30% incidence! Most with syncope, of course, never seek medical care but, despite this, approximately 1% of emergency room visits are because of an episode of syncope.[2–6]

Syncope is a syndrome of some significance. The event itself can injure the patient and, depending on the time of occurrence, for example while driving, it can be dangerous to others as well. It can be the marker for associated disease,[2–6] and may be associated with an increased incidence of sudden death. Follow-up of patients with syncope, particularly when associated with other recognizable cardiovascular disease,

---

* Example kindly provided by our colleague, William P. Mayer, M.D., Anchorage, Alaska.

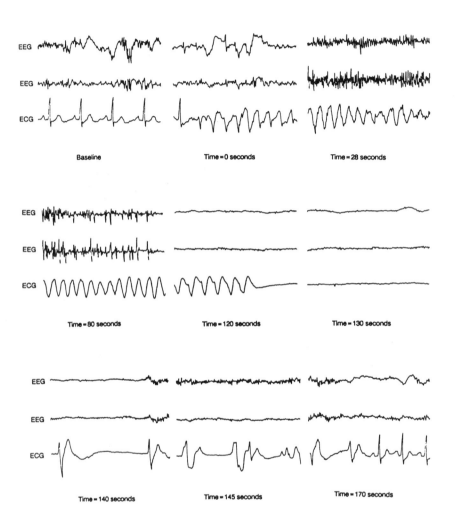

Figure 2. Ambulatory electroencephalogram (top two EEG tracings) and electrocardiogram (bottom ECG tracing) in a patient during an episode of loss of consciousness with clonic-tonic extremity motion. These are sections of a continuous recording with the times marked. Four additional EEG leads were recorded and are not pictured because of space limitations. See text for discussion of event.

has demonstrated a 20% incidence of sudden death in the next year.[3,4] Syncope can also be the marker for potentially correctable causes. Thus, recognition and evaluation of this syndrome is of some importance.

Near syncope, light-headed spells, and dizzy spells may be caused by exactly the same abnormalities that cause syncope and they may be as prognostically important. But because the explanation for those syndromes is often even less clear than that for syncope, this chapter will focus on the information available on the syndrome of syncope itself.

Syncope: Causes and Methods to Detect Them

When large populations of syncope patients are evaluated, a reasonable explanation for the event can be detected in approximately 50%.[3,4] Cardiovascular explanations predominate. A list of the causes of syncope (when they are detected) and an estimate of the frequency of each are listed in Table 2. It is often too simple to assign a single cause. Many patients have a number of problems, any one of which by itself may not cause significant decrease in cerebral perfusion, but when occurring with others can cause syncope.[4,5]

Occasional Causes

Various drugs can cause syncope and should be considered as the initial cause of *any* syndrome, including syncope. This dogmatic position is justified by the frequency with which drugs cause problems and by the reasonable possibility that stopping the drug can eliminate the problem. When drugs cause syncope, it is almost always by causing an al-

Table 2
Cause of Syncope

	Estimated Frequency
Imbalance of vascular volume and tone	70%
Cardiac causes	25%
Neurological	<5%
Drugs and Metabolic	<5%
Vascular	<5%
Hysteria	<5%

teration in intravascular volume, vascular tone, or by causing arrhythmias.

Prescription drugs and illicit drugs should be considered likely causes of syncope.[7] Of the former, anti-anginal and vasodilator agents (nitrates, Ca^{2+} channel blockers and other antihypertensive drugs) are the most common drug causes. Beta-blockers, antiarrhythmic drugs, and the phenothiazines or tricyclic antidepressants are other contributors.

Metabolic abnormalities such as hypokalemia and hypocalcemia can cause arrhythmias and thus syncope. Hypoglycemia can cause loss of consciousness but rarely the syndrome of syncope. Loss of consciousness from hypoglycemia is not sudden, but is rather preceded by weakness, diaphoresis, and tremulousness. Hyperventilation and its associated metabolic changes explain an occasional event.

Neurologic events would seem a likely explanation for syncope, but they almost never are. Intracranial bleeds, infections, and tumors cause other neurological syndromes but simply are not the explanation for the sudden complete loss of consciousness with rapid complete recovery. Seizures are neurological events, but as discussed earlier, there are advantages in terms of evaluation in considering them as a syndrome other than syncope.

Vascular stenosis is occasionally a cause of syncope, for example, with the subclavian steal syndrome. It is more important to emphasize another point about vascular stenosis: carotid artery lesions rarely cause syncope. The presence of a carotid bruit should *not* be used as an explanation for the syndrome. Stenosis of the vertebral basilar arterial system can cause collapsing episodes. Classically this does not result in syncope. An elderly patient who collapsed weeks earlier, however, may not be certain whether or not there was true loss of consciousness.

Hysteria, as an explanation, is worthy of consideration when other obvious explanations have been excluded and when the patient has demonstrated other traits that would make the explanation plausible.

Most syncope is probably caused by vascular volume or tone problems or by cardiac abnormalities. These causes will be discussed in some detail, even though the ultimate cause of any syncopal episode may go unrecognized. In those who seek medical care, an imbalance of vascular volume or tone is by far the most common cause of syncope. It also has to be the predominant mechanism in most patients never evaluated by a physician. It is a complex syndrome and often the diagnosis can be made only from a careful history; physical exam changes may have reverted to normal by the time the patient is seen.

Evidence for volume depletion may be obtained from the history.

The patient may have had the syncope on a particularly hot, dry day when they had not maintained their volume status, or, as another alternative, they may have noted 3 weeks of intermittent melena and then had a syncopal episode. Examination may reveal hypovolemia and, if so, treatment should be to replace volume appropriately.

Alteration in vascular tone may be more difficult to detect. If a patient has a chronic disease such as diabetes mellitus, Parkinson's disease, or renal failure, inadequate vascular tone should be considered a possible cause as they are associated with an increased chance of nervous system dysfunction. Other patients may have primary autonomic nervous system disease. The history and physical exam may help if there are clues suggesting a lack of appropriate sympathetic tone, such as orthostatic dizziness and hypotension, a lack of sweating, sexual dysfunction, or visual blurring.

Most often, the imbalance of vascular volume and tone appears to be "benign" and without an associated disease. It is due to an alteration in the balance of the parasympathetic and sympathetic tone, and has been called the "vasovagal" syndrome. Two mechanisms can explain most of these events. With the first, a noxious stimulus, either physical or emotional, is required. It causes inhibition of sympathetic tone by the central nervous system resulting in a relative excess of parasympathetic tone with hypotension and a bradycardia sufficient to cause syncope. The second mechanism is a reflex response to hypovolemia with decreased volume stimulating receptors, possibly in the left ventricle, which increase sympathetic tone. The central nervous system interprets this as a signal to depress sympathetic tone and increase parasympathetic tone (the Bezold-Jarisch reflex). With both mechanisms, an inhibition of heart rate may predominate in some patients while vasodepression with a decrease in arterial and venous tone is more important in others. In either case, these responses occur at exactly a time when a patient would seem to need the opposite—the result is inadequate cerebral perfusion and syncope. An interesting recent observation has suggested that the second mechanism can occur without having the heart contribute to the mechanism. "Typical" vasovagal syncope was described in a patient following a cardiac transplant—a situation where there is no cardiac innervation.[9] This suggests that the receptors stimulated by hypovolemia may not always be in the left ventricle.

A history of loss of consciousness following a noxious stimulus in a patient with no other apparent explanation is sufficient to make the diagnosis of vasovagal syncope and no other evaluation may be needed.

Unless episodes are particularly frequent, treatment is generally not required.

In attempts to better understand this syndrome of imbalance of vascular volume and tone, other diagnostic studies are being evaluated. Provocative maneuvers such as a Valsalva maneuver or carotid sinus massage may support the diagnosis, but the results should not be used by themselves as an indication for treatment. Currently, head-up tilt-table testing is being explored most enthusiastically. The early results have been informative. Various techniques have been used to perform this testing, but most include positioning a patient in the horizontal position on a tilt table until the heart rate and blood pressure have stabilized. The head of the table is then raised to an angle of 60°–80° (with a foot board to allow mild weight support and with strapping of the patient to the table). The patient is left in this position from 10 to 40 minutes with evaluation of the heart rate and blood pressure. In "normals" there is approximately a 5–10 mm Hg fall in both systolic and diastolic pressure with a 5–10 beat per minute increase in heart rate. Symptoms are rare. Abnormal responses have been noted in 30–50% of patients who have had unexplained syncope.[10–13] The blood pressure falls and the heart rate slows despite the stimulus for the opposite responses. The resultant fall in cerebral perfusion causes symptoms and syncope in these patients.

Isoproterenol has been used in order to improve the sensitivity (and possibly the specificity) of tilt table testing. If a patient has a negative response to the testing just described, the patient is then returned to the supine position and isoproterenol is administered until a stable increase in heart rate response has been achieved (between 1 and 5 mg per minute), and the tilt-testing then repeated. An abnormal heart rate and blood pressure response may be observed in up to 85% of patients who were being evaluated for unexplained syncope, compared with a similar response in less than 10% of patients who do not have unexplained syncope.

As exciting as these early findings are, they still leave many problems. Results do not prove that this is the mechanism that was the cause of syncope and therapy based on the findings is still not of proven value.

There is more to learn from the technique of tilt-table testing, such as:

1. Do the tilt-table results explain the syncope and, if so, can this testing be used to differentiate between patients who have more problems with heart rate inhibition compared to those with predominant vasodepression?

2. Does treatment work? Repeat tilt-table testing after initiation of therapy may accelerate achieving a treatment goal.

3. When is long-term treatment worth it? When syncope is due to this mechanism, it appears that events may be months or years apart. Even if a medication works, it is hard to know whether the side effects, risks, and expense are worth daily treatment.

While again it would be preferable not to have to treat patients until a definitive diagnosis has been established, this is not always possible. Some recommendations seem valid in most cases. Volume depletion should be avoided and, if possible, stimuli that initiate the symptoms should be avoided as well. The decision to treat beyond this should depend somewhat upon the frequency of the events as well as the perceived seriousness of the events, which is subjective in many cases. If there is some clue that the volume depletion and venous dilation are predominant in this syndrome, long-term use of occlusive stockings can be beneficial. In order to maintain intravascular volume, liberal sodium intake and even the use of a mineralocorticoid (such as 9-alpha fluorohydrocortisone, 1–2 mg per day) has been used. In an attempt to block the parasympathetic response, scopolamine, particularly a scopolamine patch, has been recommended. The results have been variable and the side effects and expense in many cases are real. Daily theophylline use is advocated by some, with limitations similar to those described for scopolamine.

Beta-blockade has also been advocated. This would initially seem paradoxical since a bradycardia often contributes to the syndrome. However, if the mechanism is excessive stimulation of receptors that increase sympathetic tone, blockade could potentially prevent the apparent over-reaction to a stimulus and prevent the relative imbalance of parasympathetic and sympathetic tone.[10,12,14] This form of therapy may be more applicable in the young, while elderly people may be less responsive since their β-adrenergic reaction to stimuli is diminished to begin with.[12,14]

If a bradycardia is etiologically important due to prolonged sinus node pauses or heart block, a permanent pacemaker may eliminate or minimize symptoms. Rare episodes can be treated with a basic VVI unit. Frequent and prolonged episodes are better treated with a dual chamber unit that maintains atrial-ventricular sequences with pacing.

Cardiac abnormalities are the second most important cause of syncope. Cerebral hypoperfusion can occur because of two cardiac abnormalities: obstruction to blood flow through the heart or arrhythmias.

Table 3

Cardiac Obstruction Causes of Syncope

---

1. Obstruction to left ventricular outflow
    Supraaortic valve stenosis
    Aortic valve stenosis
    Subaortic valve stenosis
    Discrete membrane
    IHSS
    Cor triatum
2. Obstruction to mitral valve flow
    Valve stenosis
    Thrombus
    Myxoma
    Cor triatrum
3. Obstruction to pulmonary blood flow
    Pulmonary hypertension
    Pulmonary emboli
4. Obstruction to right ventricular outflow
    Pulmonary artery stenosis
    Pulmonary stenosis
    Subpulmonic valve stenosis
5. Obstruction to right atrial emptying
    Valve stenosis
    Thrombus
    Myxoma

While left ventricular outflow obstruction due to aortic valve stenosis or a hypertrophic cardiomyopathy are "classic" explanations for syncope, interference with blood flow anywhere within the heart or pulmonary arterial system can be the cause (Table 3). A history of syncope occurring with or shortly after exertion should make obstruction slightly more suspect. A careful physical examination is most important for making the diagnosis. If there are clues suggesting aortic valve disease, hypertrophic cardiomyopathy, mitral or tricuspid stenosis, pulmonary hypertension, or rarely, an intracardiac tumor, further testing is appropriate.

There is some disagreement about the value of further diagnostic tests if a cardiovascular examination is normal. It is this author's opinion that an echocardiogram, while safe and always interesting, is of minimal value and the yield is simply too low.

If intracardiac obstruction is identified, treatment to eliminate it, if possible, is warranted. Other explanations for syncope, however, should not be neglected. Many patients with obstruction may have arrhythmias or hypovolemia as the more important explanation for the syncope.

Arrhythmias are the main subject of this book. They are also a likely explanation for syncope and, importantly, they are potentially correctable. Since they are often intermittent, recognition is difficult. Occasionally, they are so clearly the explanation for syncope that treatment decisions are easy. Both tachycardias and bradycardias can be clear explanations for loss of consciousness. While it is true in most cases that a heart rate exceeding 150 beats per minute is necessary to cause a loss of consciousness, associated obstructive disease, hypovolemia, or positional changes can cause syncope in patients with much slower rates. These same variables can influence the likelihood that a bradycardia will cause syncope.

A history of palpitations prior to syncope increases the chance that a tachycardia caused the event. The physical examination contributes little to making this diagnosis. The role of the carotid sinus massage remains controversial. Significant slowing of the heart rate should make sinus node disease more suspect as a cause, but treatment based on this finding alone is inappropriate. A number of testing modalities have been used to assist in the diagnosis of arrhythmias as a cause of syncope.

The electrocardiogram (ECG), while safe and inexpensive, is unlikely to demonstrate a syncopal arrhythmia but it may provide clues that an arrhythmia was the cause. Table 4 lists ECG changes that make a tachycardia or bradycardia a more likely explanation for syncope than might be true if the tracing were normal.

Table 4
Electrocardiographic Clues That an Arrhythmia Caused Syncope

Tachycardia—increased chance that this is cause if there is:
- Premature atrial or ventricular beats
- Pre-excitation
- Long QT interval

Bradycardia—increased chance that this is cause if there is:
- Atrial pauses
- First or second degree AV block
- Bundle branch block

A tachycardia might be suggested by the presence of atrial or ventricular premature beats, but these findings are so nonspecific that treatment directed against them for the purpose of preventing syncope is not appropriate. The presence of a short PR interval, especially in association with other evidence of pre-excitation (a wide QRS complex and ST-T changes, i.e., the presence of Wolff-Parkinson-White syndrome), makes it more likely that a tachycardia could explain the syncope. These patients have a high frequency of re-entry atrial tachycardia and of atrial fibrillation with a rapid ventricular response, which could explain syncope.[14] Another ominous electrocardiographic finding in a patient presenting with syncope is the presence of a long QT interval. No matter what the cause, QT interval prolongation is associated with an increased incidence of recurrent ventricular tachycardias and of sudden death. The presence of this finding is a likely explanation for the syncope, especially in the young. Unless another cause is found, most would recommend treatment, at least with β-blocking drugs.

The ECG may also give clues that bradyarrhythmias are the explanation for syncope. While prolonged sinus pauses or evidence of heart block are more clear-cut explanations for syncope, there are other clues as well. The presence of interventricular conduction delay or bundle branch block is not a reason alone to consider a pacemaker, but it is a reason to be more concerned that bradycardias (and tachycardias) are an explanation for the clinical event.

Ambulatory or Holter monitoring has been the best available method of detecting arrhythmias.[3-5] Its advantage is the capability to capture all rhythms during a certain time period. Its disadvantage is that, by necessity, the time for recording has to be relatively short—a few days at most. An event may not occur during this time. However, in the large series that has reviewed the evaluation of syncope, Holter monitoring has demonstrated arrhythmias as a likely cause in greater than 15% of cases.[3-5]

How long should monitoring be performed? Most investigators have used 24 to 48 hours but the optimal recording time is unclear. In a recent study of a population of patients with syncope of uncertain etiology, 24 hours of Holter monitoring revealed evidence of a major rhythm abnormality in 15% of patients. A second 24-hour monitor on the remaining patients provided an 11% yield, and a third 24-hour monitor provided evidence of a major rhythm abnormality in only 4% of the remaining patients. This would support the use of 48 hours of Holter monitoring as a "cost-effective" approach.[16] Of some concern is the observation that documented arrhythmias presumed to be the explanation for the syncope very rarely cause syncope during monitoring.

Event monitors are increasingly available and are continuous-loop recorders. When an event button is pushed by the patient or associate, the rhythm recorded 10–15 seconds before and after the button is pushed, is saved. Information from that tape can then be transmitted over the telephone to a recording device. This allows rhythm recording at a time the patient is symptomatic. The advantages of this approach are that the monitor can be worn for longer periods of time (a month or longer with intermittent lead changes), and analysis of large volumes of data is not necessary—only the rhythm at the time of the event is preserved. The disadvantage is that with some events, the patient or a person with them may not have time to push the button. Additionally, if the leads are not carefully applied, interpretation of the rhythm tracing may be difficult. Still, this is a particularly promising way to evaluate people with infrequent intermittent transient neurological events, including syncope (Fig. 3).

Electrophysiological testing has been enthusiastically endorsed by some as a way to define patients in whom an arrhythmia was likely. It is assumed that conduction abnormalities will not be found and that rhythms cannot be created with this test in normals, that is, in patients who have not had syncope. Thus, if an arrhythmia is created in a patient with syncope, that rhythm is considered a logical explanation for the clinical event.

While the concepts are sensible and the electrophysiological method may eventually be shown to be valuable in assessing selected patient groups, it is too early for broad-scale application. The chance of finding an abnormality on electrophysiological testing that could be considered abnormal and the potential explanation for syncope depends on the patient population studied.[17] Those with organic heart disease are much more frequently found to have abnormalities. In the studies to date, when an abnormality has been found, treatment has been initiated, with subsequent evaluation of the incidence of recurrence of syncope.[18–26] In no series to date has an abnormality been detected with patients subsequently being followed on *no* treatment or with randomization of treatment. Thus, it is unclear whether treatment based on electrophysiological study findings makes any difference in this population.[27]

Tachycardias have been considered as a likely cause of syncope when a sustained uniform (monomorphic) ventricular tachycardia can be induced during electrophysiological evaluation. Direction of therapy against that rhythm (utilizing further electrophysiology testing) has been

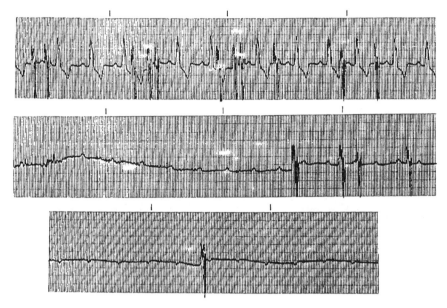

Figure 3. This tracing from an ambulatory event monitor is presented to make three points. First, in this man with syncope, known left bundle branch block, and subsequently documented complete heart block as the cause (based on this tracing), an intracardiac electrophysiological study 1 month earlier was negative. Second, these event monitors can define the cause of syncope (a family member pushed the recording button when the patient lost consciousness). Finally, it shows that while useful, the tracings may have artifacts and be difficult to read. The tracings are from a continuous recording made after the event button was pushed. The tracings were cut and mounted by a monitor-reading company before being sent to us, so the beginning of the ventricular standstill was not saved. The top tracing reveals sinus rhythm with normal conduction and artifact. Only P waves are recorded on the bottom two strips (with a change in P wave morphology; the leads were not mismounted).

thought to decrease the chance of arrhythmia and syncope recurrence. Evidence for this approach, however, is minimally supported and is controversial.[18–20] Even if it turns out that these patients will benefit, the number affected will not be large as these sustained rhythms are induced in less than 10% of patients with unexplained syncope. While it is more common to induce nonsustained ventricular tachycardia, this finding is not as acceptable as a marker and attempts to suppress it as a way to prevent recurrent syncope have not been successful. Occasionally, a supraventricular tachycardia capable of causing syncope will be induced. This is most likely in syncope patients with evidence of pre-excitation on their surface electrocardiogram.

Electrophysiological testing has also been performed as a way of detecting bradyarrhythmias. Clues for conduction abnormalities suggesting transient heart block as an explanation for syncope have included a very prolonged HV interval (>75–100 ms) and demonstration of block between the His bundle and the ventricle with atrial pacing. These findings have been used as a reason for permanent pacemaker insertion. Because of this tendency, with no available untreated group for comparison, it is difficult to know whether protection against recurrent syncope has been achieved.

The other mechanism for bradyarrhythmia, sinoatrial disease, has also been evaluated with electrophysiological testing. The sensitivity of the test in defining sinus node rhythm problems has recently been shown to be very low. In a population of patients who had demonstrated clinical sinus node and atrial bradycardias, subsequent electrophysiology testing to define evidence of disease in this area was unrevealing in most.[28]

Because of the limitations in electrophysiological testing, it is difficult to make firm recommendations. While an abnormality is more likely to be found in patients with heart disease, it is still not clear that the abnormality observed is a reason to direct treatment. At our institution, we continue to be inconsistent about the application of electrophysiology testing in the patient with syncope. When we do proceed, it is after a discussion with the patient mentioning the relatively low chance—we say under 25%—that a clear explanation for the syncope will be found. While there remains uncertainty about the value of electrophysiological test-directed treatment in preventing recurrent syncope, it may be a useful prognostic test. Those with no inducible ventricular tachyarrhythmias may have more favorable survival rates compared to those in whom these rhythms are created and treated.[19]

Signal-Averaged Electrocardiograms (SAECG) are one more way to define arrhythmias as an explanation for syncope. This technique of repetitive recording of the QRS complex filters out random electrical noise and has allowed detection of previously hidden, small electrical deflections. Most attention has been given to the events occurring at the end of the QRS complex, the "late potentials." Of interest, these late potentials are rarely found in normal subjects but are a common finding in patients who have ventricular tachycardia or fibrillation.

It is natural to think that recording of late potentials with a SAECG in patients with unexplained syncope might identify those in whom a ventricular tachyarrhythmia was the cause. Early work has suggested that this may be true.[29,30] The sensitivity and specificity of the late potential as an indication of ventricular tachycardia or fibrillation as the cause of syncope has not been defined. However, the sensitivity of the late potential as a marker for Holter-documented ventricular tachycardia (three or more beats) or for inducible ventricular tachycardia with electrophysiological testing is 75–89% and the specificity may be 90% or greater.

While the results of the SAECG cannot be used alone as a reason to direct treatment against ventricular arrhythmias, this safe, noninvasive test may become a useful screening maneuver to direct patients to intense monitoring or invasive testing.

The initial evaluation of syncope (or recurrent syncope) can provide a probable cause in up to 50% of patients. Features of the work-up and their yield is presented in Table 5. As always, the history is most important. This may be the only clue to an imbalance of vascular volume and tone. A questioning for drug use (prescribed or illicit) is essential, and the activity at the time of syncope may provide a clue as to the cause. As noted earlier, a preceding episode of stress may suggest a vasovagal etiology while exertion leading to the event may favor cardiac obstruction or an arrhythmia as a cause. Physical examination, looking for hypovolemia, autonomic nervous system dysfunction, or an obstructive cardiac process may provide the answer. It is worth re-emphasizing that if organic heart disease and possible obstruction to flow is found, it may not be this alone but rather its combination with either vascular volume distribution problems or an arrhythmia that has caused the syncope. Again, note that in the recommendations for an initial work-up an echocardiogram is not included because of its expense and low yield when the examination is normal. While an electroencephalogram is not

Table 5
Evaluation of Syncope

Initial Work-up of Syncope	Provides Diagnosis
History	25%
Physical	10%
ECG	5%
FBS, K^+, Ca^{++}	<5%
24–48 hours rhythm monitoring	15%

recommended for evaluation of syncope, if a seizure cannot be excluded as the cause of loss of consciousness, this test should be performed. If the syncope occurred with exertion, an exercise test may define the cause.

What Should be Done When the Evaluation Does Not Reveal the Cause?

If the initial evaluation of syncope is negative: STOP! This recommendation is controversial but is supportable for several reasons. The chance of recurrence is low. Approximately two-thirds of those with syncope will have no recurrence in the next 3–4 years.[3–5] Further workup is expensive, and the diagnostic yield is still questionable. Even when a test is "positive," it is often not clear that treatment alters prognosis. In addition, long-term follow-up of patients in whom no definite explanation for syncope has been found reveals that survival is excellent.[3–5] Continued testing to find the causes is not likely to lead to improved survival. Therefore, it is not clear whether the added risk and expense of a further work-up is appropriate.

All who care for patients with syncope, however, know that some patients do return with recurrent syncope and, in some (for example, public bus drivers, pilots, etc.), the initial event itself is of great significance. If a work-up is negative following initial syncope (or recurrent syncope), and the patient is discharged or followed without further management, there may be a recurrence. A repeat of the initial work-up is appropriate but of lower yield.[6] The history and physical examination are unlikely to have changed, and the electrocardiogram is less likely to give clues. With recurrent loss-of-consciousness episodes, it is time to ask, once again, whether a seizure disorder could be the cause. If an EEG and sleep-deprived EEG have not been previously obtained, they are at least worthy of consideration if there is any doubt about the type of presenting syndrome. Note that a CT or MRI scan are not recommended. They are rarely useful in the sudden loss-of-consciousness syndromes. Again, with a normal cardiac exam, it is unlikely that an echocardiogram is going to give the diagnosis although the argument can always be made that IHSS, mitral stenosis, or an atrial myxoma are being missed. It is now time to ask whether additional testing is warranted (Table 6). Since imbalance of vascular volume and tone is such a common explanation for syncope, tilt-table testing should be considered. Unrecognized and potentially treatable rhythm abnormalities remain of con-

---

Table 6
Syncope of Unknown Origin

Additonal Tests to Consider
- Tilt-table testing
- Long-term event monitoring
- Electrophysiology study
- Signal-averaged ECG

---

cern in the patient with syncope of unknown origin. Repeat Holter monitoring and event monitoring should be considered and, in some, electrophysiological testing or the SAECG may help direct management. As unsatisfying as it is to say it, individual clinical decisions will have to be made until we learn more about the role of these studies and the value of treatment.

If a patient seen in an office or emergency room because of syncope has a negative initial evaluation, and if outpatient rhythm monitoring can be instituted, hospital admission is low yield and unnecessary to protect a patient. A particularly ill patient or a patient with a likely explanation that may be dangerous or correctable may benefit from 24 to 48 hours of hospitalization.

If a definitive cause of syncope is identified, correction or treatment is essential. Clues that provide a likely explanation for syncope should preferably be used to narrow the search for the definitive cause. Treatment based on the clues alone may not work and may subject patients to unnecessary expense and risk. Many of us are responsible for patients presenting with syncope and a cardiac obstructive lesion in whom the obstruction is eliminated but syncope recurs. More commonly, we've treated frequent ectopy or nonsustained ventricular tachycardia only to find that we've exposed the patient to the risk of the drug with no beneficial effect on the syncope. A pacemaker inserted because of documented 2-second asymptomatic pauses, with the assumption that they are markers for longer symptomatic pauses at other times, may work in some, but recurrent syncope despite the treatment is not unusual. If treatment were safe, convenient, and cost-free, it should be quickly applied. Because it generally is not, its use should be reserved for documented causes when possible.

If syncope is adequately treated, a return to full employment is appropriate for most. If syncope is unexplained and a recurrence possible, patients should be advised to avoid those parts of the job in which they could hurt themselves or others if it occurred again. There are no clear guidelines for how long restrictions are advisable. We impose this restriction until a patient has been free of syncope for at least 3 months.

Since driving is so important to most patients, it is uncomfortable to discuss restrictions. Again, there are no established criteria for the time following syncope that driving should be prohibited. In the patient with unexplained syncope, we insist on 3 months of freedom from symptoms before allowing a return to driving and ask that when they begin again, they avoid expressways and high-traffic roads. In some states, the law dictates the time of abstinence from driving.

References

1. Aminoff MJ, Scheinman MM, Griffin JC, et al: Electrocerebral accompaniments of syncope associated with malignant ventricular arrhythmias. Ann Intern Med 108(6):791, 1988.
2. Stults BM, Gandolfi RJ: Diagnostic evaluation of syncope. West J Med 144:234, 1986.
3. Kapoor WN, Karpf M, Wieand S, et al: A prospective evaluation and follow-up of patients with syncope. N Engl J Med 309:198, 1983.
4. Silverstein MD, Singer DE, Mulley AG, et al: Patients with syncope admitted to medical intensive care units. JAMA 248:1185, 1982.
5. Day SC, Cook EF, Funkenstein H, et al: Evaluation and outcome of emergency room patients with transient loss of consciousness. Am J Med 73:15, 1982.
6. Kudenchuk PJ, McAnulty JH: Syncope: evaluation and treatment. Mod Concepts Cardiovasc Dis 54(5):25, 1985.
7. Davidson E, Fuchs J, Rotenberg Z, et al: Drug-related syncope. Clin cardiol 12:577, 1989.
8. Weissler AM, Boudoulas H, Lewis RP, et al: Syncope: pathophysiology, recognition and treatment. In: Hurst JM, Schlant RC, Rackley CE, et al. (eds), The Heart, 7th ed. New York, McGraw-Hill, 1990, pp 581–603.
9. Scherrer V, Vissing S, Morgan BJ, et al: Vasovagal syncope after infusion of a vasodilator in a heart transplant recipient. N Engl J Med 322:602, 1990.
10. Almquist A, Goldenberg IF, Milstein S, et al: Provocation of bradycardia and hypotension by isoproterenol and upright posture in patients with unexplained syncope. N Engl J Med 320(6):346, 1989.
11. Abi-Samara F, Maloney JD, Fouad-Tarazi FM, et al: The usefulness of head-up tilt testing and hemodynamic investigators in the workup of syncope of unknown origin. PACE 11:1202, 1988.
12. Lipsitz LA, Marks ER, Koestner J, et al: Reduced susceptibility to syncope during postural tilt in old age: Is beta-blockage protective? Arch Int Med 150:1073, 1990.
13. Ross BA: Evaluation and treatment of syncope in children. Learning Center Highlights from The American College of Cardiology, Spring 1990.

14. Guccione PT, Garson A: Relation of syncope in young patients with Wolff-Parkinson-White syndrome to rapid ventricular response during atrial fibrillation. Am J Cardiol 65:318, 1990.
15. Gibson TC, Heltzman MR: Diagnostic efficacy of 24-hour electrocardiographic monitoring for syncope. Am J Cardiol 53:1010, 1984.
16. Bass EB, Curtiss EI, Arena VC, et al: The duration of Holter monitoring in patients with syncope. Is 24 hours enough? Arch Int Med 150:1073, 1990.
17. Gulamhusein S, Naccarelli GV, Ko PT, et al: Value and limitations of clinical electrophysiology study in assessment of patients with unexplained syncope. Am J Med 73:700, 1982.
18. Morady F, Shen E, Schwartz A, et al: Long-term follow-up of patients with recurrent unexplained syncope evaluated by electrophysiologic testing. JACC 2:1053, 1983.
19. Bass EB, Elson JJ, Fogoros RN, et al: Long-term prognosis of patients undergoing electrophysiologic studies for syncope of unknown origin. Am J Cardiol 62:1186, 1988.
20. Denes P, Uretz E, Ezri MD, et al: Clinical predictors of electrophysiologic findings in patients with syncope of unknown origin. Arch Int Med 148:1922, 1988.
21. Hess DS, Morady F, Scheinman MM: Electrophysiologic testing in the evaluation of patients with syncope of undetermined origin. Am J Cardiol 50:1309, 1982.
22. Olshansky B, Meir M, Martins JB: Significance of inducible tachycardia in patients with syncope of unknown origin: a long-term follow-up. JACC 5:216, 1985.
23. Twidale N, Heddle WF, Ayres BF, et al: Clinical implications of electrophysiology study findings in patients with chronic bifascicular block and syncope. Aust NZ J Med 18:841, 1988.
24. Click RL, Gersh BJ, Sugrue DD, et al: Role of invasive electrophysiologic testing in patients with symptomatic bundle branch block. Am J Cardiol 59:817, 1987.
25. Doherty JU, Pembrook-Rogers D, Grogan EW, et al: Electrophysiologic Evaluation and follow-up characteristics of patients with recurrent unexplained syncope and presyncope. Am J Cardiol 55:703, 1985.
26. Sugrue DD, Holmes DR, Gersh BJ, et al: Impact of intracardiac electrophysiologic testing on the management of elderly patients wit recurrent syncope or near syncope. J Am Geriatr Soc 35(12):1079, 1987.
27. McAnulty JH: Syncope of unknown origin: the role of electrophysiologic studies. Circulation 75(suppl. 3):145, 1987.
28. Fujimura O, Yee R, Klein GJ, et al: The diagnostic sensitivity of electrophysiologic testing in patients with syncope caused by transient bradycardia. N Engl J Med 321:1703, 1989.
29. Kuchar DL, Thorburn CW, Sammel NL: Signal-averaged electrocardiogram for evaluation of recurrent syncope. Am J Cardiol 58:949, 1986.
30. Gang ES, Peter T, Rosenthal ME, et al: Detection of late potentials on the surface electrocardiogram in unexplained syncope. Am J Cardiol 58:1014, 1986.

Chapter 15

The Concept of Proarrhythmia

Steven P. Kutalek, Daniel J. McCormick, and R. Stephen Porter

Introduction

Despite widespread use of antiarrhythmic medications for supraventricular and ventricular arrhythmias, these agents can worsen the arrhythmias for which they are prescribed.[1-8] Antiarrhythmic drugs may increase the frequency of existing arrhythmias or potentiate the expression of new arrhythmias not previously seen in individual patients. If not fatal, these effects are frustrating to manage, providing a challenge in clinical diagnosis and therapeutic intervention. Cautious attention to the potential for proarrhythmia in patients who receive cardioactive medications improves the chances for timely and successful treatment.

Recognition of arrhythmogenic effects is straightforward when a dramatic response occurs in temporal relation to initiation, or alteration in dosage, of antiarrhythmic medications. This may involve the new onset of sustained ventricular tachycardia (VT), ventricular fibrillation (VF), complete heart block, or sudden death. Frequently, however, proarrhythmic responses occur more subtly, presenting as an increased frequency of ventricular premature complexes (VPCs), a new onset of nonsustained VT, new supraventricular arrhythmia, or progressive bradycardia.

Diagnosis and management of proarrhythmia is compounded by

From Naccarelli GV (ed): *Cardiac Arrhythmias: A Practical Approach.* Mount Kisco, NY, Futura Publishing Co., Inc., © 1991.

397

drug interactions, which may alter pharmacokinetic profiles, leading to changes in serum drug concentrations. Furthermore, drug interactions may create synergistic arrhythmogenic effects.[9] Proarrhythmia can result from treatment with noncardiac drugs and is influenced by various degrees of structural myocardial disease, metabolic dysfunction, alterations in autonomic tone, heart failure, and ischemia.

As complex as the de novo onset of arrhythmias, the origin of the proarrhythmic response is similarly not well understood. Although we can describe prevalence, recognize precipitating factors, and have formulated some concepts regarding substrate for proarrhythmia, there is as yet no unifying mechanistic explanation for its genesis. Etiologies in individual patients may be multifactorial.

Any situation in which prescribed medications aggravate underlying conditions should raise concern. This situation is especially alarming when it occurs in patients treated for cardiac arrhythmias, as exacerbations may be abrupt and difficult to control.

Scope of the Problem

Despite many years of experience with antiarrhythmic medications and an awareness that these agents can exacerbate arrhythmias,[10-15] only recently has the problem of proarrhythmia been investigated in a systemic manner. As a result of studies that have examined clinical aspects of proarrhythmia from both noninvasive and invasive advantages, some unifying factors have emerged that enable one to target populations of patients at greatest risk.

The onset of proarrhythmia in an individual patient who receives a particular medication cannot be predicted, however. Nor are we aware of the specific underlying cellular or tissue mechanisms that lead to the proarrhythmic response. Postulates include drug-induced conduction delay that can set the stage for new re-entrant circuits to develop. Additionally, there is evidence to suggest that early afterdepolarizations, which can develop with bradycardia and prolonged repolarization, play a role in proarrhythmia. This may represent the mechanism for quinidine-induced torsades de pointes that occurs at low serum concentrations of the drug. Cellular mechanisms likely involve differential binding and dissociation rates of drug onto membrane ionic channels. Drugs with potent inhibiting effects on the sodium channel that also worsen mechanical dysfunction may enhance anisotropic micro re-entry, producing arrhythmias.[16-18]

In a retrospective examination[1] of 722 antiarrhythmic drug trials in 155 patients referred for sustained and nonsustained ventricular arrhythmias, after a washout period for previously administered antiarrhythmic medications, the frequency of ventricular ectopy off drugs was recorded acutely after single-dose administration and after 48 hours on these agents. In 80 drug trials (53 patients), proarrhythmia was observed. This was defined as a fourfold increase in VPC frequency, a tenfold increase in episodes of nonsustained VT, or occurrence of sustained VT in patients in whom this arrhythmia did not occur during baseline studies. Proarrhythmia was observed with all nine drugs tested, with frequencies of 5.9–15.8% for each agent. Serum drug concentrations were within the accepted therapeutic range. The occurrence of proarrhythmia with one drug did not predict its occurrence with other drugs, nor did the presence of other toxic effects predict proarrhythmia. There was no difference in frequency of proarrhythmia among patients who presented with nonsustained VT compared with those who had sustained VT; however, it is unclear whether patients who received each drug had comparable LV contractility.

The frequency of arrhythmia exacerbation in this early study was surprisingly high and led to questions regarding the safety of widespread use of antiarrhythmic medications, especially for asymptomatic patients.

Subsequently, in a noninvasively guided study[8] of antiarrhythmic therapy in 506 patients (1268 drug trials), proarrhythmic effects (defined as spontaneous onset of new symptomatic ventricular arrhythmia after initiating drug therapy) occurred in 35 (6.9%) patients and in 43 (3.4%) drug trials. These proarrhythmic responses occurred with most drugs when used alone and with combinations that included amiodarone. The greatest frequency of proarrhythmia was observed in patients treated with encainide; many of these had rapid dose escalation during early antiarrhythmic trials. In this study, arrhythmogenic effects were higher in patients who presented with sustained VT compared with those who had nonsustained VT or VF. Proarrhythmia was also increased in patients with diminished systolic function at the basal area of the heart and characteristically occurred early after initiating antiarrhythmic therapy. Incessant VT occurred more frequently than did polymorphic VT and VF. These investigators demonstrated a high frequency of life-threatening proarrhythmic responses that can result from noninvasively guided antiarrhythmic medical therapy.

Others have examined proarrhythmic responses by invasive electrophysiological techniques.[4,6,7,19–21] In a study of 314 patients (801 drug studies) with nonsustained VT, sustained VT, or VF at presentation, proarrhythmia occurred with each of 14 drugs evaluated in 24% of drug trials.[21] Class IC agents, including flecainide and indecainide, had the highest incidence of proarrhythmia (33% and 37%). There was no significant difference in incidence of proarrhythmia in patients who received drug combinations compared with single-drug regimens, and

---

Table 1

Proposed Definitions of Proarrhythmia Comparing the Results of Noninvasive Monitoring Before and After Antiarrhythmic Drug Therapy

---

1. New onset of arrhythmia not present prior to drug therapy
   a. Bradyarrhythmias, i.e., involving sinus node, AV node, and His-Purkinje system
   b. Supraventricular extrasystoles and tachyarrhythmias
   c. VPCs
   d. Nonsustained VT
   e. Sustained monomorphic VT
   f. Sustained polymorphic VT
   g. Torsades de pointes
   h. Ventricular fibrillation
2. Increased frequency of arrhythmia on 24-hour Holter monitor*

   a.

Mean number of VPCs/hr off drug	Increase to define Proarrhythmia
1–50	×10
51–100	×5
101–300	×4
>300	×3

   b. Nonsustained VT: 10× increase in mean hourly frequency of VT complexes.
3. Spontaneous sustained VT or ventricular fibrillation which is significantly more difficult to terminate or which cannot be terminated
4. Incessant VT
5. Sudden death soon after initiating antiarrhythmic treatment or increasing dose

---

The above events are not considered to represent proarrhythmia when they occur (1) less than 72 hours after myocardial infarction; (2) greater than 30 days after initiating new antiarrhythmic medication or new dose; (3) in conjunction with electrolyte abnormalities or acute myocardial ischemia; (4) after medication has been discontinued.

VPC = ventricular premature complex; VT = ventricular tachycardia.

*Adapted from reference 43.

proarrhythmia with one agent did not predict arrhythmia exacerbation with another drug. Except for quinidine, serum drug concentrations did not correlate with proarrhythmia, nor were surface ECG changes related. Proarrhythmia was more common in patients with reduced left ventricular ejection fractions.

The severity of the proarrhythmic response in a clinical setting is evident by preliminary results of the Cardiac Arrhythmia Suppression Trial (CAST).[22] This multicenter placebo-controlled study was initiated to examine whether VPC suppression after myocardial infarction in patients with reduced LV systolic function decreases sudden death and total mortality. After an average of 10 months of follow-up, two agents selected for their potent VPC-suppressant activity, encainide and flecainide, produced an increase above placebo in death from arrhythmia or nonfatal cardiac arrest (4.5% vs. 1.2% on placebo) as well as total mortality (7.7% vs. 3.0% on placebo). Relative risks for these events on drug were 3.6% and 2.5%. Patient characteristics did not differ among the treated and nontreated groups. Of note, sudden death appeared both early and late.

Criteria for proarrhythmia remain arbitrary and speculative and do not predict a poor response to drug therapy in general. As with noninvasive studies, the definition of proarrhythmia by invasive EP guidance is not straightforward. Several criteria have been suggested (Tables 1 and 2). Which of these factors has the greatest predictive value for subsequent mortality remains unclear.

We may view proarrhythmia as a life-threatening event that can

---

Table 2
Proposed Definitions of Proarrhythmia Comparing the Results of Cardiac Electrophysiologic Testing Before and After Antiarrhythmic Drug Therapy

---

1. New induction of VT
2. Conversion of induced nonsustained VT to sustained VT or VF
3. Conversion of stable monomorphic VT to polymorphic VT or VF
4. Increase in the rate of induced VT
5. New requirement for electrical cardioversion to terminate sustained VT
6. Induction of incessant VT
7. Induction of arrhythmia with less aggressive stimulation protocol, i.e., fewer extrastimuli or at a slower paced cycle length
8. Death from induced sustained VT or VF

VF = ventricular fibrillation; VT = ventricular tachycardia.

occur unpredictably in an individual patient. Because the incidence of this adverse drug effect is high, several studies have examined patient characteristics and pharmacokinetic factors that may influence the onset or severity of proarrhythmia.

Predictors of Proarrhythmia

Aggravation or new onset of tachyarrhythmias caused by medications represents the traditional concept or proarrhythmia. As noted, such effects are surprisingly frequent. Antiarrhythmic drugs may initiate new arrhythmias not seen before in individual patients or they may aggravate pre-existing arrhythmias, by increasing tachycardia rate, increasing the frequency or duration of tachyarrhythmia episodes, or by inducing bradycardia.

Incidence of proarrhythmia varies depending on the drug given, metabolic characteristics of the individual patient, the nature of the underlying cardiovascular disease, and one's definition of the proarrhythmic response. Aggravation of ventricular arrhythmias can be especially serious if it leads to hemodynamically compromising VT or VF.

Proarrhythmic effects are dose- and concentration-related for some agents.[9,23] With digitalis, high serum concentrations are more likely to produce tachyarrhythmias and heart block than are low concentrations, although proarrhythmia can occur at any serum drug level.[10,24,25] Digitalis-induced rhythm disorders often take the form of nonparoxysmal junctional tachycardia or atrial tachycardia with block. Ventricular tachyarrhythmias and extrasystoles are also common, as are bradyarrhythmias.

Abrupt changes in serum drug concentrations induced by a rapid rate of dose escalation can be proarrhythmic, especially for class IC antiarrhythmic drugs.[8,21,23] Early trials with flecainide, indecainide, and encainide demonstrated enhancement of proarrhythmia with dose increments that occurred more frequently than every 48 to 72 hours. This produced increased VPC frequency and new onset of nonsustained or sustained VT. For drugs that exhibit extensive metabolism, rapid dose escalation may preclude achieving steady state at each dosage level. This is especially true for those agents with active metabolites such as procainamide and encainide, those with long serum half-lives, and those administered to patients with extensive renal or hepatic dysfunction.[9] Rapid dose escalation leads to difficulty in determining adequacy of cardiac effects at a given dosage, exacerbates the tendency to proar-rhythmia, and complicates subsequent control of arrhythmogenicity.

Nevertheless, for most medications, serious proarrhythmic effects do not appear to be directly related to absolute serum drug concentra-tions.[1,21] Of the 24 proarrhythmic drug trials in the electrophysiology (EP) laboratory reported by Rae and colleagues,[21] only serum concen-trations of quinidine correlated with proarrhythmia. For other antiar-rhythmic medications, proarrhythmic effects remained unrelated to serum drug concentrations. Although proarrhythmic responses in this study were not influenced by surface electrocardiographic intervals, in-cluding QRS, QTc, and JTc, excessively high serum drug concentrations can alter these intervals markedly, leading to an increased likelihood for proarrhythmia. This tendency is especially pronounced with excessive prolongation of QRS duration due to IC agents and marked increase in the JT interval with IA drugs.

The onset of proarrhythmia with one medication does not imply that the same will occur with another drug, even if both have similar electrophysiological properties, i.e., the same drug classification.[26] Fur-ther, medications that appear proarrhythmic when used alone may not have the same effect when given in combination. When combinations of antiarrhythmic drugs were administered to 40 patients who had proar-rhythmia with single agents, 55% of patients who had previously been proarrhythmic on one drug had no adverse effects while on combined therapy, despite the fact that the offending agent was included in the combination. Additionally, three patients who had no proarrhythmia on a combined regimen did demonstrate proarrhythmic effects with each agent of the combination when used alone. This lack of correlation of proarrhythmic responses observed with combined therapy as opposed to single-agent therapy appears similar for noninvasively guided drug administration.

Metabolic alterations may in themselves be arrhythmogenic, but effects are multiplied in the presence of antiarrhythmic drugs. Classic in this regard is the exacerbation of arrhythmias by digitalis at thera-peutic concentrations in the face of hypokalemia, which increases the cardiac toxicity of the drug.

Hypokalemia itself also exhibits ventricular arrhythmogenecity. Catecholamine stimulation produces intravascular depletion of potas-sium by beta-2 receptor stimulation. This, especially in concert with pre-existing hypokalemia, increases VPC frequency and is suspected to play a role in the genesis of sustained ventricular tachyarrhythmias. Cate-cholamines also alter conduction and repolarization characteristics of electrically active cardiac tissue, which may enhance the development of re-entrant circuits. They may also exacerbate or precipitate ischemia. All of these effects can aggravate or induce atrial or ventricular arrhythmias.

Virtually any electrolyte imbalance, hypoxemia, or acidosis can potentiate arrhythmias. Hypomagnesemia may be influential in arrhythmogenesis more frequently than previously recognized and has been implicated in some patients with torsades de pointes.[25] Electrolyte abnormalities should be recognized and carefully corrected in patients suspected to have proarrhythmic effects from medications.

Most antiarrhythmic medications are administered to patients with structural cardiac disease, since arrhythmias are most commonly observed in these individuals; however, significant organic cardiac disease may exacerbate the tendency to proarrhythmia.[8,21,23,27] Especially for patients with marked depression of left ventricular function, proarrhythmic effects of antiarrhythmic medications increase. This has been observed both in animal infarction models[28] as well as in humans and appears to occur for most antiarrhythmic drugs. A lower left ventricular ejection fraction has been reported in patients with proarrhythmic responses (LVEF 37%) than in patients without proarrhythmia (LVEF 43%). In the study by Rae and colleagues,[21] LVEF in patients prone to develop proarrhythmia was 27%, and in patients without proarrhythmia it was 33%.

Beyond increasing with greater degrees of left ventricular dysfunction, proarrhythmia for ventricular arrhythmias bears a relationship to the severity of the underlying arrhythmia for which therapy has been prescribed. Studies indicate that proarrhythmic effects in patients with a history of sustained arrhythmias are greater than in those in whom only nonsustained arrhythmias are recorded.[8,23,29] The actual frequency of nonsustained arrhythmias on ambulatory monitoring does not, however, appear to correlate with proarrhythmia. Thus, *severity*, in terms of type of underlying ventricular arrhythmia, rather than *frequency* of arrhythmia, plays some role in predicting proarrhythmic effects with antiarrhythmic medications.

Age, sex, cardiac diagnosis, occurrence of other side effects, and location of prior infarction do not appear related to proarrhythmia.[1–8,22,23,30] With quinidine, the presence of atrial fibrillation, hypokalemia, and congestive heart failure increases the likelihood for proarrhythmia.[31] Overall, the severity of underlying arrhythmia and the degree of left ventricular dysfunction remain the most important predictors for ventricular proarrhythmia.

Clinical Manifestations of Proarrhythmia

Proarrhythmiac responses may be classified into those that result in unanticipated bradyarrhythmias and those that result in unanticipated tachyarrhythmias. Although the onset of drug-induced pathological bradyarrhythmias is not generally thought of as a proarrhythmic response, such an effect is a real manifestation of arrhythmogenecity and may be as life-threatening as a new tachyarrhythmia.

Bradycardias

Bradyarrhythmic effects of antiarrhythmic medications most commonly involve calcium-dependent conductive tissue, i.e., sinus and AV nodes, by decreasing spontaneous automaticity or conduction. A reduction of automaticity in sinus nodal tissue can lead to profound sinus bradycardia, sinus pauses, or sinus arrest. Induced abnormalities in perinodal conduction result in sinus exit block that may be intermittent or sustained for periods long enough to produce symptoms. Additionally, a reduction of automaticity may produce excessively long escape intervals.

Bradycardia effects on the sinus node may be produced by many antiarrhythmic medications,[12,24,32,33] although severity differs among the various drugs. Pathological sinus nodal suppression is distinctly uncommon in patients with intrinsically normal sinus nodal function, despite the presence of antiarrhythmic medications in therapeutic doses. Pathological bradyarrhythmias may appear in the presence of any antiarrhythmic drug. However, in patients with dysfunctional sinus nodes, this dysfunction may not have been overtly manifest as a clinically significant abnormality before initiating antiarrhythmic therapy. Profound sinus bradycardia or sinus arrest in a patient with cardiac disease can have serious consequences. Onset may be abrupt and can occur with the first dose, but more commonly it requires drug loading before full effects are seen. Bradycardia effects may be sustained for long periods in patients who receive medications with long half-lives or who have delayed elimination secondary to altered renal or hepatic clearance. Particularly frustrating in this regard are digitalis, type IA and IC antiarrhythmics (especially disopyramide and flecainide), and amiodarone. Bradyarrhythmic effects can be quite prolonged with slow release forms of medications.

The bradycardic effects of digitalis have long been recognized.[24] Use of this agent for ventricular rate control in patients with intermittent tachyarrhythmias can lead to sinus nodal suppression, a manifestation of the "tachy-brady" form of sick sinus syndrome, even at therapeutic drug levels. Beta-adrenergic blockers may also produce profound sinus suppressant effects that can be particularly severe. Class IB drugs can affect sinus nodal function but less prominently than do other type I agents. Calcium channel blockers, especially verapamil and diltiazem, often suppress sinus nodal function, especially in patients with intrinsic sinus nodal disease. Such effects may occur at therapeutic serum concentrations.

Beyond depressant effects on sinus nodal function, antiarrhythmic medications can produce bradyarrhythmias by causing conduction block in the AV node or His-Purkinje system. Digitalis, calcium channel blockers, beta-blockers, class IC antiarrhythmics, and amiodarone exert significant slowing effects on AV nodal conduction, and even low doses in patients with native AV nodal disease can produce conduction block. Class IA antiarrhythmic medications slow conduction through infranodal tissue, delaying activation of His-Purkinje structures; heart block produced by these drugs is usually infranodal in origin. Combination drug therapy may act in both AV nodal and infranodal tissues. Similar to sinus nodal suppression, AV nodal and His-Purkinje effects may be observed with therapeutic antiarrhythmic drug concentrations in patients with native conduction system disease; however, toxic levels can produce deleterious effects even in patients with intrinsically normal cardiac electrical function.

The development of bradycardia, progressively severe sinus pauses, or conduction block while loading antiarrhythmic medications should alert one to the possibility of bradycardic proarrhythmia. Patients with known intrinsic sinus nodal or AV nodal dysfunction who require antiarrhythmic medications should be hospitalized and monitored while drugs are loaded to steady state.

Control of drug-induced bradyarrhythmias primarily involves discontinuation, or reduction in dosage, of the offending agent. In particularly severe situations, use of atropine, isoproterenol, or temporary ventricular pacing may be required. We prefer placement of a transvenous pacing wire advanced to the right ventricular apex over external transthoracic pacing in patients with bradyarrhythmias unless these disorders are very intermittent.

Extrasystoles and Tachycardias

The classic clinical presentation of proarrhythmia involves the new development, or exacerbation, of tachyarrhythmias. The onset of ventricular fibrillation due to therapy with quinidine has been evident for many years.[11,13,14,34] Likewise, new onset of nonparoxysmal junctional tachycardia, atrial trachycardia, or ventricular tachyarrhythmias as the result of digitalis therapy has also long been recognized. It is clear that many forms of tachyarrhythmia may develop as the result of therapy with antiarrhythmic drugs, when monitored noninvasively or with invasive EP testing.[20,34–42] It is the ventricular arrhythmias that hold the greatest danger for patients, since these arrhythmias have the potential to produce sudden death.

Keeping in mind the various definitions that have been suggested for proarrhythmia[21,43] with noninvasive ambulatory monitoring (Table 1) or invasive EP testing (Table 2), one can examine the spectrum of clinical presentation of ventricular proarrhythmia. Most benign in this regard is an asymptomatic drug-related increase in VPC frequency. This can occur with any antiarrhythmic drug and constitutes a less certain form of proarrhythmia than do events that are life threatening. This uncertainty is due to the inherent variability of VPC frequency on an hourly and daily basis, requiring a multifold increase in VPC frequency to define a statistically significant proarrhythmic effect.[43–46] A more marked increase in VPC frequency is required to achieve significance for patients who have low numbers of VPCs recorded off drugs. Because of intrinsic variability in incidence of nonsustained VT, a tenfold increase in frequency is required to define a proarrhythmic response. To document such proarrhythmia noninvasively, ambulatory monitoring is required for quantitation of the arrhythmia before drug administration and again after steady state serum concentrations have been achieved.

Proarrhythmia may present as sustained VT. In patients who have already had VT off antiarrhythmic medications, a *spontaneous* increase in frequency of episodes of sustained VT on drug may be difficult to differentiate from a proarrhythmic effect. Is the antiarrhythmic medication merely ineffective, or does it truly exacerbate the arrhythmia? In this situation, the clinician is faced with the decision as to whether the dosage of medication should be increased to enhance efficacy or whether the drug should be discontinued. This decision may be especially difficult if the frequency of VT off drug was high and if VT morphology is the same on drug. A new VT rate, or change in VT morphology, suggests proarrhythmia with greater certainty. In some cases, it may be necessary to discontinue the medication, then rechallenge to decide definitively whether proarrhythmia exists. As with nonsustained ventricular arrhythmia, occurrence of proarrhythmia with one medication does not imply that it will occur with another.

The onset of drug-induced incessant VT is particularly dramatic and life-threatening. Despite attempts at termination with medication, overdrive pacing, or cardioversion, VT in this situation persists, or it recurs after only a few sinus complexes. In patients with very rapid VT, hemodynamic collapse may occur. Surprisingly, however, drug-induced incessant monomorphic VT is often acutely well tolerated; VT cycle length is usually prolonged by the proarrhythmic medication. Incessant, wide complex VT appears to occur most commonly with IC and IA antiarrhythmic agents, as well as with tricyclic antidepressants. Onset may be abrupt just after initiating therapy or occur shortly after dose escalation. The arrhythmia may develop spontaneously or be initiated by exercise or programmed ventricular stimulation in the EP laboratory.

One has no choice but to discontinue the offending agent and wait for metabolism and/or excretion of active components of the drug. Use of IV xylocaine may be helpful and should be initiated and maintained unless it is involved in the proarrhythmic process. Metabolic status of the patient should be optimized. Incessant ventricular tachycardia may respond to administration of magnesium. If due to IA agents or tricyclic antidepressants, treatment of incessant VT may also be facilitated by increasing serum pH or through the use of low-dose infusions of catecholamines. Repetitive antitachycardia ventricular pacing through an indwelling transvenous right ventricular apical electrode catheter can be particularly useful for incessant VT, especially as VT frequency begins to subside concomitant with drug elimination. Repetitive overdrive pacing and IV xylocaine in combination may be effective in patients where other attempts at therapy have failed.

Beyond *exacerbation* of VPCs, nonsustained VT, and sustained VT, antiarrhythmic medications can produce *new*, life-threatening ventricular arrhythmias that have not been previously observed in a patient. Individuals with basal nonsustained ventricular ectopy off drugs may develop new sustained monomorphic or polymorphic VT, torsades de pointes, or VF. The onset of these tachycardias is sudden, often occurring with initiation of therapy (as with quinidine syncope) or within hours or days of dose escalation. One must determine whether the new arrhythmia coincidentally represents a spontaneous occurrence or whether it represents a proarrhythmic effect. Rechallenge with the medication after its withdrawal has been suggested as the only certain way to check for proarrhythmia, but this can be quite dangerous and is not generally recommended.

New sustained arrhythmias that develop late in the course of therapy, i.e., weeks or months after initiation, do not classically represent proarrhythmia, although sudden deaths occurred late in CAST.[22] Besides proarrhythmia, late occurrences can be the result of a change in the myocardial substrate or electrical condition of the heart. Alterations in hepatic or renal function can change serum drug concentrations, metabolite levels, or electrolyte balance, leading to proarrhythmia even in the late stage. Drug level and metabolite monitoring in these situations may be especially helpful to differentiate toxic effects from spontaneous changes in the ventricular arrhythmia substrate.

Torsades de pointes has long been recognized as a complication of quinidine therapy.[34] It may also occur with other antiarrhythmic agents[39,40,47,48] as well as with tricyclic antidepressants or phenothiazines. The proarrhythmic effect may be immediate, following the first dose, or it may occur as serum drug concentrations increase. Bradycardia and hypokalemia exacerbate the tendency to torsades de pointes as a proarrhythmic response, even with "therapeutic" drug concentrations. The arrhythmia may occur as a manifestation of QT prolongation with toxic concentrations of IA drugs. Torsades de pointes shows a predilection for females and may be increased in patients with congenitally prolonged QT intervals. The tendency to sustained, polymorphic ventricular arrhythmias with initiation of quinidine therapy appears more commonly in patients with atrial fibrillation, hypokalemia, and congestive heart failure.[31] This requires initiating therapy on an inpatient basis for these individuals.

Control of torsades de pointes can be difficult, but primarily requires discontinuation of the offending agent and a correction of electrolyte abnormalities. Temporary atrial or ventricular pacing or IV administration of isoproterenol should be initiated in difficult cases to increase ventricular rate, shorten repolarization time, and decrease ventricular refractory period disparity. Temporary ventricular pacing is the preferred technique for its stability if pacing is required; this can prove quite effective for acute control of drug-induced torsades de pointes. The pacing rate is initially placed at 110 to 130 bpm and "weaned" down over several days as serum drug concentrations decrease. An occasional patient will require permanent pacing to prevent bradycardic-induced ventricular tachycardia.

New onset of polymorphic VT or VF is immediately life-threatening. Fortunately, most of these episodes can be electrically converted if they occur in a monitored hospital setting. Some episodes of drug-induced VF cannot be converted, however; ischemia may play a role in these patients. Medication-induced polymorphic VT or VF may lead to sudden death on an outpatient basis and can occur with any antiarrhythmic agent, including digitalis, especially in the presence of hypokalemia.

Withdrawal of the offending agent, therapy with IV xylocaine, and temporary pacing can help to prevent recurrence in the acute situation.

Conclusion

Proarrhythmia occurs commonly and often without warning. It can result from treatment with any antiarrhythmic medication as well as other cardiac and noncardiac drugs. The risk of ventricular proarrhythmia is increased in patients with depressed left ventricular function and rapid sustained VT.

For any proarrhythmic response, the clinical impact of the drug-induced arrhythmia must be assessed.[49] Sudden onset of sustained arrhythmias present the greatest threat. Less well defined are increases in the frequency of asymptomatic arrhythmias.[8] The onset of ventricular proarrhythmia in the EP laboratory appears to hold some prognostic significance.[21]

References

1. Velebit V, Podrid P, Lown B, et al: Aggravation and provocation of ventricular arrhythmias by antiarrhythmic drugs. Circulation 65:886, 1982.
2. Ruskin JN, McGovern B, Garan H, et al: Antiarrhythmic drugs: a possible cause of out-of-hospital cardiac arrest. N Engl J Med 309:1302, 1983.
3. Podrid PJ: Aggravation of ventricular arrhythmia: a drug-induced complication. Drugs 29:33, 1985.
4. Poser R, Lombardi F, Podrid PJ, et al: Aggravation of arrhythmia induced with antiarrhythmic drugs during electrophysiologic testing. Am Heart J 110:9, 1985.
5. Torres V, Flowers D, Somberg JC: The arrhythmogenecity of antiarrhythmic agents. Am Heart J 109:1090, 1985.
6. Buxton AE, Josephson ME: Role of electrophysiologic studies in identifying arrhythmogenic properties of antiarrhythmic drugs. Circulation 73:(Suppl)II:67, 1986.
7. Podrid PJ, Lampert S, Graboys TB, et al: Aggravation of arrhythmia by antiarrhythmic drugs: incidence and predictors. Am J Cardiol 59:38E, 1987.
8. Stanton MS, Prystowsky EN, Fineberg NS, et al: Arrhythmogenic effects of antiarrhythmic drugs: a study of 506 patients treated for ventricular tachycardia or fibrillation. J Am Coll Cardiol 14:209, 1989.
9. Woosley RL, Roden DM: Pharmacologic causes of arrhythmogenic actions of antiarrhythmic drugs. Am J Cardiol 59:19E, 1987.
10. Withering W: An account of the foxglove and some of its medical uses with practical remarks on dropsy and other diseases. Birmingham, England, M. Sweeney, 1785.

11. Kerr WJ, Bender WL: Paroxysmal ventricular fibrillation with cardiac recovery in a case of auricular fibrillation and complete heart block while under quinidine sulfate therapy. Heart 9:269, 1922.
12. Epstein MA: Ventricular standstill during the intravenous procainamide treatment of ventricular tachycardia. Am Heart J 45:890, 1953.
13. Selzer A, Wray HW: Quinidine syncope: paroxysmal ventricular fibrillation occurring during treatment of chronic atrial arrhythmias. Circulation 30:17, 1964.
14. Meltzer RS, Robert EW, McMorrow M, et al: Atypical ventricular tachycardia as a manifestation of disopyramide toxicity. Am J Cardiol 42:1049, 1978.
15. Seiklos P, Chalme TM, Evans DW: Ventricular tachycardia after disopyramide. Lancet 1:98, 1978.
16. Rosen MR, Wit AL: Arrhythmogenic actions of antiarrhythmic drugs. Am J Cardiol 59:10E, 1987.
17. Hondeghem L, Katzung B: Time- and voltage-dependent interactions of antiarrythmic drugs with cardiac sodium channels. Biochem Biophys Acta 472:373, 1972.
18. Dean JW, Lab MJ: Arrhythmia in heart failure: role of mechanically-induced changes in electrophysiology. Lancet 1:1309, 1989.
19. Rinckenberger RL, Prystowsky EN, Jackman WM, et al: Drug conversion of nonsustained ventricular tachycardia to sustained ventricular tachycardia during serial electrophysiologic studies: identification of drugs that exacerbate tachycardia and potential mechanisms. Am Heart J 103:177, 1982.
20. Stavens CS, McGovern B, Garan H, et al: Aggravation of electrically provoked ventricular tachycardia during treatment with propafenone. Am Heart J 110:24, 1985.
21. Rae AP, Kay HR, Horowitz LN, et al: Proarrhythmic effects of antiarrhythmic drugs in patients with malignant ventricular arrhythmias evaluated by electrophysiologic testing. J Am Coll Cardiol 12:131, 1988.
22. The Cardiac Arrhythmia Suppression Trial (CAST) Investigators: Preliminary report: effect of encainide and flecainide on mortality in a randomized trial of arrhythmia suppression after myocardial infarction. N Engl J Med 321:406, 1989.
23. Morganroth J: Risk factors for the development of proarrhythmic events. Am J Cardiol 59:32E, 1987.
24. Reiffel JA, Bigger JT Jr, Cramer M: The effects of digoxin on sinus nodal function before and after vagal blockade in patients with sinus nodal dysfunction: a clue to the mechanisms of the action of digitalis on the sinus node. Am J Cardiol 43:983, 1979.
25. Cohen L, Ketzes R: Magnesium sulfate and digitalis-toxic arrhythmias. JAMA 249:2808, 1983.
26. Vaughan Williams EM: A classification of antiarrhythmic actions reassessed after a decade of new drugs. Clin J Pharmacol 24:129, 1984.
27. Morganroth J, Horowitz LN: Flecainide: its proarrhythmic effect and expected changes on the surface electrocardiogram. Am J Cardiol 53:89B, 1984.
28. Zimmerman JM, Bigger JT Jr, Coromilas J: Flecainide acetate is arrhythmogenic in a canine model of sustained ventricular tachycardia (abstract). J Am Coll Cardiol 5:391, 1985.
29. Morganroth J, Andersen JL, Gentzkow GD: Classification by type of ven-

tricular arrhythmia predicts frequency of adverse cardiac events from flecainide. J Am Coll Cardiol 8:607, 1986.
30. Podrid PJ: Can antiarrhythmic drugs cause arrhythmia? J Clin Pharmacol
24:313, 1984.
31. Morganroth J, Horowitz LN: Incidence of proarrhythmic effects from quinidine in the outpatient treatment of benign or potentially lethal ventricular
arrhythmias. Am J Cardiol 56:585, 1985.
32. Goldberg D, Reiffel JA, Davis JD, et al: Electrophysiologic effects of procainamide on sinus node function in patients with and without sinus node
disease. Am Heart J 103:75, 1982.
33. Hellestrand K, Nathan AW, Bexton RS, et al: Response of an abnormal sinus
node to intravenous flecainide acetate. PACE 7:436, 1984.
34. Bauman JL, Baurnfeind RA, Hoff JV, et al: Torsades de pointes due to quinidine: observation in 31 patients. Am Heart J 107:425, 1984.
35. McComb JM, Logan KR, Khan MM, et al: Amiodarone-induced ventricular
fibrillation. Eur J Cardiol 11:381, 1980.
36. Engler RL, LeWinter M: Tocainide-induced ventricular fibrillation. Am Heart
J 101:494, 1981.
37. Winkle RA, Mason JW, Friggin JC, et al: Malignant ventricular tachyarrhythmias associated with the use of encainide. Am Heart J 102:857, 1981.
38. Cui G, Huang W, Urthaler F: Ventricular flutter during treatment with amiodarone. Am J Cardiol 51:609, 1983.
39. Sclarovsky S, Lewin RF, Kracoft O, et al: Amiodarone-induced polymorphous ventricular tachycardia. Am Heart J 105:6, 1983.
40. Brown MA, Smith WM, Lubbe WF, et al: Amiodarone-induced torsades de
pointes. Eur Heart J 7:234, 1986.
41. Soyka LF: Safety of encainide for the treatment of ventricular arrhythmias.
Am J Cardiol 58:96C, 1986.
42. Herre JM, Titus C, Franz MR, et al: Inefficacy and proarrhythmia of flecainide and encainide in patients with sustained ventricular tachycardia (abstract). Circulation 78:(Suppl) II-61, 1988.
43. Morganroth J, Borland M, Chao G: Application of a frequency definition of
ventricular proarrhythmia. Am J Cardiol 59:97, 1987.
44. Morganroth J, Horowitz LN, Josephson ME, et al: Limitations of routine
long-term electrocardiographic monitoring to assess ventricular ectopic frequency. Circulation 58:408, 1978.
45. Winkle RA: Antiarrhythmic drug effect mimicked by spontaneous variability
of ventricular ectopy. Circulation 57:1116, 1978.
46. Morganroth J: Ambulatory electrocardiographic monitoring in the evaluation of new antiarrhythmic drugs. Circulation 73:II-92, 1986.
47. Olshansky B, Martins J, Hunt S: N-acetylprocainamide causing torsades de
pointes. Am J Cardiol 50:1439, 1982.
48. Kuck KH, Kunze KP, Roewer N, et al: Sotalol-induced torsades de pointes.
Am Heart J 107:179, 1984.
49. Horowitz LN, Zipes DP, Bigger JT, et al: Proarrhythmia, arrhythmogenesis
or aggravation of arrhythmia: a status report, 1987. Am J Cardiol 59:54E,
1987.

Chapter 16

Pharmacological Therapy of Arrhythmias

Gerald V. Naccarelli,
Anne H. Dougherty, Jean Nappi, and
Deborah Wolbrette

Introduction

Parenteral and oral administration of antiarrhythmic agents represent the mainstay of antiarrhythmic therapy in the acute and chronic setting. Over the last few years, multiple new oral and intravenous antiarrhythmic agents have been approved by the Food and Drug Administration (FDA) for use in the United States. In addition, several promising investigational drugs have had extensive evaluation at this time.

The purpose of this chapter is to review the electrophysiology, pharmacokinetic properties, antiarrhythmic efficacy, and adverse reaction profiles of both currently available and several investigational antiarrhythmic agents. First, we will review clinical pharmacokinetic principles pertinent to antiarrhythmic therapy and outline the classification of these agents.

Pharmacokinetic and Pharmacodynamic Principles of Antiarrhythmic Agents[1-3]

In order to use antiarrhythmic agents appropriately, a basic understanding of pharmacokinetic principles is necessary. Pharmacoki-

From Naccarelli GV (ed): *Cardiac Arrhythmias: A Practical Approach*. Mount Kisco, NY, Futura Publishing Co., Inc., © 1991.

netics is the study of the time course of drug absorption, distribution, metabolism, and excretion. Pharmacodynamics is the relationship between drug concentration at the active pharmacological site and the response. For many drugs, there is a strong correlation between plasma drug concentration and pharmacological response because the drug diffuses from plasma into the receptor site. We assume that the plasma concentrations of drugs relate directly to concentrations in the tissues where the action of the drug occurs.

The therapeutic range of a specific drug is based on studies that have provided information regarding the plasma concentrations associated with the desired pharmacological outcome, such as suppression of premature ventricular contractions (PVCs), or toxic effects of the drug. Below the therapeutic range, few desired effects of the drug are seen. It is important to note that the therapeutic range is based on population means. Individual patients may manifest the desired pharmacological response at plasma concentrations that are well below or well above the norm. This variability in response may be due to pharmacokinetic or pharmacodynamic alterations.

There are several factors that may affect the plasma drug concentration in an individual patient. Disease states may affect rate or extent of absorption. Distribution of the drug is frequently affected by alterations in protein binding. There are differences among individuals in their ability to eliminate drugs. Changes in renal and hepatic function may prolong the time it takes to remove a drug from the body. There are also specific metabolic pathways whose rates are genetically determined (pharmacogenetics). Finally, other drugs that the patient is taking can interact in any of the four phases listed above.

Mathematical principles have been applied to the process of drug absorption, distribution, metabolism, and elimination. In pharmacokinetics, the compartment model describes the body as having one, two, or more compartments. The observed drug concentrations determine the number and type of compartments since they do not represent specific body organs or tissues.

Drug absorption is usually a fairly rapid process, however, the rate of absorption and the extent of absorption are subject to change. Bioavailability is the percentage of the administered drug that reaches the systemic circulation. Once absorbed from the gastrointestinal tract, the drug goes into the portal circulation where it may be metabolized by the liver. A drug could be 100% absorbed, yet still have a bioavailability of less than 100% due to the first-pass effect of the liver. Propranolol and verapamil are examples of drugs that have a significant first-pass effect. The dose required to achieve a specific pharmacological response is much larger when given orally as compared to the intravenous administration. The rate of drug absorption is affected a great deal by the formulation of the product. Many pharmaceutical manufacturers have developed sustained release dosage forms to try to mimic the continuous administration of a drug. With this kind of preparation, patients have the benefit of a less complicated dosage regimen, taking a drug once or twice a day rather than three or four times daily. Changing the rate of absorption does not affect the rate of elimination of the drug. Because the elimination rate of the drug is not changing, sustained release preparations usually contain more of the active ingredient as compared to a conventional tablet. An additional potential benefit of slowing the rate of absorption would be the effect of minimizing the fluctuation between the peak and trough serum drug concentrations.

Once the drug is absorbed, it reaches the systemic circulation which distributes it to the various compartments. The volume of distribution does not refer to any identifiable compartment in the body. However, the volume of distribution does indicate the extent of drug distribution into body fluids and tissues. The volume of distribution is a function of the lipid versus water solubilities and the plasma and tissue protein-binding properties of the drug. Any factor that alters the volume of distribution will influence the loading dose of a drug.

In most cases, the drug behaves as though there are two or more compartments. The first compartment is a rapidly equilibrating volume, usually made up of blood and highly perfused organs. The time it takes to get 50% of the drug distributed in this initial compartment is referred to as the alpha (α) half-life (Fig. 1). The second compartment equilibrates with the drug in the initial compartment over a longer period of time.

Another important pharmacokinetic parameter is clearance, which is the ability of the body to remove drug from the blood. Clearance is not an indicator of how much drug is being removed, but it represents the volume of blood from which the drug is removed over a specific period of time. Clearance is expressed as a volume per unit of time (such as liters per minute). Body surface area, plasma protein-binding, extraction ratio, renal function, hepatic function, and cardiac output are factors that alter clearance. A drug's clearance and volume of distribution determine the rate of removal from the body.

Drugs are assumed to enter and leave the body from the initial or central compartment. Most drugs follow a first-order elimination pro-

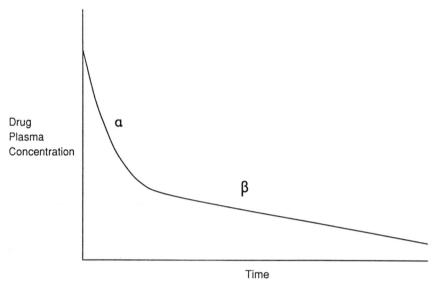

Figure 1. Schematic plot of a two-compartment model. The initial α-decay half-life is primarily due to distribution of the drug from the central to the peripheral compartments. In the β-phase, elimination of the drug from the central compartment results in a slower decline of plasma drug concentration.

cess. First-order elimination kinetics refers to a process in which the amount of drug in the body diminishes logarithmically over time. This means that the fraction of a drug in the body eliminated over a period of time remains constant. The time it takes to get 50% of the drug eliminated from this initial compartment is referred to as the beta (β) half-life. One would expect the serum drug concentration to decline by one-half over the period of time known as the elimination half-life. After a drug is discontinued, it will take approximately five half-lives before it is completely removed from the body. With drugs that follow first-order elimination, if you double the dose given, the serum drug concentrations will also double. With some drugs, this linear relationship does not hold. These particular drugs are said to follow nonlinear or dose-dependent pharmacokinetics. Nonlinear pharmacokinetics may involve absorption or distribution, but most frequently it involves the elimination process. For example, the renal tubular secretion of a compound or the hepatic metabolism may be saturable with the doses used. When this occurs, the serum drug concentration increases disproportionally in relationship to the dose given. In this situation, doubling the dose may increase serum concentrations by much more than a factor of two, thus leading to toxicity.

As successive doses of a drug are given, the drug begins to accumulate in the body. Steady state is where the rate of drug administered equals the rate of drug eliminated. For drugs that follow first-order elimination, the time to reach a steady-state equilibrium is dependent on the drug's elimination half-life. It takes one half-life to reach 50%, two half-lives to reach 75%, three half-lives to reach 87.5%, and four half-lives to reach 93.75% of the steady-state concentration. Thus, the first half-life rule can be used to estimate the time necessary to reach steady state. However, the time it takes to reach steady state varies among different drugs. Drugs that have a shorter half-life will reach steady state sooner than drugs that have a longer half-life. Reaching steady state does not ensure that the desired therapeutic response will be achieved. If the maintenance dose is too low, a subtherapeutic concentration may result. In that case, each time the maintenance dose is changed, another five half-lives must pass before the new steady-state level is reached. If it is necessary to achieve the desired pharmacological response before a period of five half-lives has passed, a loading dose may be given. Loading doses are calculated by multiplying the desired serum drug concentration and the volume of distribution.

In patients with congestive heart failure (CHF), there is a change in antiarrhythmic pharmacokinetics and drug doses may need to be altered. In CHF, the volume of distribution may be decreased by as much as 40% and drug clearances may be diminished due to decreased renal or hepatic blood flow and reduced hepatic enzyme activity. The above changes may prolong elimination half-life significantly; in some cases total daily doses need to be reduced to avoid toxicity.

Monitoring the serum concentrations of antiarrhythmic drugs is useful when certain conditions exist: (1) a good correlation exists between the pharmacological response and the serum concentration, so that one can predict response with changing concentrations, (2) the drug has a narrow therapeutic range such that toxicity is observed at doses similar to those that result in the desired response, (3) there is considerable intersubject variability in serum drug concentrations with a given dose, and (4) the desired response is not assessed by simpler means.

There are also situations where serum drug concentrations may be misleading. The stated therapeutic range may be based on a different condition than what is being treated. In the case of antiarrhythmic drugs, some therapeutic ranges are based on PVC suppression, whereas higher serum concentrations may be needed for suppression of ventricular tachycardia or prevention of sudden cardiac death. Most assays measure total drug concentration and not free drug, whereas it is the free fraction that interacts with the receptor and produces the pharmacological effect. The free fraction of the drug may differ with certain disease states (e.g., hypoalbuminemia) or be dependent on serum drug concentration. The assay may measure only the parent compound and there may be active metabolites with similar pharmacological effect to consider. In addition, these active metabolites may have different pharmacokinetic properties. Finally, most assays do not distinguish among stereoisomers even though the isomers may have quantitatively or qualitatively different pharmacological or pharmacokinetic properties. Other questions, not specifically related to assays, should also be considered if the serum drug concentration doesn't fit the clinical picture. Is the serum drug concentration at steady state? Is the patient compliant? Has a generic product with a lower bioavailability been substituted? Are the serum drug concentrations being drawn at similar times after a dose? Has the specimen been handled appropriately? Most importantly, one should keep in mind that the therapeutic range simply represents the probability that one will achieve a desired response without seeing dose-related toxicity. Each individual patient may respond differently and should be treated as such.

Antiarrhythmic Classification[4-10]

Table 1 lists a classification of antiarrhythmic drugs as proposed by Vaughn-Williams and modified over the years by Harrison and Williams. As can be seen in this table, the largest group of antiarrhythmic drugs are the sodium channel blockers. Because of the size of this class, these drugs have been subclassified into IA, IB, and IC groups based on their electrophysiological actions (see Tables 1 and 2). Some new drugs such as moricizine and recainam clearly are sodium channel blockers, but further subclassification is difficult given the current knowledge of these drugs and the limitations of this classification scheme. Acebutolol and propranolol are the two currently approved beta-blocking drugs for the treatment of ventricular arrhythmias. Intravenous esmolol has been approved as an ultra short-acting beta-blocking agent for patients with supraventricular tachycardia (SVT). Amiodarone is a class

Table 1
Vaughn-Williams Classification of Antiarrhythmic Drugs

Class	Action	Drugs
I	Sodium channel blockers	
IA	Moderate phase 0 depression Moderate conduction slowing Prolongs repolarization	Quinidine Procainimide Disopyramide
IB	Minimal phase 0 depression Shortens repolarization	Lidocaine(IV) Tocainide Mexiletine
IC	Marked phase 0 depression Marked conduction slowing Slight effect on repolarization	Flecainide Encainide Propafenone
*I	Sodium channel blockers-mechanism not clearly defined	Moricizine Recainam
II	Beta-blockers	Propranolol Acebutolol
III	Prolong repolarization	Bretylium Amiodarone Sotalol
IV	Calcium channel blockers	Verapamil Diltiazem
	Purine nucleosides	Adenosine
	Digitalis glycosides	Digoxin Digitoxin

III agent along with bretylium and sotalol. The calcium channel blockers have minimal usefulness in the treatment of ventricular arrhythmias and this is not an approved indication of this subclass of drugs. Intravenous verapamil is one of the treatments of choice for the acute treatment of hemodynamically stable paroxysmal SVT. Intravenous diltiazem is undergoing clinical investigation for the acute termination of SVT. Both oral verapamil and diltiazem have commonly been used in the treatment of SVT and for rate control in atrial fibrillation, although for diltiazem, these are not FDA-approved indications. Digitalis glycosides and purine antagonists, such as adenosine, are not classifiable in this system.

Table 3 lists the expected electrocardiographic effects of the antiarrhythmic agents. Type IA drugs predominantly prolong repolarization

Table 2
Basic Electrophysiologic Effects of Antiarrhythmic Agents

	APD	dV/DT and Conduction Velocity	Use Dependence	ERP	ERP/ADP	Sinus Node Auto-maticity	Phase 4 Auto-maticity	VFT	MSA
IA	↑↑	↓↓	intermediate	↑↑	↑	0	↓	↑	+
IB	↓	↓	fast	↓	↑	0	↓	↑	+
IC	↑↓	↓↓↓	slow	↑	↑	0↓	↓	↑	+
II	↓	0↓	NA	0↓	↑	↓	↓	↑	+
III	↑↑	0↓	intermediate	↑↑	↑	↓	↓	NA	0
IV	0	0	NA	0	0	↓	0*	0	0

APD = action potential duration; dv/dt = rate of rise phase 0 of action potential; ERP = effective refractory period; VFT = ventricular fibrillation threshold; MSA = membrane stabilizing activity.
* Decreases spontaneous depolarization in calcium channel, slow-response tissue.
↑ = increased; ↑↑ = moderately increased; ↓ = decreased; ↓↓ = moderately decreased; ↓↓↓ = greatly decreased; 0 = no effect; + = present.

and thus the QT interval. The IB drugs have a minimal effect on the electrocardiogram with a minimal shortening of the QT interval. The IC drugs, by slowing myocardial conduction, prolong the PR and QRS intervals with minimal effects on the QT interval. The beta-blocking and calcium channel blockers prolong the PR interval by slowing conduction in the AV node. Finally, sotalol and amiodarone typically prolong the PR and QRS intervals, although their primary effect is to prolong the QT interval.

Table 3
Electrocardiographic Effects of
Antiarrhythmic Agents

	PR	QRS	QT	JT
IA	↑	↑	↑↑	↑↑
IB	0	0	0↓	0↑
IC	↑↑	↑↑	↑	0
II	↑	0	0	0
III*	↑	↑	↑↑	↑↑
IV	↑	0	0	0

* Amiodarone, sotalol.
Abbreviations: same as used in Table 2.

Table 4
Antiarrhythmic Drugs: Pharmacokinetic Summary

Drug	Route of Administration	Oral Bioavailability (%)	Protein Binding (%)	Half-Life** (hrs)
Quinidine	p.o., IM, IV	80	75–95	6
Procainamide	p.o., IV	85	15	3
Disopyramide	p.o.	80	40–81	7
Lidocaine	IV	35	70	1.7
Phenytoin	p.o., IV	90	—	22
Tocainide	p.o.	95	15	13–15
Mexiletine	p.o.	85	70	10–12
Moricizine	p.o.	38	95	2–5 (9 chronic)
Flecainide	p.o.	90	40	20
Encainide	p.o.	30(85)*	70	2–3 (EM)
Propafenone	p.o.	<25	95	4–6 (EM)
Recainem	p.o.	80	15	6–10
Propranolol	p.o., IV	10	—	3–6 (p.o.)
Acebutolol	p.o.	40	25	3–4
Esmolol	IV	NA	56	9 min
Bretylium	IV	NA	—	8
Amiodarone	p.o., IV	50	90	53 days
Sotalol	p.o., IV	90	50	7–15
Verapamil	p.o., IV	16	90	5 (p.o.)
Diltiazem	p.o., IV	40	75	3.5
Adenosine	IV	NA	—	10 seconds
Digoxin	p.o., IV	70	25	36–48
Digitoxin	p.o.	95	90	7–9 days

* poor metabolizers
** parent compound
NA = not applicable
EM = extensive metabolizers

In the remainder of this chapter, we will individually review the electrophysiology, pharmacokinetics, efficacy, and adverse effect profile of the older and newer antiarrhythmic agents. Comparative pharmacokinetic data (Tables 4, 5), drug interactions (Table 6), efficacy in ventricular (Table 7) and supraventricular arrhythmias (Table 8)., hemodynamics (Table 9), proarrhythmic potential (Table 10), and toxicity (Table 11) are listed.

Table 5
Pharmacokinetic Summary

	Principal Route of Elimination	Active Metabolites	Half-Life (hrs) Active Metabolites	Steady State* (days)	Therapeutic Range (µg/mL)	Usual Maintenance Dose (mg)
Quinidine	Hepatic	3-hydroxyquinidine	NA	1–2	2–7	200–400 q.i.d.
Procainamide	Hepatic + Renal	N-acetylprocainmide	9–10	1–2	4–10	500–1500 q.i.d.
Disopyramide	Renal + Hepatic	N-monodeakyl disopyramide	NA	2	2–8	100–200 q.i.d.
Lidocaine	Hepatic	MEG + GX	NA	NA	1.5–6.0	1–4 mg/min
Phenytoin	Hepatic	No	NA	3	10–20	200–600 q/day
Tocainide	Hepatic + Renal	No	NA	2–3	4–10	300–600 t.i.d.
Mexiletine	Hepatic	No	NA	2–3	0.5–2	150–300 t.i.d.
Moricizine	Hepatic	No	NA	2	NE	200–300 t.i.d.
Flecainide	Hepatic + Renal	No	NA	4	0.4–1	100–150 b.i.d.
Encainide	Hepatic	ODE 3-mode	8–12	3–4	NE	25–50 t.i.d.
Propafenone	Hepatic	5-OH propafenone	6–12	3	NE	150–300 t.i.d.
Recainam	Renal & Hepatic	No	NA	2–3	NE	200–600 t.i.d.
Propranolol	Hepatic	No	NA	2	100–150	10–40 q.i.d.
Acebutolol	Hepatic & Renal	Diacetolol	8–13	3	NE	200–400 q/day
Esmolol	Hepatic	No	NA	NA	NE	500 µg/kg (load)
Bretylium	Renal	No	NA	NA	NE	1–4 mg/min
Amiodarone	Hepatic	Desethylamiodarone	months	months	1.5–2.5	200–400 q/day
Sotalol	Renal	No	NA	2–3	NE	80–320 b.i.d.
Verapamil	Hepatic	No	NA	1	0.1–0.4	0.1 mg/kg IV (80–160 p.o. t.i.d.)
Diltiazem	Hepatic	No	NA	1	NE	30–90 p.o. t.i.d.
Adenosine	Cellular	No	NA	NA	NE	6–12 mg IV
Digoxin	Renal	No	NA	10	0.1–2.0	.25 mg q/day
Digitoxin	Hepatic	No	NA	30	10–20	0.15 mg q/day

* Takes into account active metabolites
NE = not established
NA = not applicable

Table 6
Important Antiarrhythmic Drug Interactions

Drug	Interacts	Result
Quinidine	Digoxin	doubling of digoxin levels
Propafenone	Digoxin	"
Amiodarone	Digoxin	"
	Quinidine	15–35% increase in Na channel
	Procainamide	blocker levels
	Disopyramide	
	Flecainide	
	Warfarin	2–3× increase in prothrombin times
Disopyramide	Phenytoin	decreases disopyramide levels
Verapamil	Digoxin	increase in digoxin levels
Moricizine	Theophylline	decreases theophylline levels

Table 7
Comparative Efficacy in Ventricular Arrhythmias

	PVC/VT-NS (Holter)	Sustained VT/VF (PES)
Quinidine	65%	20–25%
Procainamide	60%	20–25%
Disopyramide	60%	20–25%
Tocainide	50%	10–15%
Mexiletine	50%	10–20%
Moricizine	65%	20%
Flecainide	75%	20–25%
Encainide	75%	20–25%
Propafenone	70%	20–25%
Recainam	65%	20%
Propranolol	45%	5%
Acebutolol	45%	5%
Amiodarone	75%	20%(60%)*
Sotalol	55%	30%

* Higher spontaneous efficacy rates despite PES inefficacy.

Table 8

Comparative Oral Efficacy and Electrophysiologic Properties in Supraventricular Arrhythmias

	PACS	AFIB	AVNant	AVNRT	AP	WPW-PSVT
Quinidine	+ +	+ +	±	+	+	+
Procainamide	+ +	+ +	±	+	+	+
Disopyramide	+ +	+ +	±	+	+ +	+ +
Tocainide	0	0	0	0	±	0
Mexiletine	0	0	0	0	±	0
Moricizine	+	NE	0	NE	+	NE
Flecainide	+ +	+ +	+	+ +	+ + +	+ + +
Encainide	+ +	+ +	+ +	+ +	+ + +	+ + +
Propafenone	+ +	+ +	+ +	+ +	+ +	+ +
Recainam	+	+ +	+	+ +	+ +	+ +
Beta-Blockers	+	+	+ +	+	0	+
Amiodarone	+ +	+ + +	+ +	+ +	+	+ +
Sotalol	+	+ +	+ +	+ +	+	+
Digoxin	0	+ *	+ +	+	±	+
Verapamil	0	+ *	+ +	+	±	+
Diltiazem	0	+ *	+ +	+	±	+

* rate control only

AFIB = atrial fibrillation; AVNant = antegrade slowing of AV nodal conduction; AVNRT = AV node reentrant tachycardia; AP = effects of accessory pathway conduction; NE = not established.

+ + + = very effective; + + = moderately effective; + = effective; ± = minimal or inconsistent efficacy; 0 = not effective.

Type IA Antiarrhythmic Agents

Procainamide (Procan-SR®, Pronestyl®, Pronestyl-SR®)[21-29]

The primary examples of the type IA antiarrhythmic agents are procainamide, quinidine, and disopyramide. Procainamide is a type IA antiarrhythmic agent useful in both atrial and ventricular arrhythmias. It is available intravenously and in oral shorter-acting and sustained release preparations. Procan-SR® is delivered via an early release wax matrix and Pronestyl-SR® as an early release inner core.

Table 9
Negative Inotropic Potential of Antiarrhythmic Drugs

Most Negative Inotropy	Disopyramide
	Verapamil
	↓
	Propranolol
	Acebutolol
↓	↓
	Flecainide
	↓
	Propafenone
	Sotalol
	Diltiazem
	↓
	Encainide
	Recainam
↓	↓
	Lidocaine
	Quinidine
	Procainamide
	Tocainide
Least Negative Inotropy	Mexiletine
	Moricizine
	Amiodarone
	Bretylium

Electrophysiology

Procainamide has electrophysiological properties similar to quinidine (see the section on quinidine). However, the electrophysiological effects are different because procainamide has fewer vagolytic effects. Typically, procainamide prolongs the AH, HV, QRS, and QR intervals. Refractory periods of the atria, His-Purkinje system, ventricle, and accessary pathways are prolonged. Similar to quinidine, procainamide may shorten the AVNERP.

Pharmacokinetics

Procainamide is 95% absorbed in the small intestine with peak levels occurring 15 minutes to 2 hours after oral administration. Bioavailability

Table 10
Proarrhythmic Potential

	Proarrhythmia Nonsustained VT Patients	Proarrhythmia Sustained VT Patients	TDP
Quinidine	+	+ +	+ + +
Procainamide	+	+ +	+ +
Disopyramide	+	+ +	+ +
Tocainide	±	+	0
Mexiletine	±	+	0
Moricizine	+	+	0
Flecainide	+	+ + +	±
Encainide	+	+ + +	±
Propafenone	+ +	+ +	±
Recainam	+	+ +	±
Beta Blockers	±	+	0
Amiodarone	±	+	+
Sotalol	+	+	+ + +

TDP = torsades de pointes; + + + = very high potential; + + = moderate potential; + = minimal potential; ± = inconsistent potential; 0 = no potential.

is about 85%. Procainamide is acetylated in the liver to an active metabolite, n-acetylprocainamide (NAPA), and the rate of acetylation is dependent on acetylation phenotype. In rapid acetylators, NAPA levels usually exceed the parent compound. NAPA is an active metabolite with 70% of the antiarrhythmic activity of the parent compound. Thirty to 60% of the drug is excreted unchanged in the urine and the remainder is excreted as NAPA. Orally, the half-life of procainamide is only 3–4 hours, thus steady state is achieved within 24 hours. NAPA has a half-life of 6 hours. Therapeutic procainamide levels are in the 4–8 μg/mL range with NAPA levels of 8–16 and combined levels in excess of 16–20 μg/mL are commonly associated with toxicity.

Dosing

Dosing with procainamide is usually initiated at about 50 mg/kg/day. Thus, sustained release therapy in a 60-kg person should be started at a dose of 750 mg q.i.d. Doses are titrated to efficacy, toxicity, and blood levels. Usually, daily doses are 500–1500 mg per dose.

Table 11
Comparative Toxicity of Antiarrhythmic Drugs

	Subjective Toxicity	End-Organ Toxicity
Quinidine	+ +	+ +
Procainamide	+	+ +
Disopyramide	+	±
Tocainide	+ +	+
Mexiletine	+ +	±
Propafenone	+	±
Moricizine	+	±
Flecainide	±	±
Encainide	±	±
Phenytoin	+ +	+
Recainam	+	±
Propranolol	+	±
Acebutolol	+	±
Amiodarone	+	+ + + +
Sotalol	+	±

+ + + = very common occurrence; + + = commonly occurs; + = occasionally occurs; ± = rarely occurs.

Intravenous procainamide requires loading doses of 10–15 mg/kg given at 25–50 mg/min depending on blood pressure. This can be followed by a 1–4 mg/min IV drip.

Efficacy

Although not FDA approved for use in treating atrial arrhythmias, IV and oral procainamide may be used to chemically convert and treat patients with ectopic atrial tachycardia, atrial flutter, atrial fibrillation, and PSVT. In atrial fibrillation and the Wolff-Parkinson-White syndrome, IV procainamide is the treatment of choice if blood pressure is stable. Procainamide is about 60% effective in suppressing PVCs, couplets, and nonsutained VT as assessed by Holter monitoring. In sustained VT, procainamide is effective in about 20–25% as assessed by programmed stimulation. The use of oral procainamide in combination with mexiletine or tocainide has demonstrated an added efficacy with a lower subjective toxicity because of lower daily doses of each prepa-

428 • CARDIAC ARRHYTHMIAS: A PRACTICAL APPROACH

ration. The response to IV procainamide in the electrophysiology laboratory appears to predict an acceptable electrophysiological response to oral procainamide and other antiarrhythmic agents. Intravenous procainamide is one of the parenteral treatments of choice for atrial and/or ventricular tachyarrhythmias. One recent study demonstrated that intravenous procainamide was superior to lidocaine in terminating sustained VT. In wide QRS tachycardias of undetermined etiology, IV procainamide is one of the drugs of choice if blood pressure is stable, since it can be effective in both supraventricular and ventricular tachyarrhythmias.

Adverse Effects

Orally, procainamide has minimal acute subjective toxicity including rare nausea, anorexia, vomiting, and rash. End-organ toxicity of concern is a rare agranulocytosis that usually occurs during the first 3 months of treatment.

The major limiting adverse reaction with procainamide has been the development of a systemic lupus-like reaction in 10–20% of patients. This is more likely to occur in slow acetylators (50% of the population). Over 70% of patients will develop a positive ANA titer within a year. This laboratory abnormality alone does not warrant discontinuation of therapy.

Procainamide has a negative inotropic effect that is mild and may be less than that of quinidine. In a 21-patient comparative study, procainamide caused less hemodynamic compromise than tocainide or encainide. Negative inotropy is most marked when the drug is rapidly infused parenterally.

Procainamide can cause high-degree AV block and widening of QRS with bundle branch block. Ventricular proarrhythmia can occur including the new onset of sustained, monomorphic VT or torsades de pointes. In renal failure, we have noted several patients to develop significantly increased levels of both procainamide and NAPA with the development of torsades de pointes.

It should also be noted that procainamide has a fairly narrow therapeutic index, indicating that the therapeutic and toxic dose may be fairly close. This pharmacological attribute may necessitate extra care in selecting both the closing interval and the type of procainamide utilized in a given clinical situation. Indeed, the narrow therapeutic range for procainamide has raised the suggestion that extreme care and caution be utilized in selection of generic alternatives.

Summary

Procainamide is an effective agent for treating supraventricular and ventricular arrhythmias. Hemodynamically, it is well tolerated. The intravenous use of this drug makes it popular in the emergency, critical care, and electrophysiology laboratory arenas. Sustained release preparations are usually prescribed to improve patient compliance and minimize generic substitution. The narrow therapeutic range for procainamide also requires caution in selected dose and in the specific preparation of procainamide being utilized.

Quinidine (Quinidex®, Quinaglute®, Cardioguin®)[10–20]

Quinidine is a type IA antiarrhythmic agent. It is manufactured as a sulfate salt (82.8% quinidine base) with long-acting trade name formulations (Quinidex®) and also as the polygalactoronate (Cardioquin®) and gluconate salts (62% quinidine base) (Quinaglute®).

Electrophysiology

Basic experiments (Fig. 2) demonstrate that quinidine reduces automaticity by raising threshold potential and decreasing the rate of rise of phase 4 depolarization. Quinidine decreases the rate of rise of phase 0 of the action potential by blocking sodium influx and thus it slows conduction. This action of quinidine is frequency-dependent with depression of V_{max} being greater at faster heart rates. Quinidine also prolongs APD, ERP, and the ERP/APD ratio.

Quinidine has vagolytic effects that can increase sinus heart rate, enhance AV nodal conduction, and shorten AV node refractory periods. Due to conduction slowing and competitive vagolytic properties, the PR and AH interval may not increase. Quinidine increases the ERP of the atria, His-Purkinje system, ventricles, and accessory pathways. Quinidine will increase the HV, QT, and QRS intervals.

Pharmacokinetics

Because quinidine has various preparations, pharmacokinetics vary. With quinidine sulfate, 95% is absorbed orally, bioavailability is about 70–90%, and peak levels occur 1–3 hours after ingestion. Twenty

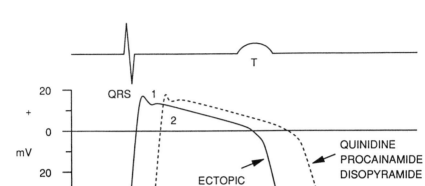

Figure 2. Transmembrane action potential of a spontaneously depolarizing fiber (solid line). Effect of type IA antiarrhythmic on action potential (broken line). Note type IA drugs, slow rate of rise of phase 0 (Na^+ channel-dependent process), prolonged action potential duration, and thus QT interval and suppressed phase 4 automaticity.

to 50% is excreted unchanged by the kidneys. Otherwise, quinidine is metabolized by hydroxylation in the liver. Both 3-hydroxyquinidine and 2'-oxoquinidine appear to have some antiarrhythmic activity. The half-life of quinidine sulfate is 5–7 hours, and thus takes about 24–36 hours to reach steady state. Therapeutic plasma levels are 2–7 μg/mL. Extended release preparations release about one-third of the dose immediately, with the remainder time-released over 6–10 hours.

Dosage

Dosage of quinidine sulfate is usually 200–600 mg q.i.d., depending on levels, efficacy, and intolerance. With most arrhythmias, we start at 300 mg q.i.d. Quinidex® is given at the same total daily dose using a b.i.d. or t.i.d. schedule. Quinaglute® doses range from 324 to 972 mg b.i.d. or t.i.d.

Efficacy

Quinidine is effective in suppressing PACs and ectopic atrial tachycardias. Quinidine has been useful in the chemical cardioversion and maintenance of patients with atrial flutter and fibrillation.

By suppressing PACs and PVCs and by slowing conduction and prolonging refractoriness of accessory pathways and the retrograde limb of the AV node, quinidine has been effective in treating PSVT secondary to AV nodal re-entrant tachycardia (AVNRT) and AV re-entrant tachycardia (AVRT). Similar to procainamide, quinidine rarely completely blocks conduction in accessory pathways with refractory periods ≤270 ms.

Quinidine is effective for the chronic suppression of ventricular ectopic activity (VEA). Based on Holter monitoring, quinidine will effectively suppress PVCs, couplets, and nonsustained ventricular tachycardia (VT) in about 60% of patients. In patients with sustained VT/VF, efficacy rates as determined by programmed stimulation are 20–25%. Patients with ejection fractions >30% appear to have higher efficiacy rates in the latter group.

Combination therapy with tocainide or mexiletine, using lower maintenance doses of both drugs, achieves added efficacy and lower toxicity. Quinidine can also be used in conjunction with amiodarone although, due to a drug interaction, quinidine doses need to be lowered by about one-third.

Adverse Effects

Subjective toxicity with quinidine is common. Approximately 10–35% of patients will develop nausea, vomiting, anorexia, or diarrhea. Some of these adverse reactions are dose-related. Fever, rash, and tinnitus can rarely occur. End-organ toxicity includes the occurrence of a rare drug-induced thrombocytopenia and granulomatous hepatitis.

Quinidine has mild negative inotropic activity, but its overall effect on cardiac output appears to be minimal. Some of its direct negative inotropic activity may be counterbalanced by its peripheral vasodilatory effects, mediated partially by α-blockade. Rarely, the vasodilatory properties of quinidine can lead to orthostatic hypotension.

Importantly, quinidine interacts with digoxin (Table 6) increasing digoxin levels by a factor of two. This occurs secondary to quinidine displacing digoxin from the tissues and by reducing renal clearance rates of digoxin. When used in combination, digoxin doses should be halved. As noted above, amiodarone also interacts with quinidine.

Due to its vagolytic effects, quinidine may cause an increase in ventricular response when used to treat patients for atrial fibrillation or flutter. Also, by slowing the atrial rate and decreasing concealed AV nodal block in the AV node, atrial flutter with 1:1 conduction can occur. Prophylactic digitalization may minimize the occurrence of this phenomenon.

Quinidine may worsen infranodal block. By slowing conduction, quinidine can be proarrhythmic with the development of new-onset monomorphic VT. Of more concern, quinidine may prolong the QT interval and cause drug-aggravated torsades de pointes in up to 5% of patients. We have noted this most commonly in patients treated for atrial fibrillation, especially if they have left ventricular dysfunction and concomitant ventricular arrhythmias. Most cases of drug-induced torsades de pointes reported in the literature have been secondary to quinidine. This is probably secondary to the fact that quinidine is more likely to cause torsades than other antiarrhythmic agents and that in the US, quinidine preparations are the most commonly prescribed antiarrhythmic agents, thus increasing the likelihood of periodic occurrences.

Summary

Quinidine has a good hemodynamic profile and versatility in treating both atrial and ventricular arrhythmias. Quinidine's usefulness has been limited by its frequent gastrointestinal side effects, rare end-organ toxicity, and incidence of torsades de pointes. Sustained-release formulations have been useful in maintaining smoother plasma concentrations and improving patient compliance via b.i.d. or t.i.d. dosing. Brand name sustained release formulations have minimized bioavailability problems encountered during various generic switchovers during short-acting therapy.

Disopyramide (Norpace®, Norpace CR®)[30–34]

Disopyramide is a type IA antiarrhythmic agent approved by the FDA in 1977 for treatment of ventricular arrhythmias. Similar to quinidine and procainamide, it has vagolytic actions.

Electrophysiology

In basic animal and human experiments, disopyramide has electrophysiological effects similar to those of quinidine and procainamide (see quinidine).

Clinically, disopyramide prolongs atrial, His-Purkinje, ventricular, and accessory pathway refractoriness. It also prolongs the HV, QRS, and QT intervals. It has minimal effect on heart rate and sinus node recovery times.

Pharmacokinetics

About 83–90% of an oral dose of disopyramide is absorbed and its bioavailability is 70–85%. Peak levels occur in 2 hours. Fifty-five percent of a dose is recovered after renal excretion unchanged in the urine while 25% is recovered as the active n-monodealkylated metabolite. Disopyramide has nonlinear pharmacokinetics with decreasing plasma protein binding as serum concentrations increase.

The half-life varies from 4 to 10 hours (averages 6–7 hours) and steady state is achieved within 40 hours. In patients with renal failure, elimination half-life is significantly increased. In patients with CHF, T½ increases to 8–10 hours. Usually therapeutic levels are in the 2–5 μg/mL range.

Dosing

Dosing ranges from 100, 150, 200 mg po q.i.d. The controlled release formulation is effective with a b.i.d. dosing schedule. We usually initiate therapy with short acting disopyramide prior to the b.i.d. conversion to the same total daily dose with the CR formulation.

Efficacy

Although disopyramide does not have an FDA-approved indication, it is very effective in treating patients with various supraventricular arrhythmias including ectopic atrial tachycardia, atrial flutter and atrial fibrillation, and PSVT associated and not associated with the WPW syndrome. Electrophysiological data suggest that disopyramide may have more potent effects than quinidine and procainamide on accessory pathway tissue.

Disopyramide is as effective as procainamide (about 60%) in suppressing PVCs, ventricular couplets, and nonsustained runs of VT as assessed by Holter monitoring. Comparative studies have shown disopyramide to be as effective as quinidine, but less effective than flecainide in a similar group of patients. In sustained VT, disopyramide is effective in 20–25% of patients as assessed by programmed stimulation.

Adverse Effects

Disopyramide's subjective toxicity is primarily secondary to its anticholinergic activity (approximately 0.6% of atropine). These include dry mouth (30%), blurred vision, urinary retention, constipation (10%), and worsening of glaucoma. Nausea, vomiting, and skin rash have also been noted. The above reactions require discontinuation in about 10% of patients. No significant end-organ toxicity has been noted with disopyramide.

Disopyramide's most important adverse reaction is worsening of CHF secondary to its significant negative inotropic activity and increase of peripheral vascular resistance. CHF occurs in 50% of patients with a prior history of CHF and only in 5% of other patients.

Disopyramide, by slowing conduction, can cause complete AV block and bundle branch block and increases in QRS interval. Slowing of conduction and prolongation of the QT interval can cause proarrhythmias such as monomorphic sustained VT and torsades de pointes.

Summary

Disopyramide is effective in treating both supraventricular and ventricular arrhythmias. Its major limitation has been its hemodynamic profile and frequent anticholinergic side effects. Because of its significant negative inotropy, this drug is rarely used in the large group of patients with arrhythmias associated with left ventricular dysfunction.

Type IA Agents: Patient Selection

All three type IA agents are useful for atrial dysrhythmias, although only quinidine has FDA approval for this indication. All are equally effective in treating ventricular arrhythmias. In patients with left ventricular dysfunction, disopyramide should be used cautiously. In patients on concomitant digoxin, we prefer procainamide or disopyramide because of the digoxin-quinidine interaction. All three drugs can be used in combination with type IB drugs if necessary.

Type IB Antiarrhythmic Agents

Lidocaine Hydrochloride (Xylocaine®)[35–39]

Lidocaine hydrochloride is a short-acting intravenous, type IB antiarrhythmic agent.

Electrophysiology

Electrophysiologically, lidocaine has characteristics of a type IB sodium channel blocking agent. Lidocaine minimally blocks the sodium channels and thus minimally slows conduction in the His-Purkinje system and myocardium with small increases in QRS duration. Lidocaine has more conduction slowing properties in ischemic tissue. Lidocaine has little to no effect on atrial tissue and AV nodal tissue and thus is ineffective in treating supraventricular arrhythmias. Lidocaine has variable effects on accessory pathway tissue. It may slow or have little effect on conduction in most patients. However, a small percentage of patients may have enhanced conduction and thus lidocaine should not be used in atrial fibrillation and antidromic conduction down an accessory pathway, since the percentage and rate of pre-excited beats may increase. Lidocaine depresses automaticity in Purkinje fibers and thus would be predicted to be efficacious in suppressing irritable ventricular foci. Its ability to slow conduction in cardiac tissue and a net increase in the ratio of the effective refractory period to action potential duration may help prevent re-entrant ventricular arrhythmias.

Pharmacokinetics

Lidocaine has poor oral absorption and 90% of an administered dose is rapidly metabolized in the liver into two major metabolites: monoethyl glycinexylidide (MEG) and glycinexylidide (GX). MEG is 80% and GX

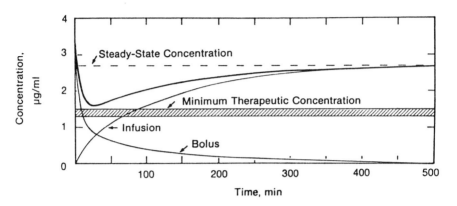

Figure 3. Lidocaine blood levels achieved with intravenous bolus, constant infusion, or bolus immediately followed by infusion. (Reproduced by permission: Harrison DC, JAMA.[39])

is 10% as potent as the parent compound. Because of these two facts, lidocaine is not useful orally and must be administered parenterally to achieve therapeutic blood levels; 70% of lidocaine is bound to plasma proteins.

Lidocaine administered as an intravenous bolus is distributed rapidly into the intravascular ($T\frac{1}{2}$ = 8 minutes) and then diffuses quickly into the peripheral compartment. Lidocaine has a half-life of $1\frac{1}{2}$ to 2 hours in the second pass of redistribution with extensive metabolism occurring hepatically. Because of this, if an infusion is started without a bolus loading dose, it takes from 20 to 60 minutes to attain therapeutic levels (see Fig. 3). If an intravenous bolus of lidocaine is given, blood levels will fall below the therapeutic range in less than 20 minutes unless a maintenance infusion is started simultaneously.

Dosing

Recommended dosing includes a loading bolus infusion of 75 mg IV followed by a 1–4 mg/min maintenance infusion. Within 15 minutes of the first bolus, a second bolus can be given to maintain levels. If maintenance infusions at higher doses are needed, patients should receive a 50–75 mg IV bolus prior to increasing the rate of the maintenance infusion in order to avoid delays in attaining higher blood levels (Fig. 3).

In patients with severe heart failure, there is decreased hepatic blood flow and thus a decreased metabolism of lidocaine. In addition, there is also a decrease in the effective central compartment of the drug. Because of this, lower doses (about ⅓ to ½) need to be used in severe CHF patients to avoid toxicity. Patients with impaired hepatocellular function also require lower doses. Elderly patients are more sensitive to the toxic effects of lidocaine. In older patients, lower loading and maintenance doses should be used. Intramuscular (deltoid) administration of a 10% solution of lidocaine can be given. The usual dose is 4.5 mg/kg bolus which will produce blood levels within 5–120 minutes. Lidopens® have been used to give this dose in high-risk patients in emergency situations.

Efficacy

Lidocaine is used as the drug of choice for the rapid suppression of PVCs and prophylaxis against the occurrence of VT/VF. In the CCU setting, the prophylactic use of lidocaine is commonly employed to suppress warning arrhythmias such as >5 PVCs/hour, multifocal or R-on-T PVCs, or complex forms such as ventricular couplets and nonsustained VT. Lidocaine can be used out of hospital both intravenously or intramuscularly as a prophylactic measure during transportation of patients to the hospital.

Adverse Effects

Lidocaine has well-described, often dose-related, adverse effects. Neurological side effects include numbness, tingling, seizures, tremors, paresthesias, disorientation, dulled sensorium, tinnitus, and drowsiness. Gastrointestinal side effects include nausea and vomiting. Lidocaine is well tolerated hemodynamically. As with all antiarrhythmic drugs, it can have some negative inotropic potential in patients with severely impaired left ventricular function. However, drug-induced hypotension is extremely rare. Lidocaine may minimally slow conduction in the His-Purkinje system. Therefore, in patients with significant His-Purkinje disease, lidocaine may induce complete AV block. However, this is extremely rare, and much more likely to occur if IA or IC agents are used. The only contraindication to the use of lidocaine is a known hypersensitivity. Therapeutic blood levels are in the 1–5 µg/mL range. Levels in excess of 5 µg/mL are commonly associated with subjective toxicity.

Summary

Lidocaine is often used as the drug of choice for the parenteral treatment of ventricular arrhythmias in the critical care and perioperative setting. The short half-life assures therapeutic concentration quickly in the emergency situation. Hemodynamically, it is well tolerated. Cardiac adverse effects are rare.

Phenytoin (Dilantin®)[40–43]

Phenytoin is an anticonvulsant that also has type IB antiarrhythmic properties. Although used as an antiarrhythmic, it does not have FDA approval for this indication.

Electrophysiology

Under conditions of a normal potassium concentration, phenytoin depresses resting membrane potential and V_{max} of the action potential. However, if potassium levels are low, phenytoin may increase RMP and V_{max}. Phenytoin shortens APD greater than ERP and thus, similar to lidocaine, can shorten the QT interval despite a net increase in ERP/APD ratio. Phenytoin decreases phase 4 automaticity of studied cardiac tissues and can suppress triggered afterdepolarizations seen with digitalis toxicity. Phenytoin enhances AV node conduction (shortens AH) and shortens the AVNFRP and may improve conduction in the setting of digitalis toxicity. Phenytoin has a depressant effect on the sympathetic centers of the central nervous system.

Pharmacokinetics

Oral phenytoin has slow oral absorption with peak levels occurring at 3–12 hours. The half-life of the drug varies between 24 to 36 hours and it takes at least 5 days for levels to reach steady state. Phenytoin is primarily hydroxylated in the liver. Subsequent glucuronidation is followed by urinary excretion. Therapeutic plasma levels are 10–20 µg/mL. Dosing includes a 1000 mg loading dose followed by 300–600 mg per day maintenance dose. Intravenous loading of 1000 mg can be obtained by infusing 10–25 mg/min under close hemodynamic monitoring.

Efficacy

Phenytoin has been used as a treatment for improving AV node function and digitoxic arrhythmias in digitalis toxicity. Phenytoin is rarely effective in treating significant ventricular arrhythmias. Phenytoin has been well studied in pediatric patients who develop ventricular arrhythmias postoperatively after repair of tetralogy of Fallot. In this setting, phenytoin remains one of the treatments of choice. Since this drug shortens the QT interval, it is one of the treatments of choice with or without beta-blockers in patients with ventricular arrhythmias associated with the prolonged QT syndrome. Combination therapy with type IA agents have not been well studied. Suppression of inducible sustained VT in the electrophysiology laboratory is 11–13%.

Adverse Effects

Intravenously, phenytoin can cause hypotension. Blood pressure monitoring and slow infusion rates are essential. Orally, the drug causes diplopia, dizziness, vertigo, ataxia, cerebellar abnormalities, nystagmus, drowsiness, skin reactions, gingival hyperplasia, and Stevens-Johnson syndrome.

Summary

Phenytoin is rarely used as a front-line antiarrhythmic. We have primarily used it in the setting of digitalis toxicity, prolonged QT syndromes, in postoperative congenital heart disease patients, and in patients who require short-term parenteral therapy when most front-line antiarrhythmics have been ineffective.

Tocainide (Tonocard®)[44–48]

Tocainide is an orally useful primary amine analogue of lidocaine.

Electrophysiology

Its electrophysiological effects in vitro are similar to those of both lidocaine and mexiletine. Tocainide shortens the effective refractory period of the ventricles and shortens the duration of the action potential. It has little effect on sinus node automaticity or intracardiac conduction. Thus, tocainide may minimally shorten the QT interval, but otherwise other electrocardiographic intervals are unaffected.

Pharmacokinetics

Tocainide has excellent oral absorption and bioavailability exceeding 95%. Peak blood levels occur 60 to 90 minutes after administration and the drug is only 10–20% protein-bound. Tocainide is eliminated by both the renal and hepatic routes. No major active metabolites exist. Its onset of action is 1–1½ hours and its half-life averages 11–19 hours with a mean of 15 hours. This prolongs in the setting of renal insufficiency. There is no important drug interaction between tocainide and digoxin. Therapeutic levels of tocainide are between 4 and 10 μg/mL.

Dosing

Oral dosing with tocainide is usually initiated at 300–400 mg t.i.d. Rarely, doses as high as 600 mg t.i.d. are required. In some cases, b.i.d. dosing may be effective.

Efficacy

Tocainide has been found to be an effective suppressor of premature ventricular beats. In patients with potentially lethal ventricular arrhythmias studied by Holter monitoring, tocainide has been found to be effective in about 50% of patients. Trials comparing tocainide to quinidine have shown these two agents to be equally effective in suppressing ventricular ectopic activity in patients with benign and potentially lethal ventricular arrhythmias. An effective response to lidocaine seems to be predictive of tocainide response. The predictive accuracy of using lidocaine response to predict tocainide is approximately 70%, although negative responsiveness seems to be more predictive. Using programmed stimulation as a measure of efficacy, tocainide is effective in less than 15% of patients with sustained ventricular tachyarrhythmias. Similar to other agents, response rates in this group of patients will be higher if efficacy is defined by Holter criteria instead of results during serial electrophysiological testing.

Combination therapy of tocainide with a type IA agent has demonstrated an added efficacy of 15–35% in patients with ventricular arrhythmias compared to either agent alone. Since lower doses of both agents are used during combination therapy, this is often associated with a lower incidence of subjective toxicity. In addition, lower doses of quinidine combined with the mild shortening of repolarization of the IB agent may minimize prolongation of the QT interval.

Adverse Effects

Similar to lidocaine and mexiletine, tocainide's side effects are primarily gastrointestinal and neurological. Gastrointestinal side effects include anorexia, nausea, vomiting, abdominal pain, and constipation. Neurological side effects include tremors, nervousness, dizziness, paresthesias, and confusion. Due to subjective intolerance which is often dose-related, tocainide has to be discontinued in 15–30% of patients. Subjective side effects can often be minimized by lowering the dose, or by taking the medication following meals. Up to 8% of patients who take tocainide get a drug-induced rash which resolves upon discontinuing the drug. Of significant concern are the rare occurrences of pulmonary fibrosis or agranulocytosis (0.2%) with tocainide. Although the incidence of these latter two severe end-organ toxicities is less than 0.05%, these problems have limited the popularity of this agent. Due to agranulocytosis and pulmonary fibrosis, the indication for this drug has been changed to a more second-line agent. From a cardiac viewpoint, tocainide is well tolerated. The incidence of drug-aggravated heart failure or arrhythmia is less than 4%. No major drug interaction problems have been reported.

Summary

Tocainide appears to be an effective agent in treating potentially lethal ventricular arrhythmias. Added efficacy and lower toxicity can be achieved when using tocainide in combination with a type IA antiarrhythmic agent. Tocainide has a narrow subjective toxic to therapeutic ratio which has limited its use in some patients. Due to rare end-organ toxicity, we have limited its use to a more second-line role. However, tocainide is very well tolerated hemodynamically and can be used safely in patients with congestive heart failure. Since tocainide is similar to lidocaine, it has no use in the treatment of supraventricular arrhythmias.

Mexiletine (Mexitil®)[49-56]

Mexiletine is a class IB oral agent that resembles lidocaine and to-cainide in structure.

Electrophysiology

Its electrophysiological/electrocardiographic effects are similar to to-cainide (Tables 1–3). Mexiletine depresses the rate of rise of phase 0 with no significant change in RMP and APD. Mexiletine has little effect on heart rate and sinus node recovery times.

Pharmacokinetics

Mexiletine is well absorbed orally with an 85% bioavailability. Hepatic metabolism is the major route of elimination and only 10–15% of the parent drug is excreted unchanged in the urine. The onset of action occurs within 1 to 2 hours and the elimination half-life averages 10–12 hours. Mexiletine is 70% protein-bound. No important drug interactions have been identified with mexiletine.

Dosing

We usually initiate mexiletine at doses of 200 mg t.i.d. Maintenance doses vary between 150 to 300 mg t.i.d. In some patients, b.i.d. dosing may be effective.

Efficacy

Similar to tocainide, mexiletine has been effective in approximately 50% of patients with potentially lethal ventricular arrhythmias studied by a Holter monitor model. Mexiletine has been shown to be comparable to quinidine in suppressing ventricular ectopic activity. Like tocainide, the addition of a type IA antiarrhythmic agent to mexiletine has demonstrated added efficacy and decreased toxicity in this group of patients. Mexiletine was not found to reduce mortality in a post-myocardial infarction population (IMPACT study), although it significantly reduced the frequency of PVCs.

Mexiletine has been more extensively studied than tocainide in patients with sustained ventricular tachyarrhythmias. In patients with recurrent monomorphic sustained VT studied in the electrophysiology laboratory, mexiletine appears to be effective in 10–15% of patients. However, efficacy rates between 20% and 30% have been demonstrated in patients with ventricular fibrillation who survived an out-of-hospital cardiac arrest. Combination therapy with type IA agents in patients with sustained ventricular tachyarrhythmias may increase the efficacy rates by an additional 15–30%.

Mexiletine is effective in treating over 70% of pediatric patients who have ventricular arrhythmias after surgery for tetralogy of Fallot. This represents a group of patients who are usually refractory to type IA agents.

Adverse Effects

Similar to lidocaine and tocainide, mexiletine has dose-related central nervous system and gastrointestinal side effects. Central nervous system toxicity includes tremors, dizziness, blurred vision, and confusion. The primary gastrointestinal side effect is nausea although vomiting and heartburn are also seen. Subjective side effects can be minimized by giving the drug with meals.

Mexiletine is relatively free of end-organ toxicity. Only rare cases of a possible drug-induced hepatitis have been reported. Therefore, from an end-organ toxicity viewpoint, mexiletine seems to be a safer drug than tocainide.

Hemodynamically, mexiletine is extremely well tolerated. No change in left ventricular ejection fraction has been noted during mexiletine therapy when compared to baseline. Mexiletine, like tocainide, seems to have minimal proarrhythmic effects. In 51 patients with sustained VT treated with mexiletine in our laboratory, no spontaneous proarrhythmia was noted. Since mexiletine and tocainide shorten the QT interval, torsades de pointes does not occur.

Summary

Mexiletine is an effective agent in treating various ventricular arrhythmias. Added efficacy is attained in combination with type IA antiarrhythmic agents. Subjective adverse effects are common. However, due to its benign hemodynamic, proarrhythmic profile and lack of end-organ toxicity, mexiletine is a safe, front-line antiarrhythmic drug.

Type IB Agents: Patient Selection

Although the treatment of arrhythmics is quite empiric, we consider using type IB agents earlier in certain situations: (1) in lidocaine-responsive patients; (2) in patients with congenital prolonged QT syndromes or in patients with a history of torsades de pointes on a type IA agent; (3) in patients with severe congestive heart failure due to a benign hemodynamic profile; (4) in patients with advanced His-Purkinje since type IB agents have minimal effects on myocardial conduction; and (5) in the outpatient setting because of the low incidence of proarrhythmia.

In patients with sustained ventricular tachyarrhythmias, we have found little use for tocainide and have found mexiletine to be more useful in patients who have survived a cardiac arrest than in patients with recurrent monomorphic sustained ventricular tachycardia especially if left ventricular function is preserved. Even though efficacy rates are less than 25%, we often use mexiletine early in our patients with sustained ventricular tachyarrhythmias either alone or in combination with a type IA antiarrhythmic primarily based on its low proarrhythmic potential and lack of end-organ toxicity.

Type IC Antiarrhythmic Agents

Flecainide (Tambocor®)[57-67]

Flecainide was the first type IC antiarrhythmic agent approved by the FDA.

Electrophysiology

Flecainide is a type IC antiarrhythmic agent that prolongs refractoriness and slows conduction in the atria, AV node, His-Purkinje system, ventricles and accessory pathways.

Pharmacokinetics

Flecainide has a bioavailability of 90–95% and a half-life averaging between 12 and 27 hours with a mean of 20 hours. Although flecainide is metabolized (70%) in the liver, 30% is excreted by the kidney. Peak blood levels are achieved in 2–4 hours. Due to its long half-life, flecainide is effective using a b.i.d. dosing schedule. Its only significant drug interaction is with amiodarone. When used in combination with amiodarone, flecainide levels may increase 15–30%.

Dosing

Flecainide is available in 100-mg tablets. We usually initiate therapy at 100 mg b.i.d. After steady state has been achieved, we increase the dose to 150 mg b.i.d. as necessary. Rarely, higher doses (200 mg b.i.d.) are required. Therapeutic levels are 0.2 to 1.0 µg/mL.

Efficacy

Flecainide has been shown to be extremely effective in decreasing the frequency of PVCs in patients with frequent ventricular ectopy. In comparative trials with quinidine and disopyramide, flecainide has been shown to be statistically superior in the suppression of PVCs, ventricular couplets, and runs of nonsustained VT. In our experience, flecainide has been useful in the control of potentially lethal ventricular arrhythmias in over 70% of patients. In patients with symptomatic ventricular arrhythmias in the post-myocardial infarction period, the CAST study demonstrated an enhanced mortality compared to placebo despite effective PVC suppression. In patients with sustained VT, the efficacy of flecainide has been comparable to type IA and slightly better than IB antiarrhythmic agents. Flecainide is effective in rendering sustained VT noninducible in 20–25% of patients studied in the electrophysiology laboratory. Efficacy rates are higher in patients with preserved left ventricular function and ejection fractions greater than 30%. In contrast to mexiletine and type IA agents, the efficacy rate of flecainide in patients who have survived a cardiac arrest is lower than that in the sustained ventricular tachycardia group, being less than 15%.

Flecainide has been demonstrated to be a very effective agent in the treatment of supraventricular arrhythmias. At this time, flecainide has the Cardio-renal Advisory Board's recommendation for approval to the FDA for treating SVT without any concomitant organic heart disease. Flecainide seems to be equally or more effective than type IA and/or II agents in the treatment of re-entrant SVT secondary to either AV node re-entry or AV re-entrant tachycardia in patients with Wolff-Parkinson-White syndrome. In primary atrial tachycardias such as paroxysmal atrial fibrillation and ectopic atrial tachycardia, flecainide seems to be equally effective and less toxic than quinidine. The use of flecainide in the conversion of chronic atrial fibrillation to sinus rhythm has been less well studied.

Adverse Effects

Subjectively, flecainide is very well tolerated. In our experience, flecainide has to be discontinued in less than 10% of patients. Noncardiac side effects which are dose-related include dizziness, visual disturbances, and headache. Of more concern are the cardiovascular adverse reactions of flecainide. Flecainide depresses left ventricular function and may cause or aggravate congestive heart failure in approximately 5% of patients. The incidence of heart failure increases to 10–20% in those patients with a prior history of heart failure. A modest increase in the incidence of heart failure was noted in the CAPS study compared to encainide and moricizine.

Of major concern is the incidence of ventricular proarrhythmia when using this drug. In patients with PVCs alone and nonsustained VT, the incidence of ventricular proarrhythmia appears to be less than 3%. However, in patients with sustained ventricular tachyarrhythmias, the incidence of proarrhythmia, including the development of incessant VT, averages between 7% and 17%, the higher incidence being noted in patients with severe organic heart disease and left ventricular dysfunction. Because proarrhythmia may only be manifested during exercise testing, it has been suggested that stress testing be made part of a normal routine asssment of efficacy with flecainide and encainide. In the CAST study, mortality was increased compared to placebo in patients treated for asymptomatic ventricular arrhythmias post-myocardial infarction. Excess mortality may have been secondary to excessive proarrhythmia in the setting of myocardial scarring. Flecainide is contraindicated in this setting. Flecainide may worsen pre-existing sinus node dysfunction and due to its potent effects on slowing His-Purkinje conduction, it may aggravate pre-existing conduction disturbances and precipitate the development of advanced AV block. Flecainide has caused acute and chronic elevation of permanent pacemaker thresholds. Flecainide may slightly increase digoxin levels. However, in our clinical experience, this has not been important enough to alter dosing.

Summary

Flecainide appears to be a very effective agent in the treatment of ventricular arrhythmias. Its long half-life and low incidence of subjective side effects make it an extremely useful antiarrhythmic agent. With its high level of efficacy and low incidence of proarrhythmia in patients with potentially lethal ventricular arrhythmias, flecainide had often been used as a front-line agent prior to release of data from the CAST study. However, the CAST data has limited flecainide to a second-line agent for ventricular arrhythmias and should be avoided in post-infarction ventricular arrhythmias. In patients with primary atrial tachycardias or re-entrant SVT, especially in those who have co-existing ventricular tachycarrhythmias, flecainide is one of our agents of choice. Flecainide can be useful for treatment of sustained ventricular tachyarrhythmias; however, due to its low efficacy in patients who have survived a cardiac arrest and the high incidence of proarrhythmia, including the development of incessant sustained ventricular tachycardia, this drug should be used cautiously under telemetry conditions in this group of patients. Flecainide's negative inotropy has limited the use of this drug in patients with severe left ventricular dysfunction.

Encainide (Enkaid®)[66-74]

Encainide is a type IC antiarrhythmic agent.

Electrophysiology

Encainide's electrophysiological and electrocardiographic effects are summarized in Tables 1, 2, and 3.

Pharmacokinetics

Encainide is a type IC antiarrhythmic agent that is well absorbed orally and is metabolized primarily in the liver. Encainide's onset of action is 1–2 hours and the half-life of the parent compound is under 3 hours. Despite this short half-life, encainide can be used very effectively on a q.i.d. 6–8 hour dosing schedule due to the effect of its active metabolites (O-demethyl-encainide and 3-methoxy O-demethyl-encainide) with half-lives of 8–12 hours. Ninety percent of patients extensively metabolize encainide to these active metabolites. In poor metabolizers, the parent compound has an extended half-life similar to that of the metabolites. Thus, regardless of the genetically determined pathway of metabolism, maintenance doses of encainide are similar in all patients. Because of the longer half-lives of the metabolites, dosing changes in encainide should be attempted only every 3–4 days.

Dosing

Encainide is available in 23, 35, and 50 mg tablets. Therapy is initiated at 25 mg t.i.d. After 3–4 days of dosing to reach steady state of the metabolites, the dose may be increased to 35 or 50 mg t.i.d. Rarely, q.i.d. dosing is required. Plasma levels are not readily available. Dose should be titrated based on efficacy, toxicity, and changes in the PR and QRS intervals.

Efficacy

Similar to flecainide, encainide has been highly effective in reducing the frequency of PVCs and in controlling nonsustained VT in those patients with potentially lethal ventricular arrhythmias. In our experience, encainide has been effective in over 70% of patients with this type of arrhythmia. Controlled studies have shown encainide to be a more effective suppressor of PVCs than either quinidine or disopyramide. Similar to flecainide, marked suppression of PVCs in post-infarction patients was associated with enhanced mortality when compared to placebo in the CAST trial. In the electrophysiology laboratory, encainide appears to be effective in controlling sustained ventricular tachycardia in approximately 20–25% of patients. In patients with preserved left ventricular function, efficacy rates are higher.

Encainide has potent electrophysiological effects and prolongs refractoriness in the atrium, AV node, ventricle, and accessory pathway. In addition, it markedly slows antegrade and retrograde conduction through the AV node, His-Purkinje system, and accessory pathway.

Because of these effects, encainide has been effective in treating over 60% of patients with re-entrant SVT. Encainide's potent effects on the accessory pathway have demonstrated this drug be effective even when other type IA sodium channel blockers have failed to control arrhythmias in this group of patients. Encainide has been less carefully studied than flecainide and propafenone in the treatment of atrial fibrillation.

Adverse Effects

Encainide has been well tolerated in the majority of patients. Although subjective side effects occur in about 10% of patients, less than 2% of patients will require discontinuation of therapy. The noncardiac side effects of headache, dizziness, diplopia, vertigo, leg cramps, and metallic taste in the mouth are dose-related and can be minimized by lowering the dose.

The most significant side effect of encainide therapy has been its potential to cause proarrhythmia. As is the case with flecainide, the incidence is less than 3–4% in patients with potentially lethal ventricular arrhythmias or simple PVCs and less in patients with SVT. The excess mortality in encainide-treated patients in the CAST study suggests an added proarrhythmia response in this setting. However, in patients with sustained VT, the incidence of proarrhythmia exceeds 10% and usually presents as a slower, incessant sustained VT. Stress testing may be a useful noninvasive screening test to unmask previously unrecognized proarrhythmia. Encainide has little adverse effect on sinus node automaticity; however, due to its potent dromotropic effects, it can cause AV block at the level of the AV node or distal to the bundle of His. Increases in pacing thresholds have been reported. Hemodynamically, encainide is generally well tolerated. However, recent evidence suggests that it may have more negative inotropic activity than procainamide.

Summary

Encainide is very effective in the treatment of patients with potentially lethal arrhythmias, and in patients with re-entrant SVT, especially those associated with Wolff-Parkinson-White syndrome. The CAST data have made this drug a second-line agent in treating chronic nonlife-threatening ventricular arrhythmias. It is contraindicated in the asymptomatic post-myocardial infarction patient with nonlife-threatening arrhythmias. Although it should be an effective agent in the treatment of atrial fibrillation unassociated with pre-excitation, more data are needed to study this indication. Hemodynamically, encainide is very well tolerated, similar to quinidine, procainamide, tocainide, and mexiletine. Therefore, encainide offers an advantage over flecainide when choosing a type IC agent in patients with left ventricular dysfunction. In patients with sustained ventricular tachyarrhythmias, encainide's proarrhythmic potential may minimize the use of this drug and careful in-hospital monitoring of patients is required.

Propafenone (Rythmol®)[75-81]

Propafenone is a new type IC-like antiarrhythmic agent with weak associated β-blocking characteristics.

Electrophysiology

Besides having type IC electrophysiological effects, propafenone also has strong membrane-stabilizing activity and weak beta-blocking effects (structure similar to propranolol). At high doses, some calcium channel blocking properties have been demonstrated in vitro.

Pharmacokinetics

Propafenone is totally absorbed then undergoes first-pass hepatic elimination via a saturable oxidative pathway. Similar to encainide, metabolism of propafenone is genetically determined and varies between patients. Ten percent of patients are poor metabolizers with a prolonged half-life of parent compound. The half-life of the parent compound ranges from 2 to 12 hours with a mean of 6 hours. Poor metabolizers often have half-lives in the 10–12 hour range. The major metabolites of propafenone are 5-hydroxy propafenone and N-debutyl propafenone. 5-Hydroxy propafenone appears to have antiarrhythmic activity. Clinical administration of propafenone is characterized by a decrease in clearance of parent compound and an accumulation of active metabolites. Although the half-life of the parent compound is only 6 hours, steady state is not usually reached for 72 hours. A therapeutic range of propafenone plasma levels has not been well established.

Dosing

The recommended starting dose of propafenone is 150 mg t.i.d. Doses may be increased up to 300 mg t.i.d. if necessary. We often used 225 mg (1½ tabs) as an intermediate dose.

Efficacy

In patients with potentially lethal ventricular arrhythmias, propafenone has been effective in controlling PVCs, couplets, and nonsustained VT in over 65% of patients. Studies have demonstrated at least equal and, in some cases, more efficacy than quinidine, mexiletine, and disopyramide. In patients with a history of sustained VT/VF, programmed stimulation studies have demonstrated propafenone to be effective in suppressing inducible VT in about 20% of patients. Similar to other type IC agents, it can profoundly slow the rate of induced and recurrent VT. As has been shown with amiodarone, induction of VT during propafenone therapy does not preclude a beneficial long-term response.

Since propafenone prolongs refractoriness and slows conduction in the atria, AV node, and accessory AV connections, similar to flecainide and encainide, propafenone is effective in treating over 50% of patients with re-entrant SVT and paroxysmal atrial fibrillation.

Adverse Effects

Subjective adverse effects with propafenone include a bitter metallic taste, nausea, vomiting, constipation, and dizziness. A drug-induced rash has been noted in about 3% of patients. Due to its beta-blocking activity, it can accentuate AV nodal block. Due to its type IC effects, it can aggravate His-Purkinje block. Propafenone has some negative inotropic activity similar to that of flecainide and therefore should be used cautiously in patients with left ventricular dysfunction. Proarrhythmia occurs in about 3% of patients treated for benign or potentially lethal ventricular arrhythmias and in 8–10% patients with a prior history of sustained VT or VF.

Propafenone interacts with digoxin and can raise digoxin levels 40–60% as can occur with quinidine and amiodarone. Propafenone appears to increase the plasma concentration of warfarin and can cause significant increase in prothrombin times.

Summary

Propafenone is a useful type IC agent with efficacy in treating paroxysmal supraventricular tachycardia, atrial fibrillation, and ventricular arrhythmias. Both its efficacy and its proarrhythmic potential are slightly less than that of other type IC agents. As with flecainide, its negative inotropic potential may minimize the use of this drug in patients with significantly diminished ejection fractions. Although the FDA has limited propafenone's approval indication to life-threatening ventricular arrhythmias, its predominant role in our practice has been in the treatment of symptomatic PVCs, potentially lethal ventricular arrhythmias, and atrial fibrillation.

Recainam[82-83]

Recainam is a propylurea compound that has class I antiarrhythmic activity. It is undergoing clinical evaluation for the treatment of various supraventricular and ventricular cardiac arrhythmias.

Electrophysiology

The electrophysiological effects of IV recainam significantly increase conduction intervals in the atria, the AV node, and His-Purkinje system. Cellular studies in canine and rabbit tissues have demonstrated that recainam reduces V_{max} and shifts the membrane responsiveness curve to the right. These properties are similar to class IC activity. Recainam also shortens ventricular muscle action potential duration (APD). In this respect, recainam resembles class IB antiarrhythmic drugs. Right ventricular refractory periods were either unchanged or shortened under the influence of recainam.

Pharmacokinetics

Recainam is 80% absorbed after oral administration and 70% is cleared by the kidney. Eighty-four percent of renally cleared recainam is recovered unchanged. No active metabolites have been identified. Approximately 15% of the drug is protein-bound. The elimination half-life of chronically administered oral recainam is longer in cardiac patients than in normal subjects (10.2 versus 6.7 hours).

Efficacy

Preliminary data show nonlinear dose proportionality in the range of 200 to 800 mg. Preliminary data in over 70 chronically treated patients with nonlife-threatening ventricular arrhythmias in a dose-ranging study have shown greater than 70% efficacy.

Therapy with oral recainam has been evaluated in over 70 patients with inducible sustained VT. Preliminary data in 44 patients receiving oral therapy demonstrated prevention of or slowing of the rate of the induced VT (by greater than 100 ms) in 23% of all patients evaluated by repeat programmed electrical stimulation (PES) testing. In a comparative study to encainide, recainam had similar rates of preventing induced sustained VT, although efficacy rates were less than 10%. Recainam appears to prolong the refractory periods of the atrial, retrograde AV node, and accessory pathway. Early studies have demonstrated efficacy in preventing the induction of PSVT and slowing SVT cycle length in those patients who are still inducible. Early studies have demonstrated up to a 60% complete or partial efficacy by electrophysiology study criteria and clinical follow-up. Similar rates of efficacy have been noted in patients with symptomatic primary atrial tachyarrhythmias.

Adverse Effects

Commonly experienced adverse experiences include gastrointestinal problems (abdominal discomfort 4%, nausea 5%), nervous system complaints (dizziness 9%, headaches 8%), and other complaints, such as fever (4%). Recainam can cause first-degree heart block, left and right bundle branch block (BBB), and arrhythmia aggravation. There has been a low incidence of arrhythmia aggravation (5%) in patients with nonlife-threatening ventricular arrhythmia with normal or mild left ventricular dysfunction.

Summary

Recainam is an investigational sodium channel blocker that appears to have usefulness in various supraventricular and ventricular arrhythmias.

Moricizine (Ethmozine®)[66,67,84–87]

Moricizine hydrochloride is a phenothiazine derivative that was developed in the Soviet Union. Recently, it has been given approval by the FDA for the treatment of life-threatening ventricular arrhythmias.

Electrophysiology

Moricizine has membrane-stabilizing activity, local anesthetic activity, and inhibits the sodium channels in phase 0 of the action potential, typical of class IA antiarrhythmic agents. However, moricizine's electrophysiological effects do not clearly define this agent into any of the subclasses as defined by Vaughn-Williams. In isolated dog Purkinje fibers, moricizine shortens phase II and phase III repolarization along with a dose-related decrease in V_{max}. In the canine model, no effects have been observed in the sinus node or the atria. In man, moricizine decreases conduction velocity through the AV node with an increase in the AH interval. It also slows conduction in the ventricular myocardium with prolongation of the HV interval, PR, and QRS intervals. There is little change in the JT interval, suggesting that the drug does not prolong ventricular repolarization. Intracardiac studies have shown that moricizine slows AV node conduction without prolonging VERP. Retrograde AV node and accessory pathway conduction is also slowed. Increases in PR and QRS duration have been noted. The QT interval does not change or may shorten. Using the Vaughn-Williams classification, moricizine has properties of type IB or IC drugs; that is, it slows conduction but does not prolong repolarization.

Pharmacokinetics

Moricizine is the ethyl ester hydrochloride of 10-(3-morpholinopro-prionyl)phenothiazine-2-carbonic acid. It is well absorbed by the gastrointestinal tract. However, due to significant first-pass metabolism, bioavailability is only 38%. Peak blood levels are reached 0.5–2 hours following oral administration. Moricizine is highly plasma-bound to protein (95%). The mean elimination half-life is 6 hours. With chronic dosing, the half-life may increase to 12 hours. Moricizine is extensively metabolized (at least 26 metabolites) with significant first-pass metabolism occurring. Two active metabolites probably have little importance since they represent less than 1% of the administered parent drug dose. About 56% of moricizine is excreted in the feces and 39% in the urine.

Dosing

Moricizine is available as 200, 250, and 300 mg tablets. The typical daily oral dosing is 200–400 mg t.i.d. We usually initiate therapy at 200 mg t.i.d. then increase by 150 mg/day at 3-day intervals.

Efficacy

In nonlife-threatening ventricular arrhythmias, moricizine is usually effective in 50–65% of patients, as assessed by Holter monitoring regardless of ejection fraction. In comparative studies, moricizine has been demonstrated to be equally effective as propranolol, quinidine, and disopyramide. In the Cardiac Arrhythmia Pilot Study (CAPS), moricizine in doses of 600–900 mg/day suppressed ventricular arrhythmias in 67% of patients entered. At the time of blinding of the CAST study in April 1989, 272 patients had been randomized to the moricizine wing of the CAST study. Different from encainide and flecainide, no excess risk of death has been observed to this point. In refractory patients with sustained ventricular tachycardia, as assessed by programmed stimulation, the response rate is less than 20%. The VT cycle length usually slows in those patients who remain inducible. The efficacy of moricizine in treating various supraventricular tachyarrhythmias has not been well established. However, moricizine has been shown to suppress retrograde AV nodal and bidirectional accessory pathway conduction.

Adverse Effects

Moricizine can cause proarrhythmia. This occurs in about 3.5% of patients. The overall incidence in patients with a history of sustained ventricular tachyarrhythmias was 4%. The most common adverse reactions include dry mouth, paresthesias, vertigo, dizziness (15%), nausea, headache, fatigue, dyspnea, palpitations, dyspepsia, diarrhea, vomiting, and sweating. Dizziness appears to be dose-related. There has been a rare occurrence of drug fever and elevation of liver function tests. No significant end-organ toxicity has been reported. Moricizine has minimal negative inotropic activity. Moricizine worsened heart failure in 12.8% of 374 patients with a prior history of heart failure and in only 0.1% of 545 patients without a history of heart failure. There is no known significant interaction with digoxin or warfarin. Cimetidine raises moricizine levels by 40% and moricizine improves the clearance and shortens the half-life of theophylline derivatives.

Summary

Moricizine appears to be a promising agent for the treatment of ventricular arrhythmias. Data are currently lacking as to its role in sustained VT and SVT. Whether this drug can alter post-myocardial infarction sudden cardiac death will be determined by the CAST trial. Subjective toxicity requiring drug discontinuation is less common than oral IA and IB agents, but more common than IC agents.

Type II Antiarrhythmic Agents

Propranolol (Inderal®, Inderal-LA®)[88-90]

Propranolol is a beta-blocker that has had FDA approval for treating supraventricular and ventricular arrhythmias since 1973. Propranolol is noncardioselective, has no intrinsic sympathomimetic activity, but does have membrane-stabilizing activity. It is available as a short-acting and long-acting (Inderal-LA®) oral preparation and also parenterally.

Pharmacokinetics

Propranolol is almost completely absorbed orally, but bioavailability is markedly reduced due to first-pass metabolic breakdown in the liver. With chronic administration, there is saturation of the hepatic system with increase in bioavailability from 10% to 20–50%. The major metabolite is 4-OH-propranolol. The half-life of propranolol is 3–6 hours with steady state being achieved within 30 hours. Inderal-LA® has a duration of action exceeding 24 hours. Although we do not routinely draw levels, the therapeutic range appears to be about 100–150 µg/mL. Intravenously, propranolol has an initial α half-life of 10 minutes followed by a β half-life of 2–3 hours. Therefore, following intravenous propranolol, systemic effects may last for hours. If short-acting levels are desired, esmolol is preferred.

Dosing

Oral dosing varies from 40 mg to 640 mg p.o. daily. Intravenously, due to bypass of first-pass metabolism, only about 10% of the dose is given (1–10 mg IV). To attain complete sympathetic blockade requires 0.15 to 0.2 mg/kg IV.

Electrophysiology

Propranolol inhibits many of the effects of beta-receptor stimulation such as blocking enhanced automaticity and adrenergic improvement in conduction velocities and shortening of refractory periods. Propranolol also blocks adrenergic activation of calcium channels. Propranolol decreases resting heart rate, prolongs sinus node recovery times, and increases PR and AH intervals. The QT interval may decrease. Propranolol prolongs refractoriness in the AV node with little effect in refractoriness of other cardiac tissues.

Efficacy

Propranolol is effective in slowing the ventricular response (especially during exercise) and rarely in terminating and preventing the occurrence of atrial flutter, fibrillation, and PSVT. Propranolol is also effective in slow sinus heart rate in patients with inappropriate symptomatic sinus tachycardia. In ventricular arrhythmias, propranolol will suppress PVCs, ventricular couplets, and nonsustained VT in 45–50% of patients. In the electrophysiology laboratory, propranolol is effective in <5% of patients with inducible sustained VT. Propranolol is the drug of choice in exercise-aggravated or induced arrhythmias and in patients with the prolonged QT syndrome. Propranolol is very effective as adjunct therapy in combination with a sodium channel blocker for both SVT and VT. Adrenergic reversal of sodium channel blockers can be blunted by propranolol. Propranolol has some role in treatment of ischemic-induced arrhythmias. Intravenously, propranolol can be used to acutely slow the ventricular response or to treat arrhythmia patients in the critical care setting.

Similar to timolol, metoprolol, and acebutolol, propranolol has been shown to significantly reduce mortality in the post-myocardial infarction period. The mechanism for this beneficial effect is unclear, although it may be a combination of anti-ischemic, antisympathetic, and antiarrhythmic properties. Propranolol minimizes the increase in the quantity of ventricular ectopic activity that has been noted 6 weeks after a myocardial infarction.

Adverse Effects

Propranolol can aggravate sinus node dysfunction, AV block, and slow heart rate. Due to its noncardioselectivity, it can cause bronchospasm or mask the sympathetic-mediated warning signs of hypoglycemia in insulin-dependent diabetics. Due to its significant negative inotropy, worsening of CHF is common. This effect is dose-related. Subjective side effects include fatigue and mental blunting.

Summary

Propranolol is effective primarily as adjunctive therapy in patients with arrhythmias. It is the treatment of choice in patients with exercise-induced and prolonged QT syndromes. The results both of the CAST and the BHAT study emphasize propranolol's importance in treating post-myocardial infarction patients at moderate to high risk for sudden cardiac death. We commonly use the once-a-day formulation for patient compliance, although it does not have FDA approval in the treatment of arrhythmias. Due to its benign proarrhythmic profile, propranolol is accepted front-line therapy in the outpatient treatment of arrhythmias.

Acebutolol (Sectral®)[90-92]

Acebutolol is a beta-blocker that has been approved for the management of ventricular arrhythmias. Acebutolol differs from propranolol in that it is more cardioselective, has intrinsic sympathomimetic activity (ISA), and is more hydrophilic. Similar to propranolol, it has membrane-stabilizing activity at higher doses.

Electrophysiology

Acebutolol has electrophysiological effects similar to those of other beta-blockers except that due to ISA, it causes less reduction in heart rate than propranolol. Acebutolol has minimal effects on atrial refractoriness. Its predominant electrophysiological effects are slowing of AV nodal conduction and prolongation of AV node refractoriness. At high levels exceeding 1000 ng/mL, acebutolol has significantly prolonged the HV interval, probably secondary to its membrane-stabilizing activity at this level.

Pharmacokinetics

Acebutolol is well absorbed from the gastrointestinal tract and is subject to extensive first-pass hepatic metabolism into the pharmacologically active N-acetyl metabolite, diacetolol. Although the T½ of acebutolol is only 3–4 hours, the T½ of diacetolol is longer (8–13 hours), making twice daily dosing an option. The drug is partially excreted in the urine.

Dosing

We usually initiate therapy with 200 mg b.i.d. and increase to 400 mg b.i.d. if necessary.

Efficacy

Acebutolol has efficacy rates similar to propranolol in suppressing ventricular ectopic activity. Acebutolol is effective in controlling about 45–50% of patients with benign and potentially lethal ventricular arrhythmias as defined by Holter monitoring. In one study, efficacy rates were similar to those of quinidine. In patients with sustained VT, acebutolol has been effective in less than 5% of patients in our experience when used as monotherapy. Similar to propranolol, acebutolol can be effective in paroxysmal SVT and controlling heart rate in atrial fibrillation. Recent data from the ASPI trial demonstrated that acetubolol reduced mortality by 48% in high-risk post-myocardial infarction patients.

Adverse Effects

The most frequent adverse reactions from acebutolol are those typically associated with beta-blockers such as depression and fatigue. Due to its ISA, symptomatic bradycardia is less common than with propranolol. Although relatively cardioselective, asthma and other bronchospastic lung disease can be exacerbated. Worsening of AV block and aggravation of heart failure due to negative inotropy may occur. Six cases of reversible hepatic toxicity represent the only known end-organ toxicity.

Summary

Acebutolol is a safe antiarrhythmic that has a role primarily in the treatment of symptomatic benign and potentially lethal ventricular arrhythmias. Its benign proarrhythmic profile makes it a logical first-line agent in the outpatient setting. Acebutolol may be preferred over propranolol when less heart rate slowing is desired.

Esmolol Hydrochloride (Brevibloc®)[93,94]

Esmolol, similar to metoprolol, is relatively cardioselective, has no ISA or membrane-stabilizing activity, and is weakly lipid soluble. After an intravenous infusion of esmolol, electrophysiological effects, as determined by a slowing in sinus cycle length and prolongation of sinus node recovery times, occur within 5 minutes. Esmolol also slows AV nodal conduction. No direct effect on atrial or ventricular refractoriness or HV interval has been noted. Less significant changes in AV nodal refractoriness have been noted.

Pharmacokinetics

Esmolol is an ultrashort-acting intravenous beta-blocker (about 1/40th the blocking potency of propranolol). The ultrashort duration of action is determined by the presence or location of an ester group added to a beta-blocker nucleus common to metoprolol. This ester group creates a molecule extremely susceptible to rapid degradation to an inactive acid metabolite and methanol by esterases in the blood and tissues. Within 24 hours of termination, up to 88% of the drug is accounted for in the urine as the clinically inactive acid metabolites. Esmolol, given IV, has a distribution half-life of 2 minutes and an elimination half-life of 9 minutes. Following a loading infusion, steady-state blood levels can be reached in 5 minutes. Following discontinuation, blood levels deplete rapidly within 10 minutes and are negligibly present within 30 minutes.

Dosing

Esmolol is usually given as a 500 μg/kg loading dose IV over 1 minute. This is usually followed by a 4-minute infusion at 50 μg/kg/min. The infusion can be increased up to 300 μg/kg/min if necessary.

Efficacy

In patients with SVT and atrial fibrillation, a slowing of mean ventricular rate is quickly achieved. In a 63-patient study, esmolol produced a therapeutic response in 72% of patients with various SVT compared to 6% on placebo. In a comparative study, a therapeutic response was noted in 72% of patients taking esmolol compared to 69% of patients taking intravenous propranolol.

Adverse Effects

Esmolol exhibits equal effects of heart rate slowing as propranolol with more rapid reversal of beta-blockade upon discontinuation. Esmolol, similar to other beta-blockers, has significant negative inotropic activity. Decreases in hemodynamics are similar to those seen after 4 mg of intravenous propranolol. Dose-related hypotension is the most common adverse effect.

Summary

Esmolol's short-acting effects make it the parenteral β-blocker of choice when a rapid therapeutic effect and rapid reversibility are desired.

Type II Agents: Patient Selection

Due to their low propensity to aggravate arrhythmias, the beta-blockers are useful front-line antiarrhythmics in the outpatient setting. In patients with exercise-induced VT and prolonged QT syndrome, the beta-blockers may be treatments of choice. Beta-blockers are also useful in digitalis-induced arrhythmias and in patients with arrhythmias and symptoms associated with the mitral valve prolapse syndrome. In patients who might benefit from beta-blocker therapy (hypertension, angina, post-myocardial infarction), especially those with concomitant supraventricular arrhythmias, beta-blockers make a logical first choice. However, we prefer propranolol, timolol, metoprolol, and acebutolol in the post-myocardial infarction setting due to their proven efficacy in this setting. In patients with lethal ventricular arrhythmias, beta-blockers are mostly useful as a second agent in combination with a sodium channel blocker. In patients with SVT, intravenous esmolol may be preferable to propranolol due to its short duration of action.

Type III Antiarrhythmic Agents

Amiodarone (Cordarone®)[95-100]

Amiodarone is an iodinated benzofuran derivative that was initially developed as an antianginal treatment due to its coronary and peripheral vasodilating properties.

Electrophysiology

Amiodarone has been subclassified as a class III antiarrhythmic agent. This is based on basic electrophysiological studies that demonstrated prolongation of repolarization similar to that of bretylium. However, more recent data suggests that amiodarone's basic electrophysiological effects are more complex since the sodium channels can be depressed in phase 0 in a use-dependent fashion, becoming more pronounced at faster heart rates. In addition, amiodarone has some sympatholytic properties. Therefore, the classification of amiodarone as a class III agent is an oversimplification of its electrophysiological properties. In vivo, amiodarone prolongs refractoriness and slows conduction in the atria AV node, His-Purkinje system, ventricles and accessory pathways. Both in vitro and in vivo, amiodarone can slow sinus node automaticity.

Pharmacokinetics

The clinical pharmacology of amiodarone is not well understood although it is best represented by a three-compartment model. Amiodarone has a large volume of distribution (500 liters) and a long half-life (average of 53 days) requiring months for blood levels to reach equilibrium. The bioavailability of amiodarone averages 30–50%. Excretion is minimal by both hepatic and fecal routes. Due to high lipophilicity, amiodarone and its metabolites are extensively distributed into fat, muscle, liver, lung, and spleen. Amiodarone is extensively metabolized to desethyl amiodarone. Amiodarone has biphasic elimination with a decrease in levels over the first 10 days after cessation of therapy followed by an increased drug concentration rebound that is thought to be from elimination of the parent compound from poorly perfused tissues. Due to the drug's long half-life, plasma levels of amiodarone and desethyl amiodarone can be measured as long as 9 months after cessation of therapy.

Dosing

Amiodarone requires a loading phase of 800–1400 mg p.o. a day for several weeks. By 4 weeks of therapy, doses average about 600 mg a day. By 4 months, most of our patients are taking 400 mg a day. In an attempt to minimize toxicity, maintenance doses ranging from 200 mg p.o. every other day to 400 mg a day are preferred. Therapeutic blood levels are in the 1.5–2.5 μg/mL range. Blood levels, along with a clinical judgment of efficacy and toxicity, are used to titrate the dose downward. Lowest doses can be used in patients with nonlife-threatening ventricular arrhythmias such as atrial fibrillation.

Efficacy

Amiodarone has been approved for the treatment of life-threatening ventricular arrhythmias. Amiodarone has been effective in over 60% of patients with refractory sustained VT. Similar efficacy rates have been noted in patients who are survivors of a cardiac arrest. Amiodarone is unique in that induction of sustained VT during serial electrophysiological testing does not preclude a beneficial clinical response. Approximately 60% of such patients will not have recurrence of their VT. Although not approved for use in patients with potentialy lethal ventricular arrhythmias, amiodarone is a very effective suppressor of ventricular ectopic activity. Similar to type IC agents, amiodarone can effectively control, as determined by Holter monitoring, 75% of patients with nonsustained VT. Trials studying the efficacy of low-dose amiodarone in the post-myocardial infarction population are in progress. Noncontrolled data suggest that low-dose amiodarone may have a beneficial effect on improving survival in patients with potentially lethal ventricular arrhythmias and dilated or hypertrophic cardiomyopathy. Well-controlled studies are looking to confirm these preliminary findings. Amiodarone, even at low doses, can be effective in controlling two-thirds of the patients with otherwise drug-refractory atrial fibrillation. Amiodarone can be effective in treating over 60% of patients with refractory primary atrial tachycardias or re-entrant SVT.

Adverse Effects

Adverse effects during amiodarone therapy are common, although they require drug discontinuation in fewer than 20% of patients. Minor side effects that seldom require drug discontinuation include corneal microdeposits, asymptomatic transient elevation of hepatic enzymes, photosensitivity of the skin, bluish-gray skin discoloration, and subjective gastrointestinal side effects. Amiodarone-induced hypothyroidism occurs in about 8% of our patients and requires the addition of thyroid replacement. Drug-induced hyperthyroidism (2%) may require discontinuatin of therapy. Other serious end-organ toxicities that may require discontinuation of amiodarone include interstitial pneumonitis (3–7%) and drug-induced hepatitis (2%). Neurological side effects include a peripheral neuropathy and myopathy that usually resolve on lowering the dose. Drug-induced bradycardia may require backup permanent pacing in up to 2% of patients.

Amiodarone is well tolerated hemodynamically with minimal negative inotropic effects. Amiodarone's vasodilating properties partially compensate for its negative inotropy. Fewer than 4% of patients will have worsening of congestive heart failure. Although amiodarone prolongs action potential duration, amiodarone-induced torsades de pointes is rare and the development of incessant sustained VT occurs in less than 4% of patients. Most case reports of amiodarone-induced torsades de pointes have occurred when amiodarone was used in combination with a type IA antiarrhythmic drug.

Amiodarone has been shown to interact with digoxin, warfarin, quinidine, procainamide, and flecainide. Digoxin levels will double, type I antiarrhythmic levels will increase 15–35%, and prothrombin times will double or triple. Concomitant use of these drugs requires lower doses and close monitoring.

Summary

Amiodarone is an extremely effective antiarrhythmic agent. Its complex pharmacokinetics require dosing with a loading phase over the first few weeks of therapy. Because of its potential for end-organ toxicity and long half-life, it is not a first-line antiarrhythmic agent. Further studies using low doses should be performed to assess its usefulness in patients with potentially lethal ventricular arrhythmias, post-myocardial infarction reduction of sudden death, and SVT. Close follow-up of patients with monitoring of liver and thyroid function tests and chest x-rays are mandatory to identify adverse reactions at an early stage. Maintenance doses of ≤400 mg per day can be useful in minimizing dose-related adverse effects.

Bretylium (Bretylol®)[101–105]

Bretylium is an intravenous, class III agent useful in the acute treatment of sustained ventricular tachyarrhythmias.

Electrophysiology

Bretylium affects the heart through direct action on the membrane and indirectly through sympathetic denervation of the heart. Initially, bretylium may release norepinephrine from adrenergic nerve endings. This may result in an increase in automaticity and conduction velocity and a decrease in the effective refractory period. After about 20 minutes, bretylium inhibits the release of norepinephrine from adrenergic nerve endings. Bretylium prolongs the action potential duration (APD) by lengthening phase II and the effective refractory period (ERP) of Purkinje fibers in ventricular muscle through a direct effect without altering the ERP/APD ratio. However, this prolongation seems to be more significant in normal tissue than in ischemic tissue (Fig. 4). Thus, bretylium may raise the ventricular fibrillation threshold by reducing the disparity of ventricular refractoriness between ischemic and nonischemic tissue. Bretylium does not usually prolong the QT interval.

Pharmacokinetics

Intravenous bretylium has a rapid onset of action that occurs within minutes. It is primarily excreted by the kidneys, with 80–90% of the

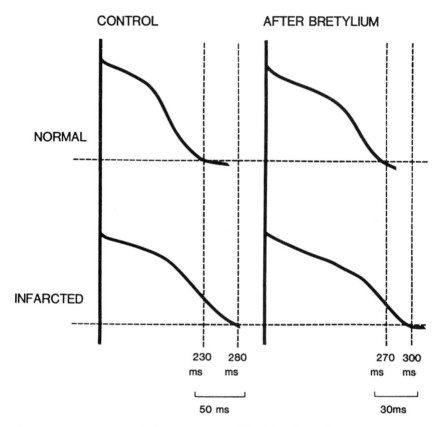

Figure 4. Action potential prolongation of Purkinje fibers in ventricular muscle by bretylium. Prolongation is more marked in normal (230 to 270 = 40 ms) than in infarcted tissue (280 to 300 = 20 ms), thus reducing the disparity of ventricular refractoriness between ischemic and nonischemic tissue.

parent compound being recovered unchanged in the urine. The half-life is 4–17 hours and therapeutic blood levels are in the range of 1 μg/mL.

Dosage

Bretylium is available in 10 cc ampules containing 500 mg of drug. The initial recommended dosage of bretylium is 5–10 mg/kg injected intravenously at a slow rate over 10–20 minutes. In life-threatening situations, 5 mg/kg of undiluted bretylium may be rapidly given intravenously. The maintenance dosage schedule is 1–2 mg/min as a continuous intravenous infusion.

Efficacy

Bretylium is a unique antiarrhythmic agent. In addition to its antiarrhythmic properties, the drug has excellent antifibrillatory properties. In multiple dog models of acute myocardial infarction, bretylium has been shown to increase the ventricular fibrillation threshold over control. Several studies have shown that defibrillation is possible with bretylium alone or with bretylium and cardioversion when lidocaine alone or cardioversion alone have failed to revert the patient to sinus rhythm. Although bretylium is antifibrillatory within minutes, one will not see any antiarrhythmic activity for 20 minutes to 2 hours. In fact, due to the initial norepinephrine release, one may note a slight increase in ventricular ectopy during the first 20 minutes. In addition to its usage as an antiarrhythmic agent in the acute treatment of ventricular tachycardia and ventricular fibrillation, bretylium has been found to be equally efficacious as lidocaine in the treatment of out-of-hospital ventricular fibrillation. In one study, bretylium was found to restore an organized rhythm in 89% of patients with ventricular fibrillation. In addition, a stable rhythm with adequate coronary perfusion was obtained in 58% of those patients receiving bretylium. This study indicated that there was no difference between bretylium and lidocaine in the establishment of an organized rhythm, the establishment of a stable perfusing rhythm, or the survival rate at the time of discharge.

Adverse Effects

Bretylium is unique in that it has no negative inotropic effects on the myocardium. Clinical studies have shown that bretylium may improve myocardial function directly by increasing the amount of calcium available for myocardial contraction from intracellular stores, and indirectly by its effects in the sympathetic nervous system.

Due to the release of norepinephrine caused by bretylium, there may be a transient increase in blood pressure, heart rate, and possibly a transient increase in blood pressure, heart rate, and PVCs during the initial 20 minutes. Later, due to some antiadrenergic effects after a dose, postural hypotension and less frequently supine hypotension may be seen. Rarely, some nausea and vomiting occur during administration of bretylium.

Summary

Intravenous bretylium is a very effective agent in the treatment of ventricular tachycardia and ventricular fibrillation. If intravenous lidocaine is not effective in stabilizing these rhythms, either bretylium or procainamide may be the second agents of choice for the treatment of these rhythms. Bretylium appears to be as effective as lidocaine in the initial management of out-of-hospital ventricular fibrillation in cardiac arrest victims.

Sotalol[106,107]

Sotalol is a unique, noncardioselective beta-blocker with type III properties. The commercially available drug is a racemic mixture of d- and l-sotalol. Sotalol has one-third the β-blocking potency of propranolol. It exhibits no intrinsic sympathomimetic or local anesthetic activity.

Electrophysiology

Sotalol prolongs repolarization in a concentration-dependent fashion resulting in increases in the QT interval and the action potential duration as determined by basic electrophysiological measurements and monophasic action potential recordings in man. Action potential lengthening may be secondary to a reduction in the delayed rectifier potassium current and a decrease in the inward rectifier current. In high concentrations, sotalol inhibits the inward sodium but not calcium currents. Sotalol slows the sinus node cycle length, and lengthens AV nodal conduction time (AH interval) and the effective refractory periods of the atria, AV node, ventricle, and accessory pathway. No effect on the HV interval has been noted. On surface ECG, PR and JTc intervals are prolonged.

Pharmacokinetics

Sotalol is nearly completely absorbed (>90%) and excreted via the kidney with minimal metabolic breakdown. Bioavailability approaches

100%. Peak blood levels are noted 2 hours after a dose and the elimination half-life varies from 7 to 15 hours. The beta-adrenergic antagonism effects of sotalol are longer than the elimination half-life.

Dosing

Oral sotalol is initiated at 80 mg b.i.d. Doses are increased to 160–480 mg b.i.d. as needed. Intravenously, sotalol is given at doses varying between 0.2 and 1.5 mg/kg.

Efficacy

Due to sotalol's effects on atrial, AV node, and accessory pathway refractoriness, it is effective in converting and maintaining in sinus rhythm patients with atrial fibrillation. Rate control is also achieved in these patients. Prevention of PSVT in AVNRT and AVRT has been demonstrated.

Sotalol appears to be effective in suppressing ventricular ectopic activity as assessed by a Holter monitoring in 50–60% of patients. In one study, sotalol was effective in 67% of patients compared to only 39% with procainamide. In comparison to propranolol (29% effective), sotalol was more effective (56%) in controlling ventricular ectopic activity as assessed by Holter monitoring. In a postmyocardial infarction study, sotalol reduced mortality by 18% (pNS compared to placebo) and reduced reinfarction rate by 41% (p < .05) during the year after infarction.

In sustained VT as assessed by programmed stimulation, sotalol was effective in suppressing VT induction in excess of 30% of patients. In a comparative study, IV procainamide was effective in 22% compared to 33% with IV sotalol.

Adverse Effects

Due to its beta-blocking properties, sotalol has some potential for negative cardiac inotropy; however, this is minimal compared to other beta-blocking agents. It seems that lengthening of action potential duration may enhance cardiac contractility. Noncardiac side effects are those typically noted of the other beta-blockers. Cardiac side effects of sotalol include hypotension, symptomatic bradycardia, or AV nodal conduction abnormalities. Ventricular proarrhythmia has occurred in 4–5%

of patients. Torsades de pointes is the most common proarrhythmia (40% of all reported proarrhythmia) with a frequency similar to the occurrence of torsades with quinidine.

Summary

Sotalol is a unique antiarrhythmic that will be useful in treating sustained VT and in atrial fibrillation. Since sotalol can cause torsades de pointes, careful dosing and observation of patients is essential.

Verapamil (Calan®, Isoptin®)[108-114]

Verapamil is a papaverine derivation that is classified as a type IV antiarrhythmic agent. Intravenous verapamil is available for the acute treatment of SVT. Oral verapamil is available in a short-acting and controlled release formulation and has some usefulness in controlling the ventricular response in atrial fibrillation and in treating re-entrant paroxysmal supraventricular tachycardia.

Electrophysiology

As a calcium channel antagonist, verapamil inhibits the slow channels by blocking the inward calcium current. The slow channels are important in the generation of the action potentials of the SA and AV node and in damaged or diseased cardiac tissue. Because of this, verapamil slows sinus rate, although this direct suppressant effect may be counteracted by its vasodilatory properties, and prolongs the AH interval and the AVNERP and AVNFRP. Verapamil has been noted to shorten the refractory period of accessory pathway tissue.

Pharmacokinetics

Although over 90% of verapamil is absorbed, only 10–20% is bioavailable due to first-pass hepatic metabolism. Only 7% of the drug is excreted unchanged in the urine. Orally, peak levels occur in 2 hours and the half-life is 3–7 hours.

Dosing

Intravenously, effects occur in 3–5 minutes and last 20–30 minutes. Intravenously, we usually dose at 0.1 mg/kg as a bolus. If continuous infusions are needed, we maintain patients at .005 mg/kg/min. Orally, the usual doses are 80–240 mg t.i.d.

Efficacy

Intravenous verapamil has been the drug of choice for the acute termination of re-entrant PSVT utilizing the AV node. Efficacy rates range from 80% to 95% for reversion to sinus rhythm. In the remainder, the ventricular rate is usually slower. IV verapamil can also be used to acutely slow the ventricular response in patients with primary atrial arrhythmias. It rarely causes acute termination of these arrhythmias. Intravenous verapamil should not be used in wide QRS tachycardias of undetermined etiology since the majority of these tachycardias are VT and verapamil may cause further hemodynamic compromise. Continuous infusions of verapamil may be useful for temporary rate control of multifocal atrial tachycardia and atrial fibrillation in the critical care setting.

Orally, verapamil is primarily useful in the additive control of the ventricular response in patients with atrial fibrillation and flutter. Oral verapamil may rarely be effective in preventing the recurrence of PSVT, although this usually requires large doses that frequently cause subjective side effects. Occasionally, the beneficial effect in AVNRT is secondary to altering of retrograde AV node conduction. Rarely, a verapamil-sensitive ventricular tachycardia is noted. This is usually in young patients with normal hearts and exercise-provoked VT.

Adverse Effects

Verapamil can cause symptomatic bradycardia, sinus arrest, and worsen AV nodal block. Due to significant negative inotropy, verapamil can depress left ventricular function and cause or worsen CHF. IV verapamil can accelerate the pre-excited ventricular response in patients with atrial fibrillation and Wolff-Parkinson-White (WPW) syndrome. Subjective toxicity includes nausea, dizziness, and constipation. Verapamil may increase the serum digoxin level during concomitant administration.

Summary

Intravenous verapamil has been the acute treatment of choice for the termination of regular, narrow QRS SVT. Its use is contraindicated in patients with atrial fibrillation and WPW and in the setting of wide QRS tachycardia of undetermined etiology. Orally, verapamil is predominantly used as adjunctive therapy to control the ventricular response in patients who have inadequate rate control with digitalis. Its use in ventricular arrhythmias is limited.

Diltiazem (Cardizem®)[114,115]

Diltiazem is a calcium channel blocker with electrophysiological effects similar to verapamil. Orally, it is approved for the treatment of angina and hypertension, although it is frequently used as adjunct therapy in rate control of atrial fibrillation. Intravenously, investigational use has proven it to be an effective drug for acutely terminating PSVT and controlling rate in rapid atrial arrhythmias.

Dosing

Oral diltiazem is used at doses of 30–90 mg t.i.d. Intravenously, the dose is 0.15–0.45 mg/kg.

Electrophysiology

Diltiazem has electrophysiological effects similar to verapamil. Due to less peripheral vasodilation, reflex changes are not as common. Because of this, diltiazem more consistently slows heart rate. Diltiazem slows conduction (AH) in the AV node and prolongs antegrade AV nodal refractoriness.

Efficacy

Continuous IV infusion of diltiazem maintained a >20% decrease in heart rate in 34 of 44 patients in atrial flutter/fibrillation.

In 14 patients with SVT and WPW, eight patients no longer had SVT induced after diltiazem. In the remainder, SVT cycle length slowed. No effect on retrograde accessory pathway conduction was noted. IV diltiazem can enhance the shortest pre-excited RR in atrial fibrillation. IV diltiazem has been effective in terminating SVT in over 80% of cases within 3 minutes.

Adverse Effects

IV diltiazem is relatively free of adverse effects. Compared to verapamil, hemodynamic compromise is less likely to occur.

Summary

Orally, diltiazem is a useful adjunct for rate control to digoxin, etc. It is more useful than verapamil in patients with CHF due to its more benign hemodynamic profile. IV diltiazem, when approved, will have efficacy rates in terminating PSVT similar to IV verapamil with better hemodynamics.

Adenosine (Adenocard®)[116–119]

Adenosine and ATP are effective in terminating PSVT. They are not classifiable within the constraints of the Vaughn-Williams classification. The effects of these drugs are mediated by extracellular purinergic receptors. ATP is metabolically broken down into adenosine, which is the active antiarrhythmic.

Electrophysiology

Adenosine has negative chronotropic and dromotropic effects on the SA and AV node. No effects on His-Purkinje conduction or ventricular refractoriness have been noted.

Pharmacokinetics

After injection, adenosine is rapidly cleared from the circulation by cellular uptake and metabolism. Adenosine enters the blood pool and metabolizes to inosine and adenosine monophosphate with an elimination half-life of <10 seconds. Onset of action is about 15–30 seconds after injection. Aminophylline counteracts the effects of adenosine. Dipyridamole, which is a potent adenosine uptake inhibitor, may potentiate the effect of adenosine.

Dosing

Adenosine is available in 6-mg vials (2 cc). Over 90% of patients will respond to a dose of 50 μg/kg (<10 mg). The current recommended dose is 6 mg IV push followed by a 12 mg IV dose if necessary.

Efficacy

Adenosine at doses of 12 mg IV is effective in terminating PSVT in 91% of cases. Conversion to NSR usually occurs in less than 1 minute. Comparing up to 12 mg IV adenosine to 7.5 mg IV verapamil, SVT was terminated in 93% and 91%, respectively. All six verapamil nonresponders converted with adenosine. Adenosine terminates SVT quicker than verapamil (median of 30 compared to 170 seconds). Adenosine has been found to be effective in terminating sustained VT in normal hearts that are catecholamine or calcium influx-sensitive. Since adenosine rarely affects VT and has a short half-life, it has been used as a diagnostic test in wide QRS tachycardia of undetermined etiology.

Adverse Effects

Dyspnea and flushing are the most common adverse effects that may occur transiently. Cardiac side effects include sinus bradycardia, sinus tachycardia, sinus pauses, and AV block. At high doses, a transient decrease in blood pressure has been noted.

Summary

IV adenosine is as effective as verapamil in terminating re-entrant SVT utilizing the AV node. Due to its brief duration of action, adverse effects are transient, but chronic therapy is not useful. Adenosine may rapidly become one of the treatments of choice in the acute termination of PSVT. Due to its short half-life, it has little use in rate control of rapid atrial arrhythmias.

Digoxin (Lanoxin®) (Lanoxicaps®) (Crystodigin®)[120–124]

Digoxin and digotoxin are cardiac glycosides, often grouped in the digitalis glycoside family. These drugs are useful in controlling the ventricular response in atrial tachyarrhythmias and also as positive inotropic agents in patients with systolic dysfunction.

Pharmacokinetics

Digoxin is 60–80% absorbed. Following drug administration, a 6–8 hour distribution phase occurs. The volume of distribution is large. Twenty to 25% of digoxin is bound to protein. The time to onset effect is $\frac{1}{2}$ to 2 hours and peak effect is 2–6 hours. Elimination of digoxin follows first-order kinetics. Since digoxin is primarily renal excreted, excretion may be diminished in patients with abnormal renal function. The half-life of elimination in patients with normal renal function is 1.5–2 days. This may be extended to 6 days in patients with significant renal dysfunction.

Digitoxin differs from digoxin in having a longer elimination half-life of 7–9 days. Over 90% is bound to tissue proteins. Digitoxin differs from digoxin that is primarily metabolized in the liver.

Electrophysiology

Digitalis glycosides cause some indirect action mediated by the autonomic nervous system secondary to vagal action. Thus, digitalis may slow sinus node automaticity and slow AV node conduction, prolonging AV node refractoriness. Directly, digoxin may increase the force velocity of myocardial systolic contractions.

Dosing

The usual maintenance dose of digoxin is 0.125–0.25 mg/day. The dose should be decreased in patients who are on co-existing quinidine, propafenone, or amiodarone. It also should be decreased in patients with renal dysfunction. Because of the long elimination half-life, it may take over a week for digoxin to reach a steady state. Orally or intravenously, patients could be more rapidly digitalized using loading doses of 8–12 μg/kg. As a general rule, in a 70-kg patient, about 1 mg is needed for initial loading. Lanoxin can be given orally, intravenously, and orally in an elixir form for pediatric patients.

For digitoxin, digitalization can occur using 0.2 mg twice daily for 4 days following maintenance doses of 0.05–0.3 mg daily, the most common doses being 0.1, 0.15, 0.2 mg daily. In patients who develop life-threatening digitalis toxicity, Digibind® can be given in an attempt to reverse some direct effects of digoxin acutely.

Efficacy

There is little proof in the literature that digoxin has significant benefit in treating ventricular arrhythmias. However, there are some minimal reports and indirect evidence that in patients with systolic dysfunction, optimizing hemodynamics may have a beneficial antiarrhythmic effect. Digoxin's primary use is controlling the ventricular rate in patients with atrial fibrillation, atrial flutter, and atrial tachycardia. Digitalis is an excellent drug for slowing conduction through the AV node and prolonging AV node refractoriness. Although rapid digitalization is often used in patients who present with new-onset atrial fibrillation in the emergency setting, placebo-controlled study has suggested that the reversion from atrial fibrillation to sinus rhythm is not more frequent with digoxin when compared to placebo. In patients with vagally induced atrial fibrillation, digitalis may make atrial fibrillation more likely to recur. Digitalis, by slowing conduction antegrade in the AV node, may be useful in slowing the ventricular response of patients with re-entrant paroxysmal supraventricular tachycardias. In rare circumstances, this effect on AV nodal conduction may be beneficial in preventing recurrences of PSVT.

Summary

Digitalis glycosides are predominently useful in treating congestive heart failure symptoms in patients with systolic dysfunction. Its main antiarrhythmic use is controlling the ventricular response in patients with atrial tachycardia. Rarely, it may be useful in the treatment of paroxysmal supraventricular tachycardia. Its use as a ventricular antiarrhythmic agent is limited. Due to the drug's inexpensive cost and once-a-day dosing, it is often a useful adjunct in patients with varying arrhythmias. However, digitalis glycosides will rarely prevent arrhythmias and are usually only used for rate control.

Choice of Antiarrhythmic Agents

For patients who are being treated for benign, symptomatic considered PVCs, we prefer to use drugs with a minimal potential for end-organ toxicity (see Table 11) and a low incidence of causing proarrhythmia (see Table 10). If beta-blockers or mexiletine are ineffective, we preferentially use type IA antiarrhythmic agents before IC drugs due to the results of the CAST study. In the post-myocardial infarction patient with ventricular arrhythmias, encainide and flecainide are now contraindicated. We avoid the use of amiodarone in this group of patients due to its end-organ toxicity.

In patients with potentially lethal ventricular arrhythmias, we prefer beta blockers or mexiletine, especially in the outpatient setting, as first-line agents due to their lack of end-organ toxicity and low proarrhythmic potential. Type IA agents alone or are also useful as front-line therapy. Combination therapy with a type IB agent can be used in more refractory patients. Other choices are type IC agents given their high efficacy and low toxicity and proarrhythmic potential in this group of patients. Again, the results of the CAST study have rendered these drugs into a second-line position. They should not be used in asymptomatic ventricular arrhythmias in the post-myocardial infarction setting. Since propafenone has a lower incidence of proarrhythmia and has not had the negative impact of CAST, we would prefer using this drug if IC therapy is required. In refractory patients we might consider amiodarone therapy if the patient had refractory nonsustained VT, especially with co-existing left ventricular dysfunction or hemodynamically compromising atrial fibrillation.

In patients with lethal ventricular arrhythmias, we prefer type IA agents and mexiletine alone or in combination as front-line agents in this group of patients. We prefer these drugs despite efficacy rates of less than 25% because of the high incidence (>10%) of drug-induced incessant ventricular tachycardia with type IC drugs in this group of patients. When available, sotalol will be a front-line agent for this indication. We reserve amiodarone for drug refractory sustained ventricular tachyarrhythmias.

In patients with primary atrial tachycardias (ectopic atrial tachycardia atrial flutter, atrial fibrillation) we prefer treatment with the type IA agents followed by type IC agents, sotalol, and if necessary, amiodarone. If suppression of the irritable focus is not attainable with the above types of therapy, we may treat the patients with digoxin, β-blockers, or calcium blockers in an attempt to attain rate control.

In patients with re-entrant supraventricular tachycardia associated with the Wolff-Parkinson-White syndrome, type IC drugs are our treatments of choice followed by the type IA agents. We prefer this approach, since it is our bias to preferentially suppress conduction in the accessory pathway rather than affecting AV nodal conduction. However, selected patients will respond to drugs that slow AV node conduction (digoxin, β-blockers, verapamil) alone or in combination with a type IA or IC sodium channel blockers.

In patients with atrial fibrillation associated with the Wolff-Parkinson-White syndrome, we prefer type IC or IA agents since they more effectively slow rapid conduction down the accessory pathway. Digoxin and verapamil are relatively contraindicated in this syndrome since accessory pathway conduction can be preferred and enhanced with these drugs.

In patients with suspected AV node re-entrant tachycardia, we prefer IC and IA agents in those patients who do not easily respond to digoxin or β-blockers.

The above recommendations should be used as guidelines in choosing an antiarrhythmic drug in a selected patient. Individual exceptions can be made depending on the clinical scenario. The type of arrhythmia, previous drug failures, co-existing disease states, concomitant medications, and left ventricular function all affect the decision in a given individual.

References

1. Woosley RL, Shand DG: Pharmacokinetics of antiarrhythmic drugs. Am J Cardiol 41:986, 1978.
2. Winter ME: Basic Clinical Pharmacokinetics, 2nd ed. Spokane, Applied Therapeutics Inc., 1988.
3. Woosley RL, Echt DS, Roden DM: Effects of congestive heart failure on the pharmacokinetics and pharmacodynamics of antiarrhythmic agents. Am J Cardiol 57:25B, 1986.

4. Vaughn Williams EM: A classification of antiarrhythmic actions reassessed after a decade of new drugs. J Clin Pharmacol 24:129, 1984.
5. Harrison DC: Antiarrhythmic drug classification: new science and practice applications. Am J Cardiol 56:185, 1985.
6. Kreeger RW, Hammill SC: New antiarrhythmic drugs: tocainide, mexiletine, flecainide, encainide, amiodarone. Mayo Clin Proc 62:1033, 1987.
7. Salerno DM: Review: antiarrhythmic drugs, 1987. Part I–J-Electrophysiology 1:217, 1987; Part II-1:300, 1987; Part III-1:435, 1987; Part IV-2:55, 1988.
8. Campbell TJ: Kinetics of onset of rate-dependent effects of class I antiarrhythmic drugs are important in determining their effects on refractoriness in guinea pig ventricle and provide a theoretical basis for their subclassification. Cardiovasc Res 17:344, 1983.
9. Hondeghem LM, Katzung BG: Antiarrhythmic agents: the modulated receptor mechanism of action of sodium and calcium channel-blocking drugs. Ann Rev Pharmacol Toxicol 24:387, 1984.
10. Naccarelli GV, Rinkenberger RL, Dougherty AH, et al: Pharmacologic therapy of arrhythmias. Hosp Practice 23(10):183, 1988.
11. Kokolow M, Ball R: Factors influencing conversion of chronic atrial fibrillation with special reference to quinidine concentration. Circulation 14:568, 1956.
12. Mason JW, Hondeghem LM: Quinidine. Ann NY Acad Sci 432:162, 1984.
13. Morganroth J, Hunter H: Comparative efficacy and safety of short-acting and sustained release quinidine in the treatment of patients with ventricular arrhythmias. Am Heart J 110:1176, 1985.
14. DiMarco JP, Garan H, Ruskin JN: Quinidine for ventricular arrhythmias: value of electrophysiologic testing. Am J Cardiol 51:90, 1983.
15. Selzer A, Wray HW: Quinidine syncope: paroxysmal ventricular fibrillation occurring during treatment of chronic atrial arrhythmias. Circulation 30:17, 1964.
16. Roden DM, Woosley RL, Primm K: Incidence and clinical features of the quinidine-associated long QT syndrome: implications for patient care. Am Heart J 111:1088, 1986.
17. Morganroth J, Horowitz LN: Incidence of proarrhythmic effects from quinidine in the outpatient treatment of benign or potentially lethal ventricular arrhythmias. Am J Cardiol 56:585, 1985.
18. Hartel G, Louhija A, Konttinen A, et al: Value of quinidine in the maintenance of sinus rhythm after electrical conversion of atrial fibrillation. Br Heart J 32:57, 1970.
19. Duff HJ, Mitchell LB, Manuari D, et al: Mexiletine-quinidine combination: electrophysiologic correlates of a favorable antiarrhythmic interaction in humans. J Am Coll Cardiol 10:1149, 1987.
20. Greenblatt DJ, Pfeifer, Ochs HR, et al: Pharmacokinetics of quinidine in humans after intravenous intramuscular and oral administration. J Pharmacol Exp Ther 202:365, 1977.
21. Waxman HL, Buxton AE, Sadowski LM, et al: Response to procainamide during electrophysiologic study for sustained ventricular tachycardia predicts response to other drugs. Circulation 67:30, 1982.
22. Giardina EG: Procainamide: clinical pharmacology and efficacy against ventricular arrhythmias. Ann NY Acad Sci 432:117, 1984.

23. Boccardo D, Pitchon R, Wiener I: Adverse reactions and efficacy of high dose procainamide therapy in resistant tachycarrhythmias. Am Heart J 102:797, 1981.
24. Halpern SW, Ellrodt G, Singh BN, et al: Efficacy of intravenous procainamide infusion in converting atrial fibrillation to sinus rhythm: relation to left atrial size. Br Heart J 44:589, 1980.
25. Marchlinski FE, Buxton AE, Vassallo JA, et al: Comparative electrophysiologic effects of intravenous and oral procainamide in patients with sustained ventricular arrhythmias. J Am Coll Cardiol 4:1247, 1984.
26. Greenspan AM, Horowitz LN, Spielman SR, et al: Large dose procainamide therapy for ventricular tachyarrhythmia. Am J Cardiol 46:453, 1980.
27. Giardina EG, Fenster P, Paul E, et al: Efficacy plasma concentrations and adverse effects of a new sustained release procainamide preparation. Am J Cardiol 46:855, 1980.
28. Myerburg RJ, Kessler KM, Kiem I, et al: Relationship between plasma levels of procainamide suppression of premature ventricular complexes and prevention of recurrent ventricular tachycardia. Circulation 64:280, 1981.
29. Lie KI, Wellens HJJ, VanCapelle FJ, et al: Lidocaine in the prevention of primary ventricular fibrillation. N Engl J Med 291:1324, 1974.
30. Morady F, Scheinman MM, Desai J: Disopyramide. Ann Intern Med 96:337, 1982.
31. Podrid PJ, Schoeneberger A, Lown B: Congestive heart failure caused by oral disopyramide. N Engl J Med 302:614, 1980.
32. Brogden LM, Todd PA: Focus on disopyramide. Drugs 34:151, 1987.
33. Koch-Weser J: Disopyramide. N Engl J Med 300:957, 1979.
34. Lerman BB, Waxman HL, Buxton AE, et al: Disopyramide: evaluation of electrophysiologic effects and clinical efficacy in patients with sustained ventricular tachycardia or ventricular fibrillation. Am J Cardiol 51:759, 1983.
35. Rosen MR, Hoffman BF, Wit AL: Electrophysiology and pharmacology of cardiac arrhythmias. V. Cardiac antiarrhythmic effects of lidocaine. Am Heart J 89;526, 1975.
36. Thompson PD, et al: Lidocaine pharmacokinetics in advanced heart failure, liver disease and renal failure in humans. Ann Intern Med 78:499, 1973.
37. Lie KI, Wellens HJJ, VanCapelle FJ, et al: Lidocaine in the prevention of ventricular fibrillation. N Engl J Med 291:1324, 1974.
38. Collingsworth KA, Kalman SN, Harrison DC: The clinical pharmacology of lidocaine as an antiarrhythmic drug. Circulation 50:1217, 1974.
39. Harrison DC: Practical guidelines for the use of lidocaine. Prevention and treatment of cardiac arrhythmias. JAMA 233:1202, 1975.
40. Bigger JT, Schmidt DH, Kutt H: Relationship between the plasma level of diphenylhydantoin sodium and its cardiac antiarrhythmic effects. Circulation 38:363, 1968.
41. Lang TW, Bernstein MD, Barbieri F, et al: Digitalis toxicity: treatment with diphenylhydantoin. Arch Intern Med 116:563, 1965.
42. Garson A, Kugler JD, Gillette PC, et al: Control of late post-operative ventricular arrhythmias with phenytoin in young patients. Am J Cardiol 46:290, 1980.
43. Epstein AE, Plumb VJ, Henthorn RW, et al: Phenytoin in the treatment of inducible ventricular tachycardia: results of electrophysiologic tachycardia.

Results of electrophysiologic testing and long-term followup. PACE 10:1049, 1987.

44. Kutalek SP, Morganroth J, Horowitz LN, Tocainide: a new oral antiarrhythmic agent. Ann Intern Med 103:387, 1985.

45. Morganroth J, Nestico FF, Horowitz LN: A review of the uses and limitations of tocainide: a class IB antiarrhythmic agent. Am Heart J 110:856, 1985.

46. Roden DM, Woosley RL: Tocainide. N Engl J Med 315:41, 1986.

47. Podrid PJ, Lown B: Tocainide for refractory symptomatic ventricular arrhythmias. Am J Cardiol 49:1279, 1982.

48. Morganroth J, Oshrain C, Steele PP: Comparative efficacy and safety of oral tocainide and quinidine for benign and potentially lethal ventricular arrhythmias. Am J Cardiol 56:581, 1985.

49. Hession M, Blum R, Podrid PJ, et al: Mexiletine and tocainide: does response to one predict response to the other? J Am Coll Cardiol 7:338, 1986.

50. Campbell RWF: Mexiletine. N Engl J Med 316:29, 1987.

51. Podrid PJ, Lown B: Mexiletine for ventricular arrhythmias. Am J Cardiol 47:895, 1981.

52. DiMarco JP, Garan H, Ruskin JN: Mexiletine for refractory ventricular arrhythmias: results using serial electrophysiologic testing. Am J Cardiol 47:131, 1981.

53. Berns E, Naccarelli GV, Dougherty AH, et al: Mexiletine: lack of predictors of clinical response in patients treated for life-threatening tachyarrhythmias. J Electrophysiol 2:201, 1988.

54. Schoenfeld MH, Whitford E, McGovern B, et al: Oral mexiletine in the treatment of refractory ventricular arrhythmias: the role of electrophysiologic techniques. Am Heart J 5:1071, 1984.

55. Duff HJ, Kolodgie FD, Roden DM, et al: Electropharmacologic synergism with mexiletine and quinidine. J Cardiovasc Pharmacol 8:840, 1986.

56. Impact Research Group: International mexiletine and placebo antiarrhythmic coronary trial. I. Report on arrhythmia and other findings. J Am Coll Cardiol 4:1148, 1984.

57. Roden DM, Woosley RL: Drug therapy: flecainide. N Engl J Med 315:36, 1986.

58. Bigger JT (ed): Symposium: flecainide acetate. Am J Cardiol 53:Supplement B, 1984.

59. Anderson JL, Pritchett ELC (ed): International Symposium on Supraventricular Arrhythmias; Focus on flecainide. Am J Cardiol 62:1D, 1988.

60. Lal R, Chapman PD, Naccarelli GV, et al: Short- and long-term experience with flecainide acetate in the management of refractory life-threatening ventricular arrhythmias. J Am Coll Cardiol 6:772, 1985.

61. Flecainide Ventricular Tachycardia Study Group: Treatment of resistant ventricular tachycardia with flecainide acetate. Am J Cardiol 57:1299, 1986.

62. Nappi JM, Anderson JL: Flecainide: a new prototype antiarrhythmic agent. Pharmacotherapy 5(4):209, 1985.

63. Lal R, Chapman PD, Naccarelli GV, et al: Flecainide in the treatment of nonsustained ventricular tachycardia. Ann Intern Med 105:493, 1986.

64. Berns E, Rinkenberger RL, Jeang M, et al: Clinical efficacy and safety of

flecainide acetate in the treatment of primary atrial tachycardias. Am J Cardiol 59:1337, 1987.

65. Anastasiou-Nana MI, Anderson JL, Stewart JR, et al: Occurrence of exercise-induced wide-complex tachycardia during therapy with flecainide for complex ventricular arrhythmias: a probable proarrhythmic effect. Am Heart J 113:1071, 1987.

66. The Cardiac Arrhythmia Pilot Study (CAPS) Investigators: Effects of encainide, flecainide, imipramine and moricizine on ventricular arrhythmias during the year after myocardial infarction. The CAPS. Am J Cardiol 61:501, 1988.

67. The Cardiac Arrhythmia Suppression Trial Investigators. Preliminary report: effect of encainide and flecainide on mortality in a randomized trial of arrhythmia suppression after myocardial infarction. N Engl J Med 321:406, 1989.

68. Naccarelli GV, Rinkenberger RL, Dougherty AH, et al: Encainide: a review of its electrophysiology, pharmacology and clinical efficacy. Clin Prog Electrophysiol Pacing 3:268, 1985.

69. Harrison DC, Morganroth J (ed): Symposium: encainide. Am J Cardiol 58:Supplement C, 1986.

70. Naccarelli GV, Wellen HJJ (ed): A symposium: the use of encainide in supraventricular tachycardia. Am J Cardiol 62:1L, 1988.

71. Jackman WM, Zipes DP, Naccarelli GV, et al: Electrophysiology of oral encainide. Am J Cardiol 49:1270, 1982.

72. Prystowsky EN, Klein G, Rinkenberger RL, et al: Clinical efficacy and electrophysiologic effects of encainide in patients with Wolff-Parkinson-White syndrome. Circulation 69:278, 1984.

73. Morganroth J, Somberg JC, Pool PE, et al: Comparative study of encainide and quinidine in the treatment of ventricular arrhythmias. J Am Coll Cardiol 7:9, 1986.

74. DiBianco R, Fletcher RD, Cohen AI, et al: Treatment of frequent ventricular arrhythmia with encainide: assessment using serial electrocardiograms, intracardiac electrophysiologic studies, treadmill exercise tests and radionuclide cineangiocardiographic studies. Circulation 85:1134, 1985.

75. Podrid PJ, Lown B: Propafenone: a new agent for ventricular arrhythmias. J Am Coll Cardiol 4:117, 1984.

76. Naccarella F, Bracchetti D, Palmieri M, et al: Comparison of propafenone and disopyramide for treatment of chronic ventricular arrhythmias: Placebo-controlled, double-blind, randomized crossover study. Am Heart J 109:833, 1985.

77. Podrid PJ (ed): Symposium on propafenone. J Electrophysiol 1:517, 1989.

78. Chilson DA, Heger JJ, Zipes DP, et al: Electrophysiologic effects and clinical efficacy of oral propafenone therapy in patients with ventricular tachycardia. J Am Coll Cardiol 5:1407, 1985.

79. Connally SJ, Kates RE, Lebsack CS, et al: Clinical pharmacology of propafenone. Circulation 68:589, 1983.

80. Ludmer PL, McGowan NE, Antman EM, et al: Efficacy of propafenone in Wolff-Parkinson-White syndrome: electrophysiologic findings and long-term followup. J Am Coll Cardiol 9:1357, 1987.

81. Siddoway LA, Thompson EA, McAllister CB, et al: Polymorphism pro-

pafenone metabolism and disposition in man: clinical and pharmacokinetic consequences. Circulation 75:785, 1987.

82. Anderson JL, Anastasiou-Nana MI, Heath BM, et al: Efficacy of recainam, a new antiarrhythmic drug for control of ventricular arrhythmias. Am J Cardiol 60:281, 1987.

83. DeBuitleir M, Kou WH, Nelson SD, et al: Electrophysiologic effects and efficacy of recainam for sustained ventricular tachycardia. Am J Cardiol 63:116, 1989.

84. Podrid PJ, Lyakishev A, Lown B, et al: Ethmozine: a new antiarrhythmic drug for suppressing ventricular premature complexes. Circulation 61:450, 1980.

85. Ruggio JM, Somberg JC: New therapy focus: ethmozine Cardiovasc Rev Reports 5:738, 1984.

86. Morganroth J, Bigger JT (ed): Pharmacologic management of ventricular arrhythmias: current status in the role of moricizine HCl. Am J Cardiol 65:10D, 1990.

87. Mann DE, Luck JC, Herre JM, et al: Electrophysiologic effects of ethmozine in patients with ventricular tachycardia. Am Heart J 107:674, 1984.

88. Beta Blocker Heart Attack Study Group: The beta-blocker heart attack trial. JAMA 246:2073, 1981.

89. Morganroth J, Lichstein E, Byington R: Beta-Blocker Heart Attack Trial: Impact of propranolol therapy on ventricular arrhythmias. Prev Med 14:346, 1985.

90. Singh SN, DiBianco R, Davidon ME, et al: Comparison of acebutolol and propranolol for treatment of chronic ventricular arrhythmia: a placebo-controlled, double-blind, randomized crossover study. Circulation 65:1356, 1982.

91. DeSoyza N, Shapiro W, Chandraratna PAN, et al: Acebutolol therapy for ventricular arrhythmias: a randomized, placebo-controlled double-blind multicenter study. Circulation 65:1129, 1982.

92. Boissel JP, Leizorowitc A, Picolet H, et al, APSI Investigators: Efficacy of acebutolol after acute myocardial infarction (the ASPI trial). Am J Cardiol 66:24C, 1990.

93. Anderson S, Blanski L, Byrd RC, et al: Comparison of the efficacy and safety of esmolol, a short acting beta-blocker with placebo in the treatment of supraventricular arrhythmias. Am Heart J 111:429, 1986.

94. Tuslapaty P, Laddu A, Murrthy VS, et al: Esmolol: A titratable short-acting intravenous beta blocker for acute critical care settings. Am Heart J 114:866, 1987.

95. Naccarelli GV, Rinkenberger RL, Dougherty AH, et al: Amiodarone: pharmacology and antiarrhythmic and adverse effects. Pharmacotherapy 5:298, 1985.

96. Singh BN, Zipes DP (ed): Proceedings of the symposium: Amiodarone: basic concepts and clinical applications. Am Heart J Vol. 106, 1983.

97. Mason JW: Amiodarone. N Engl J Med 316:455, 1987.

98. Zipes DP, Prystowsky EN, Heger JJ: Amiodarone: electrophysiologic actions, pharmacokinetics, and clinical effects. J Am Coll Cardiol 3:1059, 1984.

99. Herre JM, Sauve MJ, Malone P, et al: Long-term results of amiodarone

therapy in patients with recurrent sustained ventricular tachycardia or ventricular fibrillation. J Am Coll Cardiol 13:442, 1989.

100. Kehoe RF, Zheutlein T (eds): Amiodarone I, II, III. Prog Cardiovasc Dis 31:249, 319, 393, 1989.
101. Haynes RE, Chinn TL, Capass MK, et al: Comparison of bretylium tosylate and lidocaine in management of out-of-hospital ventricular fibrillation: a randomized clinical trial. Am J Cardiol 48:353, 1981.
102. Kerber RE, Pandian NG, Jensen SR, et al: Effect of lidocaine and bretylium on energy requirements for transthoracic defibrillation: experimental studies. J Am Coll Cardiol 7:397, 1986.
103. Heissenbuttel RH, Bigger JT: Bretylium tosylate: a newly available antiarrhythmic drug for ventricular arrhythmias. Ann Intern Med 91:229, 1979.
104. Rapeport WG: Clinical pharmacokinetics of bretylium. Clin Pharmacol 10:248, 1985.
105. Kapia GA, Lucchessi BR: Antifibrillatory action of bretylium: role of the sympathetic nervous system. Pharmacology 34:37, 1987.
106. Singh BN (ed): A symposium: controlling cardiac arrhythmias with sotalol, a broad spectrum antiarrhythmic with beta-blocking effects and class III activity. Am J Cardiol 65:IA-88A, 1990.
107. Julian DG, Jackson FS, Prescott RJ, et al: Controlled trial of sotolol for one year after myocardial infarction. Lancet 1:1142, 1982.
108. Rinkenberger RL, Prystowsky EN, Heger JJ, et al: Effects of intravenous and chronic oral verapamil administration in patients with supraventricular tachyarrhythmias. Circulation 62:996, 1980.
109. Gulamhusein S, Ko P, Carruthers SG, et al: Acceleration of the ventricular response during atrial fibrillation in the Wolff-Parkinson-White syndrome after verapamil. Circulation 65:348, 1982.
110. Sung RJ, Elser B, McAllister RG Jr: Intravenous verapamil for termination of reentrant supraventricular tachycardias: intracardiac studies correlated with plasma verapamil concentrations. Ann Intern Med 93:682, 1980.
111. Waxman HL, Myerburg RJ, Appel R, et al: Verapamil for control of ventricular rate in paroxysmal supraventricular tachycardia and atrial fibrillation or flutter: a double-blind randomized cross-over study. Ann Intern Med 94:1, 1981.
112. Buxton AE, Marchlinski FE, Doherty JW, et al: Hazards of intravenous verapamil for sustained ventricular tachycardia. Am J Cardiol 59:1107, 1987.
113. Sung RJ, Shapiro WA, Shen EN, et al: Effects of verapamil on ventricular tachycardias possibly caused by reentry, automaticity and triggered activity. J Clin Invest 72:350, 1983.
114. Shenasa M, Kus T, Fromer M, et al: Effect of intravenous and oral calcium antagonists (diltiazem and verapamil) on sustenance of atrial fibrillation. Am J Cardiol 62:403, 1988.
115. Shenasa M, Fromer M, Faugers G, et al: Efficacy and safety of intravenous and oral diltiazem for Wolff-Parkinson-White syndrome. Am J Cardiol 59:301, 1987.
116. DiMarco JP, Sellers TD, Lerman BB, et al: Diagnostic and therapeutic use of adenosine in patients with supraventricular tachyarrhythmias. J Am Coll Cardiol 6:417, 1985.
117. DiMarco JP, Sellers TD, Lerman BB, et al: Diagnostic and therapeutic use

of adenosine in patients with supraventricular tachyarrhythmias. J Am Coll Cardiol 6:417, 1985.

118. DiMarco, Sellers TD, Berne RM, et al: Adenosine: electrophysiologic effects and therapeutic use for terminating paroxysmal supraventricular tachycardia. Circulation 68:1254, 1983.

119. Griffith MJ, Linker NJ, Ward DE, et al: Adenosine in the diagnosis of broad complex tachycardia. Lancet i:672, 1988.

120. Falk RH, Knowlton AA, Bernard SA, et al: Digoxin for converting recent-onset atrial fibrillation to sinus rhythm: a randomized, double-blind trial. Ann Intern Med 106:503, 1987.

121. Mungall DR, Robichaux RP, Perry W, et al: Effects of quinidine on serum digoxin concentration: a prospective study. Ann Int Med 93:689, 1980.

122. Pick A: Digitalis and the electrocardiogram. Circulation 15:603, 1957.

123. Smith TW: Digitalis. Mechanisms of action and clinical use. N Engl J Med 318:358, 1988.

124. Lown B, Graboys TB, Podrid PJ, et al: Effect of a digitalis drug on ventricular premature beats. N Engl J Med 296:301, 1977.

Chapter 17

Cardiac Pacing I: Treatment of Bradyarrhythmias

Anne Hamilton Dougherty
and Gerald V. Naccarelli

Introduction

The first successful use of an artificial pacemaker for resuscitation was in 1931, and 17 years later, a self-contained pacemaker was implanted for continuing treatment of patients with Morgagni-Stokes-Adams attacks. Since the time of that rudimentary device, a technological revolution has resulted in the development of reliable, long-lived pacemakers whose function can be modified noninvasively by programming to adapt to the individual needs of a wide variety of patients. As a consequence, the role of pacemaker therapy has expanded from that of a strictly life-saving modality in catastrophic illness to one that also reduces morbidity in patients with less severe symptoms.

Today, over 100,000 permanent pacers are implanted yearly in the US for conditions ranging from symptomatic sinus bradycardia to potentially lethal complete heart block. In addition, pacemakers have been used for both prevention and termination of tachyarrhythmias, a subject that will be discussed in detail in Chapter 18.

From Naccarelli GV (ed): *Cardiac Arrhythmias: A Practical Approach.* Mount Kisco, NY, Futura Publishing Co., Inc., © 1991.

487

Indications for Pacing Therapy

Pacemakers are useful both for alleviation of symptoms related to bradycardia and for prevention of morbidity in patients at high risk for developing severe or debilitating bradycardia (Table 1).[1] Relevant symptoms include manifestations of inadequate cardiac output or cerebrovascular perfusion attributable to the arrhythmia, such as effort intolerance, congestive heart failure, dizziness, syncope or near syncope. Documentation of the temporal relationship between symptoms and bradycardia is essential in determining causality. The prescribing physician should also consider the overall mental, physical, and social condition of the patient, associated medical problems, availability of emergency medical care and necessity of concomitant medication which might potentially aggravate the arrhythmia in deciding whether implantation is appropriate in a particular individual.

Temporary pacemakers are frequently used when prompt resuscitation or relief of severe symptoms is necessary. They are particularly useful when the situation is likely to be self-limited, as is the case with complete heart block accompanying acute inferior myocardial infarction. Arrhythmias caused by drug toxicity, such as heart block due to digitalis or torsades de pointes due to type IA antiarrhythmic drugs, may also be amenable to stabilization with pacing during drug washout.

Temporary pacing may also be used as a diagnostic tool when the relationship between bradycardia and patient symptoms is not clear; relief of symptoms suggests a causal relationship.

Basic Principles of Pacemaker Function

Contemporary pacemaker function can be understood as the integration of its two most basic functions: myocardial stimulation (pacing) and sensing (monitoring the patient's intrinsic rhythm).

Stimulation

Stimulation of myocardium (capture) is accomplished by the application to cellular membranes of an electrical field sufficient to result in depolarization of the adjacent cells (action potential) and cell-to-cell propagation of the impulse to the remainder of the myocardium, resulting in a wide complex on the ECG. This energy is delivered as a

Table 1

Guidelines for the Implantation of Permanent Pacemakers in Adults with Bradyarrhythmias*

	Definitely Indicated	Possibly Indicated
Sinus node dysfunction	Symptomatic sinus bradycardia, sinus arrest, sinoatrial block, or asystole	Sinus node dysfunction with heart rates <40 bpm, not clearly related to symptoms
Acquired AV block	1. Intermittent or permanent complete AV block with symptoms, or with escape rate <40 bpm or periods of asystole ≥3.0 sec 2. Intermittent or permanent second degree AV block with symptomatic bradycardia 3. Atrial fibrillation, atrial flutter, or other supraventricular tachyarrhythmias with complete AV block or bradycardia unrelated to drug therapy	1. Asymptomatic complete AV block with ventricular rate ≥40 bpm 2. Asymptomatic second degree AV block at the level of the His or below
AV block associated with acute myocardial infarction	Persistent second or third degree AV block after acute myocardial infarction.	1. Persistent first degree AV block plus bundle branch block not documented prior to MI 2. Transient advanced AV block with associated bundle branch block
Bifascicular and trifascicular block	1. Bifascicular block with intermittent symptomatic complete heart block 2. Bifascicular block with intermittent symptomatic Mobitz II second degree AV block	1. Bifascicular or trifascicular block with intermittent asymptomatic Mobitz II second degree AV block 2. Bifascicular or trifascicular block with syncope of undocumented etiology 3. Pacing induced infra-His block

(continued)

Table 1 (continued)

	Definitely Indicated	Possibly Indicated
Hypersensitive carotid sinus syndrome	Recurrent syncope clearly associated with and provoked by spontaneous carotid sinus stimulation with asystole >3 seconds	Recurrent syncope without clear provocative events and with asystole >3 seconds in response to carotid sinus stimulation on exam

* Adapted from Frye, et al: Guidelines for permanent cardiac pacemaker implantation. J Am Coll Cardiol 4:434, 1984.

"square wave" pulse, usually in a fraction of a millisecond, represented on the surface ECG as a "spike" (Fig. 1). The amount of energy delivered can be adjusted by altering either the amplitude or pulse width (duration) of the stimulus. Capture threshold is the smallest stimulus that consistently results in depolarization when delivered outside of the effective refractory period of the myocardium; it can be described by a strength-duration curve (Fig. 2). Thus, capture can be optimized by increasing either pulse amplitude or pulse width, but only at the expense of accelerated battery depletion.

Capture threshold usually increases as the lead matures following implant, but stabilizes in most cases within 2–4 months (Fig. 3). Newer lead designs minimize both the acute peak and the chronic thresholds. Other conditions that may affect pacing thresholds are listed in Table 2.[2–4] Because of the frequent association between bradyarrhythmias and tachyarrhythmias, antiarrhythmic drugs are a common cause of threshold rise and may result in increased latency (interval between spike and QRS) or overt failure to capture in an established pacing system. Thus, in routine pacemaker follow-up, serial threshold testing is recommended, particularly in the first few months following implant, and with any change in antiarrhythmic therapy. Pacer output is then adjusted to a minimum, allowing for a 100% safety margin by increasing either pulse width by a factor of 3, or voltage by a factor of 2 times threshold; more generous safety margins are frequently used in the first 6–8 weeks to allow for expected threshold rise. Future generations of pacers will automatically test capture thresholds by pacing evoked response and adjusting output accordingly.

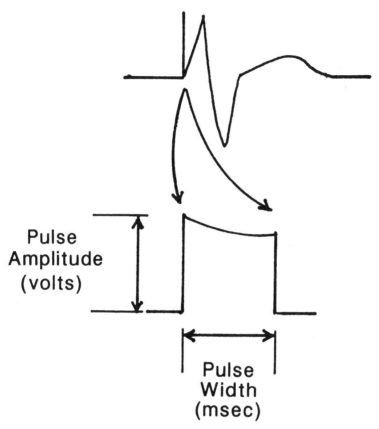

Figure 1. Representative pulse waveform for a constant voltage generator, compared to its resultant spike on the surface electrocardiogram.

Sensing

Early devices paced continually at a fixed rate independent of the patient's intrinsic rhythm. This feature resulted in competition between intrinsic and paced rhythms, as well as concern over the potential for serious tachyarrhythmias due to random pacing during the "vulnerable period." Furthermore, batteries were quickly exhausted by full-time use.

In order to promote cooperation between patient and device, and thus avoid these problems, modern pacemakers sense the intrinsic rhythm and time paced events with respect to sensed ones. Inhibition of pacer output due to sensed intrinsic complexes is the cardinal feature

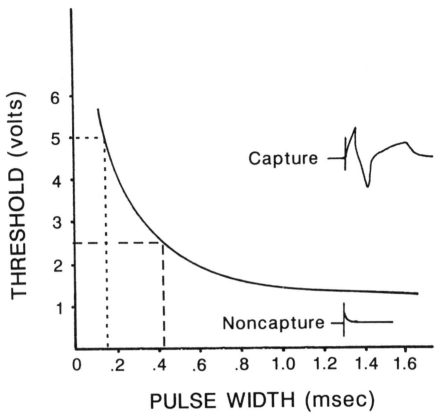

Figure 2. Strength-duration curve for a given electrode-myocardial interface. The exponential line indicates capture threshold. At 2.5 V, threshold is
0.44 ms, however, at 5.0 V, capture can be acheived with a pulse width of
only 0.15 ms in this example.

of a demand pacemaker. Sensed events may also be used to trigger
subsequent paced events; this feature is most commonly employed in
dual chambered devices in which a sensed atrial beat triggers a ventricular paced beat, thus maintaining atrioventricular (AV) synchrony.

Sensing is accomplished by monitoring the local intracardiac electrogram at the electrode-tissue interface during the patient's native
rhythm (Fig. 4). This electrogram is the potential difference between two
electrodes, both at the distal lead tip in the case of a bipolar system, and
between lead tip and pulse generator in the case of a "unipolar" system.

Table 2
Factors Potentially Affecting Capture Threshold

Increase	Decrease	No Effect
sleep	exercise	atropine
hyperkalemia	sympathetic stimuli	acetylcholine
hypoxemia	glucocorticoids	morphine
hypercarbia	isoproterenol	lidocaine
hypothyroidism	cyclopropane	tocainide
mineralocorticoids		amiodarone
parasympathetic stimuli		hypoglycemia
β-adrenergic blockers		
quinidine		
procainamide		
disopyramide		
flecainide		
verapamil		
AICD discharge		

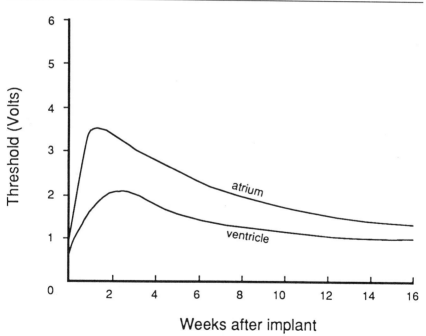

Figure 3. Expected changes in capture threshold (in volts) at a constant pulse width as the leads mature.

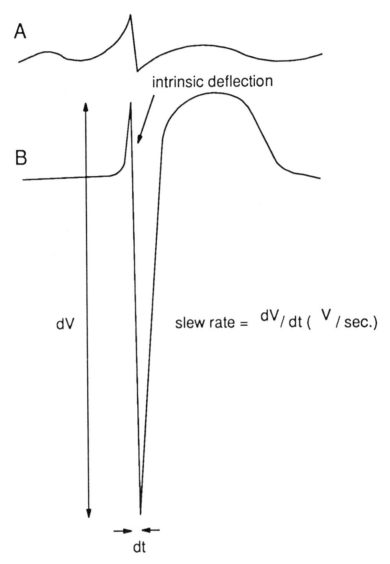

Figure 4. Acute R-wave measurement from a ventricular lead. (A) Surface electrocardiogram; (B) simultaneous intracardiac electrogram. The amplitude of the intrinsic deflection (dV) is also referred to as the R wave. The slew rate (dV/dt) is the slope of the intrinsic deflection.

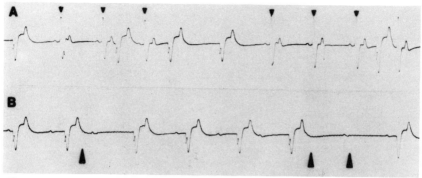

Figure 5. Sensing abnormalities in a ventricular demand pacer. (A) Undersensing. Small arrows indicate unsensed native complexes. Thus, inhibition of subsequent paced events does not occur. (B) Oversensing of myopotentials during arm exercise. Large arrows indicate the points at which myopotential noise is sensed, thus resulting in inappropriate pacer inhibition.

The amplitude of the rapid phase of the complex is commonly referred to as the "P" wave in the atrium and the "R" wave in the ventricle. Sensitivity of the pacemaker can be programmed by adjusting the number of millivolts required to register as a sensed event. Because electrical energy from other sources may also result in significant deflections, a band-pass filter is used to exclude noise and minimum slew rates (R wave slopes, dV/dt) are set to exclude T waves and far-field activity from other chambers.

Undersensing occurs when the amplitude or slew rate of the native rhythm electrogram is insufficient to meet sensing criteria (Fig. 5). Oversensing occurs when signals extrinsic to the chamber monitored are large enough to meet sensing criteria. Examples of such signals include electrograms from other chambers (crosstalk), extrinsic electromagnetic noise and skeletal muscle activity (myopotentials). Oversensing is much more likely to occur in a unipolar lead system where the sensing bipole is widely spaced across the chest, including the pectoral muscles in the field.

The Pacing System

Pulse Generators

The pulse generator consists of a power source and electronic circuitry used to time pacer output, analyze sensed events, and initiate a

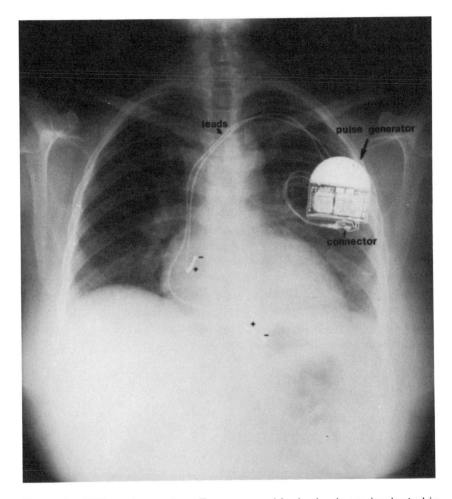

Figure 6. DDD pacing system. Transvenous bipolar leads are implanted in the right atrial appendage and right ventricular apex.

response to them (Fig. 6). When intended for permanent implantation, these elements are hermetically sealed in a titanium case with a connector for inserting the lead. Devices as small as 23 grams are now available.

Most contemporary devices use a lithium anode battery as their power source. Lithium iodide and lithium cupric sulfide are most common, and longevity with continuous use at nominal output is approximately 4–15 years. Nuclear powered devices have been used with considerably less enthusiasm. Although these may theoretically function for several decades, considerable public concern exists regarding safety from potential radiation leaks and disposal following the death of the patient. In addition, there may be a disadvantage in excessive battery life; that is, in view of rapid ongoing improvement in available technology, patients may benefit from periodic upgrading of pulse generators.

Leads

The pacing lead transmits impulses between the pulse generator and the myocardium. It is constructed of metal alloy wires insulated with either silicone or polyurethane. The electrode, usually constructed of platinum, Elgiloy, or carbon, interfaces with the myocardium. Newer designs, some incorporating steroid delivery systems in the tip, reduce the acute and chronic pacing thresholds, thus allowing the use of lower energy output and thereby improving battery longevity. Numerous lead configurations with both active and passive fixation mechanisms are available for either endocardial (transvenous) or epicardial application.

Pacing systems are available in either "unipolar" or bipolar configurations with the distal tip electrode serving as the cathode (negative) terminal in both cases. In the "unipolar" system, the titanium case of the pulse generator serves as the anode. Therefore, the electrical field through which sensing and pacing occur includes all chest tissue between the lead tip and pulse generator. In contrast, the ring anode in a bipolar system is on the lead within a couple of centimeters from the tip, creating a small electrical field. Stimulation and sensing thresholds are similar in unipolar and bipolar systems.[5,6] Although unipolar systems produce large, easily legible ECG spikes and have slightly slimmer leads, these systems are prone to uncomfortable pectoral muscle stimulation and oversensing from myopotentials and crosstalk. Bipolar systems are preferred by most experts due to the low risk of interference sensing and pocket stimulation.

Temporary Pacing Systems

Both single and dual chamber temporary transvenous pacing may be quickly established by directing leads from central veins into the right ventricular apex and/or right atrium and connecting these to an external battery-operated pulse generator. Left ventricular pacing can be accomplished by application of temporary epicardial leads at the time of thoracotomy. The duration of temporary pacing is limited by instability of lead position, predictable pacing threshold rise with time, and the risk of infection associated with an indwelling catheter.

More recently, noninvasive temporary pacing has been accomplished with external paddle-shaped electrodes applied to the chest wall. Special pulse generators capable of delivering stimuli with a pulse duration up to 20–40 ms are required to minimize chest wall discomfort. Simultaneous activation of atria and ventricles is theoretically possible and may adversely affect the hemodynamic result.

Pacing Modalities

Early pacers were designed simply to prevent asystole by ensuring a minimum ventricular rate. Although premature death was effectively prevented, many patients continued to suffer from inadequate exercise tolerance or other symptoms related to lack of an appropriate increase in heart rate with exertion and lack of AV synchrony (see section on hemodynamic considerations). As a consequence, other modes of pacing have been developed to improve the hemodynamic result. Furthermore, programmability of pacer functions and antitachycardia pacing have provided a wider selection of devices to tailor the pacer to the needs of the individual patient. A five-letter classification system for describing devices generically is shown in Table 3.[7] The first three letters are also commonly used to describe the programmed pacing mode. The first two refer to the chambers in which stimulation and sensing, respectively, are performed. The third letter indicates the response of the device to a sensed native event. Inhibition of output with resetting of timing mechanisms is the hallmark of demand pacing. A sensed event may also result in triggering of a paced event coupled to the former, as in atrial-synchronous ventricular pacing. "D" in the third position refers to the combination of atrial triggering of ventricular output and homologous inhibition with both atrial and ventricular sensing. Many possible modes exist; the most common are diagrammed in Figure 7.

Ventricular demand pacing (VVI) is extensively diagrammed in Fig. 8, which illustrates timing intervals and refractory periods. The "automatic interval" is the interval between two consecutive paced beats

Table 3
NASPE/BPEG Generic Code*

I Chamber(s) paced	II Chamber(s) sensed	III Response to sensed events	IV Programmability	V Antitachy- arrhythmia functions
O = None	O = None	O = None	O = None	O = None
A = Atrium	A = Atrium	T = Triggered	P = Rate and/or output	P = Pacing
V = Ventricle	V = Ventricle	I = Inhibited	programmable	S = Shock
D = Dual	D = Dual	D = Dual	M = Multiprogrammable	D = Dual
(A + V)	(A + V)	(T + I)	C = Communicating	(P + S)
			R = Rate modulation	

* Modified from Bernstein, et al: The NASPE/BPEG generic pacemaker code for antibradyarrhythmia and adaptive-rate pacing and antitachyarrhythmia devices. PACE 10:794, 1987.

COMMON PACING MODES

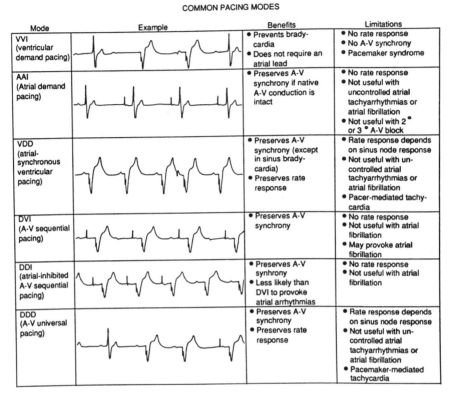

Mode	Example	Benefits	Limitations
VVI (ventricular demand pacing)		• Prevents brady-cardia • Does not require an atrial lead	• No rate response • No A-V synchrony • Pacemaker syndrome
AAI (Atrial demand pacing)		• Preserves A-V synchrony if native A-V conduction is intact	• No rate response • Not useful with uncontrolled atrial tachyarrhythmias or atrial fibrillation • Not useful with 2° or 3° A-V block
VDD (atrial-synchronous ventricular pacing)		• Preserves A-V synchrony (except in sinus brady-cardia) • Preserves rate response	• Rate response depends on sinus node response • Not useful with un-controlled atrial tachyarrhythmias or atrial fibrillation • Pacer-mediated tachy-cardia
DVI (A-V sequential pacing)		• Preserves A-V synchrony	• No rate response • Not useful with atrial fibrillation • May provoke atrial fibrillation
DDI (atrial-inhibited A-V sequential pacing)		• Preserves A-V synhrony • Less likely than DVI to provoke atrial arrhythmias	• No rate response • Not useful with atrial fibrillation
DDD (A-V universal pacing)		• Preserves A-V synchrony • Preserves rate response	• Rate response depends on sinus node response • Not useful with un-controlled atrial tachyarrhythmias or atrial fibrillation • Pacemaker-mediated tachycardia

Figure 7. Commonly used pacing modalities.

at the basic pacing rate. To calculate the automatic interval, divide 60,000 ms by the pacing rate in paces per minute (ppm), e.g.,

$$\frac{60,000 \text{ ms/min}}{70 \text{ ppm}} = 857 \text{ ms}$$

The "escape interval" is that interval between a sensed native impulse and the paced beat that follows it, providing no intervening impulses are sensed. It is the same as the automatic interval unless hysteresis, an optional feature, is used to increase the escape interval, promoting dominance of the native rhythm.

The intrinsic refractory period is the interval immediately following any impulse during which the myocardium cannot be artificially stimulated. This is a variable property of the myocardium itself which cannot

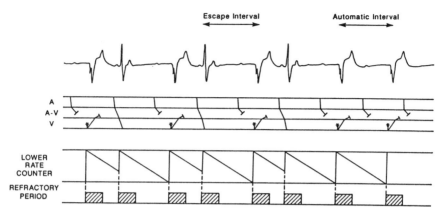

Figure 8. Representative timing diagrams for a ventricular demand (VVI) pacemaker.

be measured from the ECG, but ranges from 170 to 290 ms in normal individuals. Pacer spikes occurring during this period will not result in capture. This period should be distinguished from the pacemaker's refractory period which is the initial portion of the automatic or escape interval during which a sensed event is ignored and will not result in a pacer response. The pacer refractory period is usually programmable to a length sufficient to avoid inappropriate sensing of repolarization activity (T wave) and events in other chambers. The alert period is the remainder of the automatic interval or escape interval during which a sensed event will result in inhibition of the next stimulus and resetting of the timing mechanism.

AV universal (DDD) pacing offers the advantages of both AV synchrony and rate-responsiveness to exercise over VVI pacing, provided that the patient has normal sinus node function with an appropriate sinus tachycardia during exertion (Fig. 9). It is of limited usefulness in patients with persistent sinus bradycardia (in whom the best result will be AV sequential pacing at the lower rate limit only) and in those with uncontrolled atrial arrhythmias (in whom erratic atrial tracking rates may not accurately reflect metabolic demand).

DDD pacing requires two leads, atrial and ventricular, each of which performs the dual functions of sensing and pacing. A programmable paced AV interval is analogous to the P-R interval during sinus rhythm. Because ventricular pacing rate varies with the native atrial rate, both upper and lower rate limits are programmable. Atrial and ventricular refractory periods are usually set independently.

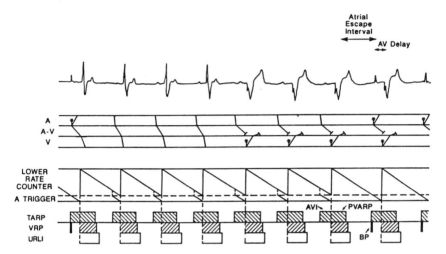

Figure 9. Representative timing diagrams for an AV universal (DDD) pacemaker.

The DDD mode combines many of the features of other types of physiological pacing. Atrial demand pacing (AAI) occurs for intrinsic atrial rates slower than the lower rate limit and ventricular pacing is triggered at the end of the AV delay if no intrinsic QRS complex intervenes (AV sequential pacing, DVI). As the intrinsic atrial rate increases above the lower rate limit, ventricular pacing is triggered, if needed, thus tracking the atrial rate up to the upper rate limit (atrial-synchronous ventricular pacing, VDD). Although atrial sensing may continue at rates above the upper rate limit, the ventricular pacing rate will not exceed that limit. Several responses are possible to sensed atrial rates above the upper rate limit: 2:1 or 3:1 block, pseudo-Wenckebach, fallback, and rate smoothing (Fig. 10).[8] The most physiological is pseudo-Wenckebach which mimics the natural response, maintaining both high ventricular rates and some degree of atrioventricular synchrony. The maximum sensed atrial rate that can be tracked during pseudo-Wenckebach behavior is determined by the total atrial refractory period (AV interval + post-ventricular atrial refractory period). At atrial rates between the upper rate limit and the maximum sensed atrial rate, the ventricular paced rate will remain near the upper rate limit. At rates exceeding the maximum sensed atrial rate, however, 2:1 or higher AV block will occur, dramatically and abruptly lowering the ventricular paced rate.

Not all patients benefit from the rate-responsive features of dual

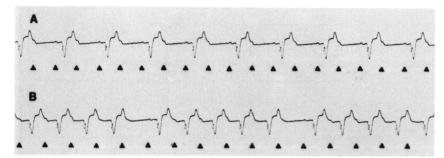

Figure 10. Examples of upper rate limit behavior in a DDD pacer. (A) 2:1 AV conduction, and (B) pseudo-Wenckebach with 6:5 AV conduction.

chamber pacing in which the intrinsic sinus or atrial rate is used as the index of metabolic need during exertion. Since that may not be an accurate indication in patients with arrhythmias, other sensing mechanisms have been sought to govern pacing rates in response to exertion (Table 4). Several such devices are now available for single chamber rate-responsive pacing (VVI-R or AAI-R) and dual chamber sensor-driven pacers are undergoing clinical investigation. Future generators may employ more than one sensor to more accurately assess metabolic need. The response of a VVI-R pacer to exertion is shown in Figure 11. Programmable parameters include lower and upper rate limits, threshold for rate change, and rate of rate change.

Table 4
Biosensors

* Atrial rate
* Mechanical vibration
* Core blood temperature
* Minute ventilation
  Mixed venous O_2 saturation
  QT interval
  Venous pH
  Stroke volume
  Right ventricular dP/dt
  Right atrial pressure
  Pacing evoked response

* Currently approved and available in U.S.

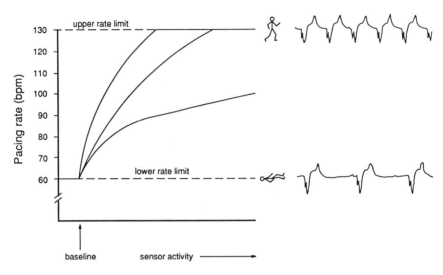

Figure 11. Rate-response to exercise in a sensor-driven pacemaker.

Magnet Function

Application of a strong magnet to the patient's chest overlying the pulse generator is a useful diagnostic maneuver for checking pacemaker function. The magnet activates a reed switch in the generator that usually turns off sensing temporarily, thus turning a demand or triggered unit into a fixed rate, asynchronous pacer (Fig. 12). Each device has a

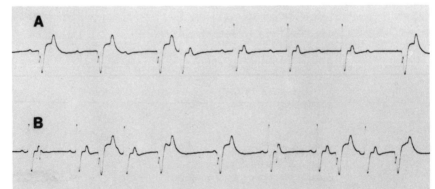

Figure 12. Magnet response in a VVI pacer. (A) Demand function. (B) Application of magnet results in temporary asynchronous pacing. Spikes occurring in the native ventricular refractory period do not result in capture.

characteristic response and magnet rate, which may change as the battery is depleted, thus serving as an indicator of impending end-of-battery-life so that elective replacement can be scheduled. Magnet application is also particularly useful for verification of capture in a demand pacer when the patient's intrinsic rate is high enough to inhibit pacing and also for determining the mode of pacing in an unknown device. Some devices have an automatic capture threshold test built into the magnet response.

Hemodynamic Considerations

The Pacemaker Syndrome

Although ventricular demand pacemakers effectively prevent bradycardia, up to 20% of patients continue to experience symptoms following implantation.[9] A pacemaker syndrome has been described that may consist of fatigue, dizziness, dyspnea, palpitations, syncope, hypotension, or uncomfortable jugular venous pulsations. Pathophysiological factors that contribute to the development of the syndrome are listed in Table 5. The atrial contribution to ventricular filling and cardiac output is at least 10% in patients with normal hearts;[10,11] in this group, intact retrograde VA conduction and lack of rate-responsiveness to exertion are primarily responsible for symptoms. In patients with diastolic or systolic ventricular dysfunction, however, the atrial contribution to ventricular filling is even more significant, and therefore the loss of atrioventricular synchrony is the major adverse factor.[12-15] Thus, patients with ventricular hypertrophy or congestive heart failure are particularly susceptible to pacemaker syndrome, as shown in Table 6. There is evidence that the syndrome is associated with excessive levels of atrial

---

Table 5
Factors Contributing to the Development
of Pacemaker Syndrome

- Fixed pacing rate
- Loss of atrioventricular synchrony
- Retrograde ventriculoatrial conduction
- Mitral or tricuspid regurgitation
- Atrial natriuretic peptide

Table 6
Clinical Conditions Predisposing to the
Development of Pacemaker Syndrome

- Active lifestyle
- Ventricular hypertrophy
- Congestive heart failure
- Intact retrograde ventriculoatrial conduction

natriuretic peptide which may be responsible for the hypotensive response.

Mild symptoms of pacemaker syndrome may be managed by reprogramming to minimize the percentage of beats paced. This can be accomplished by decreasing the programmed rate or adding hysteresis to permit emergence of the native rhythm in patients who are not pacer-dependent.

Pacemaker Prescription

Several modes of pacing offer a more favorable hemodynamic response than does VVI pacing; however, potential disadvantages still exist, particularly for those with inappropriate sinus bradycardia, atrial fibrillation, and other uncontrolled atrial arrhythmias (Table 7). Pacer prescription, then, should be tailored to the particular hemodynamic and electrophysiological needs of the individual patient. If further documentation of the potential for development of the syndrome is necessary, the hemodynamic response to temporary atrial, ventricular, and atrioventricular sequential pacing can be compared while monitoring blood pressure, pulmonary capillary wedge pressure, and cardiac output (Fig. 13). Alternatively, cardiac output can be monitored noninvasively with Doppler studies.[16] The reliability of sinus response to exertion can be tested preoperatively with treadmill exercise.

Figure 14 shows a scheme for pacemaker prescription. AAI pacing is inappropriate in patients with any evidence of AV node or His-Purkinje dysfunction. Active patients with normal ventricles should be considered candidates for sensor-driven rate-responsive ventricular pacemakers, particularly if co-existing atrial tachyarrhythmias are uncontrolled. Those with pure sinus node bradyarrhythmias may be particularly helped by AAI-R pacing.[17] Those with abnormal hearts are

Table 7
Hemodynamic Effects of Pacing Modes

Mode	Preserves AV Synchrony?	Rate-Response to Exercise?	Rate-Response Accurate in Presence of Atrial Arrhythmias?
VVI	no	no	N/A
AAI	yes*	yes**	no
DVI	yes	no	N/A
DDI	yes	no	N/A
VDD	yes***	yes**	no
DDD	yes	yes**	no
VVI-R	no	yes	yes
DDD-R	yes	yes	???

N/A = not applicable.
* only if AV conduction is preserved.
** only if sinus response to exertion preserved.
*** unless sinus bradycardia present.

most likely to benefit from DDD pacing, although sinus bradycardia and other atrial arrhythmias limit their usefulness. The presence of intact ventriculoatrial conduction should also be considered an indication for dual chambered pacing, now that fully programmable atrial refractory periods have minimized the risk of pacemaker-mediated tachycardia due to 1:1 retrograde conduction. Patients with severe neural-reflex-me-

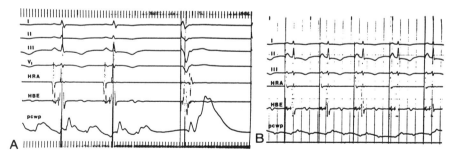

Figure 13. Hemodynamic monitoring in a patient with pacemaker syndrome. (A) VVI pacing results in retrograde VA conduction and a large cannon V wave in the left atrium, as demonstrated in the pulmonary capillary wedge pressure tracing. (B) AAI pacing in the same patient results in normalization of intracardiac pressures.

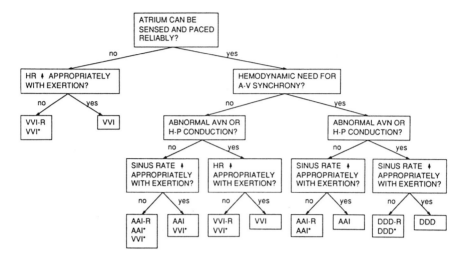

* very sedentary lifestyle or simplicity needed

Figure 14. Decision tree for pacemaker prescription. Reliable atrial pacing and sensing will not be possible in patients with atrial fibrillation or other significant uncontrolled atrial tachyarrhythmias. See text for factors determining hemodynamic need for AV synchrony.

diated syncope, such as carotid sinus syncope or vasodepressor syncope, may continue to experience milder symptoms after implant of a VVI pacer due to the concomitant vasodepressor reaction which accompanies bradycardia. Dual chamber pacing may minimize these symptoms.[18] Sensor-driven dual chamber devices are undergoing clinical trials; however, their performance in the presence of atrial tachyarrhythmias is unproven.

Pacemaker Follow-Up

Performance Monitoring

Following implantation of a permanent pacemaker, continuing surveillance is recommended to ensure optimum performance of the device, tailor its function to suit the needs of the individual, maximize battery longevity, and identify elective replacement indicators. With fully programmable devices, most malfunctions can be identified early and cor-

Table 8
Medicare Guidelines for Frequency
of Pacemaker Clinic Visits

Single-chamber devices
- 1st 6 months—twice
- Thereafter—once every 12 months

Dual-chamber devices
- 1st 6 months—twice
- Thereafter—once every 6 months

rected with noninvasive programming, thus obviating the need for operative revision in many cases.

Pacemaker clinic visits and transtelephonic monitoring are considered complementary procedures. In clinic, extensive testing can be performed, including physical exam, waveform analysis, interrogation of telemetry, detection of underlying native rhythm, magnet testing, pacing and sensing thresholds, and physical maneuvers to ensure lead stability.[19,20] Due to the rise and fall of capture thresholds as the lead matures (see Fig. 3), they should be checked frequently in the first few months following implant and after any change in medical therapy which might affect threshold. The output of the device can then be adjusted to minimize battery depletion while still maintaining an adequate capture safety margin.

Between clinic visits, pacers can be monitored transtelephonically by transmitting the ECG in demand and magnet modes. Although programming cannot be performed, some devices are capable of transmitting telemetry information which is useful in assessing battery status. The current Medicare guidelines for frequency of follow-up are described in Tables 8 and 9.[21] More frequent follow-up may be indicated if a problem is identified, or as elective replacement time nears, or if an advisory is issued regarding the generator or lead. More frequent monitoring may also be advisable in pacemaker-dependent patients.

Safety Considerations

Many patients ask if they will have to give up their microwave ovens after receiving pacemakers. In fact, modern pacers are not affected by

Table 9

Medicare Guidelines for Frequency of Transtelephonic Surveillance

Guideline I (<5 year clinical longevity)	Guideline II* (>5 year clinical longevity)
Single-chamber devices • 1st month—every 2 weeks • 2–36 months—every 8 weeks • Thereafter—every 4 weeks	Single-chamber devices • 1st month—every 2 weeks • 2–48 months—every 12 weeks • 49–72 months—every 8 weeks • Thereafter—every 4 weeks
Dual-chamber devices • 1st month—every 2 weeks • 2–6 months—every 4 weeks • 7–36 months—every 8 weeks • Thereafter—every 4 weeks	Dual-chamber devices • 1st month—every 2 weeks • 2–30 months—every 12 weeks • 31–48 months—every 8 weeks • Thereafter—every 4 weeks

* 5-year clinical longevity data exist for both pulse generator and leads.

Table 10

Potential Sources of Interference and Pacemaker Damage

Low Risk	Use with Precautions	Avoid
microwave ovens weapon detectors police radar	electrocautery cardioversion/ defibrillation AICD lithotripsy diathermal therapy therapeutic ionizing radiation electroconvulsive therapy welders jackhammers	magnetic resonance imaging betatron radiation hyperthermia

well-insulated ovens in normal use; however, many other potential sources of electromagnetic and environmental interference exist that may temporarily or permanently affect pacer function. A few potential sources of interference or damage are described in Table 10. To counter this risk, modern pacers have elaborate interference protection circuits. As a precaution, the distance between generator and interference source should be maximized, at least 5 inches from electrocautery, lithotripsy fields, and defibrillator paddles. Pacemaker-dependent patients may be programmed to a triggered (VVT) or asynchronous (VOO) mode or placed in magnet mode temporarily to protect against asystole due to oversensing when subjected to sources of potential interference.

References

1. Frye RL, Collins JJ, DeSanctis RW, et al: Guidelines for permanent cardiac pacemaker implantation, May 1984. J Am Coll Cardiol 4:434, 1984.
2. Huang SK, Hedberg PS, Marcus FI: Effects of antiarrhythmic drugs on the chronic pacing threshold and the endocardial R wave amplitude in the conscious dog. PACE 9:660, 1986.
3. Hellestrand KJ, Burnett PJ, Milne JR, et al: Effect of the antiarrhythmic agent flecainide acetate on acute and chronic pacing thresholds. PACE 6:892, 1983.
4. Nielsen AP, Griffin JC, Herre JM, et al: Effect of amiodarone on acute and chronic pacing thresholds. PACE 7:462, 1984.
5. Breivik K, Ohm O, Engedal H: Long-term comparison of unipolar and bipolar pacing and sensing, using a new multiprogrammable pacemaker system. PACE 6:592, 1983.
6. DeCaprio V, Hurzeler P, Furman S: A comparison of unipolar and bipolar electrograms for cardiac pacemaker sensing. Circulation 56:750, 1977.
7. Bernstein AD, Camm AJ, Fletcher RD, et al: The NASPE/BPEG generic pacemaker code for antibradyarrhythmia and adaptive-rate pacing and antitachyarrhythmia devices. PACE 10:794, 1987.
8. Papp MA, Mason T, Gallastegui J: Use of rate smoothing to treat pacemaker-mediated tachycardias and symptoms due to upper rate response of a DDD pacemaker. Clin Prog Pacing Electrophysiol 2:547, 1984.
9. Nishimura RA, Gersch BJ, Vlietstra RE, et al: Hemodynamic and symptomatic consequences of ventricular pacing. PACE 5:903, 1982.
10. Samet P, Bernstein WH, Nathan DA, et al: Atrial contribution to cardiac output in complete heart block. Am J Cardiol 16:1, 1965.
11. Samet P, Castillo C, Bernstein WH: Hemodynamic consequences of sequential atrioventricular pacing: Subjects with normal hearts. Am J Cardiol 21:207, 1968.
12. Benchimol A, Ellis JG, Dimond EG: Hemodynamic consequences of atrial and ventricular pacing in patients with normal and abnormal hearts. Am J Med 39:911, 1965.
13. Samet P, Castillo C, Bernstein WH: Hemodynamic sequelae of atrial, ven-

tricular and sequential atrioventricular pacing in cardiac patients. Am Heart J 72:725, 1966.

14. Kruse T, Arnman K, Conradson TB, et al: A comparison of the acute and long-term hemodynamic effects of ventricular inhibited and atrial synchronous ventricular inhibited pacing. Circulation 65:846, 1982.

15. Wish M, Fletcher RD, Cohen A: Hemodynamics of AV synchrony and rate. J Electrophysiol 3:170, 1989.

16. Stewart WJ, Dicola VC, Harthorne JW, et al: Doppler ultrasound measurement of cardiac output in patients with physiologic pacemakers. Am J Cardiol 54:308, 1984.

17. Rosenqvist M, Obel IWP: Atrial pacing and the risk for AV block: Is there a time for change in attitude? PACE 12:97, 1989.

18. Morley CA, Perrins EJ, Grant P, et al: Carotid sinus syncope treated by pacing: Analysis of persistent symptoms and role of atrioventricular sequential pacing. Br Heart J 47:411, 1982.

19. Griffin JC, Schuenemeyer TD: Pacemaker follow-up: AR introduction and overview. Clin Prog Pacing Electrophysiol 1:30, 1983.

20. Luceri RM, Hayes DL: Follow-up of DDD pacemakers. PACE 7: 1187, 1984.

21. U.S. Government Printing Office: Medicare Carriers Manual, Transmittal No. 1051, 1984.

Chapter 18

Cardiac Pacing II: Treatment of Tachyarrhythmias

Anne Hamilton Dougherty
and Gerald V. Naccarelli

Introduction

Antitachycardia devices may be designed for accomplishing any of the following strategies in managing tachyarrhythmias: prevention of arrhythmia initiation, palliation of symptoms related to arrhythmias, or termination of arrhythmia in the event of spontaneous recurrence. Most devices in current use are designed for the latter.

Overdrive pacing at a rate exceeding the sinus rate is particularly useful in suppressing arrhythmias that are bradycardia- or pause-dependent, such as torsades de pointes (Fig. 1). It may be employed on a temporary basis when the cause is reversible, as is the case in drug-induced torsades de pointes associated with antiarrhythmic or neuroleptic medications. Permanent pacemakers may be implanted for long-term arrhythmia suppression if the underlying cause is not reversible. Usually, a single-chamber atrial or ventricular demand pacer is used and programmed empirically to a rate sufficient to suppress the tachycardia. Dual chamber pacing can also be useful in maintaining atrioventricular (AV) synchrony, thus preventing many reciprocating supraventricular arrhythmias whose initiation is dependent on AV conduction delay. In

From Naccarelli GV (ed): *Cardiac Arrhythmias: A Practical Approach.* Mount Kisco, NY, Futura Publishing Co., Inc., © 1991.

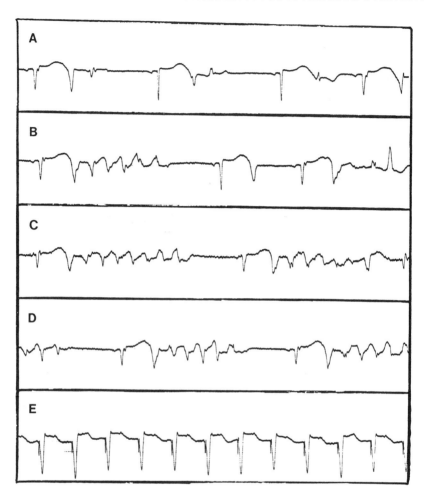

Figure 1. Pause-dependent polymorphic VT associated with QT prolongation (torsades de pointes) appears in panels A–D. Note dramatic increase in QT interval following pauses. Temporary overdrive ventricular pacing at a rate of 90 ppm suppresses the tachycardia in panel E.

an animal model, trains of subthreshold conditioning stimuli have also been used experimentally to suppress ventricular arrhythmias by lengthening the effective refractory period.[1] This technique may prove useful in preventing arrhythmias in the future. Rarely, pacemakers have been used to modify the hemodynamics of a tachyarrhythmia such that symptoms are improved without reversing the arrhythmia itself. An example of this phenomenon would be the use of rapid atrial pacing during atrial flutter or ectopic atrial tachycardia to achieve higher degrees of AV block, thus lowering the ventricular response. One-to-one ventricular conduction during atrial flutter can thus be converted to a more moderate 2:1 or 4:1 AV conduction by rapid atrial pacing at rates producing AV nodal refractoriness. Similarly, symptoms of ventricular tachycardia (VT) can occasionally be improved by rapid atrial pacing during ventricular tachycardia to maintain AV synchrony. Obviously, however, palliation is inadequate for most patients and definitive therapy is usually desirable.

Most commonly, devices have been used to terminate arrhythmias once they have occurred with either pacing or delivery of shock. Patients must be cautioned that devices of this nature do not themselves reduce the frequency of tachyarrhythmia, but can only alter the duration. Thus, symptoms including syncope may occur before the arrhythmia is actually converted. The remainder of this chapter will deal with devices designed for this purpose.

Antitachycardia Pacing

Reciprocating supraventricular and ventricular tachycardias can be induced and terminated in the invasive electrophysiology laboratory by introducing premature atrial or ventricular stimuli at critical times in the cardiac cycle (Fig. 2). The electrophysiological phenomena that are necessary to sustain such a re-entrant arrhythmia are conduction delay and unidirectional block.[2] Any two potential conduction pathways, longitudinally dissociated, with different electrophysiological properties existing between two points in the heart form the substrate for re-entry.

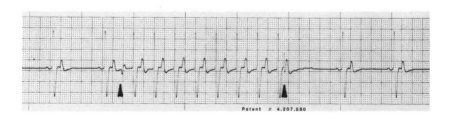

Figure 2. Arrhythmia induction with electrophysiologic testing. SVT is initiated with a single premature atrial stimulus (first arrow). The tachycardia is terminated with another atrial stimulus which is too premature to be conducted through the AV node (second arrow).

The classic example of a re-entrant arrhythmia is AV nodal re-entry tachycardia, the usual form of paroxysmal supraventricular tachycardia (SVT) in which the re-entry circuit consists of two sets of fibers within the AV junction, a fast pathway and a slow pathway, less refractory to premature stimuli than the first (Fig. 3). Premature impulses that arrive during the refractory period of the fast pathway, but beyond refractoriness of the slow one, result in unidirectional block and a detour of the impulse with conduction delay over the slow pathway. The antegrade conduction delay may be sufficient to allow the impulse to "echo" back over the no-longer-refractory "fast" limb in a retrograde manner. When the premature impulses are properly timed, the reciprocating arrhythmia can be sustained.

Similarly, the arrhythmia can be terminated by pacing stimuli timed

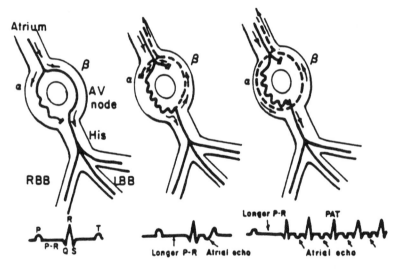

Figure 3. Mechanism of SVT due to re-entry within the AV node. The AV node consists of a slow (β) pathway and a fast (α) pathway, both of which are capable of either antegrade or retrograde conduction. The left panel shows predominant conduction over β during sinus rhythm. A premature atrial impulse (center panel) results in unidirectional block in B, shifting antegrade conduction to the α pathway, and resulting in lengthening of the P-R interval and an atrial echo beat from retrograde conduction over the β pathway which is no longer refractory. One the right, a premature atrial impulse initiates SVT. PAT = paroxysmal SVT; RBB = right bundle branch; LBB = left bundle branch. (Reproduced with permission from Josephson ME, Kastor JA: Supraventricular tachycardia: mechanisms and management. Ann Intern Med 87:350, 1977.)

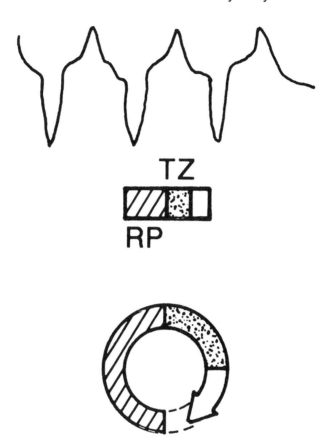

Figure 4. The termination zone (TZ) of a reciprocating tachycardia immediately follows the end of the refractory period (RP). Delivery of a premature
stimulus during this time may result in termination of the arrhythmia.

to arrive at the re-entrant circuit immediately after the refractory period
in the advancing wavefront of activation (Fig. 4). This period is called
the termination zone, or excitable gap. These principles may be applied
to the chronic treatment of any spontaneously occurring re-entrant arrhythmia, including paroxysmal SVT associated with AV nodal re-entry
or AV re-entry due to an overt or concealed accessory AV connection
in the Wolff-Parkinson-White syndrome, as well as the more rare intra-
atrial re-entrant tachycardias. Atrial flutter and sustained monomorphic
VT may also be amenable to pacing termination. Antitachycardia pacing

is not effective, however, for arrhythmias associated with abnormalities of automaticity or for fibrillation.

Slow, well-tolerated arrhythmias, which tend to have longer termination zones, are the most suitable substrates for pacing termination. Techniques that have been used include single and paired extrastimuli, bursts, and trains of extrastimuli (Fig. 5). Unfortunately, however, no technique is universally effective and any technique can actually accelerate the tachycardia or result in fibrillation in the chamber stimulated, thus potentially turning a relatively stable tachycardia into a disastrous one (Fig. 6). Bursts and trains of stimuli which tend to be the most effective also carry the highest risk of acceleration and fibrillation.[3] Overall, the success of pacing depends on the size and location of the tachycardia circuit, electrophysiological properties of intervening tissue, and tachycardia rate, as well as type of stimulation. Patients who have spontaneously varying tachycardia rates or several morphologies may need different termination algorithms for different tachycardias.

One of the most difficult problems in antitachycardia pacing has been the reliability of automatic tachycardia recognition algorithms. Those systems that rely solely on heart rate to discriminate between

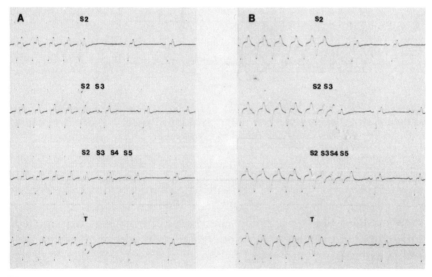

Figure 5. Techniques for tachycardia termination. (A) Atrial pacing for SVT; single extrastimulus (S_2), double extrastimuli (S_2 S_3), burst stimuli ($S_2S_3S_4S_5$) and ultra-rapid trains of stimuli (T). (B) Similar ventricular pacing techniques for VT.

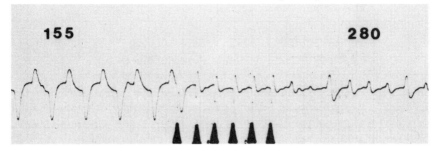

Figure 6. Acceleration of VT with termination attempts. Burst pacing (arrows) accelerates a monomorphic tachycardia from 155 bpm to 280 bpm.

sinus rhythm and tachycardia are most unreliable, particularly in active patients who may have frequent episodes of sinus tachycardia and in those patients susceptible to paroxysmal atrial fibrillation with rapid ventricular response, a rhythm that is not pacing-terminable. Overlap between sinus rates and tachycardia rates frequently occurs. Furthermore, many patients have a wide range of tachycardia rates on various occasions which makes any single recognition criterion inaccurate. To avoid this issue, manually activated devices may be used when the patient detects symptoms of tachycardia. This application is useful only if the patient is reliable and remains conscious and hemodynamically stable during the tachycardia. For automatic tachycardia recognition, suddenness of onset, beat-to-beat rate stability, and duration of tachycardia may be useful parameters in addition to high rate criteria.[4] Future devices may also be capable of analyzing the presence or absence of AV synchrony, myocardial activation sequence, and hemodynamic parameters to assist in tachycardia recognition.

Candidates must be carefully screened for suitability prior to implantation of a permanent device. A complete preoperative electrophysiological study is necessary to (1) confirm the mechanism of the arrhythmia, (2) determine both the safety and the efficacy of pacing termination techniques, and (3) evaluate the potential for concomitant arrhythmias and conduction aberrations that might require bradycardia backup pacing or concomitant defibrillator therapy. Additional maneuvers, such as exercise testing, isoproterenol infusion, and antiarrhythmic pharmacotherapy may be administered to confirm the effectiveness of detection and termination algorithms under these conditions.

Postoperative evaluation is also necessary to insure appropriateness of programming prior to discharge. Frequent post-discharge evaluation and adjustment of settings may also be necessary in some patients, particularly if concomitant anti-arrhythmic medication is prescribed or changed, thus potentially changing tachycardia rate, efficacy of termination, and pacing thresholds. Some devices allow noninvasive programmed stimulation to re-induce the tachycardia under various conditions and provide information for immediate reprogramming, if necessary. If inappropriate discharges occur during sinus tachycardia or paroxysmal atrial fibrillation, the heart rate may be suppressed with beta-adrenergic blockers, digoxin, or calcium blockers to avoid overlap with tachycardia rates.

Thus, antitachycardia pacing can be effective in patients with recurrent sustained reciprocating tachycardias associated with relative hemodynamic stability. The patient must be able to endure the initial symptoms until the tachycardia is terminated. Ideally, the tachycardia should have a distinctly abrupt onset and a rate easily distinguishable from sinus tachycardia for optimum tachycardia detection. Patients with incessant arrhythmias and those with concomitant fibrillation are not well suited for this treatment modality. Because of the risk of tachycardia acceleration and fibrillation with termination attempts, it is not usually used for treatment of VT without concomitant automatic implantable cardioverter defibrillator (AICD) implantation as backup. It is, however, a particularly useful alternative to drug therapy for young women desiring pregnancy when an ablative procedure is inappropriate or refused. Extensive preoperative screening to confirm safety and efficacy of pacing therapy is essential and close postoperative follow-up and reprogramming is necessary to insure effective operation.

Implantable Cardioverters and Defibrillators

Over 400,000 people suffer from sudden cardiopulmonary arrest each year in the United States. Of these, about one out of four are resuscitated and survive. The risk of recurrent arrest in these patients, however, is almost 50% over the next 2 years.[5-7] Those with impaired ventricular function and those in whom antiarrhythmic therapy fails to suppress arrhythmic inducibility with electrophysiological testing are particularly susceptible to recurrence.

The usefulness of shock therapy for resuscitation of these patients with ventricular fibrillation and tachycardia has been established for several decades. The principle upon which it is based is the delivery of an overwhelming amount of energy sufficient to depolarize the entire mass of myocardium in a synchronous fashion, thus allowing the re-emergence of a controlling sinus rhythm. Delivery of the shock within a few seconds of the onset of arrhythmia can also minimize the hypoxic and encephalopathic changes associated with cardiopulmonary arrest. Unfortunately, however, most arrests do not occur within immediate reach of high-level medical attention. In 1980, Mirowski and associates made available for human use an implantable device, the automatic implantable cardioverter defibrillator capable of detecting ventricular arrhythmias and delivering a 25–30 joule shock directly to the heart within 40 seconds of onset in ambulatory patients (Fig. 7). This revolutionary device has now been implanted in over 6000 patients and the improvement in survival has been clearly demonstrated (Fig. 8).[8–13] The rate of sudden death compares favorably to even those observed with surgical ablation of VT and successful medical therapy as determined by suppression of inducibility with invasive electrophysiological testing.

It is currently indicated in patients who have suffered at least one episode of cardiac arrest due to ventricular tachycardia or fibrillation not associated with an acute myocardial infarction. It has also been used in patients with recurrent sustained VT associated with syncope. Infrequency of recurrences and relative freedom from nonsustained VT and rapid supraventricular arrhythmias are desirable in order to minimize patient discomfort and preserve battery life for use in only the more serious arrhythmias.

The device is diagrammed in Figure 9. It consists of a large generator

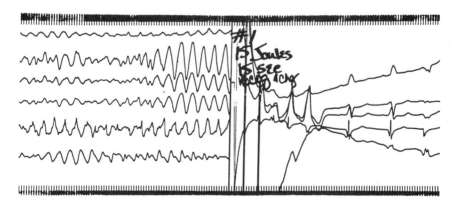

Figure 7. Intraoperative defibrillation threshold testing at AICD implantation. The upper four tracings are surface ECG leads. The lowermost two are epicardial ventricular electrograms. Ventricular fibrillation is induced at left; delivery of 15 joules terminates the arrhythmia within 15 seconds of device activation.

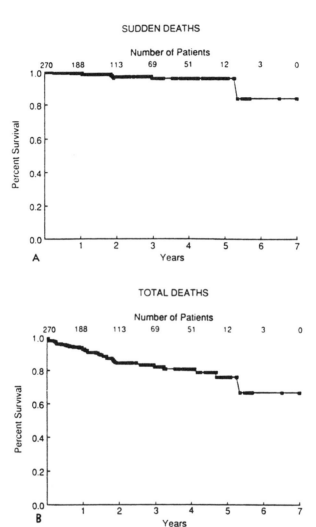

Figure 8. Actuarial analysis of survival after implantation AICD (Kaplan-Meier method). (A) Freedom from sudden death; (B) freedom from all death, including operative mortality. (Reproduced with permission from Winkle RA, Mead RH, Ruder MA, et al: Long-term outcome with the automatic implantable cardioverter-defibrillator. J Am Coll Cardiol 13:1359, 1989.)

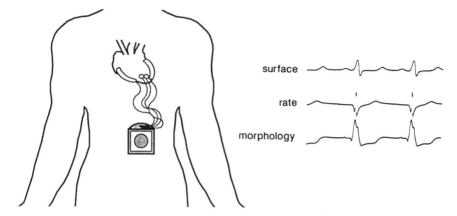

surface

rate

morphology

Figure 9. Diagram of AICD system. The generator is implanted in the abdominal wall and connected to two epicardial wire mesh patches which also sense morphology of the electrogram and to bipolar rate-sensing epicardial leads. Representative electrograms are shown at right.

(250–290 grams) implanted in the abdominal wall, connected to rate- and morphology-sensing epicardial leads and to energy-delivering electrodes. The most commonly used electrode configuration is a set of two wire mesh patches sutured to the epicardium, although a large intracardiac lead may be substituted for one of the patches. This configuration requires thoracotomy with intraoperative determination of defibrillation threshold.[14–16] In patients who are poor candidates for thoracotomy, extrathoracic subcutaneous patches have been successfully used in combination with transvenous electrodes in a few patients. Complete transvenous lead systems are also being developed, which may reduce operative morbidity and mortality substantially.

Sophisticated preoperative electrophysiological testing is necessary to optimally prescribe the device appropriate for an individual patient, particularly when nonprogrammable units are used. Tachycardia detection methods in current devices are crude when compared to those in modern antitachycardia pacers. High heart rate is the main criterion for detection and, until recently, the rate cut-off distinguishing normal rhythm from ventricular tachycardia was pre-set in the factory and not programmable thereafter. A second criterion for tachycardia detection, probability density function, has not proven to be very reliable. This feature analyzes the shape of the epicardial electrogram at the patches in an effort to detect arrhythmias of ventricular origin.

Despite their undeniable success in improving mortality, these devices are not without aggravating side effects. Operative morbidity, including wound infection, has been relatively high, presumably due to the large volume of implanted hardware. Problems in accurate tachycardia detection have also been relatively frequent, including failure to detect VT, as well as inappropriate discharge in the absence of VT. Postcardioversion arrhythmias and pacemaker-defibrillator interactions have also presented special problems.

Failure to detect VT may result from discrepancy between rate cutoff and actual tachycardia rate, undersensing of rate, narrow QRS morphology during tachycardia (when probability density function is used), or component failure. Thus, discharge might fail to occur in an episode of tachycardia one beat per minute slower than the rate cut-off (Fig. 10). Patients requiring concomitant postoperative anti-arrhythmic therapy that may slow the tachycardia rate are particularly susceptible to this problem. Failure to detect arrhythmia has also occurred when continued pacemaker spikes (due to unsensed VT or fibrillation) resulted in underestimation of heart rate by the AICD.

Similarly, inappropriate and uncomfortable discharges may occur during sinus tachycardia, paroxysmal atrial fibrillation, or any other rhythm exceeding the rate cut-off. Suppression of underlying heart rate with beta-adrenergic blockers, digoxin, or calcium antagonists may reduce the overlap with VT rates. Because the capacitors are committed to discharging once the tachycardia has been detected, but the energy delivery is delayed, episodes of nonsustained VT may trigger a discharge

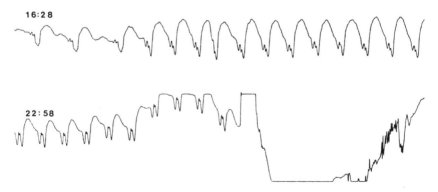

Figure 10. Holter monitor recording showing onset of slow VT (114 bpm) at 16:28. Tachycardia rate gradually accelerated to 140 bpm, finally triggering AICD discharge 6½ hours later.

several seconds later during normal sinus rhythm. Newer devices now available or undergoing investigation have programmable rate cut-offs and/or reconfirmation of arrhythmia presence prior to discharge that may minimize these nuisances.

Many patients experience significant post-cardioversion bradycardia; others have concomitant sinus node or His-Purkinje system disease requiring pacemakers for treatment of chronic bradycardia.[19,20] The combination of AICD and pacemaker presents special logistical problems. Transient pacer malfunction may follow AICD discharge, including undersensing and noncapture, which may persist up to 45 seconds. Double counting of pacer spike and QRS complex by the rate-sensing lead of the AICD can trigger an inappropriate discharge if the true heart rate is over one-half of the tachycardia rate cut-off of the device. This is particularly a problem in dual chambered devices when two pacer spikes may be detected and in any rate-responsive device in which faster paced rates are common (Fig. 11). The use of closely spaced bipolar lead configurations and maximizing the distance between electrode pairs and patches at the time of implant has helped prevent these problems.

Antitachycardia pacemakers have been used in combination with AICD for tachycardias amenable to pacing termination, thus providing relatively painless termination of slower tachycardias with backup defibrillation in the event of VT acceleration, fibrillation, or failure to convert. Extraordinary care must be taken to ensure cooperation rather than competition between the two devices.

The basic AICD now available provides approximately 100 discharges; however, battery life is highly variable. Newer devices may provide 3–5 years of use. Impending battery depletion may be detected by following capacitor charge times using serial magnet tests. This procedure is considerably less cumbersome with the new programmable units. Patients are followed at monthly or bimonthly intervals to plan elective replacement. They should be counseled to avoid strong magnetic fields that may interfere with AICD function and even disable the device.

Psychosocial factors must be considered in the rehabilitation of the AICD patient. If the arrhythmia does not result in rapid loss of consciousness prior to discharge, defibrillation is usually quite painful and may occur with little warning. Because of the potential for loss of consciousness, most agree that patients should be prohibited from driving, at least until device performance and hemodynamic consequences have been established for that individual over the course of 1–2 years.

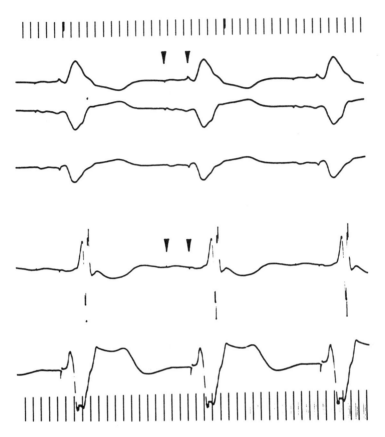

Figure 11. Intraoperative recordings from rate-sensing leads (line 4) and morphology leads (line 5) during bipolar AV sequential pacing. The distance between electrode pairs should be maximized in order to avoid sensing of pacer spikes (arrows) by the AICD.

The Ideal Antitachycardia Device

As outlined above, both antitachycardia pacemakers and AICD currently available have significant limitations. Future generations are being designed to overcome these problems. Integrated systems that combine antitachycardia pacing with backup bradycardia pacing and cardioversion-defibrillation may provide the most versatile and comfortable treatment while ensuring effective management. Features desirable in such a device are listed in Table 1. Miniaturization of circuits and particularly

Table 1

Characteristics of an Ideal Antitachycardia Device

- Flexibility in tachycardia recognition, including hemodynamic parameters
- Flexible and adaptive tachycardia termination algorithms
- Backup manual activation
- Backup bradycardia pacing
- Backup cardioversion or defibrillation
- Temporary noninvasive programmed stimulation
- Interrogation of activity
- Memory for detected events and effective termination sequences
- Programmability of output and sensitivity
- Small generator size
- Non-thoracotomy lead systems

of defibrillating capacitors and batteries will help to reduce surgical morbidity and facilitate the development of total transvenous implant techniques. Availability of such a safe but effective device would greatly expand the indication for its use. Implantation could be considered in high-risk patients prior to the occurrence of a potentially lethal arrhythmia.

Economic Considerations

Antitachycardia pacemakers and AICD devices are justifiably criticized for their expense. Initial AICD implant expenses average over $50,000 per patient. Particularly at a time when Medicare reimbursement for treatment of the most malignant arrhythmias is ridiculously meager, this form of treatment may seem extravagant to some. On the other hand, early use of this device may compare favorably to the expense of serial drug trials, especially when serial electrophysiological testing and prolonged or repeated hospitalizations are necessary to achieve reasonable arrhythmia control. The economic consequences of improved survival and productivity are very difficult to assess, but of obvious importance.

References

1. Skale BT, Kallok NJ, Prystowsky EN, et al: Inhibition of premature ventricular extrastimuli by subthreshold conditioning stimuli. J Am Coll Cardiol 6:133, 1985.

2. Josephson ME, Hastor JA: Supraventricular tachycardia: mechanisms and management. Ann Intern Med 87:346, 1977.
3. Waldecker B, Bruguda P, Zehender M, et al: Importance of modes of electrical termination of ventricular tachycardia for the selection of implantable antitachycardia devices. Am J Cardiol 57:150, 1986.
4. Pless BD, Sweeney MB: Discrimination of supraventricular tachycardia from sinus tachycardia of overlapping cycle length. PACE 7:1318, 1984.
5. Cobb LA, Werner JA, Trobaugh GB: Sudden cardiac death. II. Outcome of resuscitation: management and future directions. Mod Concepts Cardiovasc Dis 49:37, 1980.
6. Myerburg RJ, Kessler KM, Estes D, et al: Long-term survival after pre-hospital cardiac arrest: analysis of outcome during an 8-year study. Circulation 70:538, 1984.
7. Wilber DJ, Garan H, Finkelstein D, et al: Out-of-hospital cardiac arrest: use of electrophysiologic testing in the prediction of long-term outcome. New Engl J Med 318:19, 1988.
8. Mirowski M, Reid PR, winkle RA, et al: Mortality in patients with implanted automatic defibrillators. Ann Intern Med 98:585, 1983.
9. Mirowski M: The automatic implantable cardioverter-defibrillator: an overview. J Am Coll Cardiol 6:461, 1985.
10. Winkle RA, Thomas A: The automatic implantable cardioverter/defibrillator: the U.S. experience. In: Bruguda P, Wellens WJJ (eds), Cardiac Arrhythmias: Where to Go from Here? Mount Kisco, N.Y. , Futura Publishing Co., 1987, pp 663–680.
11. Annual Post-FDA Approval Report on the Automatic Implantable Cardioverter-Defibrillator (AICD) System. Cardiac Pacemakers Inc, February 15, 1988.
12. Lehmann MH, Steinman RT, Schuger CD, et al: The automatic implantable cardioverter/defibrillator as antiarrhythmic treatment modality of choice for survivors of cardiac arrest unrelated to acute myocardial infarction. Am J Cardiol 62:803, 1988.
13. Winkle RA, Mead RH, Ruder MA, et al: Long-term outcome with the automatic implantable cardioverter-defibrillator. J Am Coll Cardiol 13:1353, 1989.
14. Winkle RA, Stinson EB, Echt DS, et al: Practical aspects of automatic cardioverter-defibrillator implantation. Am Heart J 108:1335, 1984.
15. Watkins L, Mower MM, Reid PR, et al: Surgical techniques for implanting the automatic implantable defibrillator. PACE 7:1357, 1984.
16. Lawrie GM, Griffin JC, Wyndham CRC: Epicardial implantation of the automatic implantable defibrillator by left subcostal thoracotomy. PACE 7:1370, 1984.
17. Ruffy R, Smith P, Laseter M, et al: Out-of-hospital automatic cardioversion of ventricular tachycardia. J Am Coll Cardiol 6:482, 1985.
18. Marchlinski FE, Flores BT, Buxton AE, et al: The automatic implantable cardioverter-defibrillator: efficacy, complications, and device failures. Ann Intern Med 104:481, 1986.
19. Eysmann SB, Marchlinski FE, Buxton AE, et al: Electrocardiographic changes after cardioversion of ventricular arrhythmias. Circulation 73:73, 1986.
20. Waldecker B, Bruguda P, Zehender M, et. al: Dysrhythmias after direct-current cardioversion. Am J Cardiol 57:120, 1986.

Chapter 19

Nonpharmacological Treatment of Arrhythmias

Douglas L. Packer, Eric N. Prystowsky, and James E. Lowe

Introduction

The successful surgical ablation of an accessory pathway (AP) in a 33-year-old North Carolina fisherman in 1968[1] not only represented an important advancement in the treatment of patients with the Wolff-Parkinson-White (WPW) syndrome, but more importantly marked the beginning of a new era of nonpharmacological therapy for a wide variety of arrhythmias. In subsequent years, many improvements in operative techniques and myocardial preservation have allowed arrhythmia surgery to emerge from its early beginnings to become, in many cases, the gold standard of therapy. This progress has also been facilitated by improvements in electrophysiology study and mapping techniques that allow a more complete characterization of the mechanism of the underlying arrhythmia. These catheter techniques have also undergone their own evolution from strictly diagnostic to therapeutic applications. At the time of the first successful arrhythmia surgery, the concept of using simple electrode catheters or sophisticated laser technology for effective arrhythmia therapy had not yet been imagined. Today, these techniques are becoming routine and now serve as the foundation for further progress in the nonpharmacological treatment of supraventricular and ventricular arrhythmias.

From Naccarelli GV (ed): *Cardiac Arrhythmias: A Practical Approach.* Mount Kisco, NY, Futura Publishing Co., Inc., © 1991.

529

Ablation Therapy for Supraventricular Tachycardia

Treatment of the Wolff-Parkinson-White Syndrome

The greatest experience in nonpharmacological intervention has been in the operative interruption of APs in patients with the WPW syndrome. With technical improvements and accompanying surgical experience, the rate of successful ablation of an accessory connection has gone from 70%, observed in the first 100 patients operated on at Duke University,[2] to the current success rate of 98–99% in institutions where the procedure is routinely performed.[2–13] This has been accomplished with surgical mortality rates <1–2% in patients without other organic heart disease, although individuals with other pre-existing heart disease may have mortality rates up to 4–6%.[2–11] The risk of heart block associated with surgical interruption of a posteroseptal AP has also declined from a prevalence greater than 10% to 0.8–4.5%.[2–4,9,11] It has also been reported that patients with residual AP function following unsuccessful surgery may remain completely or nearly asymptomatic, perhaps due to pathway modification, although such alteration of AP characteristics may not be universally present.[2–4,8,13]

Classically, the ablative procedure involves an endocardial approach in which the atrioventricular (AV) ring on the atrial side of the annulus fibrosis in the region of the AP is incised.[14] Currently, we use an endocardial approach which has been extensively modified and improved over the years.[6] Arterial perfusion is accomplished by cannulation of the ascending aorta. The superior vena cava is cannulated through a purse-string suture placed in the right atrial appendage, and the inferior vena cava is cannulated through a purse-string suture placed over the inferior portion of the right atrium adjacent to the caval atrial junction. In the past, the heart was arrested with cold potassium cardioplegic solution for the dissection of all accessory AV connections. Presently, however, we use cardioplegic arrest only for left-sided pathways. All dissections are performed under 2.5 power optical magnification and fiberoptic-directed illumination. Dissection to eliminate right-sided accessory AV connections including those located in the posterior septal space can be carried out with the heart in sinus rhythm from within the right atrium. The area of the annulus fibrosis associated with the site of the accessory AV connection is identified and a supra-annular incision is placed 2 mm above the tricuspid valve annulus, exposing the atrioventricular fat pad containing the right coronary artery and vein.

Usually the incision is extended 3 to 4 cm on each side of the previously determined location of the AP. The AV groove fat pad containing the coronary vessels is dissected free from the top of the external wall of the ventricle to the level of the ventricular epicardial reflection throughout the extent of the supra-annular incision. All connecting accessory fibers are divided as they attach to the ventricle. After completion of the AV groove dissection, a sharp nerve hook is used to divide any remaining fibers connecting the atrium and ventricle along the tricuspid valve annulus.[6]

For posteroseptal pathways, the His bundle electrogram is identified using a hand-held mapping probe. Following identification of the His bundle, a supra-annular incision is begun just posterior to the site of the His bundle electrogram and extended in a counter-clockwise fashion onto the posterior right atrial free wall from within the right atrium as shown in Figure 1. A plane of dissection is established between the fat pad and the top of the posterior interventricular septum (Fig. 2). In the past, this dissection was carried out under cardioplegic arrest, but recently we have found that this dissction can be safely performed at normothermia with the heart beating and normally perfused. The dissection proceeds deep into the posterior pyramidal space overlying the posterior interventricular septum. The dissection is performed medially until the mitral valve annulus is visualized and posteriorly to the epicardial reflection of the ventricle at the crux of the heart as seen in Figure 3.

For left free wall pathways, the interatrial groove between the right and left atria is exposed in a manner similar to the approach used for mitral valve repair or replacement. Following completion of intraoperative mapping, the myocardium is cooled to 27°C and the heart is arrested using cold potassium cardioplegia. A left atriotomy is performed in order to expose the mitral valve (Fig. 4). Generally, patients with left free wall APs undergo the same surgical dissection regardless of the precise location of the pathway. A supra-annular incision is placed 2 mm above the posterior mitral valve annulus extending from the left fibrous trigone to the posterior interventricular septum (Fig. 5). The AV groove fat pad is entered and the atrium is disconnected from the top of the posterior left ventricle throughout the extent of the supra-annular incision. This dissection is taken to the level of the epicardial reflection of the posterior left ventricle (Fig. 6). A sharp nerve hook is used to transect any remaining fibers connecting the atrium to the ventricle along the posterior mitral valve annulus. As with other pathways, the supra-annular incision is closed with a continuous 4-0 Prolene suture

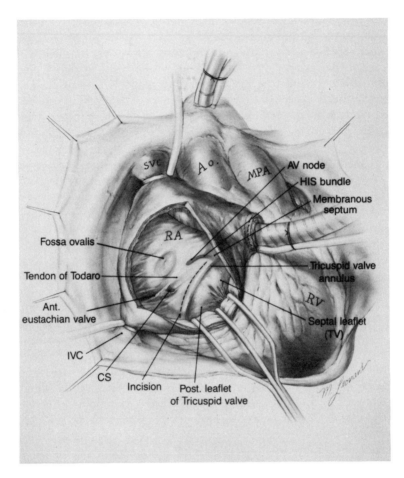

Figure 1. Surgical approach for the dissection of a posteroseptal accessory pathway. Here the right atrium has been opened for exposure of the tricuspid valve annulus with the patient on total cardiopulmonary bypass. The His bundle electrogram during sinus rhythm is first identified used a mapping probe. A supra-annular incision is then made 2 mm above the posterior tricuspid valve annulus, beginning immediately posterior to the identified His bundle region. This incision is continued in a counterclockwise direction onto the posterior right atrial free wall from within the atrium.

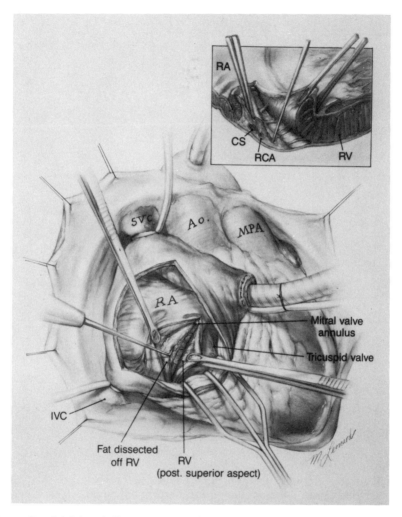

Figure 2. Additional dissection for the division of a posteroseptal pathway. Following the division of the right atrial endocardium, and while the heart is in sinus rhythm, a plane of dissection is continued between the fat pad and the superior aspect of the posterior interventricular septum. This dissection is extended deep into the posterior pyramidal space and is carried out medially to the mitral valve annulus, if visualized, and posteriorly to the epicardial reflection of the right ventricle at the crux of the heart (insert).

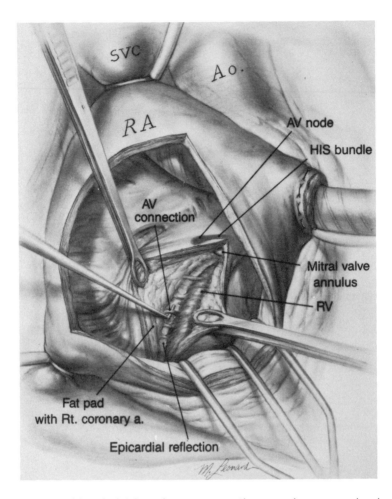

Figure 3. Additional division of accessory pathways using a nerve hook and electrocautery. Here, several accessory pathways in the posteroseptal region are depicted. The location of the normal cardiac conduction system and the medial aspect of the dissection exposing the mitral valve annulus are also shown.

followed by closure of the atrium as shown in Figure 7. Typically, dissection of left-sided APs requires only a 20- to 30-minute period of cardioplegic arrest. We continue to favor the endocardial approach because of its 99% effectiveness for the initial division of all pathways and the low intraoperative mortality of 1.0% achieved in the last 200 patients.[6]

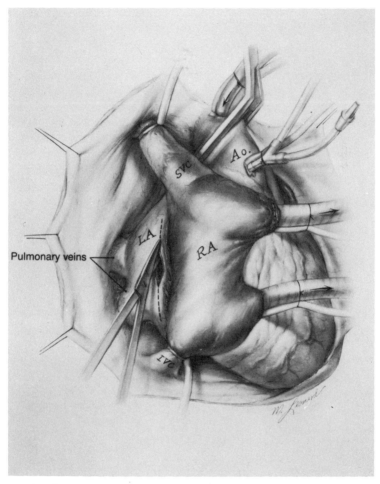

Figure 4. Surgical dissection of left free wall pathways. Following administration of cold potassium cardioplegia to achieve an arrested state, the interatrial groove is dissected and a standard left atrial incision similar to the approach taken for a mitral valve replacement is made. The pericardial reflection over the superior and inferior vena cavae is divided in order to allow rotation of the heart to the left. Here, the incision into the left atrium is depicted.

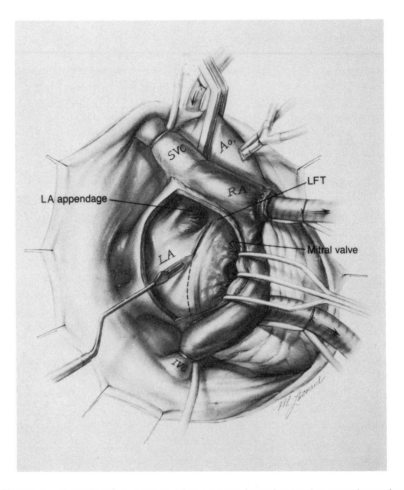

Figure 5. Additional exposure of the posterior mitral valve annulus using a modified hand-held mitral valve retractor. A supra-annular incision is then made 2 mm above the posterior mitral valve annulus, as indicated by the dashed line, beginning just below the left fibrous trigone and carried in a counterclockwise fashion to the area of the posterior interventricular septum. Thereafter, the AV groove fat pad is entered, and the left atrium is disconnected from the top of the posterior left ventricle throughout the length of the supra-annular incision.

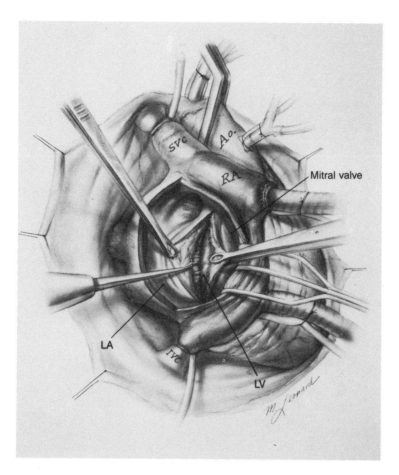

Figure 6. Depiction of several accessory atrioventricular pathways after the AV groove fat pad has been exposed. Typically, a sharp nerve hook is used to transect any such remaining fibers connecting the atrium to the ventricle along the posterior mitral valve annulus.

More recently, an epicardial technique has been reintroduced[15] for the ablation of accessory connections. Using this approach, which also requires cardiopulmonary bypass for left free wall and some posteroseptal APs, the AV fat pad and its vascular contents are mobilized from the external surface of the heart. With careful retraction of this region to avoid injury to the vascular contents, a cryothermic technique is used to deliver multiple lesions in the atrial-annular region, thus creating

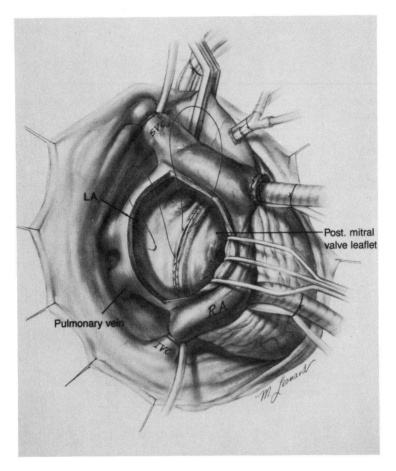

Figure 7. Closure of the left atrium. Following completion of the left-sided dissection, the supra-annular incision is closed using a continuous running 4-0 Prolene suture, followed by routine closure of the left atrium. The total cross-clamp time required for completion of left-side dissections averages 20 to 30 minutes.

transmural fibrosis and AP destruction. The success rate with this technique appears comparable to that with the endocardial approach, except in far left anterior and anteroseptal bypass tracts where the endocardial approach is superior. Additional studies will be required to determine the relative merits of each technique in other AP locations. At the present time, however, the skill of the surgeon in applying a given technique appears to be more important than the choice of one over the other.

Patients with atrial fibrillation (AF) and a rapid ventricular response rate may be at risk for degeneration of AF into ventricular fibrillation (VF). In this group, surgical treatment, which is preferred to medical therapy, is presumed to prolong life and diminish symptoms. The favorable therapeutic effect is based upon the primary removal of the AP as an avenue for rapid ventricular rates during disorganized atrial arrhythmias. There is additional evidence that bypass tract ablation not only reduces the ventricular response rate, but also decreases the frequency of episodic AF.[16,17] After surgery, a dramatic decrease in the occurrence of AF in patients with this preoperative arrhythmia[16] has been noted. Similar findings have been reported by others[17] who noted that only 16 of 169 patients with preoperative AF had recurrent AF following surgery. Interestingly, some of these patients either had unsuccessful surgery or pre-existing organic heart disease. These preliminary data also suggest that the AP may contribute to the genesis of spontaneous AF in some patients.

In addition to the potential reduction in sudden death risk, other studies have demonstrated a marked improvement in quality of life following surgery. This included a return to full-time employment following successful surgical intervention for all of their patients with preoperative disability despite medical therapy.[13] A review of the quality of life and postoperative arrhythmia status in patients having undergone AP ablation at Duke University showed that only 33 of 357 surgical patients had palpitations lasting between 1 and 5 minutes and only 27 had symptoms lasting longer than 5 minutes on follow-up over a 2-month to 18-year (mean 6-year) follow-up period.[18] Forty-eight patients had documented AF during follow-up, while only four patients whose operations had been unsuccessful had recurrent reciprocating supraventricular tachycardia related to the AP. Seventy-five percent of these patients, who typically had medically refractory arrhythmias prior to surgery, indicated that they were *completely* satisfied with the outcome of their operation, and 97% would recommend a similar procedure to other patients. In an additional study comparing long-term quality of life in 175 patients with APs treated pharmacologically and 365 treated surgically, superior outcome with operative intervention was reported.[19] Although both medically and surgically treated patients improved significantly compared with pretreatment status, a significant reduction in palpitations or documented arrhythmias has been observed in 90% of the patients undergoing surgery, while only 68% of the medically treated patients noted similar improvement. In addition, 93% of the surgical group had fewer WPW-related hospitalizations, which was also significantly better than similar improvement in 70% of medically treated patients. Arrhythmia-related activity limitations were also lower in surgical patients than in medically treated patients (2% vs. 27%). This indicates a better quality of life in surgically treated patients compared with medically treated patients. Because of improved surgical experience, low operative risk, and this significant improvement in quality of life, operative intervention need not be reserved for patients with life-threatening arrhythmias alone, but may now be recommended as an acceptable alternative to medical therapy particularly in young patients facing a lifetime of pharmacological therapy.

Catheter Ablation of Accessory Pathways

Catheter ablation techniques have also been successfully utilized to interrupt the AV conduction system in patients with supraventricular arrhythmias.[20,21] While this approach is effective in eliminating reciprocating tachycardia, its widespread application in patients with the WPW syndrome is markedly limited by the persistence of an unmodified AP, potentially capable of sustaining rapid anterograde conduction during atrial fibrillation (AF). Nevertheless, the success encountered in AV conduction system ablation provided the incentive for attempts at directly ablating APs with catheter-delivered energy. In a left free wall AP ablation attempted in eight patinets using 2–26 shocks of 40–80 joules each, delivered from unipolar or bipolar electrodes positioned in the region of the bypass tract, only one patient showed evidence of long-term conduction modification while the remaining seven patients had recurrent arrhythmias. One patient also experienced coronary sinus rupture requiring emergency operation. This potential complication and the poor overall results along with coronary sinus occlusion or mild to marked intimal hyperplasia in the left circumflex coronary artery observed in animals diminished enthusiasm for catheter ablation of left free wall APs.

Others, however, demonstrated a significantly greater success rate in the catheter ablation of posteroseptal pathways. The incidental ablation of a posteroseptal AP has been reported in a patient who underwent intentional catheter ablation of the normal AV conduction system.[21] Since this initial report, several large series documenting success rates of 67–75% have appeared in the literature, obtained with the delivery of anywhere from 1 to 10 shocks of 100–400 joules via catheters positioned at the posteroseptal AP.[23–25] The fact that at least three of these patients developed cardiac tamponade due to coronary sinus rupture requiring emergent intervention and at least one patient has died due to this complication[26] indicates that while this technique might be an alternative to both medical and traditional surgical therapy, catheter ablation of posteroseptal pathways remains experimental and should be performed only by experienced electrophysiologists with the facilities necessary to deal with potential complications.

Preliminary reports detailing successful ablation of anteroseptal and right free wall APs are also now available.[27-29] The delivery of a mean cumulative energy of 503 joules in seven patients with right anterior paraseptal APs and 608 joules in five patients with right free wall APs resulted in the elimination of pre-excitation in all but three patients with right free wall connections.[27] Of these failures, two showed pathway modification and have had no further arrhythmia recurrence in the absence of medical therapy. One has had recurrent symptoms. Others have also described the successful ablation of right free wall[28] or right anteroseptal APs[29] using radiofrequency energy. Although the numbers are small, these reports suggest that with additional technique development, more widespread use of this approach may be possible.

Unlike the preliminary results of attempted left free wall AP ablation using direct current shocks delivered via a catheter positioned in the coronary sinus, an endocardial catheter approach has been more successful. The ablation in six patients with a left free wall AP using a transseptal catheter technique has also been attempted. All of these patients remained free from arrhythmia recurrence on long-term follow-up after ablation with 480–800 cumulative joules of energy. This was accomplished without short-term evidence of damage to the coronary sinus or artery or other untoward sequelae.

Early reports also suggest that radiofrequency energy may prove more useful than direct current shocks. Early attempts to ablate accessory pathways were performed by creating a bipolar-directed field between the coronary sinuses and the mitral valve annulus.[30] Recent data suggest that left-sided pathways are ablated with a higher success rate by concentrating the lesion at the ventricular insertion side.[30] Careful catheter recordings of Kent bundle potentials improve the success rate. These initial studies together suggest that with further development, both conventional and radiofrequency ablation technique may be effective for the safe interruption of both septal and nonseptal APs. Until that time, however, surgical intervention with mortality rates <1–2% and success rates of 98% remains the gold standard of nonpharmacological therapy for these patients.

Nonpharmacological Treatment of Other Supraventricular Tachycardias

A variety of other supraventricular arrhythmias are also amenable to a nonpharmacological approach (Table 1). Another common supraventricular arrhythmia that may be refractory to medical therapy is AV nodal re-entrant tachycardia. In this rhythm disturbance, both the anterograde and retrograde components of the re-entrant circuit appear to be confined to the AV node as described in an earlier chapter. In the past, medically refractory patients required complete ablation of the AV conduction system to eliminate recurrent tachycardia. In an attempt to avoid resulting long-term pacemaker dependence, attention was directed towards the creation of sufficient AV nodal modification to eliminate tachycardia, without producing complete heart block. However, in a patient in whom attempted surgical creation of complete heart block failed, the resulting AV nodal modification successfully eliminated AV nodal re-entrant tachycardia.[32] A procedure has been developed in which the earliest site of atrial activation during tachycardia is identified using electrophysiological mapping. The right atrial wall is then incised approximately 2 mm above the tricuspid annulus from an area lateral to the coronary sinus orifice extending medially toward the apex of the triangle of Koch, onto the region of the early activtion. The coronary sinus end of the incision is dissected immediately onto the right ventricular free wall and the wall of the coronary sinus dissected from the fat in the posterior septal space. Additional dissection is dependent on the site of earliest atrial activiation observed during tachycardia map-

---

Table 1
Supraventricular Arrhythmias Amenable to
Nonpharmacological Intervention

AV re-entrant tachycardia
Atrial fibrillation using an AP for AV conduction
AV nodal re-entrant tachycardia
Ectopic atrial tachycardia
Atrial fibrillation/flutter
Inappropriate sinus tachycardia

AP = accessory pathway
AV = atrioventricular

ping. Using this surgical approach in 47 patients, freedom from recurrent arrhythmias has been observed in 45 patients at a median follow-up of 13 months.[34] Two other patients had inducible AV nodal re-entrant tachycardia although neither had spontaneous recurrences. Only one patient developed complete heart block. With a comparable procedure utilizing cryosurgical techniques to modify perinodal tissue, cryotherapy with cooling to −60° was applied around the perimeter of the AV node for 2 minutes, during which AV conduction was monitored on a beat-by-beat basis and cooling terminated if transient AV block occurred. With this technique, all eight patients undergoing this procedure showed successful AV nodal modification without the development of permanent complete heart block, and none have had recurrent AV nodal re-entrant tachycardia. Others have noted similar success.[36]

Based on this success, others have applied catheter ablation techniques to accomplish a similar closed-chest modification of the AV node. The application of such a catheter technique has been reported in 21 patients with recurrent episodes of AV nodal re-entrant tachycardia refractory to antiarrhythmic drugs. Using the local atrial activiation on the His bundle recording as a reference or guide, shocks of 160–240 joules were delivered from a distal catheter pole positioned in the perinodal region to a back paddle under the left scapula. In some patients, more than one shock was required. Tachycardia was noninducible on follow-up electrophysiological studies in 14 patients. In 16 of 21 patients, the procedure abolished the arrhythmia without the requirement for a pacemaker or subsequent drug therapy over a mean follow-up period of 14 ± 8 months. Two patients sustained complete heart block. Other attempts at AV nodal modification using both traditional electrical energy as well as radiofrequency current have produced success rates over 80% in modification of AV nodal conduction with only rare occurrence of complete heart block.[38–40]

The precise reason for the success of these surgical and catheter procedures is unclear, but could be related to modification or ablation of the retrograde connection from the AV node or His bundle to the atrium, selective modification of the anterograde slow AV junctional pathway, nonspecific trauma to the AV junction, or denervation of the AV nodal region. That the first mechanism is not universally responsible for success is the finding of presistent retrograde conduction via the AV node in at least half of the patients.[33,35] Unlike the electrophysiological findings following surgical modification, the disappearance of retrograde conduction in the majority of patients has not been demonstrated,[37] suggesting the elimination of this portion of the re-entrant circuit as the mediator of success using the catheter technique. Whether this is an absolute prerequisite to success or whether this is merely a marker indicating adequate tissue destruction is unclear, but suggests that more than one mechanism of successful ablation may be present. Modification of anterograde conduction in the AV node has also been suggested.[33–35] The possibility of nonspecific AV nodal trauma or denervation has not been thoroughly evaluated.

Ectopic Atrial Tachycardia

Unlike the typical re-entrant mechanism for most atrial tachyarrhythmias, some patients develop an abnormal automatic focus in the left or right atrium as the nidus for an ectopic atrial tachycardia. Although many of these occur only paroxysmally and may be controlled by antiarrhythmic agents, particularly the IC group, others become virtually incessant as seen in Figure 8 and can lead to a tachycardia-induced cardiomyopathy.[41,42] Using electrophysiological mapping techniques, the source of these tachycardias can be identified as the site with the earliest local activation in reference to the surface P wave as shown in Figure 9. In 68% of cases, the origin has been localized to the right atrial free wall, in the intra-atrial septum in 6%, and within the left atrium in approximately 25% of patients.[43] Following the localization of the tachycardia origin, surgical excision can be performed with a high degree of success.[42,43] In a recent review of operative procedures for ectopic atrial tachycardia,[43] the majority of patients who had undergone electrophysiologically guided operative procedures had been completely cured

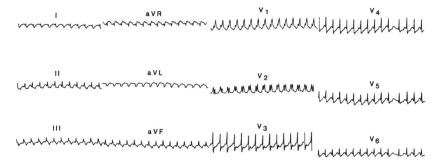

Figure 8. Twelve-lead ECG from a patient with an ectopic atrial tachycardia. Deeply inverted P waves are noted in leads II, III, and aVF, suggesting a posteroseptal or low right atrial origin.

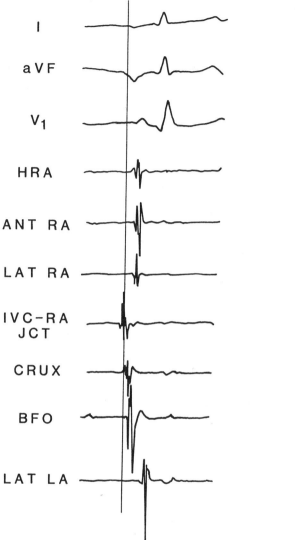

Figure 9. Composite electrograms obtained by epicardial mapping recorded of the ectopic atrial tachycardia. The earliest local atrial activation which preceded the onset of the surface P wave by 55 ms was recorded at the right atrial-IVC junction. All other areas of the right and left atria activated later than this point. Shown are leads I, aVF, and V_1 (surface electrograms) as well as epicardial electrograms from the high right atrial reference (HRA), anterior right atrium (ANT RA), lateral right atrium (LAT RA), low foramen ovale (BFO), anterior aspect of the right atrial-IVC junction (RA-IVC JCT), the crux, and the lateral left atrial (LAT LA) positions. Line indicates the onset of the surface P waves.

without the need for permanent pacemaker implantation or other post-operative antiarrhythmic therapy. If the focus cannot be precisely mapped, but is thought to reside in the left atrium, a left atrial isolation procedure has also been used to electrically disconnect the left atrium from the heart.[44]

As with other supraventricular arrhythmias, attempts have been made to ablate automatic foci using direct current shocks delivered via an endocardial catheter. Using closed-chest catheter ablation in four patients with ectopic atrial tachycardia, the two with right atrial appendage foci were succssfully ablated with 50 or 100 joules of energy, while the two with septal or free wall foci were treatment failures. This indicates, however, that additional technique development might subsequently allow a nonsurgical approach to the treatment of this form of arrhythmia, although left atrial foci are likely to remain more difficult to localize and ablate using catheter techniques.

Atrial Fibrillation

One of the most prevalent atrial arrhythmias and often the most difficult to treat is AF. In managing AF, the physician strives for a two-fold goal: (1) restoration of normal sinus rhythm, and (2) control of the ventricular response rate during AF. Although the first goal may not be possible, the second may be achieved using a variety of different pharmacological agents. Unfortunately, many patients display persistent AF with excessively rapid ventricular response rates at rest or during exercise despite medical therapy. Paradoxically, the latter patients may also have slow ventricular response rates at rest. Traditionally, surgical ablation of the AV node or His bundle region has been required in this group of medically refractory patients. Early in 1981, the original closed-chest catheter ablation technique was developed largely for this group of patients.[20,21] Several groups have demonstrated that complete heart block could be successfully created with the delivery of 200–300 joules of energy to the region of the AV conduction system as demonstrated in Figure 10. In a study comparing catheter and open surgical AV conduction system ablation, it was reported that the 88% success rate in the creation of complete heart block using a catheter approach was equivalent to the 86% success observed in patients treated with open surgical division of the AV conduction system.[45] The short-term peri-procedure complication rate was significantly lower among patients who underwent catheter ablation (12% vs. 42%), although long-term morbidity and

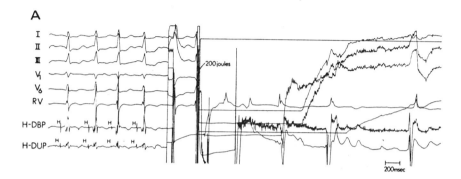

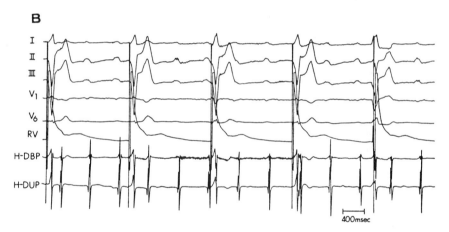

Figure 10. (A) Catheter ablation of the atrioventricular conduction system in a patient with atrial fibrillation and a rapid ventricular response rate refractory to medical therapy. A shock of 200 joules delivered from the distal pole of a catheter positioned in the region yielding the largest His bundle potential to a back plate positioned beneath the left scapula resulted in successful creation of complete heart block. Shown are surface leads I, II, III, V_1, and V_6. Also shown are the right ventricular (RV), distal bipolar His (H-DBP), and the distal unipolar His (H-DUP) electrograms. (B) Complete heart block following successful ablation of the AV conduction system. During ventricular pacing with a cycle length of 1500 ms, an atrial cycle length of 520 ms is observed with complete AV dissociation.

mortality rates were not significantly different in these patients with equivalent degrees of prior cardiac disease. The quality of life in these patients following successful catheter ablation has also been excellent compared with pre-ablation status.[46]

Similar to the observed outcome in patients with other atrial arrhythmias, recent studies indicate that AV nodal modification, while preserving conduction, may also be possible in some patients. The Catheter Ablation Registry has reported that in addition to the 70% of patients developing complete heart block, 9% although showing resumption of conduction following attempted ablation had sufficient modification of the AV conduction system to result in symptom resolution in the absence of antiarrhythmic drugs.[47] An additional 12% of patients became asymptomatic with antiarrhythmic agents previously shown to be ineffective prior to the ablation attempt.

Other techniques have been developed in the overall attempt to eliminate the effect of AF while preserving a normal sinus mechanism and avoiding pacemaker dependence. In one of these, a surgical incision in the right atrium surrounding the sinus node is made and extended down to include the region of the AV node and His bundle.[48] This effectively isolates a narrow corridor of tissue containing the sinus and AV nodes from the residual fibrillating atrial tissue, theoretically allowing the sinus node to provide continued pacemaker activity for ventricular function. Although this has not been extensively evaluated in clinical trials, it might allow the maintenance of effective sinus rhythm and preserving AV conduction, although many patients with recurrent atrial fibrillation also have deficient sinus node impulse generation as a component of a brady-tachy syndrome. Furthermore, atrial transport function remains impaired because of persistent AF outside the corridor. A modification of this procedure has also been used to isolate completely or excise the sinus node in patients with medically refractory, inappropriate sinus tachycardia.[49,50]

Ablative Therapy for Ventricular Arrhythmias

Although recent progress in the management of organic heart disease has been made, malignant ventricular arrhythmias remain a leading cause of morbidity and mortality. This is particularly true in patients with coronary artery disease, in whom improved survival following myocardial infarction has increased the prevalence of recurrent sustained ventricular arrhythmias. Traditionally, pharmacological therapy has been the mainstay of treatment for these patients. Unfortunately, the results of medical therapy in this group have been disappointing. While this reflects to some degree the inadequacy of currently available pharmacological agents, it also underscores the principle that even under the conditions of an optimal response, antiarrhythmic drugs only suppress, without eliminating the underlying arrhythmia. This problem has provided the incentive for the development of nonpharmacological therapy designed actually to cure the underlying malignant ventricular arrhythmia by permanently altering the primary substrate.

Early success of indirect surgical procedures suggested that operative techniques in patients with malignant ventricular arrhythmias might be a reasonable alternative to the pharmacological approach. In 1959, the successful application of aneurysmectomy for the treatment of ventricular tachycardia (VT) was reported. Similar success from comparable procedures was also noted by others.[52,53] It was also suggested that coronary artery bypass grafting might provide additional protection from life-threatening ventricular arrhythmias.[54] Based on these reports, additional patients underwent nondirected ventriculotomy or aneurysmectomy with or without additional coronary artery bypass grafting as primary treatment for VT. Unfortunately, the surgical success rates using these techniques were typically around 30%,[55-57] and the postoperative clinical control or partial success rates accompanying the use of previously ineffective antiarrhythmic therapy were no higher than 56%. These were achieved at a relatively high price with operative mortality rates ranging between 10% and 42%[55-57] when using the surgical and myocardial preservation techniques available in the late 1970s. Although promising in theory, these techniques proved to be of less practical value.

Directed Operative Ablation

Subsequent investigations provided both an explanation of the low success rates of these nondirected procedures, as well as a basis for a new generation of surgical techniques. Early experimental studies suggested that VT usually originates from a border zone between infarcted and normal tissue.[58-60] Later, endocardial mapping studies in humans with VT similarly demonstrated that the arrhythmia typically arises from the perianeurysmal border zone.[55,61,62] This finding suggests that the re-entrant circuit on arrhythmia focus would not necessarily be con-

Table 2
Nonpharmacological Techniques for Elimination of Ventricular
Arrhythmias

Surgical
  Ventriculotomy
  Aneurysmectomy
  Coronary artery bypass grafting
  Encircling endocardial ventriculotomy (complete/partial)
  Subendocardial resection (directed/extensive)
  Cryoablation
  Laser photocoagulation
Catheter
  Electrical ablation (at earliest ventricular activation)
  Electrical ablation (at slow conduction or mid-diastolic potentials)
  Chemical ablation (via coronary artery)

tained in tissue routinely removed during aneurysmectomy, and thus the procedure would fail.

Based on this additional understanding and building on earlier surgical experience, other procedures (Table 2) were designed primarily to interrupt the presumed re-entrant VT circuit at its origin. In 1978, a new surgical procedure, the encircling endocardial ventriculotomy (EEV), was reported.[63,64] Using this technique, the left ventrical of a patient with medically refractory VT is entered via the aneurysm or thinned zone of infarct scar. An incision perpendicular to the plane of the left ventricular wall is placed immediately outside the border of endocardial fibrosis and is continued around the entire base of the aneurysm as shown in Figure 11. The depth of the incision on the septal side of the aneurysm is approximately 1 cm while the free wall incision is carried to the level of the subepicardium, leaving a narrow bridge of subepicardium, epicardium, and overlying coronary vessels. This incision is then closed and dense scar forms. In theory, the success of this procedure depends upon the interruption of the tachycardia circuit or isolation of an arrhythmogenic focus from residual normal myocardium. The precise mechanism responsible for a favorable outcome is unclear, however, as another potential explanation in view of surgically induced changes in regional blood flow is that changes in local metabolic factors might contribute to the antiarrhythmic effect of the procedure.[65] Regardless of mechanism, initial studies demonstrated primary surgical

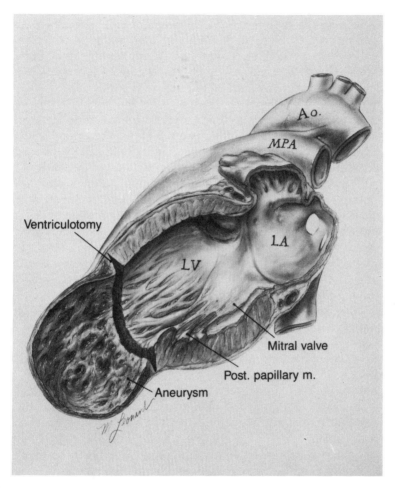

Figure 11. Encircling endocardial ventriculotomy for ventricular tachycardia. After opening a left ventricular apical aneurysm and removal of thrombus, an endocardial incision is placed above the junction of endocardial fibrosis and normal endocardium and carried around the entire base of the aneurysm as depicted. This incision, sparing only subepicardial myocardium and subepicardial blood vessels, theoretically isolates re-entrant circuits causing ventricular tachycardia from the remaining normal heart.

success rates in eliminating VT >73% with partial success rates over 90% when patients with a satisfactory postoperative response to previously ineffective antiarrhythmic therapy were included.[57,63,66]

While this was a substantial improvement over aneurysmectomy alone, other studies suggested untoward hemodynamic sequelae accompanying this procedure. It has been demonstrated that the EEV caused a profound decrease in regional blood flow in the encircled myocardium, especially in the subendocardium.[65] Furthermore, a concomitant depression of regional myocardial function in nonfibrous tissue was observed.[67] In a separate clinical study, an increase in progressive left ventricular failure was reported relative to the preoperative state in 46% of patients receiving a complete EEV compared to an 8% prevalence in those with only a partial procedure.[66] Analysis of late deaths also identified fatal left ventricular failure as a significant late complication after complete EEV.[66] Similarly, in a series of 123 ventricular arrhythmia patients, it was observed that not only was the application of the complete EEV the best predictor of VT control, but it was also a significant incremental risk factor for subsequent death. It has since been shown that a partial EEV, when guided by electrophysiological mapping, may be as effective as a complete procedure, but with lower accompanying morbidity and mortality[66] (Fig. 12). In a related procedure, a full-thickness incision used to isolate completely or disconnect the right ventricular free wall in patients with VT foci caused by arrhythmogenic dysplasia[69-70] has also been effective in several patients. Progressive right ventricular dilatation following this surgery has also been observed.[70]

Capitalizing on the relationship between the tachycardia focus and perianeurysmal subendocardial scar in patients with past myocardial infarction, additional efforts were turned towards directed endocardial excision to ablate VT.[55,62,71] A technique has been developed for the removal of the endocardium extending 2–3 cm beyond the edge of the aneurysm including any overlying scar tissue. This resection typically involved 8–25 cm^2 of endocardial tissue[55,62,71] from 25–40% of the circumference of the aneurysm, which is limited in scope compared with the EEV. In the initial report, 25 of 30 patients undergoing this procedure were shown in long-term follow-up to have a primary surgical cure, while three additional patients responded to previously ineffective antiarrhythmic agents for control of residual VT. This was accomplished with a mortality rate of only 7%. Others have described modifications of this technique in which a more extensive subendocardial resection of over 20–40 cm^2 of tissue is performed[72-77] (Fig. 13). In skilled hands,

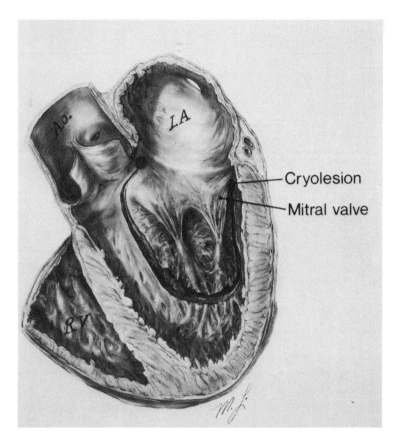

Figure 12. Partial encircling endocardial ventriculotomy and selective cryoablation for a posterobasal focus of tachycardia. Here, a partial encircling endocardial ventriculotomy with adjunctive cryolesions is shown isolating the posterior wall beginning immediately below the insertion of the papillary muscles and extending to the mitral valve annulus.

the variations on the endocardial resection theme result in overall primary surgical cure rates ranging between 73% and 92% in larger series, with a partial response or secondary clinical control rate of 82–97% when additional patients responding to previously ineffective antiarrhythmic agents are included.[56,62,73,74] Operative mortality rates range between 7% and 18%.[55,57,71–73,78,80,81] The success rates for elimination of foci in the anterior, lateral, apical, or septal portions of the left ventricle have been 85–90%, with higher failure rates ranging between 41–67% observed with resection of inferior or posterior wall VT origins.[78,79,82]

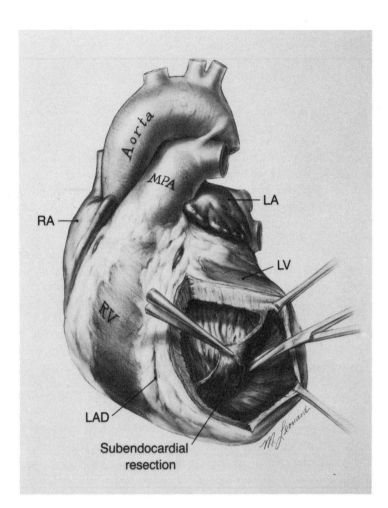

Figure 13. Subendocardial resection for the ablation of ventricular tachycardia. Here the excision of subendocardial scar tissue over a 2 to 4 cm area surrounding the origin of the arrhythmia is guided by intraoperative mapping. We and others presently perform an extended endocardial resection procedure beyond the 2 to 4 cm area of tachycardia origin in patients with anteroapical or inferoapical aneurysm associated with re-entrant ventricular tachycardia.

In part because of the latter problem, additional means besides surgical excision have been developed for the ablation of arrhythmogenic foci. In 1977, it was demonstrated that the His bundle could be ablated cryosurgically with the application of a localized freezing technique.[83] Subsequently, the successful ablation of a drug-resistant VT has been reported, suggesting a more universal application of the cryoprobe in other patients with serious VT.[84] In principle, this procedure entails the localized cooling of an area of tissue to $-60°$ to $-70°$ for a period of 2–3 minutes. This destroys underlying muscle cells, while preserving the integrity of the underlying fibrous tissue stroma.[85,86] In addition to this theoretical advantage over mechanical techniques, the cryosurgical procedure is also useful as an adjunctive measure in the ablation of foci in the posterior and inferior walls, particularly high in the interventricular septum as well as in the region of the posterior papillary muscle (Fig. 14). General application of this technique as either a primary or an adjunctive measure has resulted in improved overall clinical success rates of greater than 93% without evidence of impairment of ventricular function or significant damage to the mitral valve apparatus when cryoablation of the posterior papillary muscle is necessary.[87–89] The latter finding is particularly significant since this area is particularly prone to untoward damage accompanying extensive endocardial procedures requiring mitral valve replacement.[56,73,74]

In a parallel fashion, laser technology has been applied. As with cryoablation, laser photocoagulation is used to create discrete tissue damage and enhance the outcome of ablative therapy for arrhythmias above and beyond that possible with subendocardial resection alone. This approach is similar to cryotherapy in that the structural integrity of the affected tissues is maintained. In contrast to cryotherapy, however, laser photocoagulation can be achieved more rapidly, with more focused myocardial destruction. In addition, this may be administered to the perfused normothermic heart, allowing serial mapping, ablation, and ongoing assessment of results during the actual operative procedure. The application of neodymium:yttrium-aluminum garnet (Nd:YAG) laser photocoagulation has been describd in 15 patients with VT, many with multiple morphologies. Of the 14 operative survivors, 13 were noninducible at the time of postoperative electrophysiological evaluation. Only one recurrence of VT was reported, yielding a 93% primary success rate in operative survivors. In an additional study, the successful application of an argon laser to 6–24 cm^2 of tissue was reported in five patients with refractory sustained VT.[91] Using a map-guided approach, seven VT morphologic patterns were observed, five

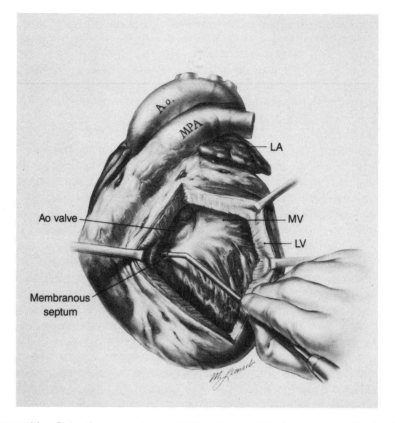

Figure 14. Selective use of cryoablation for ventricular tachycardia. Application of cryoblative techniques has proved very useful as adjunctive measures, particularly in patients with ventricular tachycardia originating high on the interventricular septum or posterior wall.

of which were located at sites deemed unresectable using standard surgical techniques. Postoperatively, both spontaneous and inducible VT was suppressed in four patients, while one additional patient responded to a previously ineffective antiarrhythmic drug. These preliminary studies indicate that laser therapy can be used effectively and safely without myocardial perforation. With additional development, this technology promises to be an important adjunct to other ablative procedures.

Role of Electrophysiological Mapping

The evolution of the surgical approach and the understanding of the mechanism of serious ventricular arrhythmias have been facilitated by the development of more sophisticated electrophysiological mapping techniques. Since the earliest applications of epicardial mapping,[92,94] these techniques have been refined to allow the identification of the focus or origin of VT and thereby direct therapy. It has been possible with endocardial catheter mapping during VT in the electrophysiology laboratory to localize the origin of the tachycardia indicated by the earliest local ventricular activation occurring before the onset of the surface QRS in 52–96% (usually about 75%) of patients.[54,61,78,79] Incomplete mapping studies in the remaining patients are due to the inability to induce tachycardia, the presence of multiple VT morphologies or VT accompanied by rapid hemodynamic deterioration, degeneration of the VT to VF, or the presence of overlying intraventricular thrombus.

At the time of surgery, intraoperative mapping is even more useful in guiding therapy. Epicardial mapping may be successfully performed in 75–95% of patients undergoing surgery. The demonstration that epicardial breakthrough of the advancing wavefront may be 5 mm to 6 cm away from the endocardial origin, however, renders this form of mapping only partially reliable in identifying the earliest VT site.[59] As a result, endocardial mapping is the gold standard for the identification of the tachycardia origin, although only obtainable in approximately 65% (range 28–90%) of patients undergoing endocardial procedures for VT,[54,65,70,71,76,78,79,95] also due to noninducibility following ventriculotomy with fortuitous division of the re-entrant circuit, hemodynamic deterioration during VT, or degeneration of VT to VF in the remaining patients. Nevertheless, with combined preoperative intracardiac catheter and operative endocardial mapping approaches, over 90% of tachycardias may be successfully mapped.[76] These techniques have revealed multiple tachycardia morphologies in 40–81% of patients[61,71,76,80,96] and have identified the most typical areas of tachycardia origin: approximately 60% are localized to the septum and 23% in the inferior or posterior wall, while 26% have shown earliest activation at the anteroapical or anterolateral margin of the anterior wall aneurysm.

While correctly identifying the origin of each tachycardia, the exact impact of mapping on the outcome or success of the surgical procedures has been debated. Although some investigators[54,55] have shown the superiority of a map-guided endocardial resection over nonguided aneurysmectomy, data contrasting the effect of map guidance during more effective subendocardial resection have been difficult to obtain. This is due in part to the relatively small size of available surgical series, the absence of randomized trials evaluating map-guided versus visually directed approaches, and the fact that even the map-guided surgical series contain visually directed procedures since some patients had noninducible or poorly tolerated arrhythmias making mapping impossible. A comparison of the primary surgical success rate of the larger series suggests that map-guided procedures result in a 65–89% primary surgical cure rate,[76–80,95] while the visually directed surgical series were less consistent with success rates of 51–92%.[71–73,75,97] Overall, complete clinical control of the arrhythmias is seen in 82–97% of both map-guided and visually directed surgical patients. Postoperative electrophysiology induction rates have also been comparable, ranging between 9% and 34% in patients having undergone map-guided therapy compared to 9–37% of patients with a visually directed procedure.

While these data only suggest an improved primary outcome with map-guided therapy, more conclusive support has been provided for the directed approach. The map-guided technique was significantly better than observed in the visually directed group, based on inducible VT at postoperative EP study. The freedom from any cardiac death at 36 months was also appreciably better in the map-guided patients than in those without map guidance. In assessing long-term freedom from VT, it was found that a negative postoperative electrophysiology study as well as a map-guided surgical approach were univariable predictors of freedom from recurrent VT. In terms of cumulative effectiveness, twice as many of the map-guided group patients remained free from recurrent tachyarrhythmias as in the nonmap-guided group. In addition, the former group also showed a greater freedom from sudden cardiac death than observed in the unguided group. Interestingly, while a negative postoperative electrophysiology study did not predict freedom from sudden cardiac death, the use of a map-guided operative procedure, in and of itself, was a significant predictor of freedom from this outcome. These data are consistent with the theoretical expectation of an improved outcome in patients with ventricular arrhythmias in whom the focus can be eliminated in a directed fashion without sacrificing other functional myocardium. The possibility of unfavorably altering overall ventricular function or damaging the mitral valve apparatus may be additional incentive to focus the ablative procedure on areas identified by mapping. These in turn would be expected to diminish the chance of postoperative heart failure, the most frequent cause of both early and late postoperative death.[79]

Predictors of Outcome

Several predictors of surgical outcome in terms of VT recurrence rates and operative mortality have been determined as listed in Table

---

Table 3
Potential Risk Factors for Recurrent VT after
Attempted Surgical Ablation*

Multiple morphologically distinct spontaneous VTs
Disparate sites of VT origin
Inferior or posterior wall VT origin
Absence of LV aneurysm

VT = ventricular tachycardia; LV = left ventricle
* Risk of recurrence may be decreased with adjunctive cryothermic ablation or laser photocoagulation.

---

3. In a study involving 100 patients, disparate sites of VT origin (>5 cm
between mapped site of origin) were identified as well as the presence
of multiple morphologically distinct spontaneous tachycardias as univariable predictors of VT recurrence. In this study, the presence of those
predictors resulted in a doubling of tachycardia recurrence: 64% surgical
failure in patients with, compared with 30% of those without disparate
sites of VT origin, and 47% failure of surgery in patients with multiple
VT morphologies compared with 25% of patients with a single VT morphology. These findings have been confirmed by the report of the In-
ternatioinal Ablation Registry involving 665 patients.[78] Importantly,
more recent studies have suggested that the application of adjunctive
cryosurgery may decrease the failure rate in patients with multiple VT
morphologies, providing that all VT morphologies are identified intraoperatively and ablated.[76,80]

As indicated, the actual location of the tachycardia origin also appears to be an indicator of outcome. Patients with a focus of VT in the
inferior or posterior wall, which are difficult to approach surgically, are
at a threefold higher risk for recurrence (41–67%)[77,78,81,88,89] compared
to those with anterior, septal, or lateral wall origins (12–15%). Here too,
adjunctive therapy has been shown to improve outcomes in the former
group. Finally, it was also found that the absence of a left ventricular
aneurysm was a predictor of failure using multivariate analysis.

In terms of risk of subsequent death, the most consistent predictor
of intra- or perioperative death is that of the preoperative clinical congestive heart failure class.[78,79] The International Ablation Registry determined that although age, global ejection fraction, VT cycle length, presence or absence of coronary artery disease, or extent of coronary artery
disease did not predict poor outcome, the severity of clinical heart failure

class did.[78] This indicator, along with bypass duration and the requirement for emergency surgery, were univariable predictors of both congestive heart failure and cardiac mortality.[79] Using a stepwise logistic regression procedure, bypass duration was the strongest independent predictor of congestive heart failure mortality, while the requirement for emergency surgery, congestive heart failure class, and bypass time (in that order) were predictive of overall cardiac mortality.[79] In addition, while global ejection fraction was not a predictor of untoward outcome, poor systolic function of the nonaneurysmal ventricular segment was the strongest and only independent predictor of operative mortality.

These predictors, along with the results of the larger surgical studies, facilitate the selection of patients most suited for a surgical procedure. Patients with refractory VT due to coronary artery disease with a ventricular aneurysm or a well-defined region of postinfarction scar may be ideal candidates for an attempt at a primary surgical cure. Patients with advanced preoperative heart failure or poor residual function in a nonaneurysmal segment, while not absolutely contraindicated as candidates for surgery, are at significantly higher risk for an operative procedure. In these patients, the potential benefit of the procedure must outweigh the risk. Patients with multiple morphologically distinct tachycardias or with posterior or inferior wall sites of origin, while at higher risk for recurrence of tachycardia, might remain acceptable candidates for surgery, given the promising results of adjunctive measures of cryoablation or laser therapy. In contrast, patients who are poor candidates for surgical resection or those with primary cardiomyopathies, primary ventricular fibrillation, or polymorphic ventricular tachycardias in the absence of a well-defined site of origin are better candidates for implantation of an automatic implantable defibrillator for medically refractory tachycardia. Patients deemed to be at higher risk for recurrent or life-threatening ventricular arrhythmias because of the presence of aforementioned predictors of recurrent VT may also benefit from placement of AICD patches at the time of primary surgery.[98,99] In this group, an AICD generator can be placed in a separate procedure if the patient remains inducible at postoperative EP testing and shows no response upon retesting of previously ineffective antiarrhythmic medications.[98]

With appropriate selection, current operative techniques including endocardial resection, cryoablation, or laser ablation, used singly or in combination, patients with VT can be expected to have primary surgical success rates of 70–90% with additional total clinical arrhythmia control or partial success rates between 80% and 95%. This translates into a 63–84% freedom from VT at 36 months[61,67] and a 63% freedom at 48 months.[61,67,79,80,95] Taking overall cardiac mortality into account, survival rates of 70–83% at 36 months[79,80] and up to 57% at 60 months should be possible. This is substantially better than the 17% 3-year survival rates initially described in patients with life-threatening ventricular tachycardia resistant to medical treatment.[100] Undoubtedly, additional refinements of these techniques will be made which, along with a better understanding of arrhythmias and mapping techniques, will result in additional improvement in arrhythmia control and diminished overall risk for an increasing number of patients in the future.

Catheter Ablation for Ventricular Tachycardia

After the delivery of energy through an endocardial catheter was shown to be highly successful in ablating the AV conduction system,[21,22] attention was turned to the similar development of a closed-chest catheter technique for the ablation of VT foci. Several series have appeared describing the application of one to four 100–400 joule shocks in a larger number of patients.[102–104] In applying this technique, electrical energy is delivered from the distal pole of a catheter positioned at the earliest site of tachycardia, identified by the position where the local endocardial electrogram precedes the onset of surface QRS by the greatest amount of time. In the majority of cases, a chest wall patch serves as the second electrode, although in some cases, the shock may be delivered between two intracardiac catheters. The primary success rate for catheter ablation of VT has ranged between 12% and 45%, while all other patients are either persistently inducible upon electrophysiological testing or have a subsequent clinical recurrent VT.[102–105] The Percutaneous Cardiac Mapping and Ablation Registry has also reported the outcome of 88 patients who underwent closed-chest catheter ablation for a VT focus.[105] Long-term follow-up indicates that, of those patients, 29 (33%) were asymptomatic without medications, although several had inducible tachycardia at postablation EP testing. An additional 33 (38%) were asymptomatic while taking antiarrhythmic medication instituted because of persistence of inducibility following the procedure. Twenty-six (29%) of this group were classified as complete failures. Based on these data, it appears that 30–40% of patients may be unsuccessfully treated using a catheter technique with energy delivered at the site of earliest local ventricular activation. As with surgery, additional patients may subsequently benefit from previously ineffective antiarrhythmic therapy.

The experimental observation that some VTs could be eliminated by cryoablation at a site of slow conduction or mid-diastolic potentials away from the earliest ventricular activation suggests that other portions of the re-entrant circuit might be amenable to ablation attempts.[106-108] In a series of 10 patients in whom 20 attempts were made to ablate 14 monomorphic VTs using one to five shocks of 50–370 joules of energy, all seven VTs in which isolated mid-diastolic potentials were targeted were successfully ablated, although one required a second attempt. It should be noted that two of seven patients had inducible sustained VT on postablation electrophysiological studies that was morphologically distinct from those observed clinically. Even counting these patients as failures, the overall success rate of VT ablation in patients with identifiable mid-diastolic potentials as a marker for a portion of the tachycardia circuit was 71%. Of the 12 attempts made to ablate seven other tachycardias by delivering shocks at the site of earliest local ventricular activation in the absence of mid-diastolic potentials, only three (25%) were successful. A similar success rate has been observed in patients in whom energy was delivered at a site of slow conduction documented by catheter mapping techniques. In contrast, 81% of those in whom the energy was delivered at the site of earliest ventricular activation showed subsequent recurrences. With the refinement of catheter ablation techniques, as well as developmentof new energy sources, the results of the closed-chest approach may improve.

Chemical Ablation of VT

The selective injection of specific cardiotoxic chemicals such as ethanol into small coronary arteries as an additional means of VT ablation is also currently under investigation. Using this approach, VT has been successfully eliminated in two patients with medically refractory incessant VT.[109] The risk of this novel technique remains unknown; chemical ablation may allow the treatment of individuals who are not candidates for any other nonpharmacological approach.

Summary

Over the past 20 years, surgical procedures for the ablation of both supraventricular and ventricular arrhythmias have been refined and new techniques utilizing energy delivered via catheters have been developed. While additional improvements in these techniques are expected in the future, current experience has already validated many of these procedures as effective modes of therapy for patients with medically refractory arrhythmias. In many cases, these nonphrarmacological techniques are already acceptable alternatives to medical therapy. With anticipated improvements, lower procedure-related complications will undoubtedly be realized and an inceasing number of patients will benefit from nonpharmacological therapy. This will in turn significantly decrease the risk of medically refractory arrhythmias, as well as the expense, potential side effects, and proarrhythmic risk accompanying medical therapy.

References

1. Cobb FR, Blumenschein SD, Sealy WL, et al: Successful surgical interruption of the bundle of Kent in a patient with Wolff-Parkinson-White syndrome. Circulation 38:1018, 1968.
2. Gallagher JJ, Sealy WC, Cox JL, et al: Results of surgery for preexcitation caused by accessory atrioventricular pathways in 267 consecutive cases. In: Josephson ME, Wellens HJJ (eds), Tachycardias: Mechanism, Diagnosis, and Treatment. Philadelphia, Lea and Febiger, 1984, pp 259–269.
3. Iwa T. Mitsui T, Misaki T, et al: Radical surgical cure of the Wolff-Parkinson-White syndrome: the Kanazawa experience. J Thorac Cardiovasc Surg 91:225, 1986.
4. Guiraudon GM, Klein GJ, Sharma AD, et al: Closed-heart technique for Wolff-Parkinson-White syndrome: further experience and potential limitations. Ann Thorac Surg 42:651, 1986.
5. Klein, GJ, Guiraudon GM, Perkins DG, et al: Surgical correction of the Wolff-Parkinson-White syndrome in the closed heart using cryosurgery: a simplified approach. J Am Coll Cardiol 3:405, 1984.
6. Lowe JE: Surgical treatment of the Wolff-Parkinson-White syndrome and other supraventricular tachyarrhythmias. J Cardiac Surg 1:117, 1986.
7. Selle JG, Sealy WC, Gallagher JJ, et al: Technical considerations in the surgical approach to multiple accessory pathways in the Wolff-Parkinson-White syndrome. Ann Thorac Surg 43:579, 1987.
8. Holmes DR, Osborn MJ, Gersh B, et al: The Wolff-Parkinson-White syndrome: a surgical approach. Mayo Clin Proc 57:345, 1982.
9. Cox JL, Gallagher JJ, Cain MD: Experience with 118 consecutive patients undergoing operation for the Wolff-Parkinson-White syndrome. J Thorac Cardiovasc Surg 90:490, 1985.
10. Packer DL, Prystowsky EN: Wolff-Parkinson-White syndrome: further progress in evaluation and treatment. Progr Cardiol 1:147, 1988.
11. Uther JB, Johnson DC, Baird DK, et al: Surgical section of accessory atrioventricular electrical connections in 108 patients. Am J Cardiol 49:995, 1982.
12. Ott DA, Garson A, Cooley DA, et al: Definitive operation for refractory

cardiac tachyarrhythmias in children. J Thorac Cardiovasc Surg 90:681, 1985.

13. Fischell TA, Stinson EB, Derby GC, et al: Long-term follow-up after surgical correction of Wolff-Parkinson-White syndrome. J Am Coll Cardiol 9:283, 1987.

14. Sealy WC, Hattler BG, Blumenschein SD, et al: Surgical treatment of Wolff-Parkinson-White syndrome. Ann Thorac Surg 8:1, 1969.

15. Gallagher JJ, Sealy WC, Anderson RW, et al: Cryosurgical ablation of accessory atrioventricular connections: a method for correction of the pre-excitation syndrome. Circulation 55:471, 1977.

16. Sharma AD, Klein GJ, Guiraudon GM, et al: Atrial fibrillation in patients with Wolff-Parkinson-White syndrome: incidence after surgical ablation of the accessory pathway. Circulation 72:161, 1985.

17. Chen PS, Pressley, JC, Tang AS, et al: New observations on atrial fibrillation before and after surgery on patients with accessory pathways. Circulation 78 (suppl II):II-41, 1988.

18. Prystowsky EN, Pressley JC, Gallagher JJ, et al: The quality of life and arrhythmia status after surgery for Wolff-Parkinson-White syndrome: an 18 year perspective. J Am Coll Cardiol 9:100A, 1987.

19. Pressley JC, German LD, Packer DL, et al: Comparison of baseline characteristics in long-term quality of life in 540 Wolff-Parkinson-White patients treated with pharmacologic versus surgical therapy. J Am Coll Cardiol 11:110A, 1988.

20. Scheinman MM, Morady F, Hess DS, et al: Catheter-induced ablation of atrioventricular junction to control refractory supraventricular arrhythmias. JAMA 248:851, 1982.

21. Gallagher JJ, Svenson RH, Castle JH, et al: Catheter technique for closed-chest ablation of the atrial ventricular conduction system: a therapeutic alternative for the treatment of refractory supraventricular tachycardia. N Engl J Med 306:194, 1982.

22. Fischer JD, Broadman R, Kim SG, et al: Attempted nonsurgical electrical ablation of accessory pathways via the coronary sinus in the Wolff-Parkinson-White syndrome. J Am Coll Cardiol 4:685, 1984.

23. Morady F, Scheinman MM, Kou WH, et al: Long-term results of catheter ablation of a posteroseptal accessory artrioventricular connection in 48 patients. Circulation 79:1160, 1989.

24. Bardy GH, Ivy TD, Coltorti F, et al: Catheter-mediated electrical ablation of posterior accessory atrioventricular pathways: developments, complications, and limitation. Am J Cardiol 61:309, 1988.

25. Ruder MA, Mead RH, Guadiani V, et al: Experience with catheter ablation of accessory pathways. J Am Coll Cardiol 9:251a, 1987.

26. Linker NJ, Ward DE, Davies MJ, et al: Fatal coronary sinus rupture following attempted catheter ablation of an accessory pathway. J Electrophysiol 3:2, 1989.

27. Warin JF, Haissaguerre M, Lemetayer P, et al: Catheter ablation of accessory pathways with a direct approach: results in 35 patients. Circulation 78:800, 1988.

28. Borggrefe M, Budde T, Martin EZ, et al: Radio-frequency catheter ablation

for drug-refractory supraventricular tachycardia. Circulation 78 (suppl 2):II-305, 1988.

29. Naccarelli GV, Rinkenberger RL, Bougherty AH, et al: Successful radio-frequency catheter ablation of right anteroseptal accessory atrioventricular connections. J Am Coll Cardiol 13:176a, 1989.

30. Kuck KH, Kunze KP, Geiger M, et al: Attempted ablation of left-sided accessory pathways by radiofrequency current. J Am Coll Cardiol 13:168A, 1989.

31. Langberg J, Griffin JC, Herre JM, et al: Catheter ablation of accessory pathways using radiofrequency energy in the canine coronary sinus. J Am Coll Cardiol 13:491, 1989.

32. Pritchett ELC, Anderson RW, Benditt DG, et al: Reentry within the atrioventricular node: surgical cure with preservation of atrioventricular conduction. Circulation 60:440, 1979.

33. Ross DL, Johnson DC, Denniss AR, et al: Curative surgery for atrial ventricular junctional ("AV Nodal") re-entrant tachydcardia. J Am Coll Cardiol 6:1383, 1985.

34. Ross DL, Johnson DC, Koo CC, et al: Surgical treatment of supraventricular tachycardia without the Wolff-Parkinson-White syndrome: current indications, techniques, and results. In: Brugada P, Wellens HJJ (Eds), Cardiac Arrhythmias: Where to Go From Here? Mt. Kisco, NY, Futura Publishing Co., 1987, pp 591–603.

35. Cox JL, Holman WL, Cain ME: Cryosurgical treatment of atrial ventricular node re-entrant tachycardia. Circulation 76:1329, 1987.

36. Wood DL, Hammill SC, Porter CJ, et al: Cryosurgical modification of atrioventricular conduction for treatment of atrioventricular node re-entrant tachycardia. Mayo Clin Proc 63:988, 1988.

37. Haissaguerre M, Warin JF, Lemetayer P, et al: Closed chest ablation of retrograde conduction in patients with atrioventricular nodal re-entrant tachycardia. N Engl J Med 320:426, 1989.

38. Kunze KP, Schlueter M, Kuck KH: Modulation of AV nodal conduction: definitive treatment for AV nodal tachycardia? Circulation 78 (Suppl II):II-305, 1988.

39. Lavergne TL, Sebag CI, Guize LJ, et al: Transcatheter radiofrequency modification of atrioventricular conduction for refractory supraventricular tachycardia. Circulation 78 (Suppl II):II-305, 1988.

40. Epstein LM, Langberg JJ, Herre JM, et al: Catheter modification of the atrioventricular node: a potential cure for atrioventricular nodal re-entrant tachycardia. J Am Coll Cardiol 13:168a, 1989.

41. Packer DL, Bardy GH, Worley SJ, et al: Tachycardia-induced cardiomyopathy: a reversible form of left ventricular dysfunction. Am J Cardiol 57:563, 1986.

42. Gillett PC, Wompler DG, Garson A, et al: Treatment of atrial automatic tachycardia by ablation procedures. J Am Coll Cardiol 6:405, 1985.

43. Lowe JE, Hendricks PJ, Packer DL, et al: Surgical management of chronic ectopic atrial tachycardia. Ann Thorac Surg (in press).

44. Williams JM, Ungerlider RM, Lauffland GK, et al: Left atrial isolation: new technique for treatment of supraventricular arrhythmias. J Thorac Cardiovasc Surg 80:373, 1980.

45. Marchese AC, Pressley JC, Sintetous AL, et al: Cryosurgical versus catheter ablation of the atrioventricular junction. Am J Cardiol 59:870, 1987.
46. Kay GN, Bubien RS, Epstein AE, et al: Effective catheter ablation of the atrioventricular junction on quality of life and exercise tolerance in paroxysmal atrial fibrillation. Am J Cardiol 62:741, 1988.
47. Evans, GT, Scheinman MM, Fox C, et al, and the Executive Committee of the Registry: Predictors of successful His ablation: a report of the percutaneous cardiac mapping and ablation registry. J Am Coll Cardiol 11:17A, 1988.
48. Defauw JJ, Van Hamel NM, Vermeulen FE, et al: Short-term results of the "corridor operation" for drug refractory paroxysmal atrial fibrillation. Circulation 78 (Suppl II):II43, 1988.
49. Lowe JE, Harwich T, Schaper J: Ultrastructure of electrophysiologically identified human sinoatrial nodes. Basic Res Cardiol 83:401, 1988.
50. Yee R, Guiraudon GM, Gardner MJ, et al: Refractory paroxysmal sinus tachycardia: management by subtotal right atrial exclusion. J Am Coll Cardiol 3:400, 1984.
51. Couch OA: Cardiac aneurysm with ventricular tachycardia and subsequent excision of aneurysm (case report). Circulation 20:251, 1959.
52. Thind GS, Blakemore WS, Zinsser AHF: Ventricular aneurysmectomy for the treatment of recurrent ventricular tachyarrhythmia. Am J Cardiol 27:690, 1971.
53. Hunt D, Sloman G, Westlake G: Ventricular aneurysmectomy for recurrent tachycardia. Br Heart J 31:264, 1969.
54. Graham AF, Miller DC, Stinson EB, et al: Surgical treatment of refractory life-threatening ventricular tachycardia. Am J Cardiol 32:909, 1973.
55. Harken AH, Horowitz LN, Josephson ME: Comparison of standard aneurysmectomy and aneurysmectomy with directed endocardial resection for the treatment of recurrent sustained ventricular tachycardia. J Thorac Cardiovasc Surg 80:527, 1980.
56. Mason JW, Stinson EB, Winkel RA, et al: Surgery for ventricular tachycardia: efficacy of left ventricular aneurysm resection compared with operation guided by electrical activation mapping. Circulation 65:1148, 1982.
57. Ostermeyer J, Breithardt G, Kolvenbach R, et al: The surgical treatment of ventricular tachycardias: simple aneurysmectomy versus electrophysiologically guided procedures. J Thorac Cardiovas Surg 84:704, 1982.
58. Wittig JH, Boineau JP: Surgical treatment of ventricular arrhythmias using epicardial, transmural, and endocardial mapping. Ann Thorac Surg 20:117, 1975.
59. Horowitz LN, Spear JF, Moore EN: Subendocardial origin of ventricular arrhythmias in 24-hour-old experimental myocardial infarction. Circulation 53:56, 1976.
60. Spielman SR, Michaelson EL, Horowitz LN, et al: The limitations of epicardial mapping as a guide to surgical therapy of ventricular tachycardia. Circulation 57:666, 1978.
61. Josephson ME, Horowitz LN, Farshidi A, et al: Recurrent sustained ventricular tachycardia. 2. Endocardial mapping. Circulation 57:440, 1978.
62. Josephson ME, Harken AH, Horowitz LN: Long-term results of endocardial

resection for sustained ventricular tachycardia in coronary disease patients. Am Heart J 104:51, 1982.

63. Guiraudon G, Fontaine G, Frank R, et al: Encircling endocardial ventriculotomy: a new surgical treatment for life-threatening ventricular tachycardias resistant to medical treatment following myocardial infarction. Ann Thorac Surg 26:438, 1978.

64. Guiraudon G, Fontaine G, Frank R, et al: La ventriculotomie circulaire d'exclusion: Traitement chirurgical des tachycardies ventriculaires compliquant un infarctus du myocarde. Arch Mal Coeur 71:1255, 1978.

65. Ungerleider RM, Holman WL, Stanley TE, et al: Encircling endocardial ventriculotomy for refractory ischemic ventricular tachycardia: II. Effects on regional myocardial blood flow. J Thorac Cardiovasc Surg 83:850, 1982.

66. Ostermeyer J, Breithardt G, Borggrefe M, et al: Surgical treatment of ventricular tachycardias: complete versus partial encircling endocardial ventriculotomy. J Thorac Cardiovasc Surg 87:517, 1984.

67. Ungerleider RM, Holman WL, Calcagno D, et al: Encircling endocardial ventriculotomy for refractory ischemic ventricular tachycardia: III. Effects on regional left ventricular function. J Thorac Cardiovasc Surg 83:857, 1982.

68. McGiffin DC, Kirkland JK, Plumb VJ, et al: Relief of life-threatening ventricular tachycardia and survival after direct operations. Circulation 76 (Suppl V):V-93, 1987.

69. Cox JL, Bardy GH, Damiano RJ, et al: Right ventricular isolation procedures for nonischemic ventricular tachycardia. J Thorac Cardiovasc Surg 90:212, 1985.

70. Guiraudon GM, Klein GJ, Gulamhusein SS, et al: Total disconnection of the right ventricular free wall: surgical treatment of right ventricular tachycardia associated with right ventricular dysplasia. Circulation 67:463, 1983.

71. Josephson ME, Harken AH, Horowitz LN: Endocardial excision: A new surgical technique for the treatment of recurrent ventricular tachycardia. Circulation 60:1430, 1979.

72. Moran JM, Kehoe RF, Lobe JM, et al: Extended endocardial resection for the treatment of ventricular tachycardia and ventricular fibrillation. Ann Thorac Surg 34:538, 1982.

73. Kron IL, Lerman BB, DiMarco JP: Extended subendocardial resection: a surgical approach to ventricular tachyarrhythmias that cannot be mapped intraoperatively. J Thorac Cardiovasc Surg 90:586, 1985.

74. Landymore RW, Kinley CE, Gardner M: Encircling endocardial resection for complete removal of endocardial scar without intraoperative mapping for the ablation of drug-resistant ventricular tachycardia. J Thorac Cardiovasc Surg 89:18, 1985.

75. Lowe JE, Sabiston DC: The surgical management of cardiac arrhythmias. J Appl Cardiol 1:1, 1986.

76. Kehoe R, Zheutlint, Finkelmeier B, et al: Visually directed endocardial resection for ventricular arrhythmia: long-term outcome and functional status. J Am Coll Cardiol 5:497, 1985.

77. Krafchek J, Lawrieg M, Roberts R, et al: Surgical ablation of ventricular tachycardia: improved results with a map-directed regional approach. Circulation 73:1239, 1986.

78. Miller JM, Kienzle MG, Harkin AH, et al: Subendocardial resection for

ventricular tachycardia: predictors of surgical success. Circulation 70:624, 1984.

79. Borggrefe M, Podczeck A, Ostermeyer J, et al: Surgical ablation registry: long-term results of electrophysiologically guided antitachycardia surgery and ventricular tachyarrhythmias: A collaborative report on 665 patients. In: Nonpharmacological Therapy of Tachyarrhythmias. Breithardt G, Borggrefe M, Zipes DP (Eds), Mount Kisco, NY, Futura Publishing Company, 1987, pp 109–132.

80. Swerdlow CD, Mason JW, Stinson EB, et al: Results of operations for ventricular tachycardia in 105 patients. J Thorac Cardiovasc Surg 92:105, 1986.

81. Garan H, Hguyen K, McGovern B, et al: Perioperative and long-term results after electrophysiological directed ventricular surgery for recurrent ventricular tachycardia. J Am Coll Cardiol 8:201, 1986.

82. Saksena S, Hussain SM, Wasty N, et al: Long-term efficacy of subendocardial resection in refractory ventricular tachycardia: relationship to site of arrhythmia origin. Ann Thorac Surg 42:685, 1986.

83. Harrison L, Gallagher JJ, Kasell J, et al: Cryosurgical ablation of the AV node-His bundle: a new method for producing AV block. Circulation 55:463, 1977.

84. Gallagher JJ, Anderson RW, Kasell J, et al: Cryoablation of drug-resistant ventricular tachycardia in a patient with a variant of scleroderma. Circulation 57:190, 1978.

85. Klein GJ, Harrison L, Idecker RF, et al: Reaction of the myocardium to cryosurgery: electrophysiologic and arrhythmogenic potential. Circulation 59:364, 1970.

86. Guiraudon GM, Jones BL, Klein GJ, et al: Feasibility of cryoablation of the posterior papillary muscle in the dog. J Am Coll Cardiol 7:236A, 1986.

87. Hargrove WC, Miller JM, Vassallo JA, et al: Improved results in the operative management of ventricular tachycardia related to inferior wall infarction: importance of the annular isthmus. J Thorac Cardiovasc Surg 92:726, 1986.

88. Caceres J, Werner P, Jazayeri M, et al: Efficacy of cryosurgery alone for refractory monomorphic sustained ventricular tachycardia due to inferior wall infarction. J Am Coll Cardiol 11:1254, 1988.

89. Caceres J, Akhtar M, Werner P, et al: Cryoablation of refractory sustained ventricular tachycardia due to coronary artery disease. Am J Cardiol 63:296, 1989.

90. Selle JG, Svenson RH, Sealy WC, et al: Successful clinical laser ablation of ventricular tachycardia: a promising new therapeutic method. Ann Thorac Surg 42:380, 1986.

91. Sakesena, Hussain SM, Gielchinsky I, et al: Intraoperative mapping-guided argon laser ablation of malignant ventricular tachycardia. Am J Cardiol 59:78, 1987.

92. Fontaine G, Frank R, Guiraudon G, et al: Surgical treatment of resistant reentrant ventricular tachycardia by ventriculotomy: the new application of epicardial mapping. Circulation 50(Suppl III):82, 1974.

93. Spurrel RAJ, Yates AK, Thornburn CW, et al: Surgical treatment of ventricular tachycardia after epicardial mapping studies. Br Heart J 37:115, 1975.

94. Gallagher J, Oldham HN, Wallace AG, et al: Ventricular aneurysm with ventricular tachycardia: report of a case with epicardial mapping and successful resection. Am J Cardiol 35:696, 1975.
95. Haines DE, Lerman BB, Kron IL, et al: Surgical ablation of ventricular tachycardia with sequential map-guided subendocardial resection: electrophysiologic assessment and long-term follow-up. Circulation 77:131, 1988.
96. Brodman R, Fisher JD, Johnston DR, et al: Results of electrophysiologically guided operations for drug-resistant ventricular tachycardia and ventricular fibrillation due to coronary artery disease. J Thorac Cardiovasc Surg 87:431, 1984.
97. Zee-Chee C-S, Kouchoukos NT, Connors JP, et al: Treatment of life-threatening ventricular arrhythmias with nonguided surgery supported by electrophysiologic testing and drug therapy. J Am Coll Cardiol 13:153, 1989.
98. Platia EV, Griffith LSC, Watkins L, et al: Treatment of malignant ventricular arrhythmias with endocardial resection and implantation of the automatic cardioverter defibrillator. N Engl J Med 314:213, 1986.
99. Manolis AS, Rastegar H, Estes NAM: Prophylactic automatic implantable cardioverter-defibrillator patches in patients at high risk for postoperative ventricular tachycardia. J Am Coll Cardiol 13:1367, 1989.
100. Graboys TB, Lown B, Podrid PJ, et al: Long-term survival of patients with malignant ventricular arrhythmias treated with antiarrhythmic drugs. Am J Cardiol 50:437, 1982.
101. Hartzler GO: Electrode catheter ablation of refractory focal ventricular tachycardia. J Am Coll Cardiol 2:1107, 1983.
102. Tonet JL, Fontaine G, Frank R, et al: Treatment of ventricular tachycardias by endocardial catheter fulguration: further experience and long-term follow-up. Circulation 78:(Suppl II):II-306, 1988.
103. Garan H, Kuchar D, Freeman C, et al: Early assessment of the effect of map-guided transcatheter intracardiac electric shock on sustained ventricular tachycardia secondary to coronary artery disease. Am J Cardiol 61:1018, 1988.
104. Morady F, Scheinman MM, BiCarlo LA, et al: Catheter ablation of ventricular tachycardia with intracardiac shocks: results in 33 patients. Circulation 75:1037, 1987.
105. Evan JT, Scheinman MM, Zipes DP, et al: Catheter ablation for control of ventricular tachycardia: a report of the percutaneous cardiac mapping and ablation registry. PACE 9:1391, 1986.
106. Fitzgerald DM, Friday KJ, Wahjayl, et al: Electrogram patterns predicting successful catheter ablation of ventricular tachycardia. Circulation 77:806, 1988.
108. Morady F, Frank R, Kou WH, et al: Identification and catheter ablation of a zone of slow conduction in the reentrant circuit of ventricular tachycardia in humans. J Am Coll Cardiol 11:775, 1988.
109. Brugada P, de Swart H, Smeets JLRM, et al: Transcoronary chemical ablation of ventricular tachycardia. Circulation 79:475, 1989.

Index